FOUNDATIONS OF GLOBAL HEALTH

An Interdisciplinary Reader

EDITED BY

PETER J. BROWN

EMORY UNIVERSITY

SVEA CLOSSER

MIDDLEBURY COLLEGE

NEW YORK OXFORD

OXFORD UNIVERSITY PRESS

Oxford University Press is a department of the University of Oxford. It furthers the University's objective of excellence in research, scholarship, and education by publishing worldwide. Oxford is a registered trade mark of Oxford University Press in the UK and certain other countries.

Published in the United States of America by Oxford University Press
198 Madison Avenue, New York, NY 10016, United States of America.

For titles covered by Section 112 of the US Higher Education Opportunity Act, please visit www.oup.com/us/he for the latest information about pricing and alternate formats.

Library of Congress Cataloging-in-Publication Data
Names: Brown, Peter J., editor.
Title: Foundations of global health : an interdisciplinary reader / edited by Peter J. Brown, Emory University, Svea Closser, Middlebury College.
Description: New York : Oxford University Press, [2019] | Includes bibliographical references.
Identifiers: LCCN 2017043138 | ISBN 9780190647940 (paperback : alk. paper)
Subjects: LCSH: World health—Textbooks. | Public health—Textbooks.
Classification: LCC RA441 .F675 2019 | DDC 362.1—dc23
LC record available at https://lccn.loc.gov/2017043138

CONTENTS

Preface: Introducing Global Health ix

PART 1 **INTRODUCING GLOBAL HEALTH** *1*

1. What Is Global Health? *2*
   Peter J. Brown and Svea Closser
   Box: What's Your Major? *4*
   Box: Portraits of Health in Five Countries *7*
   Ann Lindstrand, Staffan Bergstrom, Hans Rosling, Biritta Rubenson, Bo Stenson and Thorkild Tylleskar

SECTION 1 **Milestones in Global Health** *13*

Conceptual Tools 13

2. The Broad Street Pump *16*
   Steven Johnson
3. The Influenza Epidemic of 1918 *23*
   John Barry
4. House on Fire: The Fight to Eradicate Smallpox *30*
   William Foege
5. A Pinch, a Fist, a Cup of Water: Oral Rehydration Therapy in Bangladesh *36*
   Phillip J. Hilts
6. "Science Will Always Win in the End": The Epidemiologist Who Proved that Smoking Causes Cancer *40*
   Sir Richard Doll, Interviewed by Anna Wagstaff
7. Declaration of Alma-Ata *46*
   World Health Organization
8. AIDS in 2006—Moving toward One World, One Hope? *50*
   Jim Yong Kim and Paul Farmer

WEB RESOURCES AND CASES *53*

SECTION 2 Epidemiology and the Basic Methods of Global Health 56

Conceptual Tools 57

9. Inside the Outbreaks 59
Mark Pendergrast

10. Epidemiology and Surveillance 66
Centers for Disease Control and Prevention

WEB RESOURCES AND CASES 84

SECTION 3 Metrics and the Burden of Disease 86

Conceptual Tools 87

11. Using Evidence about "Best Buys" to Advance Global Health 93
Ramanan Laxminarayan and Lori Ashford

12. The Long Defeat 103
Tracy Kidder

13. Counting Is Complicated 112
Adeola Oni-Orisan

WEB RESOURCES AND CASES 119

PART 2 ECOLOGICAL DETERMINANTS OF HEALTH 121

SECTION 4 Water 123

Conceptual Tools 124

14. Hygiene, Sanitation, and Water: Forgotten Foundations of Health 128
Jamie Bartram and Sandy Cairncross

15. Water, Worry, and Mental Health 135
Amber Wutich and Alexandra Brewis

16. What Went Wrong in Flint 143
Anna Maria Barry-Jester

WEB RESOURCES AND CASES 151

SECTION 5 Air 153

Conceptual Tools 154

17. Indoor Air Pollution in Developing Countries 159
Nigel Bruce, Rogelio Perez-Padilla, and Rachel Albalak

18. Tobacco Industry Interference: A Global Brief 165
World Health Organization

19. The Health Consequences of Global Climate Change 175
George Luber and Stasia Widerynski

WEB RESOURCES AND CASES 186

SECTION 6 Food 188

Conceptual Tools 188

20. Clinical Medicine or Public Health? The History of Mortality Decline 195
Thomas McKeown

21. The Nature of Child Malnutrition and Its Long-Term Implications 202
Reynaldo Martorell

22. Statement to the Security Council on Missions to Yemen, South Sudan, and Kenya and an Update on the Oslo Conference on Nigeria and the Lake Chad Regions 208
Stephen O'Brien

23. Hunger in the AIDS Economy of Central Mozambique 213
Ippolytos Kalofonos

24. A Nutrition Paradox—Underweight and Obesity in Developing Countries 221
Benjamin Caballero

WEB RESOURCES AND CASES 224

PART 3 SOCIAL DETERMINANTS OF HEALTH 227

SECTION 7 Health Inequalities and the Social Gradient 229

Conceptual Tools 230

25. Social Determinants of Health: The Solid Facts 237
Richard Wilkinson and Michael Marmot, editors

26. Disease and Dying while Black: How Racism, Not Race, Gets under the Skin 245
Alan Goodman

WEB RESOURCES AND CASES 251

SECTION 8 Sex and Reproduction 254

Conceptual Tools 254

27. Why Is HIV Prevalence So Severe in Southern Africa? 260
Daniel Halperin and Helen Epstein

28. Understanding HIV/AIDS in the African Context 271
Eileen Stillwaggon and Larry Sawers

29. Why Circumcision? 284
Homa Hoodfar

30. Saving Mothers' Lives in Sri Lanka 289
Ruth Levine and the What Works Working Group

WEB RESOURCES AND CASES 297

SECTION 9 Violence *300*

Conceptual Tools *300*

31. The Global Prevalence of Intimate Partner Violence against Women *304*
K. M. Devries, J. Y. T. Mak, C. García-Moreno, M. Petzold, J. C. Child, G. Falder, S. Lim, L. J. Bacchus, R. E. Engell, L. Rosenfeld, C. Pallitto, T. Vos, N. Abrahams, and C. H. Watts

32. War and Public Health: An Overview *308*
Barry S. Levy and Victor W. Sidel

33. Beyond Happy Endings *314*
Peter Redfield

34. Structural Violence and Clinical Medicine *324*
Paul E. Farmer, Bruce Nizeye, Sara Stulac, and Salmaan Keshavjee

WEB RESOURCES AND CASES 333

PART 4 INTERVENTIONS TO IMPROVE HEALTH *335*

SECTION 10 A History of Health Institutions and Programs *337*

Conceptual Tools *337*

35. The Four 19th-Century Cultural Roots of International and Global Health: A Model for Understanding Current Policy Debates *344*
Peter J. Brown

36. Coercion and Consent in Smallpox Eradication *355*
Paul Greenough

37. Looking Back in Time from Ebola *368*
Randall Packard

WEB RESOURCES AND CASES *377*

SECTION 11 Health Systems and Aid *379*

Conceptual Tools *380*

38. A Heart for the Work *385*
Claire Wendland

39. Turning the World Upside Down *397*
Nigel Crisp

40. Why We Must Provide Better Support for Pakistan's Female Frontline Health Workers *401*
Svea Closser and Rashid Jooma

41. Are NGOs Undermining Health Systems in Mozambique? *409*
James Pfeiffer

42. The Vital Case for Global Health Investments *419*
Sten H. Vermund and Ann Kurth

43. Treating Depression Where There Are No Mental Health Professionals *424*

Vikram Patel

44. Beyond Shamanism: The Relevance of African Traditional Medicine in Global Health Policy 428

Obijiofor Aginam

WEB RESOURCES AND CASES *435*

SECTION 12 Health Communication *439*

Conceptual Tools 439

45. Riding High on Taru Fever: Entertainment-Education Broadcasts, Ground Mobilization and Service Delivery in Rural India *446*

Arvind Singhal

46. Managing Rumors and Misinformation in West Africa *453*

Amzath Fassassi

and

Ebola: Limitations of Correcting Misinformation

Clare Chandler, James Fairhead, Ann Kelly, Melissa Leach, Frederick Martineau, Esther Mokuwa, Melissa Parker, Paul Richards and Annie Wilkinson, for the Ebola Response Anthropology Platform

WEB RESOURCES AND CASES *459*

SECTION 13 Ethics, Projects and Human Rights: The Future of Global Health *462*

Conceptual Tools 463

47. The Right to Health *465*

Office of the United Nations High Commissioner for Human Rights and World Health Organization

48. Stop Trying to Save the World: Big Ideas Are Destroying International Development *470*

Michael Hobbs

49. Global Health: Your Life, Your Life Decisions, Your Moral Obligations *480*

Svea Closser and Peter Brown

Boxes: *Emily Bensen, Pam Berenbaum, Nils Daulaire, Bill Foege and Abhay Shukla*; shorter pieces by several other authors

WEB RESOURCES AND CASES *491*

Key Terms 493

PREFACE: INTRODUCING GLOBAL HEALTH

Global health is an exciting field that has gained a great deal of student interest in the past two decades. Studying the complex health and socioeconomic problems of people throughout the world, including the global majority who live in low- and middle-income countries, can help any student become a global citizen. The study of global health from an interdisciplinary perspective can be simultaneously encouraging and discouraging, in ways that we think can help students develop more nuanced perspectives on the world.

In our opinion, the true purpose of higher education is to lead us out of our self-centered universe to a place where we can perceive the world from others' perspectives and have a positive impact in the global community. Many college students need to break out of a bubble that is often characterized by great privilege. After learning about the challenges that people living in poverty face, many students have a sincere desire to do something—to make a difference in the world. Such empathy and desire to help others is a great thing. We encourage that. At the same time, students can have a certain naiveté and lack of humility in their desire to "save the world." So we also encourage the cultivation of humility and an appreciation of complexity.

As teachers, we are excited about students' interest in and enthusiasm for global health and social justice. We too are aspiring global citizens, and we are deeply committed to helping improve the health and well-being of others throughout the world. But we can only do this in our own small ways. With this book, for example, our modest goal is to help others learn about the health problems and living conditions of people living in the "majority world."

It is necessary to learn not only about the world's complex and interwoven problems but also about successful solutions. Some are quite simple, like oral rehydration therapy (ORT), which has saved the lives of millions of children from dehydration caused by diarrhea. ORT is as inexpensive as it is effective. ORT is one of the simplest solutions in global health, not requiring trained healthcare personnel to implement. Some solutions are more complex, like the worldwide eradication of smallpox in 1979 (although that remarkable success took nearly 200 years between the discovery of a vaccine, the mobilization of global resources and the eradication of the disease).

Global health is an inspiring and encouraging field. This book will help you understand the *tremendous progress* that has been made during the last 20 years in terms of the health and welfare of your fellow global citizens. The tools of global public health have played an important role in those improvements, as can be seen in the progress made under the United Nations' Millennium Development Goals between 2000 and 2015. Globally, life expectancy has increased, child mortality rates have decreased, access to education and medical care has improved, and significant progress has been made in combatting some age-old scourges of humankind. This remarkable progress has been made possible, in part, by the unprecedented increases in the amount of money invested in health and development programs. Although the generosity of rich individuals and nations is important, the real work in improving health and welfare across the world is done by local health workers and local communities.

Global health is also inspiring because of the people working in this field. Many are veritable heroes, dedicated to reducing individual suffering and fighting for social justice. Some work in situations like the 2014 Ebola epidemic, whereas others work in refugee camps in war-torn areas. Others—such as researchers, program managers and logisticians—devote their lives to improving health in ways that are less dramatic but no less important. For them, people cannot be reduced to mere numbers, spreadsheets or economic calculations. If you are searching for personal heroes and role models, global health is a good place to look.

On the other hand, global health can be discouraging and depressing. The problems are large and complex; the interaction of poverty and poor health is strong. Disease and suffering are so widespread and historically intractable that it can seem like nothing can be done to end them. It is easy to become overwhelmed by scope and complexity of the problems and their requisite solutions. These do not simply disappear when they are glossed over as simple "challenges." Moreover, there is a danger of becoming cynical and thinking that ideas like "Make Poverty History" are just empty slogans.

Witnessing the suffering of others can be heartbreaking, and progress is always slower than we would wish. In global health, it is often the case that we have the appropriate biomedical knowledge and technologies to save lives, but we fail in "delivering the goods." We live in a world where Coca-Cola is ubiquitous, but life-saving vaccines and medicines can be scarce. We live at a time of unprecedented prosperity and profoundly unequal distribution of wealth. In this book we do not avoid or skate over these issues. Instead, we raise them as important topics for examination and discussion. We think that global health practitioners who are prepared for the deeply complex problems they will face will be less likely to become disillusioned or cynical when they confront them in their careers.

Global health is not a particular discipline but rather a set of wicked problems. Thus, to design and implement solutions to those problems, global health must be multidisciplinary. Look at the Box in Chapter 1, on page 4 "What's Your Major?"; it should give you an idea of what multidisciplinarity is about. In short, you do not have to be a doctor or a health professional to make a big difference in improving the health and well-being of people. Every academic field of study provides ideas and skills to contribute to global health. Although many people working in global health have graduate degrees like a

MPH, MD, RN or PhD, it is remarkable to see the wide variety of undergraduate majors they had. Areas as diverse as chemistry and theater have a great deal to offer.

We need to be honest about our prejudice in terms of academic discipline. We are both medical anthropologists who are interested in applying social science to public health problems. By its very nature, Anthropology is interdisciplinary, combining biological, cultural, archeological/historical and linguistic approaches for studying human similarities and difference. The idea is to get the "big picture" of humanity. Similarly, we hope that the multidisciplinary approach of this book will provide you with the big picture of global health. We think that it is important to know the history of these approaches, the theories, the tools, and the critical skills for being able to read the professional literature *before* you start any professional training. We believe that, on the most basic level, global health should be a valuable addition to the education of all global citizens.

What do we, as editors, hope you will begin to learn with this book? There are certain skills in interpreting quantitative information and statistics (numeracy) that we think every informed citizen should master. There needs to be an appreciation of the complexity of gathering and critically interpreting global health data.

Thinking historically is also fundamental to critical thinking. Historical case studies of successes and failures can illuminate contemporary global health issues. We believe that students of global health need to have a thorough understanding of successful global health interventions. These can serve as inspiration for future successes and are important to counter the cynical dismissal of international aid for health and development programs. However, it is also important to learn about programs that did not work even though the failures are seldom discussed.

We also hope you learn that there are multiple levels of causation for health problems and that solutions become more difficult to find as one moves "upstream." Finally, we hope you gain an appreciation for new technologies for improving the human condition, while still realizing that they are not panaceas.

The Consortium of Universities for Global Health has released a set of competencies that students of global health should know. This book brings students to what Consortium of Universities for Global Health describes as "Level 2" competencies, appropriate for students considering future study in global health or preparing for a summer field experience. It also includes much information that goes beyond this into "Level 3" competencies to prepare students to work in the field—for example, understanding the factors underlying the movement of health-care workers globally, and applying issues of social justice and human rights to public health work.

We structured this book in a way that is different from other texts, which often progress disease by disease. Instead, we present the book in four main parts, each of which is divided into subsections. In the first part, you will be introduced to the field of global health. The second and third parts of the book examines the ecological and social determinants of health. The fourth part considers interventions to improve global health. As you can see the by the table of contents, the introductory part has three sections, dealing with some milestones in global public health, the basic epidemiological tools of global health and measuring disease burden. The second part of the book covers the ecological determinants of health: air, water, and food. The third part of the book focuses on the social determinants of health: social inequalities, sex and reproduction and violence. The final part on interventions and programs has four parts: historical programs, health systems and aid, health communication efforts and global health ethics.

In total, there are thirteen sections, and each one is introduced with a series of conceptual tools to orient you to the take-home messages of each section. Each section is followed by a list of resources for further exploration through Internet resources, audio-visual materials and case studies for problem-based learning. We encourage you to explore these resources through this book's companion website (www.oup.com/us/brown-closser).

The resources in the "case studies" sections of this book can be used in many different ways; when we teach we like to use them for discussion in small groups in class. For those case studies that simply pose a problem without asking specific questions, we have found that asking students to write policy briefs with a solution can be a great assignment. The section of the UN's Food and Agriculture Organization's Food Security Communications Toolkit (available for free online) that focuses on policy briefs is an excellent resource for students who might be writing a policy brief for the first time.

This volume is a collection of 49 separate readings that can be read in any order. For each reading there is an introduction, a handful of discussion questions to consider while reading and a context box that explains who the author is, where the article appeared and the correct way to cite it. There is a glossary in the back that includes key terms (bolded in the text).

Understanding global health challenges and their potential solutions requires multiple viewpoints—from history and international economics to disease ecology and health bureaucracies. This book is designed to showcase the value of a variety of disciplinary perspectives and to stimulate discussion about ethical issues. We think this approach can help prepare students for lives of effective action in a deeply complex world.[1]

[1] Since we started writing this book, there was a change in the presidency of the United States, and there are now many questions about the country's future direction. We agree with Vermund and Kurth (Reading 42) that continuing and expanding global health is of vital interest to the United States.

ACKNOWLEDGMENTS

First, we must thank Jennifer Barr for her wonderful work in proofing, glossary writing and general editing. Her useful comments truly improved the book.

Second, we thank the hundreds of undergraduate students whom we have taught in global health courses at Middlebury and Emory over the years. Their interest and enthusiasm is inspiring. Quite a few continued their studies in public health and now have impressive careers. As most professors know, we learn a great deal from our students.

At Middlebury, Yasmine Gilbert and Hannah Blair were extremely helpful student assistants. Yasmine successfully countered our combined forces of disorganization and, with unfailing good cheer, kept us focused and moving forward. We are grateful. Students in the Spring 2017 Global Health course at Middlebury contributed to the glossary, including Cameron Pierce, Sarah Lake, Elissa Denunzio, Jared Whitman, Sophie Kapica, Tegan Whitney and Jeremy Carter. At Emory, Saleem Hadera served as an undergraduate student assistant.

The many contributors to this volume generously provided their time and knowledge toward our shared goal of educating students. We appreciate their thoughtful work.

PJB thanks current Emory graduate students in medical anthropology and global health who have helped by reading alternative articles, sharing concepts and working as teaching assistants, including Jen Barr, Bisan Salhi, A. G. Tribble, Amanda Maxfield, Kaitlin Banfield, Tatenda Mangurenje and Tenzin Namdul. PJB is also honored to have worked with Emory alumni, especially ones dually trained in Anthropology and Public Health who become inspirational colleagues: Svea Closser, Casey Bouskill, Cameron Rollins, Sarah Willen, Aun Lor, Dredge Kang, Erin Finley, Alexa Dietrich, Vinay Kamat, Emily Mendenhall, Kate Sabot, Bonnie Fullard, Brandon Kohrt, Daniel J. Smith, Leandris Liburd, Elizabeth Whitaker, Thom McDade, Chris Kuzawa, Tassi Hirshfield, Howard Chiou, Kenneth Maes, Jennifer Tookes, Jed Stephenson, Jo Weaver, Jessica Gregg, Amy Patterson, Kendra Hatfield, Jen Kuzara, Ron Barrett, Matseliso Molapo, Deanne Dunbar, Gayatri Reddy, Mark Padilla, Daniel Lende, Michelle Parsons, Melissa Melby, Matt Dudgeon and Bethany Turner. PJB is grateful for his Emory colleagues in Medical Anthropology and Public Health, including Craig Hadley, Peggy Barlett, Melvin Konner, Chikako Osawa de Silva, Michelle Lampl, Kate Winskell, Jim Lavery, Carlos del Rios, Mimi Kaiser, Roger Rochat, Richard Levinson, Deb McFarland, Dabney Evans, Stan

Foster, Jim Curran and Jeff Koplan. PJB also wants to thank Svea for being such a wonderful co-author. SC thanks the many collaborators who have taught her so much, particularly Peter Brown, Judith Justice, Anat Rosenthal, Kenneth Maes and Erin Finley. At Middlebury, Pam Berenbaum's, Rebecca Tiger's and Michael Sheridan's conversations have enriched how she thinks about the field.

We thank our families for their support, encouragement and patience. Betsy Brown warmly opened her home to SC on many occasions, and her great companionship and wonderful food made these visits very special. Kaif Rehman cheerfully embraced beach vacations dominated by conversations about chapter introductions (maybe because he had no choice, but we appreciate it anyway). Svea thanks Bruce and Sally Closser for their warm enthusiasm. She is grateful, as always, for Matt Luck's unfailing support. Finally, Peter thanks Betsy, the long-time love of his life, for everything.

The authors and OUP also wish to thank the following reviewers:

Violeta Aguilar-Figuly, *Miami Dade College*
Susan E. Bell, *Drexel University*
Bria Dunham, *Boston University*
Audrey Giles, *University of Ottawa*
M. Cameron Hay-Rollins, *Miami University*
Cheryl Killion, *Case Western Reserve University*
Ann Magennis, *Colorado State University*
Meredith Marten, *University of West Florida*
Laura E. Nathan, *University of California, Berkeley*
Carole A. Pepa, *Valparaiso University*
Bernardo Ramirez, *University of Central Florida*
Monika Sawhney, *Marshall University*

PART 1

Introducing Global Health

1 WHAT IS GLOBAL HEALTH?

A Definition of Health

Health is not easy to define. When you see a friend, a typical greeting in English might be, "How are you?" Are we asking for a self-assessment of their health? Do you really want an answer? Most of the time, your friend will just say "fine," and that ends the ritualized greeting. Sometimes, the person will talk about a recent illness or current problem. Occasionally, they might unload on you with a series of physical, social, and emotional complaints and worries. All of those are appropriate answers, and all of them are about health. Health, after all, is about life.

In the United States, the **Centers for Disease Control and Prevention** (CDC) conducts an annual survey of over 400,000 Americans called the Behavioral Risk Factor Surveillance Survey (BRFSS). They ask many questions, such as whether you smoke cigarettes (and how many a day), use seat belts, exercise, eat vegetables, and so forth. But the first question they ask is: "How would you rate your general health today? Excellent, Very Good, Good, Fair, or Poor?"

After the survey is conducted, **epidemiologists** analyze the data. When they look at which survey respondents died within the year after the survey, those who answered "fair" or "poor" are the most likely to die; the correlation is very strong. Thus, we can conclude that those people are indeed unhealthy.

While lots of people tend to think of health exclusively in terms of the physical body, the most accurate definition of the concept is a three-pronged one, a bio-psycho-social model of health. This is because every human being is simultaneously a physical organism (a body), a self-aware individual (mind), and a member of a number of social groups (like family or school). A majority of people would also argue that everyone also has a spiritual dimension, but there is disagreement about that.

In 1946, the **World Health Organization** (WHO) was formed as part of the United Nations. The founding charter of the WHO provides the most widely held definition of health:

> *Health is a state of complete physical, mental and social well-being and not merely the absence of disease or infirmity.*[1]

There are several things worth noting in this classic definition. First, health does include medical issues like the absence of disease; this means that issues like access to clinical health-care services are important.

Second, the emphasis on well-being—both mental and social—points to the obvious reality that all humans are more than just their corporeal bodies. Think about this in terms of yourself—you are much more than your body. Do you just think of yourself as the sum total of your bones, organs, and tissues? Thus, it is difficult to overemphasize the importance of mental health, both for individuals and worldwide. Mental health problems include common "mental disorders" like anxiety and depression, as well as psychotic diseases like schizophrenia.

But this WHO definition also goes beyond these narrow definitions of mental health. Your personal well-being is dependent on external factors: Do you live in a war zone? Is there enough money to get food? Is your country in political turmoil? Do you have access to a safe shelter? Your well-being also includes small-scale social factors and internal feelings—like your love for others, your social support, and your hope for the future. Many people include their faith or spirituality as important contributors to their well-being.

In the end, all aspects of health are highly valued by all people of the world—irrespective of nationality, religion, or ethnicity.

Three Levels of Health

There are three levels of health: individual health, population health, and global health. In general, the fields of **medicine** and health care deal with individual health. Most medical doctors wait for sick patients come to them for help, and then the doctor treats them in the clinic. Sometimes that treatment might include information on what to expect or advice on how to prevent a reoccurrence. Often, the treatment is expensive and needs to be performed in the hospital or clinic.

Population health is the bailiwick of **public health**, a discipline with roots in both social reform movements and in science. These practitioners, often employed in government agencies, keep track of how groups of people are doing: they discover and examine the rates of diseases or deaths in a particular city, state, or category of people. People working in population health strive to prevent health problems through activities like education, vaccination programs, or enforcing health and safety standards (e.g., they monitor the sanitary conditions of restaurants).

Because public health focuses on health at the population level, it is theoretically and methodologically distinct from medicine, which focuses on the individual. Public health and medicine have very different goals, theories, and educational trajectories; the standard pre-med curriculum at the undergraduate level is helpful for medical school, but it is not the best preparation for a career in public health. Table 1 shows the major differences between public health and medicine. These boundaries are not rigid: For example, doctors frequently practice preventative medicine, and public health professionals might include treatment for a disease as part of their plan for controlling it.

Still, these characteristics mean that careers in public health and medicine are quite different. Doctors and nurses, for example, care for individual patients. Caring for individual human beings can be very rewarding, in part, because cures can be easy to identify and patients are sometimes so grateful after they are healed. Public health professionals, on the other hand, might spend their entire career in front of a computer doing statistics or in conference rooms trying to shape policy. They have less of a personal connection to the people their work might affect. They work to *prevent* or *manage* health problems, so there are no grateful individuals who can thank them.

TABLE 1.1 Major Differences between Public Health and Medicine.

Public Health	Medicine
Preventative	Curative
Populations	Individuals

But those in public health might argue that their work has a much larger impact in the long run. They may spend years figuring out how to decrease cigarette smoking, and as a result, fewer people smoke and fewer people die of lung cancer. But there is often nothing outwardly heroic or glamorous in this day-to-day work (except that it takes courage and fortitude to "take on" Big Tobacco corporations).

In addition, people working in public health would argue that their work is more economically efficient—they can have a greater health impact per dollar spent on their work because health care and hospital treatment is so expensive. Benjamin Franklin said that "an ounce of prevention is worth a pound of cure"—but who knows if he got the exact proportions correct?

The cartoon in Figure 1.1 comes from an epidemiology course at the CDC decades ago. Take a look at it.

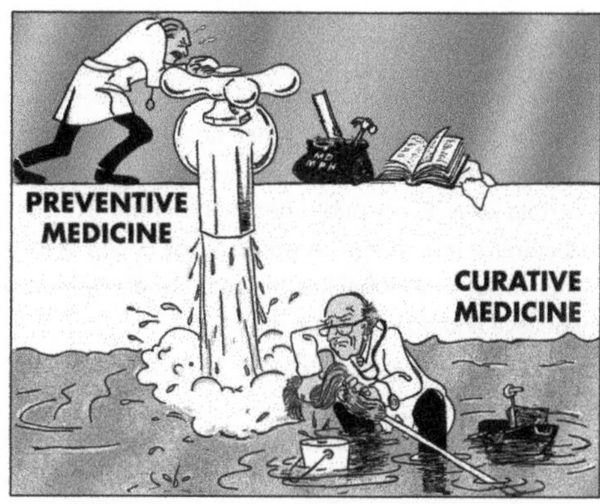

FIGURE 1.1. Cartoon from Lecture on Preventive Medicine.

Source: Centers for Disease Control and Prevention, *c.* 1980. Courtesy of Eugene Gangarosa.

WHAT'S YOUR MAJOR? ALL DISCIPLINES CONTRIBUTE TO GLOBAL HEALTH

Undergraduates sometimes ask each other, "What's your major?" American colleges and universities have an amazing number of majors and minors available to undergraduate students. In our own colleges, Emory has around 120 options, and Middlebury has more than 60. (Note: more is not necessarily better.) We have stated that global health is more of a set of problems than a single discipline. We have also said that the solutions to global health problems require the skills and insights of people from a wide variety of disciplines. One does not have to become a doctor or work in the health sciences to make important contributions to efforts in global health.

We were once challenged by colleagues to defend our assertion that global health is everyone's concern—no matter what you study. For some majors or minors, the connection is more obvious, but for others, it's more challenging to articulate. But whatever your undergraduate major or minor is, you can make a difference in global health during your lifetime (even if it is simply through donation). What's your major? And how could it connect to global health?

Accounting

There is a good deal of money spend in global health—around $200 billion every year. Those funds need to be managed efficiently and accounted for. Problems with financial corruption occur in all sectors of economies, but it has been particularly challenging in global health.

Anthropology[i]

People's ideas, beliefs and values—their culture—influence their behavior and consequently their health. Anthropologists can help global health workers understand why local people act certain ways. Every public health intervention involves a cross-cultural interaction. Anthropologists can also offer insights about why global health practitioners believe what they believe and do what they do.

Art

Studio Art is relevant to global health. Health communication requires capturing people's attention; posters, for example, are a classic health education medium. There are NGOs who provide art therapy to treat child victims of trauma.

[i] The two editors are trained in both anthropology and public health. We could describe how anthropologists can and do contribute to global health for pages and pages.

Biology

Health and disease are biological processes, although not exclusively so (see the WHO definition of health). Advancements in biomedicine most often depend on discoveries in molecular biology, genetics, biochemistry, and so forth. Humans live in a world of microbes both inside and outside of their bodies; microbiologists are essential for understanding those little critters. Human biologists do basic science related to immunology, endocrinology, growth, and aging.

Business

The skills of business are at the core of successful global health programming and advancement. These include management, marketing, logistics, finance, human resource management, and public relations. Even the most basic management skills—like running an effective meeting—are necessary for making progress. The best NGOs can be considered as "social businesses" where the final bottom line is the improvement of human well-being rather than making a profit. Global health research and programming needs to be run efficiently and without wasting often scarce resources.

Chemistry

Some parts of chemistry are related to the development of pharmaceuticals and many chemists work for "big pharma." While many of the medicines needed to treat the diseases that plague low- and middle-income countries were discovered many years ago, new diseases are emerging, and old ones are gaining resistance, requiring the development of new drugs. When HIV/AIDS emerged, it represented a huge challenge to chemists, biochemists, and biomedical scientists, but they very quickly (in historical terms) developed effective antiretroviral drug therapies ("the triple cocktail"), saving millions of lives. Other chemists work in terms of understanding and assessing environmental contaminants, such as industrial wastes that cause cancer, and work to help clean contaminated sites.

Communication

There are a variety of different media that are produced and examined by communication majors—radio, TV, film, posters, and so forth. Global health education and outreach uses all of them in their programs. Health education is a necessary (but not sufficient) cause of behavior change.

Ecology and Environmental Science

Ecologists study the interrelationships between organisms. Therefore, disease ecology plays a role in understanding the chain of infection and therefore designing disease control measures. But health problems are not limited to infectious agents. Environmental Science students learn about water and air pollution as well as ways to sustain a health ecosystem.

Economics

It is impossible to separate global health from issues of economics and economic development. Poverty is associated with poor health status, and poor health contributes to ongoing poverty. Conversely, economic improvements improve population health. The field of economics is necessary for understanding factors like income inequality, health-care financing, and consumer behavior.

Education

Education, especially the education of girls, is a fundamental goal of the UN development plans. It is known that mothers' literacy and education has a strong positive effect on the health of their children. Interestingly, we do not know exactly how this happens. Education majors most often become teachers, and the field of education works to improve the effectiveness of educational systems. Such improvements are important in all parts of the world.

English

English majors learn to think critically and write clearly. These are important skills for people working everywhere. With globalization, English has become the near-universal language of international communication.

History

Global health problems must be understood in historical context. The biomedical solutions to most infectious disease were discovered decades and even centuries ago. Therefore, the historical question is why those solutions have not spread to the rest of the world. The answers lie in the history of imperialism, colonialism, war, and capitalist exploitation. Epidemic diseases have greatly affected human history from the bubonic plague, to the conquest of the Americas, to the influenza pandemic following World War I, and examining these historical precedents can help us prepare for the future.

Languages

To be an effective global health practitioner in the field, one must speak different languages. While many languages spoken by local people in low- and middle-income countries might not be taught to undergraduates, it is clear that that knowing another language is extremely useful.

Math and Statistics

Quantification is central in all of global health. Statistical skills are more important than pure mathematics in this field. However, important new metrics, like disability-adjusted like years lost (DALYs), are based on mathematically complex algorithms. Epidemiology is based on statistics, and every student in public health graduate school is required to take courses in biostatistics.

Medicine

If you study in the United States, you cannot have a major in medicine or surgery. Why not? Many countries do have an education system in which students directly study medicine right out of high school. What might be the advantage of studying an arts and science discipline before learning a profession?

Nutrition and Exercise Science

These majors are not found at all colleges and, in some places, used to be called physical education. But these areas of study are critical for improving global health because of the contemporary epidemic of noncommunicable diseases like cardiovascular disease. Good nutrition and physical activity are requirements for health. The challenge is to make these available to people throughout the world and to get them to change their behavior.

Philosophy and Ethics

There is a field called Bioethics, of which global health ethics is one part. There are important questions that need to be asked and discussed: Is it ethical to conduct research—for example, in drug testing—in low-income countries when the same research would not be approved in the United States? How far may governments go in limiting privacy and freedom of movement in the name of infectious disease control? Is there a human right to health care?

Political Science

Politics might be considered the key for achieving real progress in global health and economic development. Departments of Public Health are parts of political structures,

continued

and most of the financing of programs is through public funds. International political cooperation is necessary when there are disease outbreaks that can spread across national boundaries. In an unequal globalized world, what are the responsibilities of rich nations to the poor?

Psychology

There is no global health without mental health. Clinical psychology has brought tools like cognitive behavioral therapy to relieve suffering and disability from common mental disorders like depression. Global health researchers have shown that such tools can work with minimally trained community members. Psychological research explores the way people think and reasons they behave in certain ways. For example, why do people do things that are bad for their health, such as smoking, unsafe sex, drunk driving, or being a couch potato?

Religion

Religion is a universal aspect of human societies. Religious beliefs can influence behaviors in ways that often enhance people's health. Religious beliefs can also be harmful for health, for example, in religiously motivated armed conflicts. To make global health programs work well, it is essential to be respectful of other people's religious traditions and cultures. Many practitioners of global health go into the field because of personal religious motivations.

Sociology

As the fundamental social science, Sociology is necessary for understanding inequalities, especially health inequalities, in regard to social class, race/ethnicity, and gender. Sociologists are interested in groups and group behavior including institutions like those involved in global health. The quantitative methodological tools of sociology are similar to those of epidemiology.

Theater and Film

Successful health communications require the combination of education and entertainment. In many parts of the world, some of the most successful techniques for health education about complex issues—for example, social stigma suffered by people with HIV/AIDS—is theater and film. In some countries, street theater has been used to involve local youth in a health cause and to promote awareness of health messages.

Urban Planning

More and more people around the world are living in cities. Urban planners can lay out cities that promote healthy behaviors, such as ensuring there are sidewalks and road crossings to promote walking. They can also plan cities to be healthier habitats, with green spaces and trees to mitigate air pollution and improve the mental health of residents.

Zoology

In many parts of the world, humans and animals live in close proximity. Infectious diseases like HIV become serious human problems when they jump between species. The chain of infection often involves animals (this includes the complex chain of influenza), and there is the need for zoologists and other animal scientists to control such diseases.

After you finish this course in global health, see if you can expand this list. The idea is that global health is multidisciplinary to its core.

It seems to have been drawn by someone working in public health, not a doctor working in curative medicine. What is going on here? What is the water a metaphor for? Where is the water coming from? Why is he pushing the faucet in that direction? Why would public health professionals argue that their approach to improving health is superior? What might a doctor say? What do you think?

The third level of health is **global health**. This involves understanding the causes of health problems for people all over the world—and then solving those problems. The field of global health is based in public health, but understanding the impacts of global forces and population-level interventions on community health requires a multidisciplinary approach. The tools of global health include not only clinical medicine but also tools from many other disciplines as well (see the "What's Your Major" box).

Global health belongs to everybody. Unlike most disciplines, global health is really a ***collection of problems*** having to do with health in all parts of the world. Many of these health problems relate to preventable causes of death or disability; these health issues keep people from living long, productive, and enjoyable lives. Solutions to these problems must come from work bringing together researchers, practitioners in the field who deliver the goods, and people in communities most affected by a given health issue.

In addition to involving different stakeholders, solving global health problems also requires using a variety of theoretical and methodological perspectives. For example, people attempting to slow the spread of HIV include scientists working on vaccine development; researchers studying the political dynamics of health aid in Mozambique; and community workers investigating how gay Latino men in the United States navigate their social circles. These people are frequently in conversation with one another and must reach across disciplinary lines to comprehend various facets of the larger problems. These people might be trained in the biosciences, social sciences, business, or the humanities. Examine the box entitled "What's Your Major?" Many fields of study provide skills that can contribute to solving complex global health problems.

Global health professionals also come from diverse backgrounds across the world: the field has been shaped in profound ways by the work of researchers and practitioners from low-and middle-income countries, as well as those from rich countries (who tend to have more access to funding, though not necessarily better ideas). Because diseases do not respect national or ethnic borders in our global village, health problems like new "emerging" diseases must be understood and dealt with in specific local contexts, but the problems need to be the concern of everyone.

Health and Wealth

There is a strong relationship between health and wealth. The poorer you and your family are, the worse your health and lower your life expectancy will be. This is a simple fact that is true both between countries and within countries. Wealth is one of the key social **determinants of health**, the topic of Section 6 of this book. The box entitled "Portraits of Health" illustrates some of the reasons for this relationship between health and wealth. The stories it tells are fictional, but the problems those stories describe are very real.

PORTRAITS OF HEALTH IN FIVE COUNTRIES

Family in a High-Income Country (Daily Income about US$50 per Person)

The Swedish family gathers after the evening meal to discuss the 20-year-old daughter's holiday plans. Anna has just finished upper secondary school and has not yet decided whether she wants to start university studies after the summer holiday. But, just in case, she has applied for the favorable public loans that enable young people from all socio-economic backgrounds to study at universities. Her main concern is not about her future but that she is leaving home in less than one week for her first holiday trip without her parents. She is going to travel by train through Germany, France, Spain, and Portugal together with her cousin. She had planned to do this trip with her boyfriend, but he left her for another girl two months ago. Her mother is not happy about Anna's holiday plans. She worries that her daughter may lose the medicines she needs to take daily to treat her asthma. It may be difficult to find the same brands of tablets and inhalation sprays in foreign countries. Anna comforts her mother by telling her that she will take enough medicine with her, medicine that she buys at highly subsidized prices in Sweden. Her mother also worries that her daughter will not eat enough. In her early teens, Anna suffered a mild form of anorexia nervosa. The daughter knows about her mother's secret worries, and to comfort her further she promises to call home daily on her mobile telephone, which she will take with her. Her father suggests that it will be cheaper for her to send SMS messages. He reluctantly allows Anna to borrow his digital camera. The father reminds Anna to send postcards to her grandmother. The 80-year-old has been admitted to a public nursing home due to advanced Alzheimer's disease. Anna cannot see the point of sending postcards to her grandmother, as she does not remember anything. However, Anna knows her father has a bad conscience for not visiting his mother every week, so she promises to send postcards to the nursing home. After all, her father has agreed to lend her his new digital camera! The daughter is also reminded by her mother to take enough disposable contact lenses. For cosmetic reasons, she uses lenses instead of glasses to correct for her short-sightedness. Anna is happy that she can leave her parents just to enjoy

continued

traveling to foreign countries. Anna has earned part of the money needed for the travel by working during the holidays, but most of the money is a gift from her grandfather, who said that his pension was high enough to share some of it with his beloved granddaughter.

Family in a Middle-Income Country (Daily Income about US$10 per Person)

The Brazilian family in a small town in central Brazil gathers for the evening meal. The 20-year-old daughter, Ana, is upset because her father has said that he is unable to pay for her planned university studies. She was involved in a traffic accident last year, and her father explains the lack of money by reference to the high cost of her treatment. She underwent an operation for fractures of both legs. Her father took her to a private hospital, which he believed would provide better care than the cheaper government hospital. Since childhood Ana wears glasses to correct her short-sightedness. She hates the glasses for cosmetic reasons, but the family cannot afford to buy her contact lenses. Ana often takes her glasses off so that she will look better when she is walking around town. Her father claims that the accident occurred because she was not using her glasses that day. Ana says the car hit her because the driver was drunk. Regardless, glasses, the treatment of her fractures, and installation of a new bathroom in the house was what this family's economy could afford, says the father. Ana must now start earning her own money.

To find a job, she has been offered the opportunity to stay with her cousin's family in Rio de Janeiro. This is on the understanding that she helps to care for the sick grandmother, who lives with the cousin's family. The 66-year-old had one leg amputated last year due to complications from diabetes, and since then she has had to take regular medication against depression. Ana is told that it is a good offer to go to Rio. The cousin's family has a new DVD player, something that her own family has not yet been able to afford to buy. Ana is reluctant to leave her hometown because of her new boyfriend, whom she has not yet introduced to her parents. She would really like to study at the university in her hometown instead of working and caring for her sick and sad grandmother.

Family in a Low-Income Country (Daily Income about US$2 per Person)

The Indian family gathers for the evening meal on the veranda outside their small house in rural India. Ana's family lives in a village in the state of Uttar Pradesh.

The 20-year-old daughter, Ana, is visiting her parents today to show them her second child, a baby who was born the year before. Ana says she wants to listen to her father's radio. Her husband's family has a radio, but because her last delivery was costly for her and her husband, they have been unable to afford batteries for the radio for several months now. She is still weak following the delivery and has developed a cough in recent months. The cough syrup she was prescribed at the public health center did not cure her. The eight-kilometer walk today from the village where she lives with her husband's family has tired her. The hidden aim of her visit to her parents is to discuss whether they can help to pay for medicines to treat her cough and her weakness. She and her husband hope that her parents will help to pay for good medicines. She looks at her small family and thinks: "Well, at least I still have two healthy children and a kind husband, although we are so poor that we only get enough food to eat every second day." She thinks that it is a shame that she should be a burden to them. How long will her husband put up with her if she remains sick?

She cannot read, as she had to leave primary school after only one year. Her father said there was no point in continuing, since she could not see what the teacher wrote on the blackboard. The family could never afford to buy glasses for her short-sightedness. The teacher had told her father that glasses were the only thing the clever little girl needed to learn to read and write. Her younger brother, went to school long enough to learn to read. He is now reading the text on the bottle of cough syrup that she has been taking every day for a week, without any effect. Her parents are very concerned about her health, but no one realizes that, in addition to anemia, she has pulmonary tuberculosis. The latter diagnosis was missed due to the limited diagnostic resources at the health center where she was very briefly examined.

Her grandmother died some years ago, after coughing blood for many months. The family thinks she died from tuberculosis, but she was never taken to the clinic for diagnosis. She was instead given traditional medicines at home. Tuberculosis is considered to be a shameful sign of poverty. Consequently, the word "tuberculosis" is never mentioned in the family discussion. The family knows the possible significance of chronic coughing but use an old Hindi word for chronic cough when talking about Ana's disease. Her mother says she should be taken to a private doctor. Her father says it is too expensive; it would be cheaper to take her to a traditional Ayurvedic clinic. The herbal treatment given at that clinic cured his back pain last year, and he thinks it also may cure his daughter's cough. He is willing to pay for traditional treatment but not for consultation with a private doctor. The reason for his reluctance is that doctors always prescribe very expensive medicines. Ana knows precisely what she would do if she had her own money and the right to decide for herself. But this is not the case, and she does not want to embarrass her husband by begging her father for more money. She will try the herbal medicine, but the tuberculosis bacteria will continue to destroy her lungs and infect her children. Ana does not have any other choice, not even to cry. But she has a secret determination: "I must survive this disease, to make it possible for my daughter to go to school!"

Family in a Collapsed Country (Daily Income Less Than US$1 per Person)

The family in Liberia lived in a rural village not far from the capital Monrovia during the recent period when the political and administrative functions of this West African country collapsed during a prolonged armed conflict. Liberia is presently in the process of regaining peace and basic public functions.

The young Liberian woman, Ana, had never been to school. This had always saddened her. This story begins when her parents returned to what used to be their home before the war. Ana's father had been in hospital close to the capital for two months. He suffered severe injuries during the fighting that took place between two armed gangs in their village two months ago. After the fight, the victorious armed gang started to burn down all the houses in the village. While trying to stop them from burning the family house down, her father was badly cut with a large knife. His right elbow joint was cut open, but he managed to escape to his family, who were already hiding in the forest. The mother told Ana to remain with her small brothers in the hiding place in the forest while she tried to help her husband to get to a hospital. They knew of a hospital supported by a humanitarian relief organization. It was situated a few day's walk away. Ana's mother had heard that this hospital also treated poor people who could not pay. Her father reached the hospital in time and recovered, following amputation of his right arm above the elbow. He now thanks God that he is alive and still has his left hand.

Ana lived in the forest with her brothers while their parents were at the hospital. They ate from the family's cassava field. This productive root crop protected them from starvation. During the second week of hiding, her youngest brother suddenly developed a high fever, and she had to return to their village with her sick brother on her back to look for treatment. The older brothers had to follow. On the path, they met a passing gang of armed teenagers, who raped Ana in front of her brothers. She had not recognized the kind of people who were approaching in time to be able to hide. Once, the imam in their village had said that her problem in recognizing people was because she was short-sighted. The family could never afford to buy her the glasses that the imam said she needed.

Following the rape, she managed to get back to their village with her sick brother. However, the man who owned a bicycle and used to bring and sell modern tablets against malaria had left the village, as had the traditional healer who sold herbal medicine against fever. As the sun set and in the darkness of the night, she could do nothing but sit beside her young brother and try to comfort him. His fever became worse; he got convulsions and died in the middle of the night. The next morning, some old women who had remained in the village helped her to bury the little body. She now shows her parents the grave, where they all pray together.

Ana is relieved that her parents do not blame her for her brother's death. Although her parents are kind, she does not want to tell them that she was raped. Despite all the tragedies that have affected them, Ana and her mother are comforted by the reunion of the family, and they cook a full meal for everyone. They have not eaten much in recent weeks, because one night someone stole almost all the cassava plants in their field. The children have been extremely hungry, but tonight they will be able to eat well. The parents have brought back a sack of maize flour that they were given when leaving the hospital. Ana's two surviving brothers have managed to catch two small birds. Ana fries the birds over the fire, while her mother prepares the maize porridge. She and her brothers are allowed to eat as much as they want. In silence, they watch their father learning to eat with his left hand. The father thinks: "Had we fled in time to the neighboring country, we would have avoided all these sufferings." Ana thinks that she is pregnant, as she has not had any bleedings since the rape. It saddens her immensely that this is not the child of the man she loved. He was killed in the war last year. What she will not know until several years later when peace has returned to her country is that she was infected with HIV during the rape. She and her only child will only have a few years to live together.

Ann Lindstrand, Staffan Bergstrom, Hans Rosling, Biritta Rubenson, Bo Stenson, and Thorkild Tylleskar. *Global Health: An Introductory Textbook*. Enskede, Sweden: Studentlitteratur, 2011, pp. 15–18

Examine Figures 1.2 and 1.3 carefully. They both illustrate the close relationship between health and wealth from an international viewpoint. You might notice some differences between the figures even though they illustrate the same story. Figure 1.2 uses life expectancy at birth as a measure of health, and both axes have a simple arithmetic scale. In Figure 1.3 (from the famous Gapminder website, https://www.gapminder.org), income is in a logarithmic scale. The first figure shows a very strong relationship between wealth and health for countries with lower per capita incomes, and then the curve levels off as the average life expectancy reaches a biological maximum, meaning that the human organism simply can't live any longer. The second figure shows the same relationship, even though it looks like a straight line (this is because of the logarithmic scale). This is useful because it is easier to see how particular countries fare.

The World Bank's categorization of countries by wealth are

- low-income economies have a gross national income (GNI) per capita of around $1,000 or less in 2015;
- lower middle-income economies have a GNI per capita between $1,000 and $4,000;
- upper middle-income economies have a GNI per capita between $4,000 and $12,000; and
- high-income economies enjoy a GNI per capita of $12,000 or more.

You can see that these wealth categories are highly correlated with health outcomes.

Global Health: A New Field?

The mid-1990s saw a huge increase in the interest of rich nations in funding health programs in low- and middle-income countries. Some of this new interest was linked to the global rise of HIV/AIDS and other emerging diseases. The change was also linked to the process of globalization, including increased flows of ideas and products. Countries recognized that the health problems of "over there" could very quickly become the health problems of "right here."

For this new era of global engagement of health, the new term "global health" arose, replacing the older term "international health" that was used throughout the Cold War era. The change to "global health" was meant to reflect the fact that the distinction between domestic and international health problems is

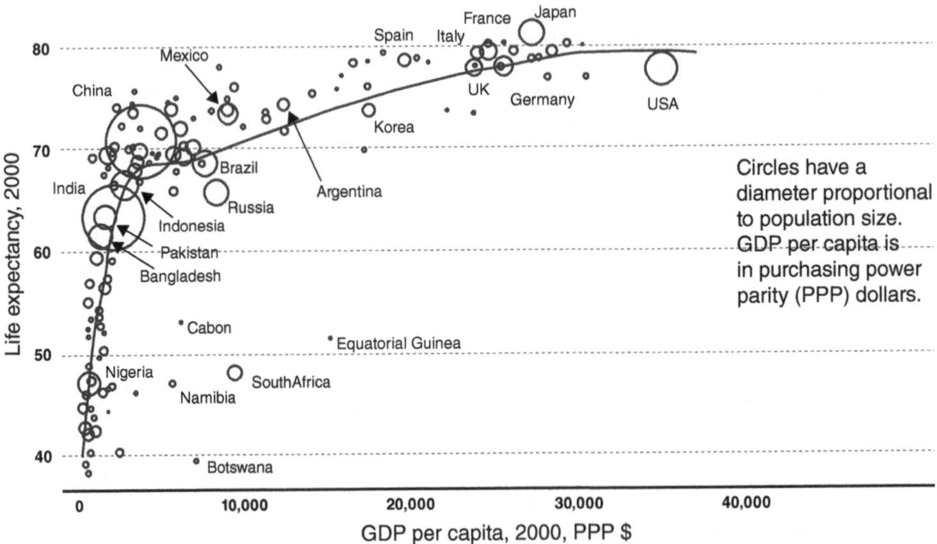

FIGURE 1.2 Average Life Expectancy and National Income per Capita (Arithmetic Scale).
Source: World Health Organization Commission on Social Determinants of Health. *Closing the Gap in a Generation,* http://apps.who.int/iris/bitstream/10665/43943/1/9789241563703_eng.pdf.

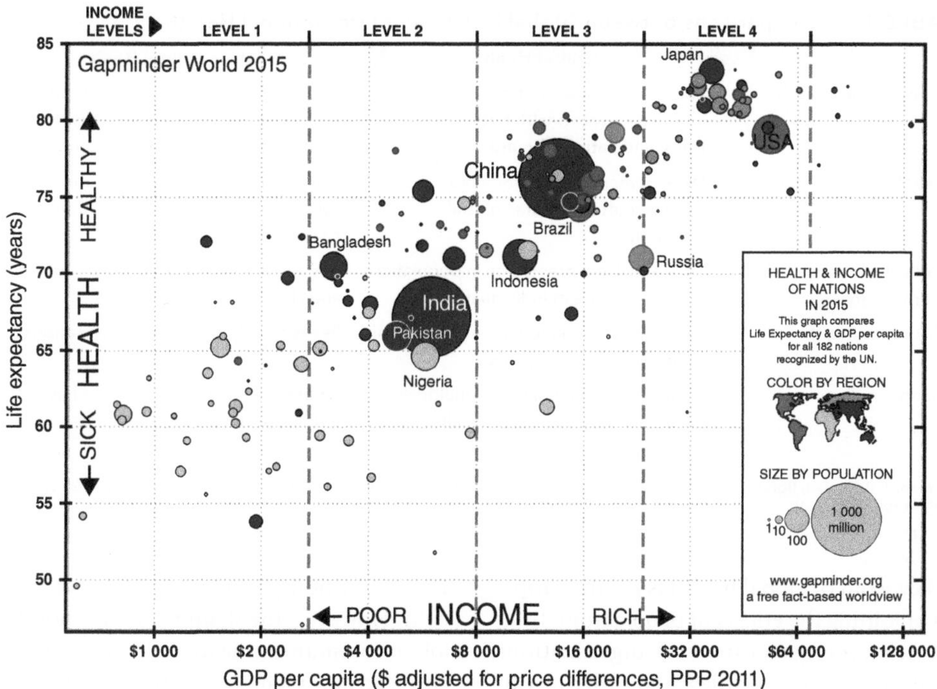

FIGURE 1.3 Life Expectancy and National Income per Capita (Logarithmic Scale).
Source: Free material from gapminder.org.

anachronistic. In other words, you can practice global health without a passport, because there are a lot of commonalities and connections between health problems in both high- and low-income countries.

The differences between global health and international health are summarized in Table 1.2. One important thing to recognize is that both of these fields include a combination of preventive measures and curative clinical medicine. In other words, the cartoon of the flood from the open faucet may represent a false dichotomy, representing public health and clinical health as distinct and separate, when they often overlap. Public health emphasizes primary prevention, or actions that will reduce the risk of people getting sick in the first place, but global health includes clinical action too.

The new term "global health" represented more than just a new way of talking; it marked a new philosophical orientation that had palpable effects. In general, global health is different from international health in at least five ways:

1. A new emphasis on nonpaternalistic partnerships between international donors and local recipients/communities;
2. An increase in the influence of nongovernmental organizations and a decrease in the influence of international organizations like the WHO;
3. Significant funding for research into new technologies to address the often-neglected health problems of the poorest people globally;
4. A recognition that health problems transcend national boundaries in a time of rapid travel and migration; and
5. Simultaneous support by both political conservatives concerned with biosecurity and political progressives interested in social justice and human rights.

TABLE 1.2 Comparisons between Global Health and International Health.

	Global Health	International Health
Geographical reach	Focuses on issues that directly or indirectly affect health but that can transcend national boundaries	Focuses on health issues of countries other than one's own, especially those of low-income and middle-income
Level of cooperation	Development and implementation of solutions often requires global cooperation	Development and implementation of solutions usually requires binational cooperation
Individuals or populations	Embraces both prevention in populations and clinical care of individuals	Embraces both prevention in populations and clinical care of individuals
Access to health	Health equity among nations and for all people is a major objective	Seeks to help people of other nations
Range of disciplines	Highly interdisciplinary and multidisciplinary within and beyond health sciences	Embraces a few disciplines but has not emphasised multidisciplinarity

Source: J. P. Koplan, Bond, T. C., Merson, M. H., et al. "Towards a Common Definition of Global Health. *The Lancet*, 2009, 373(9679): 1993–1995.

One key word of global health is **partnership**—the idea of joining the efforts of people from different countries, nongovernmental organizations, private companies, universities, and other institutions. As will be described in detail in Section 11, this ideal of partnership is not yet a reality on the ground, especially in terms of equal partnerships between people from the **Global North** and the **Global South**. It is hard to have equal partnerships when there are so many differences in access to resources like money.

In 2008, a number of leaders from the Consortium of Universities for Global Health suggested a definitive definition of the field:

> Global Health is an area for study, research, and practice that places a priority on improving health and achieving equity in health for all people worldwide. Global health emphasizes transnational health issues, determinants, and solutions; involves many disciplines within and beyond the health sciences and promotes interdisciplinary collaboration; and is a synthesis of population-based prevention with individual-level clinical care.[2]

This definition provides an inclusive view of the field. However, the definition does not do a good job in communicating the field's impressive and exciting achievements so far and the substantial contribution that it can make for all of humanity in the future. In Section 1 of this book, there are many examples of famous public health interventions—the success stories of the past that shape the way people in global health think about what they do moving forward. These successful cases of global health interventions show that although the causes of health problems are often very complex, committed and thoughtful people have made real impacts on population health.

1 World Health Organization. *Closing the Gap in a Generation.* Geneva: World Health Organization; 2008. http://apps.who.int/iris/bitstream/10665/43943/1/9789241563703_eng.pdf.
2. Koplan, J. P., Bond, T. C., Merson, M. H., et al. Towards a common definition of global health. *The Lancet.* 2009;373 (9679):1993–1995. doi:10.1016/S0140-6736(09)60332-9.

SECTION

1

Milestones in Global Health

This section of the book describes famous global health interventions—the success stories that shape the way people in global public health think about what they do. The people whose work is described in this section are heroes of global health; they devised solutions to health problems that saved many lives and changed the landscape of the field of public health. Some of these solutions are simple, like oral rehydration therapy, which has saved the lives of millions of children from dehydration caused by diarrhea. Oral rehydration therapy is extremely effective yet inexpensive; it does not require trained health-care personnel or special equipment. Some solutions are more complex and expensive, like the worldwide eradication of smallpox in 1979 (although that remarkable success took nearly 200 years between the discovery of a vaccine and the eradication of the disease).

These successful cases of global health interventions show that although the health challenges that they faced were often enormous, thoughtful, committed, and hard-working individuals were able to improve the lives of billions of people and make historic contributions to how we think about and do global health.

›› CONCEPTUAL TOOLS ‹‹

- **Global health involves understanding the causes of health problems for people all over the world—and then solving those problems.** The field of global health is based in public health, but understanding the impacts of global forces and population-level interventions on community health requires a multidisciplinary approach.
- **History is important.** There is much to be learned by studying the history of international and global health—both the successes and the failures. If you are in a Masters of Public Health program, you probably will not study the history of the discipline much, because public health training primarily emphasizes the

acquisition of specific and concrete skills such as surveying or program design. We believe, however, that it is invaluable to understand the historical trajectory of global health. Understanding the milestones mistakes of the past century and a half are vital to being more reflexive, more ethical, and more effective practitioners.

- **There is a generally positive historical trend in health since 1850.** As stated by the famous health statistician Hans Rosling, the general trend is for societies to change from being poor and sick to being wealthier and healthier. This trend, which is sometimes called the "great escape" from poverty and disease, had until recently primarily been seen in wealthy countries. The majority of the world is still undergoing this transition. Over the past 40 years, there has been an accelerated pace of improvements in health, particularly in low- and middle-income countries, because of improvements in living conditions, new technologies, and collaborative work in global health.
- **Epidemics, famines, wars, and colonialism have negatively affected the trend toward improved health in human history.** These are some of the major reasons for the striking inequalities in today's world. Global health's history is tightly linked to the world's political-economic changes, including today's context of globalization.
- **The threat of future epidemics still exists, and future epidemics may spread very quickly because of rapid global travel.** Epidemics have changed human history in the past. One of the most thoroughly studied global pandemics is the influenza of 1918. This is seen in Reading 3 and in Figure CT1.1. An ongoing challenge to global public health is the identification of new emerging infectious diseases through surveillance and their subsequent control. The future threats and the current need for investments in global health to prevent such a disaster are discussed in Reading 42.
- **The historic advancement of health—including the decline of mortality in the 19th century—was not simply due to clinical biomedicine.** Rather,

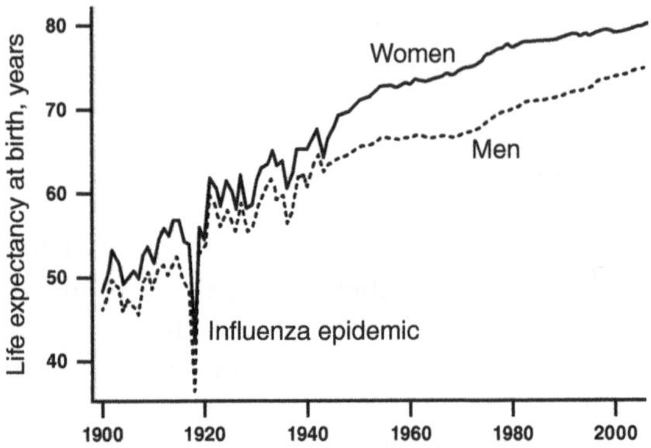

FIGURE CT1.1 Life Expectancy for Men and Women in the United States.

Source: Angus Deaton. (2013). *The Great Escape: Health, Wealth, and the Origins of Inequality.* Princeton, NJ: Princeton University Press.

nonmedical changes in environmental conditions like clean water, sanitation, nutrition, and housing were extremely important.

- **Diseases do not recognize political borders.** In our globalized world, diseases can spread quickly across international political borders. The historical record indicates that quarantines between countries do not work very well. As such, the distinction between domestic health and international health is to a large degree an illusion.
- **Health risks can spread globally—even when they are caused by behaviors rather than diseases.** Noncommunicable diseases—like heart disease, some cancers, obesity, and diabetes—are global problems. Cigarette smoking, the largest single preventable cause of death in the world, was invented in the United States and spread throughout the world in the 20th century. Many chronic diseases are linked to the Western obesogenic diet (a diet that predisposes people to become overweight or obese) that started in wealthier countries and is spreading globally.
- **Vertical programs are public health programs focused on just one disease.** Many of the programs described in this section were vertical; they focused on cutting global transmission of a disease like smallpox or HIV and didn't worry about other diseases. Vertical programs have some major strengths: they allow focus and clarity in goals and they can be very appealing to donors. But they also have strong critics, because they can ignore a community's most pressing health needs while they focus on their disease of choice. These debates are explored in depth in Sections 10 and 11.
- **Eradication is the permanent and total obliteration of a disease from the face of the earth.** It means that no one will ever get that disease again, because the agent that causes the disease is gone forever. Smallpox is the only human disease to ever be eradicated. The smallpox virus is extinct in the wild, so nobody can contract the disease (though it still exists in some labs).
- **The most common goal in public health is disease control.** Unlike eradication (see Reading 4), the goal in disease control is to bring transmission down to a level deemed acceptable. Of course, what is seen as acceptable varies in different times and places. The concepts of eradication and control are explored in depth in Section 10.
- **HIV/AIDS is the global health challenge of our times.** Because the HIV/AIDS pandemic catalyzed a new era of global health, it represents a historic milestone in the development of the field of Global Health. The huge amounts of funding for HIV/AIDS issues—and the associated successes and failures—is addressed in a number of articles in this book, including Chapters 8, 23, 27, and 28.

2 THE BROAD STREET PUMP

This is an iconic story featuring an epidemic of cholera in a particular neighborhood of London and an extremely clever and persistent physician who wanted to explain that epidemic and do something to stop it. This is the origin story of the science of ***epidemiology*** *and its heroic father figure, Dr. John Snow. Although he was best known at the time as a pioneer of anesthesiology, John Snow was a born scientist, not the laboratory type, but an observer, record-keeper, and analyst of what he saw in the real world. In this case, he actually studied a cholera outbreak in his own neighborhood.*

The setting, a mid-19th century slum in Soho near the Golden Square in London, would be considered rather disgusting by modern standards; the neighborhood was smelly, poor, crowded, and unhealthy. In many ways, it was like the slums of modern-day megacities in low-income countries. More than 127 people died in that neighborhood in a period of three days in September 1854; more than 800 people died over a period of three weeks. In terms of space, these deaths were highly concentrated—they were primarily within a radius of 250 yards.

Snow wanted to know the cause of the disease, which spread so rapidly yet was mostly limited to a restricted area. He wanted to know what the deceased had in common. Snow counted the dead from that localized epidemic in what would become the basic categories of ***descriptive epidemiology****: time, place, and person. By looking very carefully at place—where people had died—he determined that the disease was coming from a public water source: the Broad Street pump.*

At that time, the scientific dogma about the easily observed poor health of poor people and neighborhoods was that disease was spread by stinky, foul air called "miasma." As a scientific skeptic, Snow hypothesized that the disease was spread by contaminated water, but the medical authorities were slow to believe him. Therefore, it took a good deal of effort and epidemiological data—some of it shown in a famous map he made of cholera deaths—for Snow to convince the local commissioners to remove the handle from the pump within a week of the beginning of the outbreak. While the commissioners did not really believe Snow, they were desperate to do something.

The commissioners and the scientific community were slow to abandon the miasma theory of disease, despite the fact that Snow conducted other convincing studies during later outbreaks. In the summer of 1858, when hot weather baked the untreated sewage in the River Thames, it created a stench so bad that half the government and city shut down; this was an historic event called "The Great Stink." John Snow's brilliant epidemiological work proved that cholera outbreaks were the result of sewage-polluted drinking water. However, it was probably "The Great Stink" that really motivated the politicians to fund a huge, modern sewage system for the city, consequently cleaning up the Thames.

As you read this selection, consider the following questions:

- **In your opinion, why should this story be considered a milestone of Global Health?**
- **The author argues that the truly historic part of this story is removal of the pump handle. Why?**
- **Why did Snow look for anomalies like the work house and the brewery? How did these observations add to his evidence that cholera was waterborne?**
- **What were some of Snow's personal characteristics that made him skeptical about the miasma theory? How was his work with ether gas for anesthesiology relevant?**

CONTEXT

Steven Johnson is a best-selling writer of nine books about the intersection of science, technology and personal experience. This book was on the *New York Times* bestseller list for over a year. The book reveals some important aspects of Snow's investigation that were not widely known. Specifically, Johnson traced the role of Reverend Henry Whitehead, a local priest who knew the neighborhood well. While Whitehead initially did not believe Snow, he greatly aided the research by gaining community cooperation.

Sunday, September 3

The Investigator

By Sunday morning, a strange quiet had overtaken the streets of Soho. The usual chaos of the streetsellers had disappeared; most of the neighborhood's residents had either evacuated or were suffering behind their doors. Seventy of them had perished over the preceding twenty-four hours, hundreds more were at the very edge of death. Out in front of 40 Broad, the pump attracted only a handful of stragglers. The most common sight on the streets were the priests and doctors making their frantic rounds.

Word of the outbreak had traveled through the wider city and beyond. The chemist's son who had enjoyed his pudding days before on Wardour Street died on that Sunday at his home in Willesden. The entire city held its breath as it took in refugees from the embattled neighborhood, waiting to see if the outbreak in Golden Square would be re-created on a larger scale in the coming days. Seventy deaths in a single parish was not an uncommon number to hear in an age of cholera epidemics. But it normally took months for the disease to chalk up so many victims. The Broad Street strain of cholera—whatever it was, wherever it had come from—had managed that terrible feat in a single day.

While the disease had remained largely confined to an area of roughly five square blocks, the rest of Soho was on high alert. Many packed their bags and visited friends or family who lived in the country or other parts of the city; some locked the doors and shuttered the windows. The vast majority steered clear of the Golden Square neighborhood at all cost.

But one Soho regular had been following the case closely from his residence at Sackville Street on the southwestern edge of the neighborhood. Sometime near dusk he set out from his home, marching through the empty streets, directly into the heart of the outbreak. When he reached 40 Broad, he stopped and examined the pump for a few minutes in the fading light. He drew a bottle of water from the well, stared at it for a few seconds, then turned and made his way back to Sackville Street.

We don't know exactly what sequence of events turned John Snow's interest toward cholera in the late 1840s. For this working physician and researcher, of course, the disease would have been a constant presence in his life. There may in fact have been a direct link to his practice as an anesthesiologist, since chloroform had been (wrongly) championed as a potential cure for cholera by some early adopters who were less rigorous in their empiricism than Snow. Certainly, the outbreak of 1848–1849, the most severe British outbreak in more than a decade, made cholera one of the most urgent medical riddles of its time. For a man like Snow, obsessed with both the practice of medicine and the intellectual challenge of science, cholera would have been the ultimate quarry.

There were practically as many theories about cholera as there were cases of the disease. But in 1848, the dispute was largely divided between two camps: the contagionists and the miasmatists. Either cholera was some kind of agent that passed from person to person, like the flu, or it somehow lingered in the "miasma" of unsanitary spaces. The contagion theory had attracted some followers when the disease first reached British soil in the early 1830s. "We can only suppose the existence of a poison which progresses independently of the wind, of the soil, of all conditions of the air, and of the barrier of the sea," *The Lancet* editorialized in 1831. "In short, one that makes mankind the chief agent for its dissemination." But most physicians and scientists believed that cholera was disease spread via poisoned atmosphere, not personal contact. One survey of published statements from U.S. physicians during the period found that less than five percent believed the disease was primarily contagious.

Snow's detective work into cholera began when he noticed a telling detail in the published accounts of the 1848 epidemic. Asiatic cholera had been absent from Britain for several years, but it had recently broken out on the Continent, including the city of Hamburg. In September of that year, the German steamer *Elbe* docked in London, having left port at Hamburg a few days earlier. A crewman named John Harnold checked into a lodging house in Horsley-down. On September 22, he came down with cholera and died within a matter of hours. A few days later, a man named Blenkinsopp took over the room; he was seized by the disease on September 30. Within a week, the cholera began to spread through the surrounding neighborhood, and eventually through the entire nation. By the time the epidemic wound down, two years later, 50,000 people were dead.

In the weeks after the Horsley-down outbreak, as the cholera began its fatal march through the wider city and beyond, Snow embarked on a torrid stretch of inquiry: consulting with chemists who had studied the rice-water stools of cholera victims, mailing requests for information from the water and sewer authorities in Horsley-down, devouring accounts of the great epidemic of 1832. By the middle of 1849, he felt confident enough to go public with his theory. Cholera, Snow argued, was caused by some as-yet-unidentified agent that victims ingested, either through direct contact with the waste matter of other sufferers or, more likely, through drinking water that had been contaminated with that waste matter. Cholera was contagious, yes, but not in the way smallpox was contagious. Sanitary conditions were crucial to fighting the disease, but foul air had nothing to do with its transmission. Cholera wasn't something you inhaled. It was something you swallowed.

Snow built his argument for the waterborne theory around two primary studies, both of which showcased talents that would prove to be crucial five years later, during the Broad Street outbreak. In late July of 1849, an outbreak of cholera killed about twelve people living in slum conditions on Thomas Street in Horsleydown. Snow made an exhaustive inspection of the site and found ample evidence to support his developing theory. All twelve lived in a row of connected cottages called the Surrey building, which shared a single well in the courtyard they faced. A drainage channel for dirty water ran alongside the front of the houses, connecting to an open sewer at the end of the courtyard. Several large cracks in the drain allowed water to flow directly into the well, and during summer storms, the entire courtyard would flood with fetid water. And so a single case of cholera would quickly spread through the entire Surrey building population.

The layout of the Thomas Street flats provided Snow with an ingenious control study for his inquiry. The Surrey building backed onto a set of houses that faced another courtyard known as Truscott's Court. These abodes were every bit as squalid as the Surrey building, with the exact same demographic makeup of poor working families living within them. For all intents and purposes, they shared the same environment, save one crucial difference: they got their water from different sources. During the two-week period that saw the deaths of a dozen residents in the Surrey building, only one person perished in Truscott's Court, despite the fact that both groups lived within yards of each other. If the miasma were responsible for the outbreak, why would one squalid, impoverished group suffer ten times the loss of the one living next door?

Snow introduced his theory of cholera in two forms during the second half of 1849: first as a self-published thirty-one-page monograph, *On the Mode and Communication of Cholera*, intended for his immediate peers in the medical community, and then as an article in the *London Medical Gazette*, targeted at a slightly wider audience.

The reaction to Snow's argument was positive but skeptical. "Dr. Snow deserves the thanks of the profession for endeavouring to solve the mystery of the communication of cholera," a reviewer wrote in the *London Medical Gazette*. But Snow's case studies had not convinced: "[They] furnish no proof whatever of the correctness of his views." He had convincingly demonstrated that the South London neighborhoods were more at risk for cholera than the rest of the city, but it did not necessarily follow that the water in those neighborhoods was responsible for the disparity. Perhaps there was special toxicity to the air in those zones of the city that was absent in the slums to the north. Perhaps cholera was contagious, and thus the cluster of cases in South London simply reflected the chain of infection thus far; if the initial cases had unfolded differently, perhaps the East End would have been attacked more grievously, and South London left relatively unscathed. There was a correlation between water supply and cholera—that much Snow had convincingly proved. But he had not yet established a cause.

The *Gazette* did suggest one scenario that might settle the matter convincingly:

> The *experimentum crucis* would be, that the water conveyed to a distant locality, where cholera had been hitherto unknown, produced the disease in all who used it, while those who did not use it, escaped.

That passing suggestion stayed with Snow for five long years. As his anesthesia practice expanded, and his prominence grew, he continued to follow the details of each cholera outbreak, looking for a scenario that might help prove his theory. He probed, and studied, and waited. When word arrived of a terrible outbreak in Golden Square, not ten blocks from his new offices on Sackville Street, he was ready. So many casualties in such a short stretch of time suggested a central contaminated water source used by large numbers of people. He needed to get samples of the water while the epidemic was still at full force. And so he made the journey across Soho, into the belly of the beast.

Snow's expectation was that contaminated water would have a cloudiness to it that was visible to the naked eye. But his initial glance at the Broad Street water surprised him; it was almost entirely clear. He drew samples from the other pumps in the area: Warwick Street, Vigo Street, Brandle Lane, and Little Marlborough Street. All were murkier than the Broad Street water. The Little Marlborough Street sample was worst of all. As he drew the water there, a handful of local residents on the street remarked that the pump water was notoriously poor—so poor, in fact, that many of them had taken to walking the extra blocks to Broad Street for their drinking water.

As Snow hurried back to his home on Sackville Street, he turned over the clues in his mind. Perhaps the Broad Street pump was not the culprit after all, given the lack of particles in the water. Perhaps one of the other pumps was the culprit? Or perhaps some other force was at work here? He would have a long night ahead of him, analyzing the samples, taking notes. He knew an outbreak of this magnitude could supply the linchpin for his argument. It was just a matter of finding the right evidence, and figuring out how to present that evidence in a way that would persuade the skeptics.

Wednesday, September 6

Building the Case

A hundred yards west of the Broad Street pump, in the dark alley of Cross Street, a tailor lived in a single room at number 10, sharing the space with his five children, two of whom were fully grown. On warm summer nights the heat in their cramped living space could be unbearable, and the father would often wake after midnight and send one of the boys out to fetch some cool well water to combat the sweltering air. They lived only two blocks from the pump at Little Marlborough Street, but that water had such an offensive smell that they regularly walked the extra block to Broad Street.

The tailor and his twelve-year-old boy had been struck in the first hours of the outbreak, and both were dead by Saturday. Snow had found their address listed in the inventory of deaths that Farr had supplied him. Several other deaths were recorded on Cross Street as well. The location had caught Snow's eye when he first arrived back at the pump to survey the surrounding streets, armed with the addresses of the dead. Almost half the deaths Farr had recorded were linked to addresses within his line of sight; and half the remaining ones came from residences that were only a matter of steps from Broad Street itself. The Cross Street deaths were unusual, though: to make it to the Broad Street pump from there, you had to wind your way through two small side streets, then take a right onto Marshall Street, then another left, and then walk a long block down Broad Street. To get to the Little Marlborough pump, though, you simply strolled down the alley, walked two short blocks north, and you were there. It was within your line of sight if you stood at the very end of Cross Street.

Snow had noticed another element while scanning Farr's records: the deaths on Cross Street were much less evenly distributed than the ones in the immediate vicinity of the pump. Almost every house along Broad Street had suffered a loss, but there were only a handful of isolated cases on Cross Street. This is what Snow was looking for now. He could see at a glance that he'd be able to demonstrate that the outbreak was clustered around the pump, yet he knew from experience that that kind of evidence, on its own, would not satisfy a miasmatist. The cluster could just as easily reflect some pocket of poisoned air that had settled over that part of Soho, something emanating from the gulley holes or cesspools—or perhaps even from the pump itself. Snow knew that the case would be made in the exceptions to the rule. What he needed now were aberrations, deviations from the norm. Pockets of life where you would expect death, pockets of death where you would expect life. Cross Street was closer to Little Marlborough, and thus should have been spared in the outbreak, according to Snow's theory. And indeed, it had largely been spared, but for the four cases Farr had reported. Could those cases have some connection to Broad Street?

Sadly, by the time Snow arrived at 10 Cross to interview the tailor's surviving children, he was too late. He learned from a neighbor that the entire family—five children and their father—had died in the space of four days. Their late-night thirst for Broad Street water had destroyed them all.

In his mind Snow was already drawing maps. He'd imagined an overview of the Golden Square neighborhood, with a boundary line running an erratic circle around the Broad Street pump. Every person inside that border lived closer to the poisoned well; everyone outside would have had reason to draw water from a different source. Snow's survey of the neighborhood, based on Farr's initial data, revealed ten deaths that lay outside the boundary line. Two of them were the tailor and his son on Cross Street. After a few hours of conversation, Snow determined that three others were children who went to school near Broad Street; their grieving parents reported that the children had often drunk from the pump on their way to and from school. Relatives confirmed that three other casualties had maintained a regular habit of drawing water from Broad Street, despite living closer to another source. That left two remaining deaths outside the border with no connection to Broad Street, but Snow knew that two cholera deaths over a weekend was well within the average for a London neighborhood at that time. They might easily have contracted the disease from a different source altogether.

Snow knew that his case would also revolve around the inverse situation: residents who lived near the pump who survived, because, for one reason or another, they had opted not to drink from the poisoned well. He reviewed Farr's list again, looking this time for telltale absences. There were a handful of deaths reported at 50 Poland Street. On its own, this was a predictable number: Poland Street lay immediately to the north of the pump, well within Snow's imagined border. But in scanning the list, Snow realized that the number was strikingly low, because 50 Poland Street was the address of the St. James Workhouse, home to 535 people. Two deaths was routine for a household of ten living off of Broad Street. A population of five hundred living close to the pump should have seen dozens of death. As Whitehead had already learned from his daily rounds, the workhouse—despite its destitute and morally suspect inmates—had been something of a sanctuary from the outbreak. When Snow interrogated the workhouse directors, an explanation immediately jumped out at him: the workhouse had a private supply from the Grand Junction Water Works, which Snow knew from his earlier research to be one of the more reliable sources of piped water. The workhouse also had its own well on the premises. They had no reason to venture out to the Broad Street pump for water, even though it lay not fifty yards from their front door.

Snow noticed another telling absence on Farr's list. With seventy workers, the Lion Brewery at 50 Broad was the second-largest employer in the immediate vicinity. Yet not a single death was recorded for that address in Farr's list. It was possible, of course, that the workers had gone home to die, and so Snow paid a visit to the Lion's proprietors, Edward and John Huggins, who reported with some bafflement that the plague had passed over their establishment. Two workers had reported mild cases of diarrhea, but not a single one had shown severe symptoms. When Snow inquired about the water supply on the premises, the Hugginses replied that, like the workhouse, the brewery had both a private pipeline and a well. But, they explained for the benefit of the teetotaling doctor, they rarely saw their men drink water at all. Their daily rations of malt liquor usually satisfied their thirst.

Later, Snow would visit the Eley Brothers factory, where he found the situation much more dire. The proprietors reported that dozens of their employees had fallen ill, many of them dying in their own homes over the first few days of the epidemic. When

Snow noticed the two large tubs of water that the brothers kept on premises for their employees to drink from, he scarcely needed to ask where the water had originated.

By the end of the day, Snow had built a convincing statistical case against the pump. Of the eighty-three deaths recorded on Farr's list, seventy-three were in houses that were closer to the Broad Street pump than to any other public water source. Of those seventy-three, Snow had learned, sixty-one were habitual drinkers of Broad Street water. Only six of the dead were definitively not Broad Street drinkers. The final six remained mysteries, "owing to the death or departure of every one connected with the deceased individuals," as Snow would later write. The ten cases that fell outside the imagined boundary line surrounding the Broad Street pump were equally telling: eight appeared to have a connection to Broad Street. Snow had established new causal chains back to the pump water, beyond the list of Farr's addresses: the proprietor of the coffeehouse who often sold sherbet mixed with Broad Street water told Snow that nine of her customers had died since the outbreak began. He had drawn the telling contrast between the Lion Brewery and the Eley Brothers factory; he had documented the unlikely safe haven of the Poland Street Workhouse. It was, on the face of it, a staggering display of investigative work, given the manic condition of the neighborhood itself. In the twenty-four hours since he'd received Farr's early numbers, Snow had tracked down intimate details of behavior from the surviving family and neighbors of more than seventy people. The fearlessness of the act still astonishes: as the neighborhood emptied in terror from the most savage outbreak in the city's history, Snow spent hour after hour visiting the houses that had suffered the worst—houses that were, in fact, still under assault. His friend and biographer Benjamin Ward Richardson later recalled: "No one but those who knew him intimately can conceive how he laboured, at what cost, and at what risk. Wherever cholera was visitant, there was he in the midst."

Friday, September 8

The Pump Handle

On Thursday night, the board of governors of St. James Parish had held an emergency meeting to discuss the ongoing outbreak and the neighborhood's response. Halfway into the meeting, they received notice that a gentleman wished to address them. It was John Snow, armed with his survey of the past week's devastation. He stood before them, and in his odd, husky voice told them that he knew the cause of the outbreak, and could prove convincingly that the great majority of cases in the neighborhood could be traced to its original source. It is unlikely that Snow went into the intricacies of his broader case against the miasma theory—better to go straight to the telling patterns of death and life, leave the philosophizing for another day. He explained the dismal ratios of survival among the people living near the pump, and the unusual exemptions granted to people who had not drunk the water. He told the Board of Governors of deaths that had transpired far from Golden Square, connected to the area only by the consumption of Broad Street water. He may have told them of the brewery of the workhouse on Poland Street. Death after death after death had been linked to the water at the base of the Broad Street well. And yet the pump remained in active use.

The members of the Board were skeptical. They knew as well as any other locals how highly regarded the Broad Street water was—particularly as compared to the other nearby pumps. But they also knew firsthand the smells and noxious fumes that were rampant in the neighborhood; surely these were more responsible for the outbreak than the reliable Broad Street water. Yet Snow's argument was persuasive—and, besides, they had few other options. If Snow was wrong, the neighborhood might go thirsty for a few weeks. If he was right, who knew how many lives they might save? And so, after a quick internal consultation, the Board voted that the Broad Street well should be closed down.

The following morning, Friday, September 8, exactly a week after the outbreak had first begun its awful rampage through Soho, the pump handle was removed. Whatever menace lay at the bottom of the well would stay there for the time being.

The deaths in Soho would continue for still another week, and the final reckoning of the assault of the Broad Street well on the neighborhood would not be calculated for months. The removal of the pump handle was generally ignored by the newspapers. On Friday, the *Globe* had published an upbeat—and typically miasmatic—account of the present state of the neighborhood: "Owing to the favourable change in the weather, the pestilence which has raged with such frightful severity in this district has abated, and it may be hoped that the inhabitants have seen the worst of the visitation. Yesterday there were very few deaths, and this morning no new cases were reported." On the following day, however, the news appeared to be less encouraging:

> We regret to announce that after the account was written which appeared in The Globe of yesterday, there were several severe and fatal cases of cholera, and that seven or eight were reported on Saturday morning, although the wisest precautions were adopted to arrest the progress of the disease. The neighbourhood of Golden-square presented . . . a most melancholy and heart-rending appearance. There was scarcely a street free from hearses and mourning coaches, and the inhabitants of the district, appalled by the calamity which has visited them, crowded the streets to witness the last sorrowing act of duty towards their neighbours and friends. A vast number of the tradespeople left their shops and fled from the place, the closed shutters bearing the announcement that business had been suspended for a few days. Messers Huggins, the brewers, with praiseworthy forethought, have issued an announcement that the poor . . . may obtain any quantity of hot water for cleansing their dwellings, or other purposes, at any hour of the day or night, an act of humanity and kindness of which a large number have availed themselves.

Dozens would die over the next week, but clearly the worst was over. When the final numbers were tallied, the severity of the outbreak shocked even those who had lived through it. Nearly seven hundred people living within 250 yards of the Broad Street pump had died in a period of less than two weeks. Broad Street's population had literally been decimated: ninety out of 896 residents had perished. Among the forty-five houses extending in all directions from the intersection of Broad and Cambridge streets, only four managed to survive the epidemic without losing a single inhabitant. "Such a mortality in so short a time is almost unparalleled in this country," the *Observer* noted. Past epidemics had produced higher body counts citywide, but none had killed so many in such a small area with such devastating speed.

The removal of the pump handle was a historical turning point, and not just because it marked the end of London's most explosive outbreak. History has its epic thresholds where the world is transformed in a matter of minutes—a leader is assassinated, a volcano erupts, a constitution is ratified. But there are other, smaller, turning points that are no less important. A hundred disparate historical trends converge on a single, modest act—some unknown person unscrews the handle of a pump on a side street in a bustling city—and in the years and decades that follow, a thousand changes ripple out from that simple act. It's not that the world is changed instantly; the change itself takes many years to become visible. But the change is no less momentous for its quiet evolution.

And so it was with the Broad Street well that the *decision* to remove the pump handle turned out to be more significant than the short-term effects of that decision. Yes, the Broad Street outbreak would burn itself out over the next few days, as the last victims died off and other, more fortunate, cases recovered. Yes, the neighborhood would slowly return to normalcy in the weeks and months that followed. These were real achievements that arose from that pump handle being removed, even if the water in the well had potentially been purged of *V. cholerae* by the time Snow made his case to the Board of Governors. But the pump handle stands for more than that local redemption. It marks a turning point in the battle between urban man and *Vibrio cholerae*, because for the first time a public institution had made an informed intervention into a cholera outbreak based on a scientifically sound theory of the disease. The decision to remove the handle was not based on meteorological charts or social prejudice or watered-down medieval humorology; it was based on a methodical survey of the actual social patterns of the epidemic, confirming predictions put forward by an underlying theory of the disease's effect on the human body. It was based on information that the city's own organization had made visible. For the first time, the *V. cholerae*'s growing dominion over the city would be challenged by reason, not superstition.

3 THE INFLUENZA EPIDEMIC OF 1918

This article is about a shocking epidemic of influenza that spread across the world between 1918 and 1920. Often called the "Spanish flu," the epidemic was terrible and terrifying.[1] *It infected some 500 million people worldwide—one-third of the globe's population at the time—and killed somewhere between 20 and 50 million. This deadly strain of flu spread to all continents in a very short period, spreading through populations in waves. The largest number of dead were in poor countries, like India, where malnutrition was common because of colonial policies. However, the best historical information is from the United States, where roughly a half of a million citizens died. There are many stunning photographs of the epidemic with people wearing face masks and ambulances collecting the dead (see the Web Resources at the end of this section). Particularly devastating was the fact that a large proportion of the dead were young adults in the prime of their lives.*

The 1918 flu epidemic occurred before the invention of antibiotics or influenza vaccines. Of course, good nursing care meant that most victims did not die, but the case-mortality rate (the percentage of the sick who died) was extremely high, and there was not much doctors could do; death often happened because bacterial pneumonia followed the initial influenza.

This reading goes into detail about the wide variety of clinical symptoms the disease presented with. More important, it describes the human suffering involved in the epidemic—including the fear and the panic. This epidemic and panic also occurred in the chaotic context of World War I, when the initial outbreak was a military secret. Historical studies have shown that US cities that quickly enforced "social distancing" public interventions—like the closing of schools and banning of assemblies—had much lower rates of infection and death.

This historic epidemic reminds us of the important role of infectious disease as a factor shaping world history. This was the topic of a classic book by William H. McNeil, Plagues and Peoples, *which demonstrated how global history might be seen in terms of the "confluence of disease pools"—when populations with different disease experiences began to come into contact. For example, one reason why Europeans were able to expand into the Americas was the fact that they introduced a number of diseases to which the natives had no immunities; the result was that roughly 90% of the indigenous populations (including Aztec, Maya, and Inca peoples) died within a relatively short period of time. In another example of historically important epidemics, the "Black Death" (Bubonic plague) in 14th-century Europe killed around 25 million people over a four-year period; some historians say that the severe population crash ultimately resulted in major cultural changes, including the Italian Renaissance.*

Is such a catastrophe possible, even in today's context of modern technological medicine? The movie Contagion, *which is a dystopic portrayal of the chaos and fallout of a massive outbreak, may be fictional, but epidemiologists agree that the idea of a disease "jumping" from one species to another is a realistic scenario. Another possible source for a disease that could start a pandemic is through the basic evolutionary process of natural selection. For example, some tuberculosis bacteria have evolved to be resistant to our current antibiotics. We often forget that humans live in a world of microbes; they are all around us and inside our guts, and they are constantly evolving.*

[1] Peter Brown's grandfather remembered the epidemic and talked about it often. The experience influenced his grandfather's decision to become a pharmacist, and he witnessed the amazing antibiotic revolution during the mid-20th century.

People working in global health are trying to prevent future pandemics—this book describes a range of activities that can protect populations. Some people working in public health improve environmental conditions to prevent transmission of a range of diseases. Others use epidemiological surveillance to track new threats. Others prepare and plan for response in the case of epidemics.

As you read this article, consider the following questions:

- **Why did the 1918 flu epidemic surprise physicians? What did they mean that the disease was "interesting"?**
- **List some of the particular nonbiological factors that made the 1918 flu epidemic worse.**
- **Why does the author keep saying "This was just influenza"?**
- **Given the state of medical knowledge at the time, what could be done to attenuate the effects of the epidemic? What is "social distancing"?**
- **Why are epidemics global rather than local problems?**
- **How can a society prepare for a disaster like the 1918 flu epidemic? In your opinion, would hospitals and health-care workers be able to handle the surge in demand—or would there be a meltdown?**
- **Today, only some people have access to annual flu immunizations, antibiotics, breathing machines, and other technologies of modern medicine. How might this shape the risks we all face from infectious disease?**

CONTEXT

This reading is from the historian John Barry's award-winning book, *The Great Influenza: The Story of the Deadliest Pandemic in History*. The book details the complexities and context of the epidemic from an American perspective. It describes a milestone in the historical development of biomedicine. Barry is a distinguished scholar at Tulane University. One of his earlier books concerned the great Mississippi flood of 1827. His historical research has had direct policy relevance, both for public health and environmental protection.

This was influenza, only influenza.

This new influenza virus, like most new influenza viruses, spread rapidly and widely. As a modern epidemiologist already quoted has observed, *Influenza is a special instance among infectious diseases. This virus is transmitted so effectively that it exhausts the supply of susceptible hosts*. This meant that the virus sickened tens of millions of people in the United States—in many cities more than half of all families had at least one victim ill with influenza; in San Antonio the virus made more than half the entire population ill—and hundreds of millions across the world.

But this was influenza, only influenza. The overwhelming majority of victims got well. They endured, sometimes a mild attack and sometimes a severe one, and they recovered.

The virus passed through this vast majority in the same way influenza viruses usually did. Victims had an extremely unpleasant several days (the unpleasantness multiplied by terror that they would develop serious complications) and then recovered within ten days. The course of the disease in these millions actually convinced the medical profession that this was indeed only influenza.

But in a minority of cases, and not just in a tiny minority, the virus manifested itself in an influenza that did not follow normal patterns, that was unlike any influenza ever reported, that followed a course so different from the usual one for the disease.

Generally in the Western world, the virus demonstrated extreme virulence or led to pneumonia in from 10 to 20 percent of all cases. In the United States, this translated into two to three million cases. In other parts of the world, chiefly in isolated areas where people had rarely been exposed to influenza viruses—in Eskimo settlements of Alaska, in jungle villages of Africa, in islands of the

Pacific—the virus demonstrated extreme virulence in far more than 20 percent of cases. These numbers most likely translate into several hundred million severe cases around the world in a world with a population less than one-third that of today.

This was still influenza, only influenza. The most common symptoms then as now are well known. The mucosal membranes in the nose, pharynx, and throat become inflamed. The conjunctiva, the delicate membrane that lines the eyelids, becomes inflamed. Victims suffer headache, body aches, fever, often complete exhaustion, cough. As one leading clinician observed in 1918, the disease was "ushered in by two groups of symptoms: in the first place the constitutional reactions of an acute febrile disease—headache, general aching, chills, fever, malaise, prostration, anorexia, nausea or vomiting; and in the second place, symptoms referable to an intense congestion of the mucous membranes of the nose, pharynx, larynx, trachea, and upper respiratory tract in general, and of the conjunctivae." Another noted, "The disease began with absolute exhaustion and chill, fever, headache, conjunctivitis, pain in back and limbs, flushing of face. . . . Cough was often constant. Upper air passages were clogged." A third reported, "In nonfatal cases . . . the temperature ranged from 100 to 103F. Nonfatal cases usually recovered after an illness of about a week."

Then there were the cases in which the virus struck with violence.

To those who suffered a violent attack, there was often pain, terrific pain, and the pain could come almost anywhere. The disease also separated them, pushed them into a solitary and concentrated place.

In Philadelphia, Clifford Adams said, "I didn't think about anything. ... I got to the point where I didn't care if I died or not. I just felt like that all my life was nothing but when I breathe."

Bill Sardo in Washington, D.C., recalled, "I wasn't expected to live, just like everybody else that had gotten it. . . . You were sick as a dog and you weren't in a coma but you were in a condition that at the height of the crisis you weren't thinking normally and you weren't reacting normally, you sort of had delusions."

In Lincoln, Illinois, William Maxwell felt "time was a blur as I was lying in that little upstairs room and I . . . had no sense of day or night, I felt sick and hollow inside and I knew from telephone calls my aunt had, I knew enough to be alarmed about my mother. . . . I heard her say, 'Will, oh no,' and then, 'if you want me to . . .' The tears ran down her face so she didn't need to tell me."

Josey Brown fell ill working as a nurse at the Great Lakes Naval Training Station and her "heart was racing so hard and pounding that it was going to jump out" of her chest and with terrible fevers she was "shaking so badly that the ice would rattle and would shake the chart attached to the end of the bed."

Harvey Cushing served in France. On October 8, 1918, he wrote in his journal, "Something has happened to my hind legs and I wobble like a tabetic"—someone suffering from a long and wasting illness, like a person with AIDS who needs a cane—"and can't feel the floor when I unsteadily get up in the morning. . . . So this is the sequence of the grippe. We may perhaps thank it for helping us win the war if it really hit the German Army thus hard [during their offensive]." In his case what seemed to be the complications were largely neurological. On October 31, after spending three weeks in bed with headache, double vision, and numbness of both legs, he observed, "It's a curious business, unquestionably still progressing . . . with considerable muscular wasting. . . . I have a vague sense of familiarity with the sensation—as if I had met [it] somewhere in a dream." Four days later: "My hands now have caught up with my feet—so numb and clumsy that shaving's a danger and buttoning laborious. When the periphery is thus affected the brain too is benumbed and awkward."

Cushing would never fully recover.

And across the lines lay Rudolph Binding, a German officer, who described his illness as "something like typhoid, with ghastly symptoms of intestinal poisoning." For weeks he was "in the grip of the fever. Some days I am quite free; then again a weakness overcomes me so that I can barely drag myself in a cold perspiration onto my bed and blankets. Then pain, so that I don't care whether I am alive or dead."

Katherine Anne Porter was a reporter then, on the *Rocky Mountain News*. Her fiancé, a young officer, died. He caught the disease nursing her, and she, too, was expected to die. Her colleagues set her obituary in type. She lived. In *Pale Horse, Pale Rider* she described her movement toward death: "She lay on a narrow ledge over a pit she knew to be bottomless . . . and soft carefully shaped words like oblivion and eternity are curtains hung before nothing at all. . . . Her mind tottered and slithered again, broke from its foundation and spun like a cast wheel in a ditch. . . . She sank easily through deeps and deeps of darkness until she lay like a stone at the farthest bottom of life, knowing herself to be blind, deaf, speechless, no longer aware of the members of her own body, entirely withdrawn from all human concerns, yet alive with a peculiar lucidity and coherence; all notions of the mind, all ties of blood and the desires of the heart, dissolved and fell away from her, and there remained of her only a minute fiercely burning particle of being that knew itself alone, that relied upon nothing beyond itself for its strength; not susceptible to any appeal or inducement, being itself composed entirely of one single motive, the stubborn will to live. This fiery motionless particle set itself unaided to resist destruction, to survive and to be in its own madness of being, motiveless and planless beyond that one essential end."

Then, as she climbed back from that depth, "Pain returned, a terrible compelling pain running through her veins like heavy fire, the stench of corruption filled her nostrils, the sweetish sickening smell of rotting flesh and pus; she opened her eyes and saw pale light through a coarse white cloth over her face, knew that the smell of death was in her own body, and struggled to lift her hand."

These victims came with an extraordinary array of symptoms, symptoms either previously unknown entirely in influenza or experienced with previously unknown intensity. Initially, physicians, good physicians, intelligent physicians searching for a disease that fitted the clues before them—and influenza did not fit the clues—routinely misdiagnosed the disease.

Patients would writhe from agonizing pain in their joints. Doctors would diagnose dengue, also called "breakbone fever."

Patients would suffer extreme fever and chills, shuddering, shivering, then huddling under blankets. Doctors would diagnose malaria.

Dr. Henry Berg at New York City's Willard Parker Hospital—across the street from William Park's laboratory—worried that the patients' complaints of "a burning pain above the diaphragm" meant cholera. Noted another doctor, "Many had vomiting; some became tender over the abdomen indicating an intra-abdominal condition."

In Paris, while some physicians also diagnosed cholera or dysentery, others interpreted the intensity and location of headache pain as typhoid. Deep into the epidemic Parisian physicians still remained reluctant to diagnose influenza. In Spain public health officials also declared that the complications were due to "typhoid," which was "general throughout Spain."

But neither typhoid nor cholera, neither dengue nor yellow fever, neither plague nor tuberculosis, neither diphtheria nor dysentery, could account for other symptoms. No known disease could.

In *Proceedings of the Royal Society of Medicine*, a British physician noted "one thing I have never seen before—namely the occurrence of subcutaneous emphysema"—pockets of air accumulating just beneath the skin—"beginning in the neck and spreading sometimes over the whole body."

Those pockets of air leaking through ruptured lungs made patients crackle when they were rolled onto their sides. One navy nurse later compared the sound to a bowl of rice crispies, and the memory of that sound was so vivid to her that for the rest of her life she could not tolerate being around anyone who was eating rice crispies.

Extreme earaches were common. One physician observed that otitis media—inflammation of the middle ear marked by pain, fever, and dizziness—"developed with surprising rapidity, and rupture of the drum membrane was observed at times in a few hours after the onset of pain." Another wrote, "Otitis media reported in 41 cases. Otologists on duty day and night and did immediate paracentesis [insertion of a needle to remove fluid] on all bulging eardrums.

. . ." Another: "Discharge of pus from the external ear was noted. At autopsy practically every case showed otitis media with perforation. . . . This destructive action on the drum seems to me to be similar to the destructive action on the tissues of the lung."

The headaches throbbed deep in the skull, victims feeling as if their heads would literally split open, as if a sledgehammer were driving a wedge not into the head but from inside the head out. The pain seemed to locate particularly behind the eye orbit and could be nearly unbearable when patients moved their eyes. There were areas of lost vision, areas where the normal frame of sight went black. Some paralysis of ocular muscles was frequently recorded, and German medical literature noted eye involvement with special frequency, sometimes in 25 percent of influenza cases.

The ability to smell was affected, sometimes for weeks. Rarer complications included acute—even fatal—renal failure. Reye's syndrome attacked the liver. An army summary later stated simply, "The symptoms were of exceeding variety as to severity and kind."

It was not only death but these symptoms that spread the terror.

This was influenza, only influenza. Yet to a layperson at home, to a wife caring for a husband, to a father caring for a child, to a brother caring for a sister, symptoms unlike anything they had seen terrified. And the symptoms terrified a Boy Scout delivering food to an incapacitated family; they terrified a policeman who entered an apartment to find a tenant dead or dying; they terrified a man who volunteered his car as an ambulance. The symptoms chilled laypeople, chilled them with winds of fear.

The world looked black. Cyanosis turned it black. Patients might have few other symptoms at first, but if nurses and doctors noted cyanosis they began to treat such patients as terminal, as the walking dead. If the cyanosis became extreme, death was certain. And cyanosis was common. One physician reported, "Intense cyanosis was a striking phenomenon. The lips, ears, nose, cheeks, tongue, conjunctivae, fingers, and sometimes the entire body partook of a dusky, leaden hue." And another: "Many patients exhibited upon admission a strikingly intense cyanosis, especially noticeable in the lips. This was not the dusky pallid blueness that one is accustomed to in a failing pneumonia, but rather [a] deep blueness." And a third: "In cases with bilateral lesions the cyanosis was marked, even to an indigo blue color. . . . The pallor was of particularly bad prognostic import."

Then there was the blood, blood pouring from the body. To see blood trickle, and in some cases spurt, from someone's nose, mouth, even from the ears or around the eyes, had to terrify. Terrifying as the bleeding was, it did not mean death, but even to physicians, even to those accustomed to thinking of the body as a machine and to trying to understand the disease process, symptoms like these previously unassociated with influenza had to be unsettling. For when the virus turned violent, blood was everywhere.*

In U.S. Army cantonments, from 5 percent to 15 percent of all men hospitalized suffered from epistaxis—bleeding from the nose—as with hemorrhagic viruses such as Ebola. There are many reports that blood sometimes spurted from the nose with enough power to travel several feet. Doctors had no explanation for these symptoms. They could only report them.

"15% suffered from epistaxis. . . ." "In about one-half the cases a foamy, blood-stained liquid ran from the nose and mouth when the head was lowered. . . ." "Epistaxis occurs in a considerable number of cases, in one person a pint of bright red blood gushing from the nostrils. . . ." "A striking feature in the early stages of these cases was a bleeding from some portion of the body. . . . Six cases vomited blood; one died from loss of blood from this cause."

What was this?

"One of the most striking of the complications was hemorrhage from mucous membranes, especially from the nose, stomach, and intestine. Bleeding from the ears and petechial hemorrhages in the skin also occurred."

One German investigator recorded "hemorrhages occurring in different parts of the interior of the eye" with great frequency. An American pathologist

* Many mechanisms can cause bleeding in mucous membranes, and the precise way the influenza virus does this is unknown. Some viruses also attack platelets—which are necessary for clotting—directly or indirectly, and elements of the immune system may inadvertently attack platelets as well.

noted: "Fifty cases of subconjunctival hemorrhage [bleeding from the lining of the eye] were counted. Twelve had a true hemoptysis, bright red blood with no admixture of mucus. . . . Three cases had intestinal hemorrhage. . . ."

"Female patients had a hemorrhagic vaginal discharge which was at first considered to be coincident menstruation, but later was interpreted as hemorrhage form the uterine mucosa."

What was this?

Never did the virus cause only a single symptom. The chief diagnostician in the New York City Health Department summarized, "Cases with intense pain look and act like cases of dengue . . . hemorrhage from nose or bronchi. . . . Expectoration is usually profuse and may be blood-stained . . . paresis or paralysis of either cerebral or spinal origin . . . impairment of motion may be severe or mild, permanent or temporary . . . physical and mental depression. Intense and protracted prostration led to hysteria, melancholia, and insanity with suicidal intent."

The impact on the mental state of the victims would be one of the most widely noted sequelae.

During the course of the epidemic, 47 percent of all deaths in the United States, nearly half of all those who died from all causes combined—from cancer, from heart disease, from stroke, from tuberculosis, from accidents, from suicide, from murder, and from all other causes—resulted from influenza and its complications. And it killed enough to depress the average life expectancy in the United States by more than ten years.

Some of those who died from influenza and pneumonia would have died if no epidemic had occurred. Pneumonia was after all the leading cause of death. So the key figure is actually the "excess death" toll. Investigators today believe that in the United States the 1918–19 epidemic caused an excess death toll of about 675,000 people. The nation then had a population between 105 and 110 million, compared to 285 million in 2004. So a comparable figure today would be approximately 1,750,000 deaths.

And there was something even beyond the gross numbers that gave the 1918 influenza pandemic terrifying immediacy, brought it into every home, brought it into homes with the most life.

Influenza almost always selects the weakest in a society to kill, the very young and the very old. It kills opportunistically, like a bully. It almost always allows the most vigorous, the most healthy, to escape, including young adults as a group. Pneumonia was even known as "the old man's friend" for killing particularly the elderly, and doing so in a relatively painless and peaceful fashion that even allowed time to say good-bye.

There was no such grace about influenza in 1918. It killed the young and strong. Studies worldwide all found the same thing. Young adults, the healthiest and strongest part of the population, were the most likely to die. Those with the most to live for—the robust, the fit, the hearty, the ones raising young sons and daughters—those were the ones who died.

In South African cities, those between the ages of twenty and forty accounted for 60 percent of the deaths. In Chicago the deaths among those aged twenty to forty almost quintupled deaths of those aged forty-one to sixty. A Swiss physician "saw no severe case in anyone over 50." In the "registration area" of the United States—those states and cities that kept reliable statistics—breaking the population into five-year increments, the single greatest number of deaths occurred in men and women aged twenty-five to twenty-nine, the second-greatest number in those aged thirty to thirty-four, the third-greatest in those aged twenty to twenty-four. And more people died in *each* of those five-year groups than the total deaths among *all* those over age sixty.

Graphs that correlate mortality rates and age in influenza outbreaks always—always, that is, except for 1918–19—start out with a peak representing infant deaths, then fall into a valley, then rise again, with a second peak representing people somewhere past sixty-five or so. With mortality on the vertical and age on the horizontal, a graph of the dead would look like a U.

But 1918 was different. Infants did die then in large numbers, and so did the elderly. But in 1918 the great spike came in the middle. In 1918 an age graph of the dead would look like a W.

It is a graph that tells a story of utter tragedy. Even at the front in France, Harvey Cushing recognized this tragedy and called the victims "doubly dead in that they died so young."

In the American military alone, influenza-related deaths totaled just over the number of Americans killed in combat in Vietnam. One in every sixty-seven soldiers in the army died of influenza and its complications, nearly all of them in a ten-week period beginning in mid-September.

But influenza of course did not kill only men in the military. In the United States it killed fifteen times as many civilians as military. And among young adults still another demographic stood out. Those most vulnerable of all to influenza, those most likely of the most likely to die, were pregnant women. As far back as the year 1557, observers connected influenza with miscarriage and the death of pregnant women. In thirteen studies of hospitalized pregnant women during the 1918 pandemic, the death rate ranged from 23 percent to 71 percent. Of the pregnant women who survived, 26 percent lost the child. And these women were the most likely group to already have other children, so an unknown but enormous number of children lost their mothers.

The most pregnant word in science is "interesting." It suggests something new, puzzling, and potentially significant. Burt Wolbach, the brilliant chief pathologist at the great Boston hospital known as "the Brigham," called it "the most interesting pathological experience I have ever had."

The epidemiology of this pandemic was *interesting*. The unusual symptoms were *interesting*. And the autopsies—and some symptoms revealed themselves only in autopsy—were *interesting*. The damage this virus caused and its epidemiology presented a deep mystery. An explanation would come—but not for decades.

In the meantime this influenza, for it was after all only influenza, left almost no internal organ untouched. Another distinguished pathologist noted that the brain showed "marked hyperemia"—blood flooding the brain, probably because of an out-of-control inflammatory response—adding, "the convolutions of the brain were flattened and the brain tissues were noticeably dry."

The virus inflamed or affected the pericardium—the sac of tissue and fluid that protects the heart—and the heart muscle itself, noted others. The heart was also often "relaxed and flabby, offering strong contrast to the firm, contracted left ventricle nearly always present in post-mortem in patients dying from lobar pneumonia."

The amount of damage to the kidneys varied but at least some damage "occurred in nearly every case." The liver was sometimes damaged. The adrenal glands suffered "necrotic areas, frank hemorrhage, and occasionally abscesses. . . . When not involved in the hemorrhagic process they usually showed considerable congestion."

Muscles along the rib cage were torn apart both by internal toxic processes and by the external stress of coughing, and in many other muscles pathologists noted "necrosis," or "waxy degeneration."

Even the testes showed "very striking changes . . . encountered in nearly every case. . . . It was difficult to understand why such severe toxic lesions of the muscle and the testis should occur. . . ."

And, finally, came the lungs.

Physicians had seen lungs in such condition. But those lungs had not come from pneumonia patients. Only one known disease—a particularly virulent form of bubonic plague called pneumonic plague, which kills approximately 90 percent of its victims—ripped the lungs apart in the way this disease did. So did weapons in war.

An army physician concluded, "The only comparable findings are those of pneumonic plague and those seen in acute death from toxic gas."

Seventy years after the pandemic, Edwin Kilbourne, a highly respected scientist who has spent much of his life studying influenza, confirmed this observation, stating that the condition of the lungs was "unusual in other viral respiratory infections and is reminiscent of lesions seen following inhalation of poison gas."

But the cause was not poison gas, and it was not pneumonic plague. It was only influenza.

4 HOUSE ON FIRE: THE FIGHT TO ERADICATE SMALLPOX

*Within the field of global health, the **eradication** of smallpox was more than just a major success—it was the equivalent of landing an astronaut on the moon. Considered the most important and iconic success in the history of international health, it is the example that all students should know about. To date, smallpox is the only disease ever eradicated (if you do not count the laboratory samples at the Centers for Disease Control in Atlanta and the equivalent institution in Russia).*

Smallpox was a horrible disease—your skin would break out in fever and a rash, especially around your face and hands. The rash would turn into painful pustules, which then scabbed over and filled with pus. The sufferer began to stink of rotting flesh. There is no cure for this infectious disease. About 30% of those afflicted died, and the survivors were scarred for life with disfiguring pockmarks.

*Smallpox was declared eradicated in 1980 after an intensive effort coordinated by the World Health Organization (WHO). But the story actually began nearly than 200 years earlier with Edward Jenner's discovery of **vaccination**. For centuries prior to Jenner's discovery, people practiced **inoculation**, in which people were intentionally exposed to a particular disease (often a milder strain). Just like survival from a disease gives one immunity from it, inoculation prevented reinfection. However, inoculation was often a risky process, and people died from this attempt to cure.*

*What Jenner discovered in 1796 was the phenomenon of **vaccination**. The immunological concept behind vaccination is the creation of immunity for one disease (such as smallpox) by exposing a person to a related but much less dangerous disease (in this case, cowpox—in fact, the term "vaccination" comes from the Latin* vacca, *meaning cow). By using a similar disease instead of the same one, Jenner discovered a safer process than inoculation. This discovery led to the development of routine childhood immunization for a range of diseases; these "shots" should be considered the most powerful technology ever used in public health. Vaccination was the key technology behind smallpox eradication.*

In this reading, one of the heroes of the worldwide smallpox eradication campaign, William Foege, describes how the WHO decided to take on the challenge of worldwide smallpox eradication. The notion was suggested by the Russians, but its feasibility depended on new technologies like a freeze-dried vaccine and international funding and political support. The disease itself had certain biological characteristics that made it more likely for the campaign to be a success.

*However, one of the most important lessons of this story is how the strategy changed and was refined over time—even after the campaign began. Initially, the strategic plan focused on the idea of mass vaccination in a population to achieve **herd immunity**; if you vaccinate enough people in a population, then the disease can no longer affect that population.*

However, this plan was later changed based on experience and careful observation. Instead of mass immunizations, workers would find active cases of smallpox, rush there, and then vaccinate everyone who may have come in contact with the person or were within a large radius of the sick person. This strategy was initially tried out because of a shortage of vaccine. But it turned out to be the most effective strategy. Good surveillance and communication could discover when and where an outbreak started, and then personnel could be sent directly to the problem. It is analogous to a firefighter's approach: find out when a house is on fire, get there quickly, and stop it from spreading by robbing the burnable "fuel" in its path. Instead of trying to vaccinate thousands of people at a

Excerpts from *House on Fire*, by Bill Foege. Berkeley: University of California Press, 2012.

time, the surveillance and containment strategy focused on those most at risk.

Vaccinators used a simple technology for performing the vaccinations—the bifurcated needle. It is almost like a sewing needle, with a sharp eye section holding the correct dose of vaccine. The technological solution was old and relatively simple, but reaching everyone in the world who needed this vaccine at the right time was an amazing feat. Some people thought that the project was impossible. Also, as this reading describes, many people were skeptical that surveillance—containment could work, which made carrying out the project on a large scale with collaborators across the world even more challenging.

This reading begins with a description Foege's experiences in India, specifically the impoverished state of Bihar. He writes of the detailed logistical issues involved in running the eradication campaign. In reading other accounts of this global health milestone, it is clear that the "smallpox warriors" were persistent, innovative, and very lucky. In a future reading (Chapter 36) we will return to questions about the ethics of some of the techniques used by the smallpox warriors in getting their mission accomplished.

As you read this selection, consider the following discussion questions:

- **What biological characteristics of smallpox made it a good candidate for eradication?**
- **Why was smallpox chosen as a target for eradication?**
- **Why did it take almost 200 years for Jenner's discovery to spread throughout the world? After all, Thomas Jefferson wrote a fan letter to Jenner, envisaging the eradication of the disease.**
- **Why did Foege think that the combination of surveillance and containment would be better than mass vaccination for eradicating smallpox? (After all, mass vaccination was how many endemic diseases have been eliminated from the United States.)**
- **Why was surveillance so important in the story of smallpox eradication? What is necessary to have a good surveillance system?**
- **When is changing a strategy in the middle of a campaign a good idea? In what way was the final strategy like the game "Whack a Mole"?**

CONTEXT

William Foege is the former director of the Centers for Disease Control and the chief adviser to the global health efforts of the Bill and Melinda Gates Foundation. He was a leader of the smallpox eradication project in Nigeria and India, in which he pioneered the strategic shift described here. He is an inspirational individual and orator.

A Young Physician Speaks Up

With a profound sense of resignation, Sharma, Dutta, and I entered the meeting room on that hot, sticky Monday morning for the monthly routine. After seven months of intensive activities in Bihar (India), the staff in the field had increased, and eighty or ninety people crowded the room. Ceiling fans provided some air movement, but when the room temperature exceeds body temperature, even air movement doesn't yield much comfort. But these were field-workers, accustomed to hardship, and I watched with appreciation and some awe as they pressed on despite the heat.

I sat at the front table with Sharma, Dutta, and Achari (director of the smallpox eradication program for the state of Bihar), gazing at this roomful of very weary faces. The meeting opened with the usual greetings, followed by reviews of the world smallpox situation and the situation in the rest of India, a description of the programs in key states, and a summary of new and potentially useful ideas that had come out of other state meetings. Finally, we got to the review of the smallpox situation in Bihar, including the pressures that were on the minister of health to change the strategy. We shared the fact that the minister was preparing to ask us to change the strategy and return to mass vaccination. We also shared our discouragement in being unable to change his mind.

The minister suddenly appeared, flanked by an entourage, and strode to the front table. He was given the floor immediately, and he described the problem as he saw it. Bihar was now faced with fifty-seven hundred pending outbreaks involving every district of the state. He saw no alternative but to revert to mass vaccination, and to do it quickly, before the backlog of unvaccinated children increased even more. At meeting's end, he declared, we would return to the strategy of mass vaccination in Bihar. We all knew this was coming, yet hearing the words actually uttered was shocking. Their impact began to sink in, and the room became very quiet.

One of the field-workers, a young Indian physician, raised his hand. He looked too young even to be a medical school graduate, and he was very thin, the epitome of a dedicated field-worker. He did not appear to have the needed gravitas for the moment, and I worried that a mistake was in the making. But the physician stood and, with great deference, addressed the minister. He was shaking as he described himself as just a poor village man. But, he said, when he was growing up, there were things you could depend on. For example, if a house is on fire in a village, no one wastes time putting water on the other houses, just in case the fire spreads. That is the mass vaccination strategy. Instead, as in the surveillance/containment strategy, they rush to pour water where it will do the most good—on the burning house.

Despite the heat of the day, a chill went up my spine as this man condensed all the work, discussions, discoveries, and massive human effort of the previous seven months into a few words and the indelible image of a house on fire.

The minister hesitated and stared at the group for some time. And then the unimaginable happened. He changed his mind on the spot. This man of public authority, who over the weekend had resisted the combined persuasive powers of Drs. Sharma, Dutta, and myself, this man who had entered the meeting room thirty minutes earlier with such presence and purpose, now seemed subdued, almost bewildered. He pointed out the great personal and political risk of his changing his mind. But he said, in a small voice, "I'll give you one more month."

Soon after, other things began to go right. A railway strike was settled that same day, and other groups withdrew their strikes and strike threats. The monsoons arrived, and with them, a decrease in the transmission potential of smallpox.

The search conducted during the first week of June finally brought good news and the information we needed to influence politicians. The number of outbreaks decreased by over a third from a month earlier (2,622 to 1,678), the number of pending outbreaks did not increase (remaining at slightly more than 4,000), and even the intensity of cases per outbreak seemed to be declining as the number of cases found dropped from over 14,000 in the April/May search to about 7,500 in the June search. The change was sufficiently dramatic that we had no problem convincing the politicians—including Bihar's minister of health.

Anyone who has lived in India or Africa through the dry season knows the incredible surge of emotions and energy that accompanies the first rain. People dance in the villages and celebrate. This was the feeling of the smallpox workers when the smallpox problem in Bihar finally began to decline in June 1974.

From mid-1974 until the end of the year was the best time to be working on smallpox in India. Once the decline began, it was dramatic. In July, three states—Bihar, Uttar Pradesh, and West Bengal—reported 95 percent of all smallpox cases in India, with Bihar accounting for two thirds of them. But with Bihar containing over eight hundred outbreaks a week in May and June, the totals of pending outbreaks in India fell rapidly, from a peak of over eight thousand in May to fewer than six thousand in July.

The work became easier as it became more predictable. With fewer surprises, the approach became one of overkill in both surveillance and containment. Nor was this the time to determine minimum inputs needed or assess maximum efficiencies across various approaches. Instead, having worked so hard to get to the current position, everyone now went overboard. Much of the work was of low efficiency. Indeed, much of it was redundant, some outright unproductive, but we were in no mood to take chances. Watch guards at each smallpox house were doubled, and searches

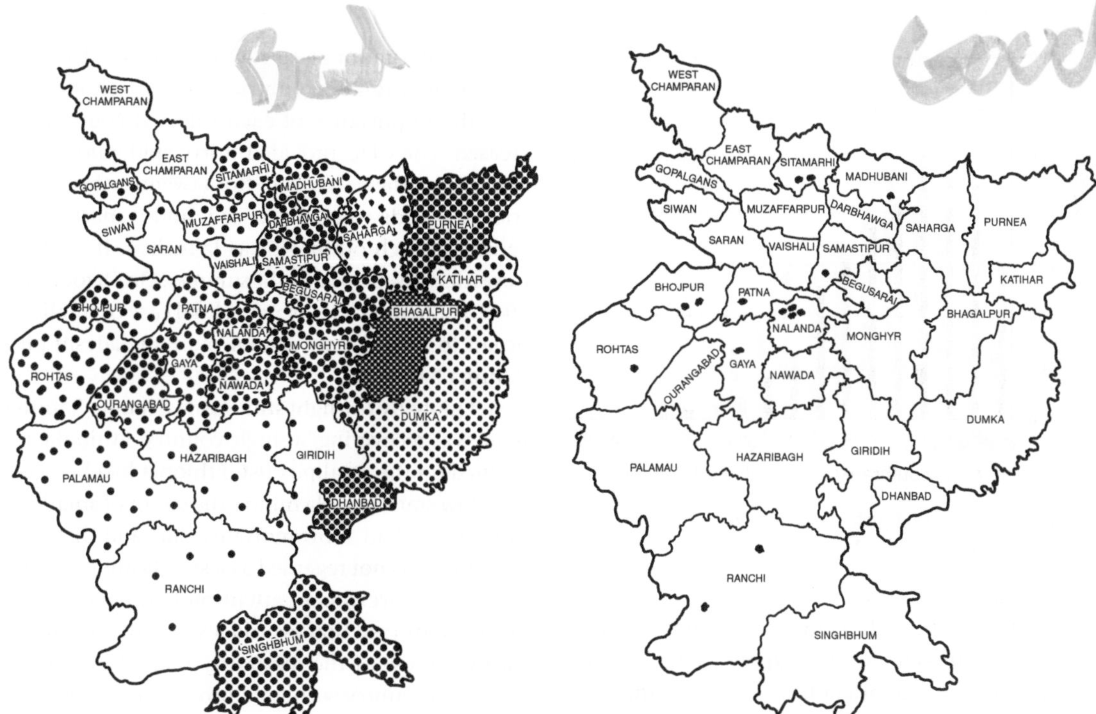

FIGURE 4.1 New Smallpox Outbreaks in Bihar, India, 1974 and 1975 Compared.

Left: New outbreaks detected in the fourth search, January 28–February 2, 1974. Right: New outbreaks detected in the sixteenth search, January 27–February 1, 1975.

were repeated. The vaccination circle gradually increased from the infected household itself to surrounding houses and then the entire village. Over one thousand outbreaks per month were being removed from the pending numbers for the country as a whole. The system was becoming more efficient at the same time as the size of the problem was decreasing.

Finally, the ultimate search tool was deployed. As the number of cases declined, India began to offer a reward for the reporting of previously unknown cases of smallpox. The reward started small, at Rs. 10 (less than US $1.50), but even that amount was large enough to cause immediate problems. When new cases were reported to health workers, the health workers wanted to claim the reward themselves. The problem was solved by providing the reward to both the person who made the report and the health worker who forwarded the report. The health worker could not claim the reward until the informant had been identified.

As the number of cases declined, the reward was increased incrementally until, at about the time of India's last cases, the reward had been increased to US$1,000.

The reward was advertised, and the general public was quick to recognize the potential bounty. Surveys were conducted to determine the percentage of people who knew about the reward and about where to report a suspected case of smallpox to collect the reward. One survey late in the campaign revealed that more people knew about the smallpox reward than knew the name of the prime minister.

Operation Smallpox Zero

The last case was reported in May. And on June 12, 1975, Nicole Grasset was able to send a letter to all smallpox workers in the country to say that smallpox transmission had been broken the previous month.

It seemed almost anticlimactic. A virus that for millennia had spread such despair, inspiring religious ritual and even the worship of a goddess, was

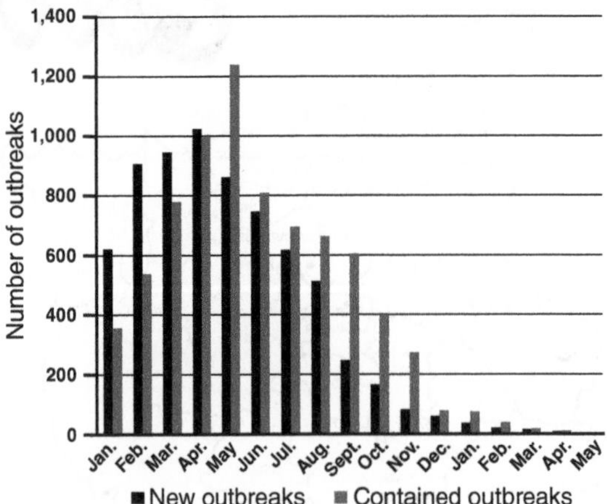

FIGURE 4.2 Total Outbreaks per Week in India, January 1974 to May 1975.

suddenly gone from the country. In twenty months, the surveillance/containment approach had proved itself ideally suited for eradicating a virus that had eluded the best efforts of mass vaccination programs for 175 years. It was the right tool for the task.

The Eradication of Smallpox Worldwide

India was one of the toughest chapters in the global fight against smallpox, but victory over smallpox in India was not the end of the story. As the last cases of smallpox were being subdued in India, Bangladesh workers were in the middle of a nightmare.

Earlier, the program in Bangladesh had been ahead of the program in India, and this information had even been used to encourage Indian workers at state meetings. In October 1974, as India still struggled with almost 1,000 outbreaks, Bangladesh had only 91 outbreaks on the books. But that month, a flood in Bangladesh, the worst in decades, decimated entire villages. People left their homes in search of food, relief, and shelter. The smallpox virus went with them, and by the end of January the outbreak count had increased from 91 to 572. This problem, already of enormous proportions, was then made worse when the government bulldozed urban slums, sending tens of thousands of refugees from urban areas to other parts of the country. The president of Bangladesh declared a national emergency.

The international community responded, not least because as more countries became free of smallpox, the importance of each infected country increased. The CDC provided thirty epidemiologists, and thirty others were sent from twenty other countries. Rewards were advertised, and a massive response to each outbreak was launched. It worked. Cases decreased through the summer. On October 16, 1975, the first vesicles of Asia's final case of smallpox began to form on a two-year-old Bangladeshi girl, Rahima Banu.

Yet globally the fight still wasn't over. As Rahima Banu was recovering, a single country, Ethiopia, remained on the smallpox list. Ethiopia had been off to a slow start. Variola minor, the strain of smallpox in Ethiopia, had a low mortality rate, and therefore smallpox was not regarded as a significant problem. Moreover, government attention had been on the political unrest that would eventually result in the overthrow of the monarchy in 1976. But now, as the last country with smallpox, Ethiopia could no longer ignore the problem. WHO helped arrange for supplies, helicopters, and several dozen foreign advisors. By early 1976, after a herculean effort, the country had become free of smallpox except for an area in the Blue Nile Gorge and in the desert of the south. By August, Ethiopia had eliminated the last cases.

It seemed to be time for the world to celebrate. But Murphy's Law (anything that can go wrong will go wrong) operates no less frequently in public health programs than elsewhere. At the last moment the tenacity of this virus, combined with the movement of people, again intervened. Drought in the south forced some Ethiopians to seek refuge in Somalia. In September 1976, smallpox cases were reported in Mogadishu, Somalia's capital. Six months later, outbreaks were occurring around the country. National and international resources descended on the problem areas. Two dozen WHO epidemiologists and thousands of Somalian health workers carried out the now-familiar surveillance/containment procedures under what some consider the most difficult conditions of a hard decade. Again the strategy worked.

In early October 1977, a couple with two small children, both with smallpox, approached the hospital in Merka, Somalia. They asked Ali Maow Maalin, an employee, for directions to the infectious disease ward. A considerate person, he took them to the ward rather than directing them. Although he had been vaccinated, it was evidently not an effective take. Two weeks later, on October 26, 1977, he developed the last smallpox rash that Africa would ever see. He recovered without transmitting the virus. The global chain of smallpox transmission was finally broken. Smallpox had been eliminated from the world because of a plan. It did not happen by accident.

There was yet a final irony. After ten months of worldwide freedom from smallpox, the country that had provided the vaccine to the world had two final cases. Both were due to a virus that escaped from a laboratory—demonstrating again the challenge of containing this tenacious virus. On August 11, 1978, a woman in Birmingham, England, developed the first symptoms of smallpox and died a month later. Her mother developed symptoms on September 2, 1978, but recovered.

In medicine, the medical practitioner is obliged to apply the best knowledge of the times to each patient. In public health, the obligation is to apply the best knowledge to the entire human community. The purpose of public health is to promote social justice. By 1978, public health achieved its first complete success in social justice, applying the knowledge required for smallpox control to eliminate a disease for current humanity and for all future generations. Humanity will continue to hold its collective breath, hoping for the wisdom that prevents the virus from ever being released again—intentionally or unintentionally.

5 A PINCH, A FIST, A CUP OF WATER: ORAL REHYDRATION THERAPY IN BANGLADESH

This reading is about a "simple solution" to the huge challenge of infant diarrhea dehydration death. It refers to an important invention for child survival—oral rehydration therapy (ORT)—a life-saving home-based therapy that was developed at the International Centre for Diarrheal Disease Research in Matlab, Bangladesh (once known as the "Cholera Lab"). Most childhood diarrhea is caused by bacteria transmitted through ***fecal-oral transmission****. Most often such infections are self-limiting, but the body's reaction to the sickness—diarrhea—can cause life-threatening dehydration. In the past, diarrhea dehydration was considered the largest single cause of infant death in the world, and it is still in the top-five causes of child death. But such deaths are avoidable with proper treatment.*

Before ORT, a child with severe dehydration would need to be taken to a clinic and given intravenous transfusions. This was expensive and required clinical infrastructure and personnel. Such therapy was simply impossible for poor families in much of the world, and these were the children most at risk of death. The critical discovery made by the International Centre for Diarrheal Disease Research in Bangladesh was that rehydration could be successfully accomplished orally *by getting the sick baby to drink a mixture of clean water, sugars, and potassium. Oral administration of the solution meant that the therapy could be accomplished at home. The use of ORT is common now, even in rich countries like the United States, where it is marketed under brand-names like Pedialyte.*

Like many challenges in global health, the primary issue was not the technology but the delivery *of that knowledge and technology to the people who need it most. This is an issue of "scaling up" an intervention like ORT.*

This reading is about a historical global health milestone when a Bangladeshi nongovernmental organization named the Bangladesh Rural Advancement Committee (BRAC) took on a 10-year project to teach women in every household in this densely populated country (12 million mothers) how to mix the ORT solution with commonly available ingredients. The decision to teach a homemade mixture was controversial in Global Health institutions like the WHO. They preferred the distribution and sale of packets of oral rehydration ingredients to be mixed with water. As the reading indicates, an incorrect recipe can cause as much harm as no therapy at all. But BRAC decided to follow this challenging strategy. The BRAC story of ORT is one of repeated failures and program adjustments; it is also one of inspired community health workers who worked to improve the lives of the poor in their own communities. It is an example of "health by the people."

BRAC is an amazing nongovernmental organization created in 1971 by the ex-businessman and Bangladeshi patriot Fazle Hasan Abed. BRAC's accomplishments, in many areas beyond health including education and micro-credit, are chronicled in the Ian Smilie's book Freedom from Want: The Remarkable Success Story of BRAC, the Global Grassroots Organization That's Winning the Fight Against Poverty *(2009).*

This project benefited greatly from international cooperation and the leadership of an American physician, Richard Cash. This is a global health story in which millions of children's lives have been saved. UNICEF estimates that ORT currently saves 1 million lives a year worldwide.

As you read this article, consider the following questions:

- **Does ORT cure diarrhea? If not, why does it save lives?**
- **BRAC kept evaluating the knowledge of mothers trained with ORT, and at first the results were a miserable failure. Why didn't they give up? What changes did they make to improve the results—and ultimately achieve a 98% success rate?**
- **This 10-year project cost about $9.3 million dollars. Is this cheap or expensive? Why?**
- **Recent research has indicated that the mothers who were taught about ORT in the BRAC project have taught their daughters about the life-saving therapy. What are the implications of that?**
- **Why did the WHO and UNICEF object to BRAC's decision to teach how to make ORT rather than distribute packets? Might the appropriateness of the ORT strategy depend on the local socio-economic context?**

CONTEXT

This reading is adapted from a companion volume to the video series *Rx for Survival: the Global Health Challenge* produced by PBS. Philip Hilts was a former reporter for the *New York Times* covering issues in public health. He also served as director of the Knight Science Journalism Program at MIT.

A Pinch, A Fist, A Cup of Water

For the BRAC leaders, as they sat in the village of Sulla in rural Bangladesh discussing their strategy, it was clear that the high death rate from diarrhea would continue. They walked through the problems.

Bags of saline were sold by local doctors in Bangladesh, but the price was one hundred taka per bag, and five to ten bags would be needed to treat each patient. At the time, the average income in the villages was about fifteen hundred taka per family per year, and the average child had three bouts of serious diarrhea per year, so the bags could quickly bankrupt a family. Packets of soluble salts were also beginning to be manufactured; couldn't they be mixed at home? They were cheaper than saline, and in theory could be sold in Bangladeshi villages, where the women would then buy them in emergencies, take them home, and mix them in water to give to their sick babies. But no distribution system was in place, and if the government were to buy the packets for distribution, it would take hundreds of millions of packets to cover the country. And in the end, would the marketed packets reach the ones who needed them most? The instructions on the packets might or might not be clear; but in any case, 80 percent of the women intended to use them were illiterate. And finally, even with relatively inexpensive packets, it would still have to be the mothers who would diagnose the problem, buy the salts, mix them in water at home, and give the solution to their babies.

It was clear that the center of the problem were questions about the mothers, not the solution. Why not acknowledge it and deal with it?

"From the beginning we had this sense that you must trust people," said Abed. "Trust the mothers. We had a great belief that illiterate people, any human beings, trained to do certain things could be very good at it. Put in a position to help their own communities, they could do it." In the long run many of the most basic problems came down to whether they should "get local people to do something, or get professionals to come in and do it for you. We are too poor to hire professionals everywhere, all the time."

After thinking it through, they decided the first issue was the mothers' ability to mix the solution.

Directions that called for using a teaspoon would be no help; the village people don't have or use teaspoons routinely. Sugar was to be used, but which sugar? Refined white sugar was not commonly available and was expensive. What the villagers more often had was *gur*, a brown sugar made from local cane or date juice. Analysis soon showed that *gur* was actually better than refined sugar because it often contained small amounts of potassium and bicarbonate—which were ingredients in the official oral rehydration solution.

So Abed started from scratch, in his own kitchen, with ingredients from the street. He took local salt, *lobon, gur,* and a tin cup common in the villages, a *seer.* After Abed and his wife cooked up dozens of batches of differing measures, they were sent to the Cholera Research Laboratory. The homemade concoction that proved closest to the official WHO formula was the following: a pinch of salt (in Bangladesh, it's a three-finger pinch using the index finger, middle finger, and thumb), two small scoops of *gur,* and half a *seer* of water. Later it was modified slightly in the field, because women use their hollowed palms to measure scoops. One "fist" was about two scoops.

After much more work, the formula finally became a simple chant: "a pinch, a fist, and half a *seer.*" The mixture was dubbed "*lobon-gur* solution" and the first great trial of the fundamental question—could illiterate mothers be taught to make and use *lobon-gur* successfully?—began in Sulla, Bangladesh, in February 1979.

BRAC carefully selected teachers (the first two were young village women, Hemlata Sarkar and Shwapna Bowmick), wrote and tested a teaching method several times, and only gradually spread the experiment from Sulla to other villages. Routinely, they took samples from the solutions made by mothers and sent them to the Cholera Research Laboratory for analysis.

Doctors in Bangladesh felt their turf was the treatment of human illness and that BRAC's experiments were now starting to invade that territory. One official from the World Health Organization rushed to Bangladesh to try to get the government to greatly expand its anti-diarrhea program to head off BRAC. But that program was poorly planned and did not take into account the scale and difficulties of the problem.

BRAC went ahead, and over the next year young women trainers in groups of six moved through 662 villages, a few weeks in each village, attempting to train 58,000 mothers in the new treatment method.

One thing distinctive about this project when compared to many "development" projects over the years is that it was carried out entirely locally, by people who had become deadly serious about making it work. So the many mistakes and repeated trouble in this or that part of the program were confronted, not ignored. That doing and redoing turned out to be the most difficult part. After the first thirty thousand women were trained, and their competence had been checked and rechecked by visits from monitors, Abed said, they reached a first plateau. It was thrilling to have built the project up so far, especially as it was under fire even as it carried on.

"This was our first opportunity to scale-up programs from small areas to the whole nation," he said. "When we got done teaching the first thirty thousand mothers, we went back to check how we had succeeded. But we found that of all the women who had been taught the method, only six percent were using it when their children became sick. I was very disappointed. Disheartened. Why should we be going from house to house teaching women to do this if then they are not going to use it?"

Abed and the other leaders of BRAC believed in it. It was technically sound and medically potent, truly lifesaving. "We decided there must be something wrong with our teaching. The commitment we had was not being transmitted, somehow."

They heard of one case when a mother with a very sick baby was visited by a young BRAC worker. The worker quickly suggested running down to the medicine shop for some diarrhea medicine, saying, "It will be quicker."

Abed, talking about it now, looks down at his desk. "So we found out that some of our workers didn't believe in what they were teaching. They thought our homemade solution was crude, second-rate."

Abed realized their earlier explanations had been too sketchy and had not caught the imaginations of their workers. So he rounded up all three hundred workers of the time and started from the beginning, explaining why this solution was lifesaving and that anything else, short of intensive hospital treatment, could be deadly. They explained the infections that cause diarrhea and the reaction of the bowel; they gave details of why sugar and salt were crucial. They talked about the number of deaths of children in the villages in which they were working.

"Once workers became convinced this was the best therapy, their whole attitude changed, their behavior changed. They became committed," he said.

In all BRAC work, that is now a vital test of whether a project will succeed or fail. Do the workers understand it? Are they excited, committed?

When they went back a little while later to check again, "we found things had improved a little—now twenty-one percent of mothers were using the method. But again, we were not very happy."

There was another element they hadn't considered enough. They decided to bring in some anthropologists to talk to the mothers and other villagers about BRAC and diarrhea and their lives in general.

"We found that the women were not the only ones we had to convince. They were not the sole decision makers in the house or in the village," he said. There were the husbands and brothers, who would say, "Don't use that cheap method, I don't trust it." And there were the local traditional healers who advised against using the BRAC method. So they added to their effort visits to the men in the villages, talks in the marketplace, and later added even radio advertising.

This round of effort pushed the rate of usage up over 50 percent, Abed said. Still not enough.

On further probing they found some of the workers were doing their teaching in too rote a fashion when they were tired, and some even cheated, skipping the teaching and mixing up solution themselves and sending for tests as if the mothers had made it. So a further round of fixes went in. They set up monitoring and paid the rehydration teachers not on the basis of houses covered, or sessions with mothers, but on the basis of a sampling of the actual performance of the mothers. For each mother who could answer questions and make an effective *lobongur* solution, the worker would get paid a certain amount. For each mother who was taught but did not perform well, the BRAC workers earned less.

And on it went. "The commitment grew, and the teachers began to get more creative and involved," Abed said. Eventually they were able to get the quality of teaching up and routinely get mothers to make the solution right over 98 percent of the time. The rate of death from diarrhea began to drop across the nation.

"I have seen a lot of bad development projects," Abed said. "It is not that the people doing them are not sincere. They are. But in many cases, whether they come from outside the country or from inside, they expect to work a project for three years, do the best they can, and then go on to something else.

"But in BRAC we were there for the long haul. We were committed to building the country forever. We wanted to make sure things really change. We were totally results-oriented from the beginning. That made quite a lot of difference."

The project took ten years, but by the time it was over it was firmly rooted in the national psyche. Entrepreneurs soon began to take advantage of it, and started importing and selling packets of rehydration salts throughout the nation and in all the village medicine shops. Mothers could now make their own or, if they could afford it, buy the salts and work from there. The treatments of deadly diarrhea were now in their hands. The whole BRAC project from 1979 to 1990 cost about $9.3 million.

By 1990, the word had spread, and oral rehydration was being used in dozens of countries around the world. In 1991, one of the worst epidemics of cholera since the nineteenth century struck South America and Mexico. But the usual rate of death—one-third to one-half—did not materialize. In this epidemic millions of packets of salts were flown in and put in the hands of local medical people and villagers. The death rate when the epidemic died down proved to be nearer 1 percent than 50 percent. The transmission of Bangladesh's success was, in fact, another kind of globalization.

SIR RICHARD DOLL, INTERVIEWED BY ANNA WAGSTAFF

6 "SCIENCE WILL ALWAYS WIN IN THE END": THE EPIDEMIOLOGIST WHO PROVED THAT SMOKING CAUSES CANCER

The milestones in global health described in earlier chapters concerned historical epidemics of ***infectious diseases****. By the mid-20th century, rates of those communicable diseases had fallen drastically in wealthy countries. Part of the reason for this was better science. Improved theories (e.g., the germ theory) and technologies (e.g., the microscope, vaccines, and methods for culturing pathogens) resulted in incredible advances in health and medicine.*

At the same time, improvements in living conditions also reduced rates of infectious disease in wealthy populations. During the last century, many countries experienced an ***epidemiological transition*** *in which the overall* ***mortality*** *rate declined, and the primary causes of death changed from infectious diseases to noncommunicable* ***chronic diseases*** *like heart disease or cancer.*

However, poor populations in low- and middle-income countries have not experienced this epidemiological transition completely, and still experience these infectious diseases—particularly socioecomically disadvantaged groups. Low-income countries are also seeing rising rates of many chronic diseases that are common to the higher income countries, causing them to suffer under the ***dual burden*** *of both infectious and chronic disease.*

Smoking causes cancer. That sounds simple, obvious, and boring. However, it was not long ago that most American men smoked cigarettes—including most medical doctors. People generally thought that the causal connection between tobacco and lung cancer was unproven. After all, it is clear that not everyone who smokes cigarettes gets cancer, and laboratory rats exposed to tobacco do not always develop cancer. On the other hand, cigarette smoking can be enjoyable, relaxing, and "cool"—but they are extremely addictive.

Big tobacco companies profited greatly with the rising popularity of cigarettes. To protect their profits, those companies paid scientists to conduct studies that obfuscated the emerging evidence showing that cigarettes were dangerous and addictive; they were paid to create a smokescreen of doubt. The question of the time was what scientific evidence is necessary to demonstrate causation? What is the relationship between correlation and convincing evidence of causation. Proof of causation depends of a number of factors, including: strength *of the association,* temporality *(the risk factor should come before developing the disease),* consistency *of the association,* specificity, dose effect *(more exposure to a risk factor leads to more disease),* plausibility, coherence *(epidemiological findings in the real world should match up with what is observed in the laboratory),* experiment, *and* analogy *(similar risk factors cause similar health outcomes).*

Understanding the causation of chronic diseases is often more complicated than infectious diseases because there can be multiple risk factors, as well as a time lag between exposure and the appearance of a disease. It was not until the 1950s that epidemiologists began to develop the analytical methods for untangling the causes of chronic disease. Epidemiology is the methodological backbone of global health, but epidemiological methods of proof remained controversial around the middle of the last century; in some sense, these methods can remain controversial when scientific facts become politicized and some parties have strong financial interests.

This reading is an interview with a famous epidemiologist, Sir Richard Doll, who advanced the science of public health by conducting studies linking lung cancer and cigarette smoking. Together with his mentor Austin

Originally published in *Cancer World* magazine, European School of Oncology, www.cancerworld.net.

Bradford Hill, he designed case-control studies and then cohort studies that conclusively showed that cigarette smoking causes cancer. These epidemiological study designs use different methods to compare rates of a particular risk factor (in this case, smoking) among people who do and do not develop a given disease (in this case, cancer). These study designs are described in detail in Chapter 10. However, even with the striking evidence from these analytical strategies evidence, convincing the scientific and medical communities—and especially the public—was not easy.

Ultimately, as Doll says, scientific facts did win out. Tobacco companies lost cases in US courts and paid large penalties. Public health authorities and antitobacco advocates were able to regulate smoking in public places, increase taxes on cigarettes, require warning labels on packaging, and ultimately eliminate cigarette advertising from airwaves. Consequently, smoking rates—and lung cancer deaths—declined drastically. This was a significant victory for population health. Most important, health education efforts assured that the dangers of cigarette smoking were universally understood in society. Cigarette smoking is addictive, even though it is pleasurable. It is perhaps the only consumer product that can kill you if used regularly as the manufacturers intended.

However, that is not the end of the story. Tobacco companies then started focusing on low- and middle-income countries and started aggressively marketing their products—even to children. Moreover, the largest nation in world, China, had a state-run tobacco company and a charismatic leader who was a chain-smoker. As explained later in this book, cigarette smoking is one of the largest preventable causes of death in today's world. In the world of global health policy, a major victory came about with the World Health Organization Framework Convention on Tobacco Control in 2003 that was signed by 168 countries. Nevertheless, people in global health must continue to battle the economic interests of the tobacco industry and its political power throughout the world.

As you read this article, consider the following questions:

- **Why was the creation of an epidemiological research design and method of statistical analysis so important?**
- **Why do people smoke if they know it is bad for their health and potentially lethal?**
- **Is it true that cigarettes are the only legal commodity that, if used as the manufacturers intended, can kill their consumers?**
- **Why was the connection of cigarette smoking and cancer so controversial? What scientific evidence is necessary to demonstrate causation?**
- **Why is cigarette smoking popular? What might be the effect of advertising?**
- **Why is smoking still one of the largest preventable causes of death in the world more than 50 years after this scientific discovery?**
- **What do you think about Doll's comments about the relative unimportance of secondhand smoke?**

CONTEXT

This interview was conducted in 2004, when Sir Richard Doll was 92 years old. He died in 2005. The questions were asked by a writer for *Cancer World*, a magazine for the cancer research community. Since the epidemiology of chronic noncommunicable disease is a relatively new discipline, this interview has particular importance as an oral history document.

In 1950, Richard Doll showed the world that smoking causes lung cancer. Today, aged 92, a word from him can still cause anxiety in the Nokia boardroom or have us counting our portions of fruit and veg. He carries the responsibility lightly, because he believes in the power of evidence. After all, when it comes to the causality of cancer, he wrote the rules.

Lung cancer had been rising sharply for decades before your groundbreaking report showed, with only a one in a million scintilla of doubt, that smoking is a cause of lung cancer. Why did such a strong association take so long to identify?

RICHARD DOLL Cigarette smoke had first been suspected in the 1920s, but some pathologists tried to produce skin cancer in mice by smearing them with cigarette smoke tar. When there was no response, smoking was ruled out as a possible carcinogen, and researchers turned their attention to other possible causes.

The technique of testing for carcinogens by exposing animals to them had only been introduced in about 1919, in Japan, and for the next two or three decades, scientists thought that's the way we discover the causes of cancers, by getting suspect materials and putting them on the skin of mice.

I myself did not expect to find smoking was a major problem. If I'd had to bet money at that time, I would have put it on something to do with the roads and motorcars.

Was yours the first epidemiological study on lung cancer?

Richard Doll There were a few others, but we were the first to have sufficient confidence in our findings to state that "We conclude that smoking is a cause and an important cause of the disease."

A couple of very primitive studies had been carried out in Germany, but they were very flawed. For example, one used the average age of lung cancer patients as a basis for selecting control patients—so if the average age of the lung cancer patients was 54, they interviewed a lot of people aged 54. You really need to have the separate experiences of a 70-year-old and a 30-year-old, you can't assume that the experience of a 54-year-old is representative.

Then there was a US study that came out about the same time as ours and had similar findings, but because they had used less rigorous techniques, they were more cautious about drawing conclusions from their data, and merely concluded that there was an association they'd found which might imply causality.

The trouble was that, until then, epidemiology had been concerned almost entirely with infectious diseases, which required very different methods and tended to look at differences between entire populations—differences in rainfall, temperature, things like that. With cancer and chronic diseases, you need to compare individuals with the disease against those without. There are all sorts of biases that can affect this kind of epidemiological study, and that was not understood at the time. A person being interviewed, for instance, will tend to overemphasise something that they think might be useful. It took some time to establish and find techniques to eliminate all the biases that can affect the results.

We were confident of our data because we had taken steps to ensure that our results were robust. Chance you could cut out immediately, because you were talking about odds of less than one in a million of getting our results by chance. Then you had to show that your results weren't biased, and then you had to show that the results were not due to what is now called confounding; that it was not smoking that caused the disease, but smoking was associated with something else that did. For example lung cancer is associated with drinking alcohol—smokers tend to drink more alcohol.

Then we checked our results against ecological evidence, to see what sense it made in the world at large. If smoking is the cause, we ought to find that wherever the disease was common, smoking should be common, and vice versa. So where people didn't smoke there shouldn't be much lung cancer. And that's what we found when we looked round the world.

Was the medical world convinced?

Richard Doll Not at all. Sir Harold Himsworth, the Secretary of the Medical Research Council (MRC), who had commissioned the study, accepted the results straight off. But most cancer research workers did not accept it, and in fact they advised the Department of Health that they shouldn't take any action because they were uncertain about what it meant.

It wasn't until 1957, when the Government asked the MRC for a formal opinion as to whether our conclusion was correct or not, that the MRC formally considered it and said it was correct and advised the Government to that effect. The result was that the Minister of Health in 1957 called a press conference to announce the results of the MRC consultation. He announced that the MRC had advised them that smoking was the cause of the great increase in lung cancer. While he was reporting this to the media, he was smoking a cigarette himself!

One of the problems we found in trying to convince the scientific community was that thinking at that time was dominated by the discovery of bacteria such as diphtheria, typhoid, and the tubercle, which had been the basis for the big advances in medicine in the last decades of the 19th century.

When it came to drawing conclusions from an epidemiology study, scientists tended to use the rules that had been used to show that a particular germ was the cause of an infectious—Koch's three postulates. Koch was a great German pathologist who discovered the tubercle bacillus, and one of his postulates was that you must always find the organism in every case of the disease.

When we did our study on lung cancer and smoking, 50 years later, a number of scientists thought this applied to the cause of chronic diseases. A lot of people said, "Smoking can't be the cause of lung cancer because I have seen a case in a non-smoker, and therefore by Koch's postulate smoking is not the cause."

But, of course, nobody was saying it was *the* cause; what we were saying is that it is *a* cause. People didn't realise that these chronic diseases could have multiple causes. And smoking is only one cause of lung cancer—it happens to be much the most important cause, however.

How did you convince the doubters?

Richard Doll When we saw that, apart from Sir Harold Himsworth and one or two others, practically no-one believed our conclusions, we thought it's no good repeating the study. So we designed another one, using a different method. We decided to look at people's smoking habits and see whether that could predict who would contract lung cancer.

We chose doctors as our sample, principally because they were easy to follow up, and we planned to do the study for five years. But within two and a half years, we already had 37 deaths from lung cancer—none in non-smokers, and a high incidence in heavy smokers. The association was very clear. It turned out to have been very fortunate to have chosen doctors, from a number of points of view. One was that the medical profession in this country became convinced of the findings quicker than anywhere else. They said, "Goodness! Smoking kills doctors, it must be very serious," and, of course, a very high proportion gave up.

After five years we had around 70 cases, but by this time, our results were beginning to show that smoking was also associated with a number of other diseases, particularly with heart disease, so we decided to continue the study, though this had never been the initial plan.

Your findings have implications for us all. Do you get drawn in to discussions about people's lifestyles?

Richard Doll My job has been to try to find out what the causes are, or what is the efficient treatment. If I then go round telling people what they should do, I may get prejudiced because I'm committed to a particular opinion, and as a scientist you must always be prepared to change your mind if the evidence changes.

I am now committed to the viewpoint that people shouldn't smoke, but that's 50 years after the first observation. I never gave any advice for the first 30 years. But it is so established now that there is no question of my being prejudiced.

People can also over-react. Radiation is an example—people are ridiculously frightened of it. I also think we've gone too far in eliminating asbestos—I mean the less dangerous white type, which carefully handled probably does more good than harm. Several hundred British sailors died in the Falklands War who needn't have, because they hadn't got the adequate fire control that you had with asbestos.

Fifty years ago you showed the world that smoking can kill. Why do you think so many youngsters are still not getting the message?

Richard Doll Young people will always behave a bit recklessly. That's why it's so important that we now can show that giving up smoking early in life is really effective. I think we're going to save more lives by persuading people to give up than we are by stopping people from starting.

Obviously you try to educate children and young people, but you know you are not going to win with all of them. Even my own children smoked. My son smoked from about age 12 to 16. My daughter didn't stop till she was 30.

Did you personally come up against the tobacco industry?

Richard Doll What you've got to remember is that the directors of the tobacco companies in 1950 were responsible people, insofar as the directors of any firm were, and they were horrified by the idea that what they were selling was killing people. They made serious efforts, perfectly reasonably, to disprove the claim, but their own statistical advisor after a few years told them that it was a waste of time and that he was convinced that smoking caused lung cancer.

I remember he rang me up and said that he agreed with my findings and that he was going to have to leave his job.

He wanted to take the opportunity of his final two weeks' of expenses allowance to invite me and my wife out to dinner. As it happened, his employers accepted his advice, and he agreed to continue working for them on the basis that they would never publicly deny that smoking caused lung cancer.

It's a different case with today's directors of the tobacco industry. They have gone into it knowing perfectly well that they are selling something that is a lethal material, and they are to my mind thoroughly immoral people. But that wasn't true of the directors of 1950.

The tobacco industry in America did not react at all in the same way, and they tried to get a colleague of mine, Ernest Wynder, sacked from his job with the Sloan-Kettering. They put pressure on the Director not to allow Wynder to publish anything that claimed smoking caused disease, and the Director did try to suppress his studies. Wynder, however, responded by setting up his own organisation and getting support from somebody else to carry on doing the research. So when he published his results, they didn't have the Sloan-Kettering stamp. Sloan-Kettering came out of it very badly.

However, despite this sort of pressure, the leading epidemiologists in America all got together fairly early on—in the late 1950s—and said they regarded it as proved that smoking causes disease. The trouble was the American law courts. The industry made it so expensive to sue them that it wasn't for some years that you got very wealthy groups of lawyers who were prepared to take them on. The industry could make it so expensive by raising objections and making it last a very long time.

Did you feel a sense of triumph when the courts finally found against the mighty tobacco industry?

RICHARD DOLL Science will always win in the end.

Your discovery that smoking causes lung cancer was the preventive equivalent of the 'magic bullet'. Are there any more major factors that we don't yet know about?

RICHARD DOLL No there are not. We've eliminated so many causes of cancer. What people don't realise now is how many occupational cancers there used to be. They've all been cleared up. 2-naphthylamine, for instance, which was used in dyes and in the preparation of rubber, led to a very high incidence of bladder cancer among those who worked with it. That's gone. Road workers would get skin cancer from tar, or lung cancer from the fumes. Many oils used for lubricating machinery would result in skin cancer or cancer of the scrotum. Asbestos. All these work-related cancers have now been eliminated. We've also made huge strides identifying which cancers have an infectious origin. We now know, for instance, that cervical cancer has a viral origin, and we shall have a vaccine against it in a few years' time. We are beginning to find other cancers with viral origins. Hepatitis B and C are major causes of liver cancer in many parts of the world, the Epstein Barr virus causes some rare cancers in the Far East, but is also responsible for some cases of Hodgkin's disease. And we now know that gastric cancer, which dropped dramatically in incidence during the last century, is largely caused by the helicobacter pylori bacterium. What we're left with now are the smaller risk factors, such as alcohol for breast cancer, which can only be detected by collaborative studies looking at populations of tens of thousands rather than the hundreds that we used to use. This sort of work has been pioneered by Richard Peto, whom I brought with me from London when I took up my position of Regius Professor at Oxford University. This has to my mind been his really major contribution. These large-scale studies were undreamed of until he demonstrated the possibility by collaborating with different people in different countries.

The increased effectiveness of new treatments can also be too small to measure except through this sort of study. Tamoxifen, for instance, was not being used in this country until Peto's collaborative analysis in 1988. The evidence was all there but it was in little bits and contradictory. It wasn't until the evidence was all put together that you could say "Look! It's absolutely clear that giving women tamoxifen after the operation reduces their mortality by about 10–15%. You saw a very clear answer, and people changed their habits overnight. Very few people had been using it, or they had only been using it for a year. After this study everyone started using it and they realised they had to continue using it for up to five years.

What do you see as your legacy to the world of epidemiology?

Richard Doll Sir Austin Bradford Hill has largely been forgotten about nowadays because he is dead. But he was my boss and my teacher, and the methods and techniques we developed together in order to find out why lung cancer was increasing so dramatically are still used to this day.

Bradford Hill later codified these into what he termed "nine guidelines", (often wrongly referred to as "criteria") which are universally accepted now. They are cited in courts of law.

I wrote an article about three years ago on proof of causality—proof that something is actually a cause of a disease—which made use of what I'd learnt from Bradford Hill, and which is now used as a reference point for epidemiologists.

And of course our report that established smoking as an important cause of lung cancer was very important. That was the first serious epidemiological study ever done into cancer, at a time when there were probably no more than a dozen of us working on this issue worldwide. Looking back with the benefit of more than 50 years' hindsight, I can honestly say that we did a good job.

7 DECLARATION OF ALMA-ATA

This is a very important document in the history of global health. The 1978 World Health Organization (WHO) conference on **primary health care** *(PHC) produced this milestone declaration. The conference was held in Alma-Ata, Kazakhstan. Like many international agreements, the wording is very careful because it is the result of negotiations, so read it carefully. Despite the style of the rhetoric, it is a powerful, persuasive, and passionate document stating that health is a human right and that the growing inequalities in the health status between different countries is completely unacceptable. Referring to a "new international economic order," it states that the right to health is a common concern to all countries—rich and poor alike. The declaration is a strong political statement, but in this book, we argue that global health has always been political, and that practitioners of global public health must constantly identify conditions that are unacceptable.*

The declaration on PHC states that all people have the right to participate in their o[illegible]lth and that healthcare cannot simply be a privi[illegible]es. This theme was emphasized by a volume [illegible]udies of community-based health care called Health by the People *that was edited by Kenneth W. Newell in 1975. These case studies—one of which described the "barefoot doctors" of rural communist China—identified the core reasons for the success of ground-level systems of basic health care and preventive medicine.*

The bedrock of these systems are **community health workers** *(CHW). CHWs are members of local communities who have been trained in basic healthcare delivery. A CHW might bandage a wound, deliver a baby, give advice to a new mother, treat diarrhea, instruct how to build a sanitary latrine, vaccinate people, or set a broken bone. They address what they can, but if needed, they also will make referrals to higher-level health care. But CHWs ideally do more than just provide basic care. As this document suggests, they can provide a bridge between communities and health systems. And, they can be a cornerstone of community participation in health, spurring activism for the right to health. This is a lot for one person to do, and these are ideals—but they are powerful ideals that many people in global health are working toward.*

PHC is a so-called horizontal approach to global health delivery. It is meant to include everyone and not be limited to specific health problems chosen by outsiders (e.g., a disease-eradication program). As described in this document, PHC programs are designed to be "available, accessible, and acceptable." These programs require continuing financial investments, but the idea is that many common health problems can be most effectively addressed at the community level, not in expensive tertiary hospitals.

The declaration of Alma-Ata also states that it is the responsibility of all governments to provide adequate health systems and social measures to maintain their populations' health. In other words, it is the responsibility and purpose of each nation to ensure that its citizens live with conditions in which it is possible to be healthy. Such conditions include the basics of adequate food, clean air and water, security, and basic health care. Guaranteeing such conditions for all is not an easy task, and it requires political will to accomplish. This may be considered an idealistic position, since most national leaders are primarily concerned with the maintenance of power, rather than securing health rights for those with the least power. For example, the fact that there is a debate over the Affordable Care Act (Obamacare) in the United States illustrates that the values laid out in this declaration are not supported by everyone.

The largest portion of the declaration is the definition of PHC in Section 7. That definition includes a minimum set of requirements, including (i) treatment of common

WHO Regional Office for Europe, 1978. Alma-Ata Declaration. Copenhagen: WHO. http://www.euro.who.int/en/publications/policy-documents/declaration-of-alma-ata,-1978

diseases and injuries; (ii) provision of essential drugs; (iii) health education; (iv) maternal and child health care; (v) control of endemic diseases; and (vi) food, clean water, and sanitation. The declaration also makes the case that health is not a separate sector—it must be integrated with economic development, agriculture, and social justice. That's a tall order. But even if achieving these things is very difficult, this document provides a moral compass that many people in global health find very powerful.

The catch phrase for Alma-Ata was "Health for All by the Year 2000!" At that time, the millennium seemed a long time in the future, and the ambiguity of that lofty goal was later an issue of contention. We will return to these issues in Section 10 while discussing the history of global health.

As you read this historical document, consider the following questions:

- **In your opinion, what is the "new international economic order" that the declaration is referring to? Is it globalization? Was does that term mean?**
- **How can an international "declaration" be a historical milestone? How is this document different from the other global health milestones you have read about?**
- **In your opinion, is this declaration overly idealistic? Why wasn't it possible to achieve the goals of PHC in the years between 1978 and 2000?**
- **How is it different from the United Nations' Millennium Development Goals for 2015 and Sustainable Development Goals for 2030?**
- **Why is this approach considered "horizontal"? In your opinion, what are the advantages of horizontal programs over vertical programs like smallpox eradication or oral rehydration solution that focus on just one disease? What are the disadvantages?**
- **The declaration of a United Nations agency like the WHO does not have any funding or executive "teeth" to it, so the problems identified in the document still exist over 40 years later. So, in your opinion, what's the point of it?**

CONTEXT

The Declaration of Alma-Ata was adopted at the International Conference on Primary Health Care (PHC), at Alma-Ata, Kazakh Soviet Socialist Republic, now Almaty, Kazakhstan. The conference brought together 134 countries and 67 international organizations. In addition to this brief declaration, the conference documents included detailed reports of the discussions and plans for the future. In this same year, 1978, the WHO's Malaria Eradication Program failed, and smallpox was successfully eradicated (see Reading 4).

The International Conference on Primary Health Care, meeting in Alma-Ata this twelfth day of September in the year Nineteen hundred and seventy-eight, expressing the need for urgent action by all governments, all health and development workers, and the world community to protect and promote the health of all the people of the world, hereby makes the following

Declaration:

I

The Conference strongly reaffirms that health, which is a state of complete physical, mental and social wellbeing, and not merely the absence of disease or infirmity, is a fundamental human right and that the attainment of the highest possible level of health is a most important world-wide social goal whose realization requires the action of many other social and economic sectors in addition to the health sector.

II

The existing gross inequality in the health status of the people particularly between developed and developing countries as well as within countries is politically, socially and economically unacceptable and is, therefore, of common concern to all countries.

III

Economic and social development, based on a New International Economic Order, is of basic importance to the fullest attainment of health for all and to the reduction of the gap between the health status of the developing and developed countries. The promotion and protection of the health of the people is essential to sustained economic and social development and contributes to a better quality of life and to world peace.

IV

The people have the right and duty to participate individually and collectively in the planning and implementation of their health care.

V

Governments have a responsibility for the health of their people which can be fulfilled only by the provision of adequate health and social measures. A main social target of governments, international organizations and the whole world community in the coming decades should be the attainment by all peoples of the world by the year 2000 of a level of health that will permit them to lead a socially and economically productive life. Primary health care is the key to attaining this target as part of development in the spirit of social justice.

VI

Primary health care is essential health care based on practical, scientifically sound and socially acceptable methods and technology made universally accessible to individuals and families in the community through their full participation and at a cost that the community and country can afford to maintain at every stage of their development in the spirit of self-reliance and self-determination. It forms an integral part both of the country's health system, of which it is the central function and main focus, and of the overall social and economic development of the community. It is the first level of contact of individuals, the family and community with the national health system bringing health care as close as possible to where people live and work, and constitutes the first element of a continuing health care process.

VII

Primary health care:

1. reflects and evolves from the economic conditions and sociocultural and political characteristics of the country and its communities and is based on the application of the relevant results of social, biomedical and health services research and public health experience;
2. addresses the main health problems in the community, providing promotive, preventive, curative and rehabilitative services accordingly;
3. includes at least: education concerning prevailing health problems and the methods of preventing and controlling them; promotion of food supply and proper nutrition; an adequate supply of safe water and basic sanitation; maternal and child health care, including family planning; immunization against the major infectious diseases; prevention and control of locally endemic diseases; appropriate treatment of common diseases and injuries; and provision of essential drugs;
4. involves, in addition to the health sector, all related sectors and aspects of national and community development, in particular agriculture, animal husbandry, food, industry, education, housing, public works, communications and other sectors; and demands the coordinated efforts of all those sectors;
5. requires and promotes maximum community and individual self-reliance and participation in the planning, organization, operation and control of primary health care, making fullest use of local, national and other available resources; and to this end develops through appropriate education the ability of communities to participate;
6. should be sustained by integrated, functional and mutually supportive referral systems, leading to the progressive improvement of

comprehensive health care for all, and giving priority to those most in need;

7. relies, at local and referral levels, on health workers, including physicians, nurses, midwives, auxiliaries and community workers as applicable, as well as traditional practitioners as needed, suitably trained socially and technically to work as a health team and to respond to the expressed health needs of the community.

VIII

All governments should formulate national policies, strategies and plans of action to launch and sustain primary health care as part of a comprehensive national health system and in coordination with other sectors. To this end, it will be necessary to exercise political will, to mobilize the country's resources and to use available external resources rationally.

IX

All countries should cooperate in a spirit of partnership and service to ensure primary health care for all people since the attainment of health by people in any one country directly concerns and benefits every other country. In this context the joint WHO/UNICEF report on primary health care constitutes a solid basis for the further development and operation of primary health care throughout the world.

X

An acceptable level of health for all the people of the world by the year 2000 can be attained through a fuller and better use of the world's resources, a considerable part of which is now spent on armaments and military conflicts. A genuine policy of independence, peace, détente and disarmament could and should release additional resources that could well be devoted to peaceful aims and in particular to the acceleration of social and economic development of which primary health care, as an essential part, should be allotted its proper share.

The International Conference on Primary Health Care calls for urgent and effective national and international action to develop and implement primary health care throughout the world and particularly in developing countries in a spirit of technical cooperation and in keeping with a New International Economic Order. It urges governments, WHO and UNICEF, and other international organizations, as well as multilateral and bilateral agencies, nongovernmental organizations, funding agencies, all health workers and the whole world community to support national and international commitment to primary health care and to channel increased technical and financial support to it, particularly in developing countries. The Conference calls on all the aforementioned to collaborate in introducing, developing and maintaining primary health care in accordance with the spirit and content of this Declaration.

JIM YONG KIM AND PAUL FARMER

8 AIDS IN 2006—MOVING TOWARD ONE WORLD, ONE HOPE?

A single disease, Acquired Immune Deficiency Syndrome (AIDS), killed roughly 35 million people between 1981 and 2015. This disease is caused by a tiny retrovirus called the **human immunodeficiency virus (HIV)***. Currently, about 40 million people in the world are infected with it. At the beginning of this pandemic, the only thing that could be done to stop the spread of the virus was to educate people on how to prevent HIV transmission. But in the three decades since HIV was first identified, an HIV infection has changed from an immediate death sentence into a manageable chronic disease, given adequate medical care.*

Alan Brandt from the Harvard School of Public Health has argued that HIV/AIDS played a critical role in the transformation of "international health" to "global health." The HIV/AIDS crisis caused this shift in five ways:

- *First, it brought* **public health** *and* **medicine** *together. Reducing the impact of HIV/AIDS involves both prevention through public health measures, and clinical medical interventions including antiretroviral therapies and treatment of opportunistic infections.*
- *Second, HIV/AIDS demonstrated that diseases do not recognize national borders, so that population health has to be a global concern rather than a local issue.*
- *Third, the HIV/AIDS crisis provoked widespread activism aimed at accelerating drug development research and, more important, the distribution of that life-saving medicine to infected people who could not afford it. There are some excellent documentaries about these activist movements in the Web Resources for this section.*
- *Fourth, that advocacy was effective in bringing unprecedented levels of funding and attention for research and health care delivery through* **partnerships** *including new global institutions (UNAIDS), national governments, private companies, nongovernmental humanitarian organizations, and universities.*
- *Finally, the HIV/AIDS crisis, along with disasters like famines, brought worldwide attention to the terrible social injustices of inequalities in health and wealth. That attention was linked to an ethos of optimism and commitment to improving the lives of the world's poor.*

This article was written by two friends who are inspirational leaders in the global health movement. They are both physicians, anthropologists, and co-founders of a nongovernmental organization called Partners in Health. Dr. Jim Kim is currently the president of the World Bank. At the time that this article was written, Kim was director of a WHO/UNAIDS project called "3 by 5," which aimed to increase the number of HIV-infected people being treated by anti-retroviral therapies drugs from about 400,000 in 2003 to 3,000,000 in 2005. This was a very ambitious goal, but the initiative did scale up ART treatment by 300% over the two years – an impressive accomplishment.

Paul Farmer is a physician, scientist, author, and advocate for social justice in health and health care, especially for the poor. When they study global health, many students read a book called Mountains beyond Mountains *by Terry Kidder that describes the early career of Farmer and his work in Haiti and elsewhere; the book's hero-worshipping title describes him as "a man who would cure the world." Chapter 12 ("The Long Defeat") is an excerpt from that book.*

Farmer and Kim's example is inspirational and sometimes controversial, but there is no doubt that the relentless advocacy of Partners in Health provoked changes in WHO policy in two areas: the standardization

Jim Young Kim and Paul Farmer. "AIDS in 2006: Moving Toward One World, One Hope?" *New England Journal of Medicine*, 2006, 355(7): 645–647.

of anti-retroviral therapies for HIV treatment in low-resource settings and the recognition of the necessity of appropriate treatment for people with multidrug-resistant tuberculosis (MDR-TB).

This article summarizes what Kim and Farmer learned from their HIV/AIDS experiences throughout the world. They argue for free treatment, strengthening of health systems, more doctors and funding, and more research for vaccines, diagnostics, and therapeutics. Farmer boils this down to the four Ss necessary for good clinical care: staff, stuff, space, and systems. Finally, Farmer and Kim argue that the underlying problems of health are linked to extreme poverty—an argument that runs throughout this book. While written at a historic time over a decade ago, the challenges still remain.

As you read this article, consider the following questions:

- **In what ways may the HIV/AIDS crisis and related activism might have influenced cultural changes in the United States—for example, attitudes about homosexuality?**
- **From a historical perspective, do you think that governments and health institutions moved quickly or slowly in response to the HIV/AIDS epidemic? Why?**
- **Why is HIV/AIDS associated with stigma? How might that stigma make prevention, testing, and treatment more difficult?**
- **Has HIV/AIDS been seen as an "exceptional" disease—one that has received undue attention and research? After all, many other easily preventable diseases cause as much or more death and suffering but do not get much attention or funding.**
- **Is HIV infection simply the result of the poor choices of individuals?**

CONTEXT

This is an editorial before the annual International AIDS Conference, held in Toronto that year.

For the past two decades, AIDS experts—clinicians, epidemiologists, policymakers, activists, and scientists—have gathered every two years to confer about what is now the world's leading infectious cause of death among young adults. This year, the International AIDS Society is hosting the meeting in Toronto from August 13 through 18. The last time the conference was held in Canada, in 1996, its theme was "One World, One Hope." But it was evident to conferees from the poorer reaches of the world that the price tag of the era's great hope—combination antiretroviral therapy—rendered it out of their reach. Indeed, some African participants that year made a banner reading "One World, No Hope."

Today, the global picture is quite different. The claims that have been made for the efficacy of antiretroviral therapy have proved to be well founded: in the United States, such therapy has prolonged life by an estimated 13 years[1]—a success rate that would compare favorably with that of almost any treatment for cancer or complications of coronary artery disease. In addition, a number of lessons, with implications for policy and action, have emerged from efforts that are well under way in the developing world. During the past decade, we have gleaned these lessons from our work in setting global AIDS policies at the World Health Organization in Geneva and in implementing integrated programs for AIDS prevention and care in places such as rural Haiti and Rwanda. As vastly different as these places may be, they are part of one world, and we believe that ambitious policy goals, adequate funding, and knowledge about implementation can move us toward the elusive goal of shared hope.

The first lesson is that charging for AIDS prevention and care will pose insurmountable problems for people living in poverty, since there will always be those unable to pay even modest amounts for services or medications, whether generic or branded. Like efforts to battle airborne tuberculosis, such services should be seen as a public good for public health. Policymakers and public health officials, especially in heavily burdened regions, should

[1] Walensky RP, Paltiel AD, Losina E, et al. The survival benefits of AIDS treatment in the United States. J Infect Dis 2006;194:11–9.

adopt universal-access plans and waive fees for HIV care. Initially, this approach will require sustained donor contributions, but many African countries have recently set targets for increased national investments in health, a pledge that could render ambitious programs sustainable in the long run.

As local investments increase, the price of AIDS care is decreasing. The development of generic medications means that antiretroviral therapy can now cost less than 50 cents per day, and costs continue to decrease to affordable levels for public health officials in developing countries. All antiretroviral medications—first-line, second-line, and third-line—must be made available at such prices. Manufacturers of generic drugs in China, India, and other developing countries stand ready to provide the full range of drugs. Whether through negotiated agreements or use of the full flexibilities of the Agreement on Trade-Related Aspects of Intellectual Property Rights, full access to all available antiretroviral drugs must quickly become the standard in all countries.

Second, the effective scale-up of pilot projects will require the strengthening and even rebuilding of health care systems, including those charged with delivering primary care. In the past, the lack of a health care infrastructure has been a barrier to antiretroviral therapy; we must now marshal AIDS resources, which are at last considerable, to rebuild public health systems in sub-Saharan Africa and other HIV-burdened regions. These efforts will not weaken efforts to address other problems—malaria and other diseases of poverty, maternal mortality, and insufficient vaccination coverage—if they are planned deliberately with the public sector in mind.[2] Only the public sector, not nongovernmental organizations, can offer health care as a right.

Third, a lack of trained health care personnel, most notably doctors, is invoked as a reason for the failure to treat AIDS in poor countries. The lack is real, and the brain drain continues. But one reason doctors flee Africa is that they lack the tools of their trade. AIDS funding offers us a chance not only to recruit physicians and nurses to underserved regions, but also to train community health care workers to supervise care, for AIDS and many other diseases, within their home villages and neighborhoods. Such training should be undertaken even in places where physicians are abundant, since community-based, closely supervised care represents the highest standard of care for chronic disease,[3] whether in the First World or the Third. And community health care workers must be compensated for their labor if these programs are to be sustainable.

Fourth, extreme poverty makes it difficult for many patients to comply with antiretroviral therapy. Indeed, poverty is far and away the greatest barrier to the scale-up of treatment and prevention programs. Our experience in Haiti and Rwanda has shown us that it is possible to remove many of the social and economic barriers to adherence but only with what are sometimes termed "wrap-around services": food supplements for the hungry, help with transportation to clinics, child care, and housing. In many rural regions of Africa, hunger is the major coexisting condition in patients with AIDS or tuberculosis, and these consumptive diseases cannot be treated effectively without food supplementation.[4] Coordination among initiatives such as the President's Emergency Plan for AIDS Relief, the Global Fund to Fight AIDS, Tuberculosis, and Malaria, and the World Food Program of the United Nations can help in the short term; fair-trade agreements and support of African farmers will help in the long run.

Fifth, investments in efforts to combat the global epidemics of AIDS and tuberculosis are much more generous than they were five years ago, but funding must be increased and sustained if we are to slow

[2] Walton DA, Farmer PE, Lambert W, Léandre F, Koenig SP, Mukherjee JS. Integrated HIV prevention and care strengthens primary health care: lessons from rural Haiti. J Public Health Policy 2004;25:137–58.

[3] Behforouz HL, Farmer PE, Mukherjee JS. From directly observed therapy to *accompagnateurs*: enhancing AIDS treatment outcomes in Haiti and in Boston. Clin Infect Dis 2004; 38:Suppl 5:S429-S436.

[4] Paton NI, Sangeetha S, Earnest A, Bellamy R. The impact of malnutrition on survival and the CD4 count response in HIV-infected patients starting antiretroviral therapy. HIV Med 2006;7:323–30.

these increasingly complex epidemics. One of the most ominous recent developments is the advent of highly drug-resistant strains of both causative pathogens. "Extensively drug-resistant tuberculosis" has been reported in the United States, Eastern Europe, Asia, South Africa, and elsewhere; in each of these settings, the copresence of HIV has amplified local epidemics of these almost untreatable strains. Drug-resistant malaria is now common worldwide, extensively drug-resistant HIV disease will surely follow, and massive efforts to diagnose and treat these diseases ethically and effectively will be needed. We have already learned a great deal about how best to expand access to second-line antituberculous drugs while increasing control over their use[5]; these lessons must be applied in the struggles against AIDS, malaria, and other infectious pathogens.

Finally, there is a need for a renewed basic-science commitment to vaccine development, more reliable diagnostics (the 100-year-old tests widely used to diagnose tuberculosis are neither specific nor sensitive), and new classes of therapeutics. The research-based pharmaceutical industry has a critical role to play in drug development, even if the overall goal is a segmented market, with higher prices in developed countries and generic production with affordable prices in developing countries.

There has been a heartening increase in basic-science investments for tuberculosis and malaria; funding for HIV research at the National Institutes of Health remains robust. Yet the fruits of such research will not arrive in time for those now living with, and dying from, AIDS and tuberculosis. New tools to prevent, diagnose, and treat the diseases of poverty will be added to the stockpile of other potentially lifesaving products that do not reach the poorest people, unless we develop an equity plan to provide them. Right now, our focus must be on improving access to the therapies that are available in high-income countries. The past few years have shown us that we can make these services available to millions, even in the poorest reaches of the world.

The unglamorous and difficult process of increasing access to prevention and care needs to be our primary focus if we are to move toward the lofty goal of equitably distributed medical services in a world riven by inequality. Without such goals, the slogan "One World, One Hope" will remain nothing more than a dream.

[5] Gupta R, Kim JY, Espinal MA, et al. Responding to market failures in tuberculosis control. Science 2001;293: 1049–51.

SECTION 1 CASES FOR TEACHING AND LEARNING

The following are web resources that instructors or students can use to enhance learning. The cases are introductory and do not require a background in public health. Many of these cases investigate health issues described in this section about historical milestones in global health and can supplement the readings.

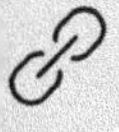

Visit the companion website, www.oup.com/us/brown-closser, for direct links to these featured online resources.

Marcia Harrison-Pitaniello et al., *Campus Outbreak! Modeling Seasonal Influenza*

This PowerPoint-based case study introduces the idea of mathematical modeling for predicting the spread of influenza and evaluating the effects of potential interventions. Students can use an online tool to explore different outcomes.

Jaclyn McLean and Ram Veerapaneni, *Cancer Cluster or Coincidence?*

This case highlights the different approaches of public health and medicine. Students consider whether a cluster of cancer cases is worth investigating.

Andrea Nicholas and Isabella Villano, *Disease along the River: A Case Study and Cholera Outbreak Game*

This simulation game illustrates the epidemiology and prevention of cholera.

Annie Prud'homme-Généreux and Carmen Petrick, *Why Was the 1918 Influenza So Deadly? An Intimate Debate Case*

In this classroom debate, students explore the social as well as the biological causes of the 1918 flu pandemic.

Oregon State University, *John Snow and the Cholera Epidemic*

This case study brings students through the steps of John Snow's outbreak investigation. It was designed for juniors and seniors in high school but is useful for teaching first-year college students or could be adapted for older students.

SECTION 1 VIDEOS AND WEB RESOURCES

Visit the companion website, www.oup.com/us/brown-closser, for direct links to the online resources featured below.

Rx for Survival: A Global Health Challenge

This six-part video series includes extensive footage and commentary on many of the milestones in this book, including John Snow's famous experiments; the development of ORS; and the eradication of smallpox. Many other parts of this video fit nicely with other sections of this book. For example, the episode "Back to the Basics" covers the determinants of health. (6 hours, but does not need to be viewed in its entirety)

100 Objects that Shaped Global Health – Johns Hopkins Bloomberg School of Public Health

This website presents 100 objects, from the bifurcated needle to the birth certificate, that have shaped public health.

Smallpox Eradication

Demon in the Freezer – Errol Morris

In this New York Times "Op-doc," renowned documentary filmmaker Errol Morris interviews D. A. Henderson and others involved in smallpox eradication about the decision not to destroy stocks of smallpox in labs in the United States and USSR post-eradication. (18 minutes)

Learning from Smallpox: How to Eradicate a Disease – Julie Garon and Walter A. Orenstein

A TED-Ed video briefly describing how smallpox was eradicated, what is necessary for eradication, and where we're headed with eradication efforts for the future. This pro-eradication viewpoint can be compared with other, more critical perspectives in this book. (5 minutes)

AIDS Activism

How to Survive a Plague (2012)

This searing and fascinating documentary follows the history of ACT UP during the height of the AIDS epidemic in the United States. It is well worth watching, especially for those students who may not be aware of the history of LGBTQ activism in the United States.

Fire in the Blood (2013)

This documentary explores the global movement for access to affordable anti-retroviral therapy.

1918 Flu

There are dozens of excellent documentaries on the Internet featuring interviews with survivors and many vintage photographs. Here are a few resources:

1918 and Bird Flu – Nova Science Now

A brief, entertaining introduction to the 1918 flu epidemic that makes connections to current concerns with bird flu. (13 min)

Influenza Archive – University of Michigan

This website features documents and photographs from the 1918 flu epidemic in a number of American cities.

1918 Flu Pandemic Song

This light-hearted entertaining song emphasizes the connection between WWI and the influenza epidemic. (2 min)

The 1918 Influenza Pandemic in America: the Struggle Against the Spanish Flu

This documentary is a bit older, but it has a collection of very interesting interviews with survivors of the 1918 flu. (56 min)

Smoking and Cancer

Last Week Tonight with John Oliver (2015)

Excellent activist (and entertaining) review of Big Tobacco's pressure on low- and middle - income countries of their expanding market.

Thank You for Smoking (2005)

Satirical comedy about Big Tobacco's chief representative and lobbyist obfuscating the truth. While this movie is fictional, it reflects the truth that much of the tobacco industry's work is about advertising (a great topic for student research papers).

SECTION 2

Epidemiology and the Basic Methods of Global Health

This section of the book deals with epidemiology, the primary method used in global health research. During your classes in global health, you will probably be exposed to many charts, graphs, and tables. Pay attention to these numbers because they are important. Morbidity and mortality statistics, in reality, represent actual human beings and their very real suffering. The numbers and the statistical analyses might seem dry to some students, but the primary way that we know things in population health is to collect quantitative data.

Epidemiologists study the distribution of disease and death in populations in regard to time, place, and person. If they are dealing with an outbreak of a disease but they do not know the cause, they can use that epidemiological data to figure out the cause—or at least make a good guess (hypothesis) about it.

There are only two articles in this section. The first is about how disease outbreaks are investigated by epidemiologists from the Centers for Disease Control and Prevention. It describes the disease detectives of the Epidemic Intelligence Service. Their work can be rather exciting when they are asked to unravel a medical mystery—especially when there can be so much at stake with a possible epidemic. Other times, their work involves the slow grind of millions of data points and the slow work of convincing stakeholders to take action based on data.

The second article is actually a basic learning module created by the Centers for Disease Control Prevention. In general, physicians do not get a lot of training in epidemiology, and the logics of problem solving for a single individual and that of problem solving for a population are very different. But learning the basics of epidemiology is essential for everyone involved in global health because of global health's interdisciplinary nature. That reading is a bit longer than most of the selections in this book.

» CONCEPTUAL TOOLS «

- **Global health is not a single academic field but rather a set of complex problems that require the efforts of people from a wide variety of disciplines and with many different skills.** You do not have to become a doctor to make a contribution to improvements in global health. The problems and solutions are complicated. It is an interdisciplinary field that requires people trained in just about everything – from anthropology to zoology (see "What's Your Major" in Chapter 1).
- **There are important differences between health and medicine.** "Health" refers to a state of well-being either for an individual or a population. In many ways, health is an ideal goal rather than a specific thing. "Clinical medicine" refers to diagnosing and treating health problems, like diseases, that affect individuals. Access to clinical medicine is only one of many determinants of health.
- **Health must be understood on both a population level and an individual level.** The field of global health nearly always refers to large groups of people—entire populations who can be analyzed in terms of variations in social and geographical categories. Measuring population health is a fundamental goal of epidemiology.
- **There are at least three levels of causation for health problems: the individual biological level, an individual behavioral level, and a macro political-economic-ecological level.** Understanding both the causes of health problems and the solutions to them requires addressing all three of these levels.
- **Epidemiology is the study of factors affecting the health and illness of populations.** It provides the foundational method for public health and preventive medicine. Epidemiology allows scientists to understand the causation (etiology) of health problems. It, therefore, provides the logic for designing public health interventions.
- **There are two basic types of epidemiology: descriptive and analytic.** Descriptive epidemiology describes the distribution of cases (people who got sick) and controls (people who did not get sick) in regard to time, place, and person (TPP). Analytic epidemiology uses the TPP data and examines it in relation to exposure to various things to determine the cause (etiology) of an outbreak or disease cluster.
- **Surveillance is a cornerstone of an effective public health infrastructure**. Systematically measuring the health of a population provides the information necessary for knowing how serious a health problem is, ascertaining whether new health problems are developing, and gauging the effectiveness of health interventions. Surveillance systems, including periodic surveys, produce the data for Epidemiology. Collecting quality global health data is difficult.
- **Global health statistics must be taken with a "grain of salt."** Both medicine and population health studies use a lot of numbers to describe realities on the ground, and they use statistical analysis to better understand what those numbers actually mean. While experimental studies in laboratories can produce precise measurements, this is much more difficult in studies of populations (or maybe even impossible!). This is especially the case when considering data that come from areas of the world with weak surveillance systems. However, even if the numbers represent estimates and the data collection methods have weaknesses, the *general trends* described in the numbers must be taken seriously. Collection of this data requires a great deal of work.

- **There are many different ways to measure population health.** There are diverse metrics used in global health, and they emphasize different things.
- **Epidemiologists measure both morbidity and mortality when evaluating the burden of disease.** "Morbidity" refers to people who are sickened or injured by a particular health problem; "mortality" refers to people who are killed. Both measures are useful in particular situations. For example, in describing the impact of polio, a disease that paralyzes but, in most cases, is not deadly, "morbidity" is generally used. On the other hand, in evaluating the impact of treating HIV-positive people, looking at mortality would be the more useful measure, since you would want to know whether treatment keeps HIV-positive people alive.

  The burden of disease may be described in terms of prevalence (percentage of a given population affected by a disease at a single point in time) or incidence (number of *new cases* in a given population in a given time period).
- **In its simplest sense, epidemiological reasoning involves a 2×2 table.** There are two rows and two columns. Everyone in the study is put in a box depending on whether they were exposed or not exposed to something that might cause a disease (like moldy potato salad) and whether they got sick with a particular disease (like gastroenteritis). If the cells for disease/exposed and not exposed/no disease are larger than would be expected by chance, then the potato salad is probably the culprit in the gastroenteritis outbreak. More information on some very basic analyses using these **2×2 tables** is in Chapter 10.

TABLE CT2.1 A 2 × 2 Table.

	Disease	No Disease
Exposed		
Not Exposed		

- **Demography is the science of counting people.** It counts the number of individuals in a given group of people, as well as the numbers of births, deaths, and people who migrate. Demographers use these data to create mathematical models to predict future trends like population growth or migration rates.

  People in global health must consider *rates* of health problems, which requires both a numerator and a denominator. In other words, not only do you need to know how many sick people there are in a population, you can't make conclusions or plan an intervention without also knowing about how many people there are in the population as a whole. Demography is necessary for knowing that number. Population size and density is also very important for understanding factors like the demand for food, shelter needs, and economic development.
- **The terms "endemic," "epidemic," and "pandemic" are often confused.** An endemic disease exists permanently in a particular region or population, although its prevalence may increase or decrease for different reasons. An epidemic is an outbreak of a disease—an appearance of a greater number of cases than expected. By definition, an epidemic attacks many people at the same time, and depending on the epidemic, may spread between communities. A pandemic is a global outbreak involving many people on multiple continents.

MARK PENDERGRAST

9 INSIDE THE OUTBREAKS

An especially exciting part of epidemiology is the solving of medical mysteries through a type of systematic detective work in the field. These are called outbreak investigations. They focus on unexpected—and sometimes unexplained—clusters of disease that occur in a particular time and place. There is a corps of field epidemiologists called the Epidemic Intelligence Service (EIS), headquartered at the Centers for Disease Control and Prevention in Atlanta, Georgia, that can be called upon to perform these investigations in the United States (and sometimes in other countries).

EIS officers can be sent into the field at any time to do an investigation using the tools of epidemiology. As part of their work, EIS officers often interview patients in person and inspect local conditions. They are sometimes called "shoe-leather epidemiologists" because of this.

The information they collect provides clues for understanding the causes of a disease outbreak and, hopefully, stopping the epidemic. The 2011 film Contagion *depicts an EIS officer investigating an outbreak that becomes an extremely serious epidemic. That film drew inspiration from some real outbreaks, including the 1918 influenza pandemic (Reading 3) and the H1N5 ("bird flu") influenza threat of 1997, described in this reading.*

The case of the "church supper," also described in this reading, is a famous one for teaching field methods in epidemiology. The bacteria got into one of the food items at the potluck—and an EIS officer figured out the source using epidemiological methods. Note that the analytical tools used were not mathematically complicated. They are the same concepts and tools that are described in the next reading (10). Using the link in the cases listed at the end of this section, you can work through this classic outbreak investigation yourself (though in this case, the culprit might not be the potato salad)!

Just as John Snow is considered the father of epidemiology (see Reading 2), the father of the EIS was Alexander Langmuir. As you see in this reading, Langmuir emphasized infectious disease, and his approach to epidemiology was straightforward. He encouraged his EIS officers to do studies and then make recommendations as quickly as possible.

As you read these cases, consider the following questions:

- **The metaphor of the river and the people drowning in it is a common one in global public health. In your opinion, is it an apt metaphor? Does it denigrate curative medicine (i.e., the "lifeguards")?**
- **From its inception, the EIS has intentionally used military language; most EIS officers are members of the Commissioned Corp of the US Navy. Why is this the case? What are reasons for the association with military security?**
- **What is epidemiology?**
- **Why is the triad of person, place, and time important?**
- **The H1N5 outbreak of bird flu created a good deal of fear throughout the world. Why? Was it really necessary to kill all those chickens?**
- **Does the life of an EIS officer sound exciting to you? Why or why not?**
- **Currently, EIS officers apply epidemiology to noninfectious disease. How could you use EIS-style epidemiology for problems like cancer and heart disease?**
- **What is the connection between the EIS and the Cold War? You can see Reading 35 for more information on the Cold War.**
- **During the last decade, there have been many "disease detective" learning challenges**

Revised from *Inside the Outbreaks: The Elite Medical Detectives of the Epidemic Intelligence Service* by Mark Pendergrast. Boston: Mariner Books, 2011.

designed for younger students (e.g., Science Olympiads). Why are outbreaks a good way to teach about scientific critical thinking?

CONTEXT

Mark Pendergrast modified and amplified material in this chapter from his book, *Inside the Outbreaks: The Elite Medical Detectives of the Epidemic Intelligence Service* (Boston: Mariner Books, 2011).

Mark Pendergrast is a well-known independent science writer. His books cover a wide variety of topics from the science and history of coffee and Coca-Cola to the questions of how false memories of witnesses are created—and the way they can destroy lives of those accused of crimes. His book *Inside the Outbreaks* (2011) is based on extensive research and interviews with EIS officers, past and present.

The Parable of the Clinician and the Epidemiologist

A lazy brown river flows through the middle of town. It usually carries branches and leaves, swirling them slowly in its current, or perhaps the occasional bottle, bobbing along. But today it also carries bodies, bodies of people. Many are dead, but some are still alive, gasping for air, thrashing the water, but unable to speak or swim.

Approaching the river to enjoy their lunch hour on its banks, two doctors are horrified by what they see. They begin to haul the people out of the river and to revive them as best they can. There are no signs of violence, but the victims' eyes are glazed, their weak pulses racing.

The doctors cannot keep up with the flow of bodies that continue to float down the river. It is all they can do to save a few. They watch helplessly as the others drift beyond them.

Suddenly, one of the doctors lets the old man she has just dragged from the water drop onto the ground. She begins to run away. "What are you doing?" yells the other doctor. "For God's sake, come back and help me save these people!"

Without stopping, she yells back over her shoulder. "I'm going upstream to find out why they're falling in."

Biowarriors

For over half a century, Epidemic Intelligence Service officers, working out of the CDC (Centers for Disease Control and Prevention) in Atlanta, Georgia, have been the largely unheralded foot-soldiers of disease diagnosis and prevention who are sent into the heart of an epidemic, be it Salmonella spread at a church picnic in Peoria or Ebola killing villagers in Africa.

Since its founding by Alexander Langmuir as a service/training program for young epidemiologists in 1951, the Epidemic Intelligence Service has sent out over 3,000 officers to combat every imaginable human (and sometimes animal) ailment, now including chronic disease, environmental issues, and societal problems. Suitcases packed, vaccinations ready, the mantra "time-place-person" on their lips, these young doctors—and veterinarians, dentists, statisticians, nurses, microbiologists, academic epidemiologists, sociologists, anthropologists, and now even lawyers—call themselves "shoe-leather epidemiologists."

Appropriately, the EIS logo features the sole of a shoe, a prominent hole worn through the bottom, superimposed over the earth. EIS officers—at first men, but now more than half women—have ventured over the globe to combat diseases, sometimes dumped from airplanes whose pilots immediately took off for fear of contamination, sometimes in Jeeps mired in muddy rice paddies, sometimes on bicycles wheeled through favelas, sometimes aboard fragile boats tossed on stormy seas or struggling up the Amazon, sometimes on dogsleds over the tundra, sometimes atop elephants and camels. Always on call, often working 20-hour days during their two-year EIS stint, they have occasionally caught the bugs they were studying, but, astonishingly, only one officer has thus far died in the line of duty—in an airplane crash.

Epidemic Intelligence Service officers have not served without controversy. They have been accused of using strong-arm tactics during global smallpox eradication, of being secret government agents causing rather than curing AIDS and syphilis, of being "the feds" running rough-shod through the states, of ignoring the pleas of the sick while merely counting the dead, of being swayed by political pressure, of grandstanding for the media, of focusing on the wrong issues, of crying wolf over epidemics that never occurred, of taking too long to identify the cause of real epidemics. Some of the criticisms have had some substance; most have not.

For the most part, EIS officers have performed their tasks—difficult, dangerous, or dead-end, confusing, exciting, or tedious—without fanfare or notice. They have saved uncountable lives in the process, preventing disease from spreading uncontrolled and diagnosing problems before they got out of hand. They may have saved your life, though you probably will never know it.

Of all U. S. government agencies, the Epidemic Intelligence Service has been one of the most independent, iconoclastic, and compassionate. The EIS has carried on and developed the tradition of field epidemiology begun in the mid-19th century by John Snow, among others. By going door-to-door and mapping London cases during an 1854 cholera outbreak, Snow noted that infections in one area centered around the Broad Street pump, but that employees at a nearby brewing company, which had its own spring water (and beer), remained well. Snow concluded that an infectious agent (bacteria had not yet been discovered) must be in the public water supply. He advised authorities to remove the handle of the Broad Street pump, and the epidemic ceased. As EIS founder Alexander Langmuir put it, such "direct field observations, orderly arraying of evidence, and incisive inductive reasoning have set a pattern for all epidemiologists to emulate today."

Epidemics can be regarded as natural experiments that allow epidemiologists to learn about risk factors and causation. Young, energetic EIS officers, supported by excellent supervision and labs, can take full advantage of such circumstances. One or two enterprising officers, allowed the flexibility to pursue every lead, can sometimes be more effective than too many investigators, just as too many cooks can spoil the proverbial broth.

Early EIS officers employed simple descriptive epidemiology, looking for the frequency and pattern of an outbreak by examining a particular time period in a well-defined place and population. Over time, the EIS methodology became more sophisticated, employing case-control studies, computing odds ratios, and utilizing other complex statistical analyses such as multivariate regression.

The first EIS officers were mostly young white male U. S. physicians. Over time, the selection process has evolved so that about 15% of each class come from other countries, over half are female, and many are Ph.D.s or have other non-M.D. training. The age of the typical EIS recruit has moved from 27 to 34. Many arrive in the EIS with extensive experience and education in public health.

Cold War, Hot Pathogens

"Using modern laboratory techniques, many pathogenic agents may be grown in almost limitless quantities, and may be dispersed into the air as single cells." Alexander Langmuir, 41, leaned over the lectern at the Kansas City Medical Center on a cold February day in 1951. As the chief epidemiologist for the Communicable Disease Center (CDC) in Atlanta, Georgia, Langmuir had been invited to give an in-service training lecture in public health and preventive medicine. Now he was scaring the hell out of the assembled doctors and nurses.

He enjoyed it. A big man in every way, over six feet tall, he bent over the audience, his balding dome seemingly alight with special knowledge, his booming baritone filling the hall. "The purposeful creation of such clouds is biological warfare."

In these early days of the Cold War era—as the Korean War raged, Russia amassed nuclear weapons, and Communist China joined the North Koreans in their fight—Langmuir's terrifying message was not unusual. The newspapers and magazines had been full of headlines about biological warfare since 1946, as in *Newsweek*'s Jan. 14, 1946, "Armies of Germs" or *Time*'s Aug. 12, 1946, "Planned Pestilence." But with the new war beginning in June 1950, fear and rhetoric escalated. "Germ Warfare in Korea?" asked a *Science News Letter* headline the month after the war began.

Then in June 1951, reports came back from Korea that young American soldiers were dying of a mysterious infection that first gave them high fever, aches, nausea, and vomiting, after which their blood vessels turned to sieves, and they bled internally and often externally. Dubbed Korean hemorrhagic fever, it laid 25,000 United Nations (mostly American) troops low and killed nearly 3,000 of them during the course of the conflict. Surely this must be a horrible new biological warfare agent let loose by the Communists? In later years, Langmuir told colleagues that fear of the new epidemic disease solidified funding for his new trainees. (Korean hemorrhagic fever was caused by a virus, not bioterrorists. But EIS officers would later investigate a real bioterrorist who sent anthrax letters in 2001.)

What did you need to fight epidemics? Epidemiologists, of course. But as Langmuir advised, "one urgent problem arises, namely, the dearth of trained epidemiologists. This dearth exists even in peacetime. Defense needs exaggerate this deficiency." Brilliantly, Langmuir named his new program the Epidemic Intelligence Service, deliberately employing a military term and implying a comparison with the recently-created Central Intelligence Agency.

Only three years old when Langmuir arrived there in 1949, the fledgling CDC was the revamped and rechristened unit formerly called Malaria Control in War Areas (MCWA), based in Atlanta, Georgia, because so many troops training in the Southeast had been plagued with malaria. Langmuir was impressed with the can-do, unstuffy attitude at the CDC, with its mandate to move beyond malaria and address all infectious diseases.

In 1949, Langmuir thought that infectious diseases could be fought on broad fronts with the power of epidemiology, which stems from the Greek, meaning "upon, or among, the people." On the surface a dull statistical exercise, epidemiology permitted disease detectives to solve medical mysteries and to save hundreds, thousands, even millions of lives. While clinical doctors worked with patients one-on-one, epidemiologists treated entire populations.

Among his many definitions of epidemiology, one of Langmuir's earliest was that it is "the science concerned with understanding the factors related to the occurrence and distribution of disease in the population. Epidemiology must consider both the sick and the well in their relation to each other and to their environment." He espoused what came to be called a cohort study of a carefully defined group of people (*Who attended the church supper?*) comparing their behavior (*What did they eat? Where did they go? Who did they associate with?*) and looking for key differences between those who had become ill and those who had not. Sometimes through such comparisons, the cause of an epidemic suddenly became obvious. It was the potato salad!

Langmuir stressed the importance of simple mathematics—long division, to be precise. To find the rate of a given disease in a particular population, you needed a numerator (number of ill over a defined period of time) and a denominator (the population at risk over the same time span). "Stripped to its basics," he said, "epidemiology is simply a process of obtaining the appropriate numerator and denominator, determining a rate, and interpreting that rate." Thus, the three essential elements were time (*When were people exposed and when did they become ill?*), person (*Who was affected in what defined population?*), and place (*Where did the epidemic take place?*).

But how do you know that an epidemic is actually occurring? First, you need to establish what the "normal" rate of disease for that area might be. Langmuir introduced another military term to epidemiology, talking about the importance of routine disease surveillance to establish such baseline data and to look for anomalous blips.

Traced on a time-line tracking the number of accumulating daily cases, most epidemics form a classic epidemic curve, a bell shaped hump. In the simplest version, an outbreak begins in a particular community with an index case, spreads to others, reaches a peak, and then gradually burns itself out, as susceptibles either survive and become immune or die. Just by looking at this epi-curve, the disease detective could deduce a fair amount. A common source epidemic, such as bad potato salad at a picnic, would have a sudden onset, sharp peak, and rapid resolution among a limited population, whereas an ongoing problem such as a contaminated water supply might affect an entire community for a longer time, unless some diagnosis and intervention halted it. Once a likely moment of exposure was determined—i.e., the time of the picnic in a common source exposure—the epi-curve also revealed the average incubation period, the time between the infection and the disease onset.

The EIS officers were assigned around the country in carefully selected state and city health departments, research universities and hospitals, the headquarters of the CDC in Atlanta, or in a CDC branch. All were on call 24 hours a day, their bags packed. Langmuir took pride in a swift response to a call for help. "State health officers were astounded to find bright, young, responsive epidemiologists in their offices the next morning, or sometimes the same day that they called," he recalled. "Each epidemic aid call was an adventure and a training experience, even the false alarms."

The Classic Church Supper

"My God, I'm coming down with typhoid!" In the summer of 1952, Harold Nitowsky, the 26-year-old son of a Brooklyn tailor, was sweating with fever in a fleabag hotel room in remote Trinidad, Colorado, where he had been sent from the CDC Kansas City field station to investigate a typhoid epidemic. But his fever soon subsided, and he continued to pursue the source of the epidemic. Typhoid, a particularly nasty variant of the Salmonella bacterium, was rare in the United States, and carriers—like the infamous "Typhoid Mary" Mallon—had to register with state health departments. Such carriers were never supposed to handle food, because typhoid is spread by fecal-oral contact, and unless their hands are washed very thoroughly, typhoid carriers can contaminate what they prepare for others to eat.

If not countered by antibiotics or a vaccine, typhoid is a vicious disease that causes a rash, tender spleen, high fever, slow pulse, nausea, and diarrhea. That is what six people who had eaten at a local church potluck supper were going through, and Nitowsky was there to sort out the mystery. He contacted everyone who had attended the supper, asking them to recall what they had eaten. "They weren't sure about this strange young man with the Russian name asking all these questions during the Cold War." His parents had, in fact, come from Poland in the early 20th century, classic immigrants in search of a better life.

Nitowsky made a chart with the different food and drink items running down a page on the left, and two columns marked ILL and NOT ILL at the top. Basically, this was a combined form of what epidemiologists call a 2 × 2 table, where two opposite conditions for each food item (or whatever variable is being examined) are listed on two sides of a four-part square: Ate – Didn't Eat on the left side, and Ill – Not Ill across the top. There are four possible permutations. 1) People ate a particular item and got ill. 2) They ate it and did not get ill. 3) They didn't eat it and got ill. 4) They didn't eat it and didn't get ill. From the results, the epidemiologist can ascertain how strong an association the illness has with a particular food item.

Some who had contracted typhoid had eaten pickles; some had not. What did that tell him? But Nitowsky didn't need fancy math to solve the mystery. One food item leaped from the page. The carrot salad, made by a woman we will call Mabel, had a very high food specific attack rate, which simply means the percentage of those eating this food who became ill. When her stool sample was tested, the matronly, well-meaning Mabel turned out to be an unregistered, unrecognized typhoid carrier. "She was very upset," Nitowsky recalls, "but there was nothing to be done. She had to be registered and avoid serving food to others. And I cautioned her to be very careful washing her hands."

This Is How It Begins

In May of 1997, a three-year-old boy died of influenza in Hong Kong. When the local laboratory couldn't identify the strain, it sent it to a Dutch lab, which finally determined in August that it was an H5N1 strain. That seemed impossible, since no human had ever caught flu with this hemagglutinin protein, which afflicted only poultry. Indeed, an H5N1 epidemic in Hong Kong's rural New Territories in March 1997 had killed thousands of chickens on three farms.

EIS alum Keiji Fukuda, the epidemiology section chief of the CDC Influenza Branch, was not expecting any urgent calls in August. The flu assignment, which the EIS alum had taken on the previous year, was considered a backwater, though Fukuda—born in Japan but raised in Vermont—took it very seriously, knowing that flu killed some 35,000 U. S. citizens every year. Prior to taking on flu, Fukuda had spent several years investigating chronic fatigue syndrome and Gulf War syndrome, both politically sensitive and possibly psychosomatic. "At least you're dealing with a real disease now," his EIS officer Carolyn Bridges teased. Since the swine flu panic of 1976, nothing extraordinary had happened in the Influenza Branch. Even though another worldwide influenza pandemic would inevitably occur at some point—there had been pandemics in 1918, 1957, and 1968—few worried about it.

When he got the call about the boy with the bird flu, the normally unflappable Fukuda thought, *This is how it begins.* Carolyn Bridges was in the middle of a major research project (a cost-benefit analysis of giving the flu vaccine to healthy working adults), so he asked Catherine Dentinger, an EIS nurse practitioner assigned to hepatitis, to fly with him to Hong Kong. "I knew virtually nothing about flu," she recalls, "but I got a sense that Keiji, a very quiet guy, had the weight of the world on his shoulders."

Arriving in Hong Kong on August 20, they could find no evidence that the boy had contact with the sick chickens in the New Territories, but they discovered that pet chicks and ducklings at his day care center had died shortly before he became ill. Fukuda, Dentinger and two other CDC staff collected blood samples from about 2,000 possible contacts, finding antibodies to H5N1 in nine people, including one of the child's doctors and a classmate, as well as five poultry workers in the New Territories. None had become ill. After two-and-a-half weeks, the CDC team flew home. *This is probably some odd, sporadic thing,* a relieved Fukuda thought.

Then in late November 1997, the Hong Kong lab identified another H5N1 sample from a two-year-old boy who had been hospitalized briefly but recovered. Fukuda headed for Hong Kong again, this time taking second-year EIS officer Carolyn Bridges with him. By the time they arrived in Hong Kong on Saturday, December 6, two more H5N1 cases had been identified—a 13-year-old girl struggling for her life on a respirator, and a 54-year-old man who had died that day. Fukuda called the CDC for backup, and within a few days EIS officers Tony Mounts and Seymour Williams arrived with two other staff.

Over the next three weeks, there were 14 more cases. The 13-year-old died on December 21. Two days later a 60-year-old woman died. Avian flu attacked a fourth New Territories chicken farm and was identified in chickens in the live markets inside Hong Hong. On Christmas Day, hearing of several possible new cases, the frantic CDC team worried that the epidemic might be spinning out of control. The two previous pandemics had begun in southern China; the 1968 variety had even been called the Hong Kong flu. Were they at Ground Zero, witnessing the birth of a new pandemic? Perhaps most ominously, H5N1 was killing otherwise healthy adults, as had the lethal 1918 influenza.

People weren't supposed to catch flu directly from chickens. In theory, the flu virus had to mutate within another intermediary such as a pig. The CDC team pondered whether mice or cats might harbor the virus but found no evidence. Meanwhile, 10% of the chickens in the Hong Kong markets tested positive for H5N1. "There were poultry stalls on every block," Carolyn Bridges recalls. "People would either have the birds slaughtered at the stall or bring them home to fatten them up." Savvy customers blew on the feathers to see how meaty the fowl were—a good way to aerosolize the virus.

The biggest concern was whether human-to-human transmission was taking place. "The population density of Hong Kong is amazing," Bridges observes. "If this flu could easily jump from human to human, it would just explode." In the worst-case scenario, a person might simultaneously contract H5N1 and H3N2, the common human virus, and the adaptable microbes would trade genes, with a resulting strain that could spread simply and quickly. With the regular Hong Kong flu season due to begin in February, such a viral reassortment was a real possibility.

The EIS officers were particularly concerned about the case of a five-year-old girl, whose grandmother scavenged dead chickens from the market next to their high-rise apartment building. The girl's two-year-old cousin then tested positive for H5N1. Did he catch it from the five-year-old? Looking for evidence of human-to-human spread, Bridges interviewed and drew blood from close household contacts of cases, people who shared a tour bus with the 54-year-old man who had died, and health care workers exposed to H5N1 patients.

Seymour Williams studied cohorts of a day care case, while Tony Mounts looked for risk factors in a case-control study. A case-control study is a quick, down-and-dirty epidemiological investigation tool. "Cases" are the people who have contracted the illness being investigated. Carefully chosen "controls" are associated people who are very similar to cases but who did not contract the illness. By comparing them, it is sometimes possible to determine what sets them apart and what exposure or behavior caused the illness.

On Sunday, December 28, 1997, the 18th victim, a 34-year-old woman, was hospitalized, and the desperate Chinese authorities decided to kill all of the birds in chicken farms, wholesale markets, and live bird stalls in Hong Kong. It took three days to slaughter 1.6 million birds. In the ensuing weeks, no new cases occurred, though two more women in intensive care died. Thus, six out of 18 hospitalized patients died, yielding a 33% mortality rate.

The distraught poultry workers objected to the slaughter, pointing out that they themselves weren't sick. In January, as her fellow EIS officers returned to Atlanta, Carolyn Bridges drew blood from the poultry workers, finding that 10% of them had antibodies to H5N1. Her other studies found that six of 51 household contacts and one tour bus occupant tested positive, as did eight of 217 exposed health care workers. She concluded that the bird flu had indeed been transmitted from person to person, but that it required extremely close contact. Tony Mounts' case-control study showed that the primary risk factor for contracting H5N1 was recent exposure to live poultry—not exposure to someone else with the infection.

Bridges and Fukuda finally flew back to Atlanta at the end of January 1998, after two months of frenetic, frantic activity. No one knew whether H5N1 would return to infect humans again. "The only predictable thing about flu is that it is unpredictable," Bridges concluded. "However long I study this organism," Fukuda added, "it may well be completely elusive to me in the end."

The EIS Legacy

In 500-plus interviews over five years, EIS officers told me surprisingly similar stories about their experience: *The EIS changed my life, shaped my career, gave me a worldview. Those were the best two years of my life.* Of course, not every former officer felt that way, and some expressed unhappiness with their assignment, supervisor, or other frustrations or obstacles they encountered. But for the overwhelming majority, the Epidemic Intelligence Service was transformative. EIS officers now apply epidemiological investigative methodology to chronic, noninfectious diseases caused by human behavior such as smoking, eating habits, nutritional deficiency, and lack of exercise.

For an obscure government program, the Epidemic Intelligence Service has produced remarkable results. Perhaps it has done so in part by remaining relatively small, nimble, and flexible. Early on, Alexander Langmuir learned that sending out one or two officers was usually more effective than throwing an unwieldy team into the field. One of the lessons of the EIS history is the impact that one person can have, often as a result of an outbreak he or she happened to investigate. As just one example, EIS officer Henry Falk identified vinyl chloride as a liver carcinogen and consequently pioneered environmental work at the CDC. Put creative, intelligent, well-trained, motivated individuals into the right environment, and the unanticipated outcome can save lives and lead to vital careers. Then clone the program in other countries, seek out more such trainees, and send them out. EIS officers and alums have been able to have an impact far beyond their original numbers.

The EIS program and its offspring have influenced and defined how field epidemiology and public health are practiced globally. EIS officers and alums have literally left their footprints all over the world, giving real meaning to the logo with the hole in the shoe. They face daunting obstacles against impossible odds, and they certainly cannot solve all of the world's health problems. Like most public health programs, the EIS is underfunded and must function as part of a political system that can impinge on its activities. But EIS officers, true to their mission, do not give up.

Future EIS officers will never lack for challenges in this troubled world that is increasingly a global village, connected by jets, cell phones, and the Internet, but with incredible inequities, poverty, inaccessible care for millions, and new diseases about to emerge from invaded ecosystems, while global warming heats the stew. But it is comforting to know that idealistic, enthusiastic EIS officers will be spanning the globe, fighting to make the earth a safer, healthier home.

10 EPIDEMIOLOGY AND SURVEILLANCE

Epidemiology is primarily the study of the distribution and determinants of health in specific populations. The field emphasizes methods for knowing things in population health—what are the main health problems of a group? What groups of people are at the greatest risk for which diseases? Why? What causes those diseases? Are things getting better or worse for this group of people? This kind of information is absolutely critical for designing and evaluating programs to improve health. Such information must be collected in a systematic way, and analyses must be rigorous to avoid false conclusions.

When you study global health, there are many charts, tables, graphs, maps, and statistics. You need to learn how to read them and critically evaluate them. There is a classic book from the 1950s called How to Lie with Statistics *that has basic information of how people—like advertisers or pharmaceutical companies—can make seemingly convincing arguments to the unsuspecting. Just like we need to fact-check our politicians, it is important to be a critical consumer of information. Too many people tend to skip over the numbers when reading or listening; in studying global health you will need to look at all numbers critically, especially when the question involves the concept of "risk." Too many Americans are relatively* innumerate; *they studied arithmetic and mathematics in school, but they cannot use those skills in everyday life. For the ordinary citizen, epidemiology and statistics are more useful than more advanced subjects like Calculus.*

In global health, it is difficult and complicated to collect excellent reliable data (see Reading 13). Epidemiologists must design the methods for collecting data, often through surveys, so that the information they analyze is representative of the population they are trying to understand. The classic epidemiological investigation is that of a sudden "outbreak," as described in the stories of the Epidemic Intelligence Service in the previous reading by Pendergast (Reading 9). Outbreak investigation must follow a particular procedure starting with affirming that the outbreak exists and creating an operational definition of the illness. Next, data must be collected about the behavior, exposures, and sociodemographic characteristics of both the cases (people who got sick) and controls (see Conceptual Tools for this section).

The following reading, which is really a quick training module designed by the Centers for Disease Control and Prevention, explains the basic analytical techniques of descriptive epidemiology, analytic epidemiology, and risk assessment. Descriptive epidemiology concerns the distribution of illness in a population in terms of time, place, and person. Analytic epidemiology uses that data to determine the cause of the outbreak, or at least to generate hypotheses about the cause.

The point of an outbreak investigation, as well as the point of epidemiology in general, is not simply to understand a disease and its spread but also to control risk factors to stop the transmission or development of the disease. Epidemiologists study things that have serious consequences for people's health. The job of the epidemiologist is not completed until the community is informed about what is going on and how they can protect themselves. In outbreak situations, there is often social panic that needs to be kept under control. This is especially the case when an outbreak is continuing to spread while the investigation is ongoing.

Most noncommunicable diseases have multiple causes that are related in complex ways. When studying these diseases, epidemiologists must decipher which risk factors contribute the most to the illness. Understanding basic epidemiological terms and methods is important so that you can be informed and be a cautious consumer of popular health reporting.

Excepts from *Principles of Epidemiology in Public Health Practice*, by Centers for Disease Control and Prevention, 3d ed. Atlanta: CDC, 2006, updated May 2012. https://www.cdc.gov/ophss/csels/dsepd/ss1978/ss1978.pdf.

As you read the following module, consider the following questions:

- **Why do epidemiologists need to focus on *rates* of disease based on both a numerator and a denominator? In your opinion, which of the two numbers is more important?**
- **Why might a 2×2 table be the simplest way to explain the fundamental logic of epidemiology? Why does this require some understanding of basic statistics?**
- **Why do you think that epidemiological findings are often reported in the form of graphs and tables?**
- **Can you think of some reasons why an epidemiological study may be wrong or biased?**
- **What is a "sample size" of a study? How might it affect the confidence that a scientist can have in his or her results?**

CONTEXT

This chapter is made up of excerpts from a self-study training manual for learning the fundamentals of Epidemiology and Biostatistics. The entire course is available online from the Centers for Disease Control and Prevention at https://www.cdc.gov/ophss/csels/dsepd/ss1978/ss1978.pdf.

Recently, a news story described a neighborhood's concern about the rise in the number of children with asthma. Another story reported the revised recommendations for who should receive influenza vaccine this year. A third story discussed the extensive disease-monitoring strategies being implemented in a city recently affected by a massive hurricane. A fourth story described a finding published in a leading medical journal of an association in workers exposed to a particular chemical and an increased risk of cancer. Each of these news stories included interviews with public health officials or researchers who called themselves epidemiologists. Well, who are these epidemiologists, and what do they do? What is epidemiology?

Students of journalism are taught that a good news story, whether it be about a bank robbery, dramatic rescue, or presidential candidate's speech, must include the 5 W's: what, who, where, when and why (sometimes cited as why/how). The 5 W's are the essential components of a news story because if any of the five are missing, the story is incomplete.

The same is true in characterizing epidemiologic events, whether it be an outbreak of norovirus among cruise ship passengers or the use of mammograms to detect early breast cancer. The difference is that epidemiologists tend to use synonyms for the 5 W's: diagnosis or health event (what), person (who), place (where), time (when), and causes, risk factors, and modes of transmission (why/how).

Definition of Epidemiology

The word epidemiology comes from the Greek words *epi*, meaning on or upon, *demos*, meaning people, and *logos*, meaning the study of. In other words, the word epidemiology has its roots in the study of what befalls a population. Many definitions have been proposed, but the following definition captures the underlying principles and public health spirit of epidemiology:

> *Epidemiology is the **study** of the **distribution** and **determinants** of **health-related states or events** in **specified populations**, and the **application** of this study to the control of health problems.*

The Epidemiologic Approach

As with all scientific endeavors, the practice of epidemiology relies on a systematic approach. In very simple terms, the epidemiologist:

- **Counts** cases or health events, and describes them in terms of time, place, and person;
- **Divides** the number of cases by an appropriate denominator to calculate rates; and
- **Compares** these rates over time or for different groups of people.

Before counting cases, however, the epidemiologist must decide what a case is. This is done by developing a case definition. Then, using this case definition, the epidemiologist finds and collects information about the case-patients. The epidemiologist then performs descriptive epidemiology by characterizing the cases collectively according to time, place, and person. To calculate the disease rate, the epidemiologist divides the number of cases by the size of the population. Finally, to determine whether this rate is greater than what one would normally expect, and if so to identify factors contributing to this increase, the epidemiologist compares the rate from this population to the rate in an appropriate comparison group, using analytic epidemiology techniques. These epidemiologic actions are described in more detail below. Subsequent tasks, such as reporting the results and recommending how they can be used for public health action, are just as important, but are beyond the scope of this lesson.

Defining a case

Before counting cases, the epidemiologist must decide what to count, that is, what to call a case. For that, the epidemiologist uses a **case definition**. A case definition is a set of standard criteria for classifying whether a person has a particular disease, syndrome, or other health condition. Some case definitions, particularly those used for national surveillance, have been developed and adopted as national standards that ensure comparability. Use of an agreed-upon standard case definition ensures that every case is equivalent, regardless of when or where it occurred, or who identified it. Furthermore, the number of cases or rate of disease identified in one time or place can be compared with the number or rate from another time or place. For example, with a standard case definition, health officials could compare the number of cases of listeriosis that occurred in Forsyth County, North Carolina, in 2000 with the number that occurred there in 1999. Or they could compare the rate of listeriosis in Forsyth County in 2000 with the national rate in that same year. When everyone uses the same standard case definition and a difference is observed, the difference is likely to be real rather than the result of variation in how cases are classified.

Using counts and rates

As noted, one of the basic tasks in public health is identifying and counting cases. These counts, usually derived from case reports submitted by health-care workers and laboratories to the health department, allow public health officials to determine the extent and patterns of disease occurrence by time, place, and person. They may also indicate clusters or outbreaks of disease in the community. Counts are also valuable for health planning. For example, a health official might use counts (i.e., numbers) to plan how many infection control isolation units or doses of vaccine may be needed.

However, simple counts do not provide all the information a health department needs. For some purposes, the counts must be put into context, based on the population in which they arose. Rates are measures that relate the numbers of cases during a certain period of time (usually per year) to the size of the population in which they occurred. For example, 42,745 new cases of AIDS were reported in the United States in 2002. This number, divided by the estimated 2002 population, results in a rate of 15.3 cases per 100,000 population. Rates are particularly useful for comparing the frequency of disease in different locations whose populations differ in size. For example, in 2003, Pennsylvania had over twelve times as many births (140,660) as its neighboring state, Delaware (11,264). However, Pennsylvania has nearly ten times the population of Delaware. So a more fair way to compare is to calculate rates. In fact, the birth rate was greater in Delaware (13.8 per 1,000 women aged 15–44 years) than in Pennsylvania (11.4 per 1,000 women aged 15–44 years).

Rates are also useful for comparing disease occurrence during different periods of time. For example, 19.5 cases of chickenpox per 100,000 were reported in 2001 compared with 135.8 cases per 100,000 in 1991. In addition, rates of disease among different subgroups can be compared to identify those at increased risk of disease. These so-called high risk groups can be further assessed and targeted for special intervention. High risk groups can also be studied to identify risk factors that cause them to have increased risk of disease. While some risk factors such as age and family history of breast cancer may not be modifiable, others, such as smoking and unsafe sexual practices, are. Individuals can use knowledge of the modifiable risk factors to guide decisions about behaviors that influence their health.

Descriptive Epidemiology

As noted earlier, every novice newspaper reporter is taught that a story is incomplete if it does not describe the what, who, where, when, and why/how of a situation, whether it be a space shuttle launch or a house fire. Epidemiologists strive for similar comprehensiveness in characterizing an epidemiologic event, whether it be a pandemic of influenza or a local increase in all-terrain vehicle crashes. However, epidemiologists tend to use synonyms for the five W's listed above: case definition, person, place, time, and causes/risk factors/modes of transmission. Descriptive epidemiology covers **time**, **place**, and **person**.

Compiling and analyzing data by time, place, and person is desirable for several reasons.

- First, by looking at the data carefully, the epidemiologist becomes very familiar with the data. He or she can see what the data can or cannot reveal based on the variables available, its limitations (for example, the number of records with missing information for each important variable), and its eccentricities (for example, all cases range in age from 2 months to 6 years, plus one 17-year-old.).
- Second, the epidemiologist learns the extent and pattern of the public health problem being investigated—which months, which neighborhoods, and which groups of people have the most and least cases.
- Third, the epidemiologist creates a detailed description of the health of a population that can be easily communicated with tables, graphs, and maps.
- Fourth, the epidemiologist can identify areas or groups within the population that have high rates of disease. This information in turn provides important clues to the causes of the disease, and these clues can be turned into testable hypotheses.

Time

The occurrence of disease changes over time. Some of these changes occur regularly, while others are unpredictable. Two diseases that occur during the same season each year include influenza (winter) and West Nile virus infection (August–September). In contrast, diseases such as hepatitis B and salmonellosis can occur at any time. For diseases that occur seasonally, health officials can anticipate their occurrence and implement control and prevention measures, such as an influenza vaccination campaign or mosquito spraying. For diseases that occur sporadically, investigators can conduct studies to identify the causes and modes of spread, and then develop appropriately targeted actions to control or prevent further occurrence of the disease.

In either situation, displaying the patterns of disease occurrence by time is critical for monitoring disease occurrence in the community and for assessing whether the public health interventions made a difference.

Time data are usually displayed with a two-dimensional graph. The vertical or y-axis usually shows the number or rate of cases; the horizontal or x-axis shows the time periods such as years, months, or days. The number or rate of cases is plotted over time. Graphs of disease occurrence over time are usually plotted as line graphs (Figure 10.1) or histograms (Figure 10.2).

Sometimes a graph shows the timing of events that are related to disease trends being displayed. For example, the graph may indicate the period of exposure or the date control measures were implemented. Studying a graph that notes the period of exposure may lead to insights into what may have caused illness. Studying a graph that notes the timing of control measures shows what impact, if any, the measures may have had on disease occurrence.

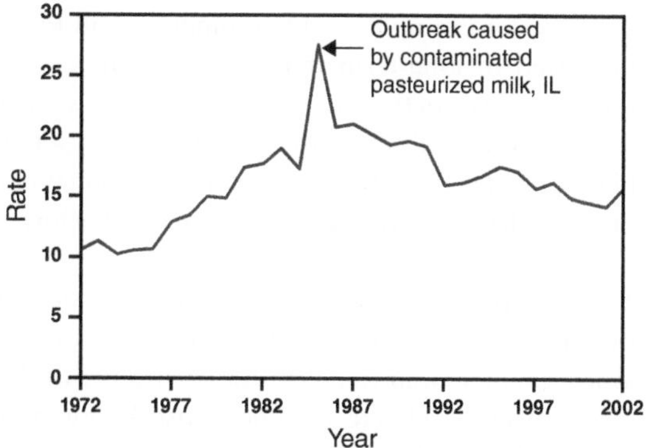

FIGURE 10.1 Reported Cases of Salmonellosis per 100,000 Population, by Year—United States, 1972–2002.

Source: Centers for Disease Control and Prevention. *"Summary of Notifiable Diseases–United States, 2002." MMWR*, 2002, 51(53): 59.

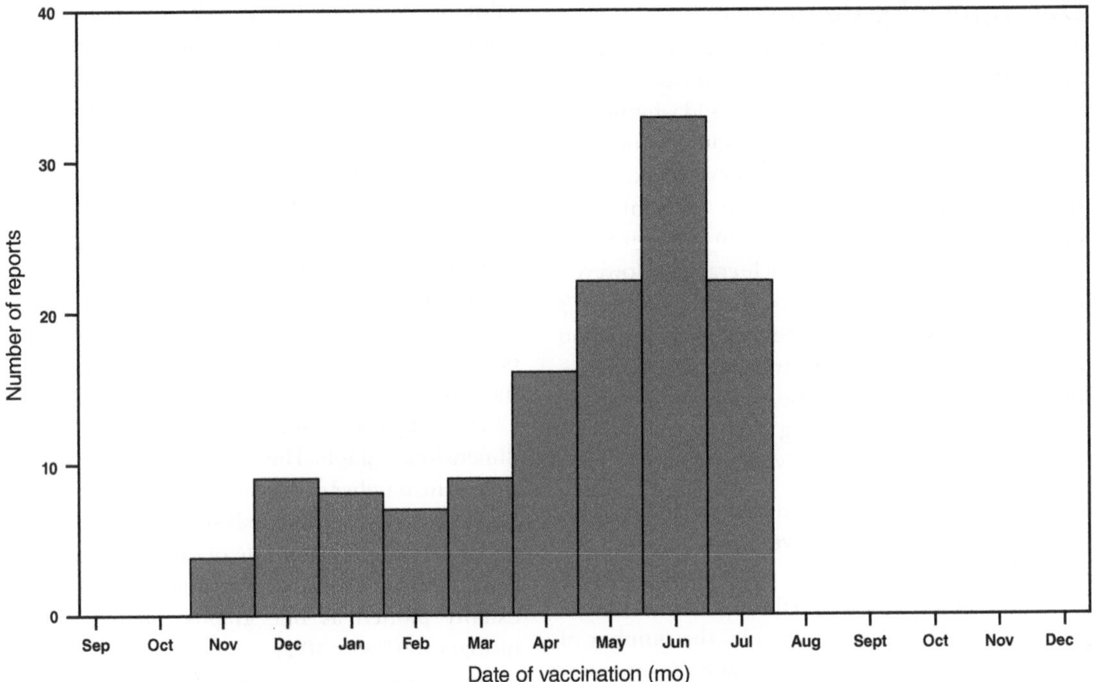

FIGURE 10.2 Number of Intussusception Reports After the Rhesus Rotavirus Vaccine-Tetravalent (RRV-TV) by Vaccination Date—United States, September 1998–December 1999.

Source: W. Zhou, Pool, V., Iskander, J. K., English-Bullard, R., Ball, R., Wise, R. P., et al. "Surveillance Summaries, January 24, 2003." *MMWR*, 2003, 52(SS1): 1–26.

As noted above, time is plotted along the x-axis. Depending on the disease, the time scale may be as broad as years or decades, or as brief as days or even hours of the day. For some conditions—many chronic diseases, for example—epidemiologists tend to be interested in long-term trends or patterns in the number of cases or the rate. For other conditions, such as foodborne outbreaks, the relevant time scale is likely to be days or hours. Some of the common types of time-related graphs are further described below.

Secular (long-term) trends. Graphing the annual cases or rate of a disease over a period of years shows long-term or secular trends in the occurrence of the disease (Figure 10.1). Health officials use these graphs to assess the prevailing direction of disease occurrence (increasing, decreasing, or essentially flat), help them evaluate programs or make policy decisions, infer what caused an increase or decrease in the occurrence of a disease (particularly if the graph indicates when related events took place), and use past trends as a predictor of future incidence of disease.

Seasonality. Disease occurrence can be graphed by week or month over the course of a year or more to show its seasonal pattern, if any. Some diseases such as influenza and West Nile infection are known to have characteristic seasonal distributions. Seasonal patterns may suggest hypotheses about how the infection is transmitted, what behavioral factors increase risk, and other possible contributors to the disease or condition. Figure 10.3 shows the seasonal patterns of rubella, influenza, and rotavirus. All three diseases display consistent seasonal distributions, but each disease peaks in different months—rubella in March to June, influenza in November to March, and rotavirus in February to April. The rubella graph is striking for the epidemic that occurred in 1963 (rubella vaccine was not available until 1969), but this epidemic nonetheless followed the seasonal pattern.

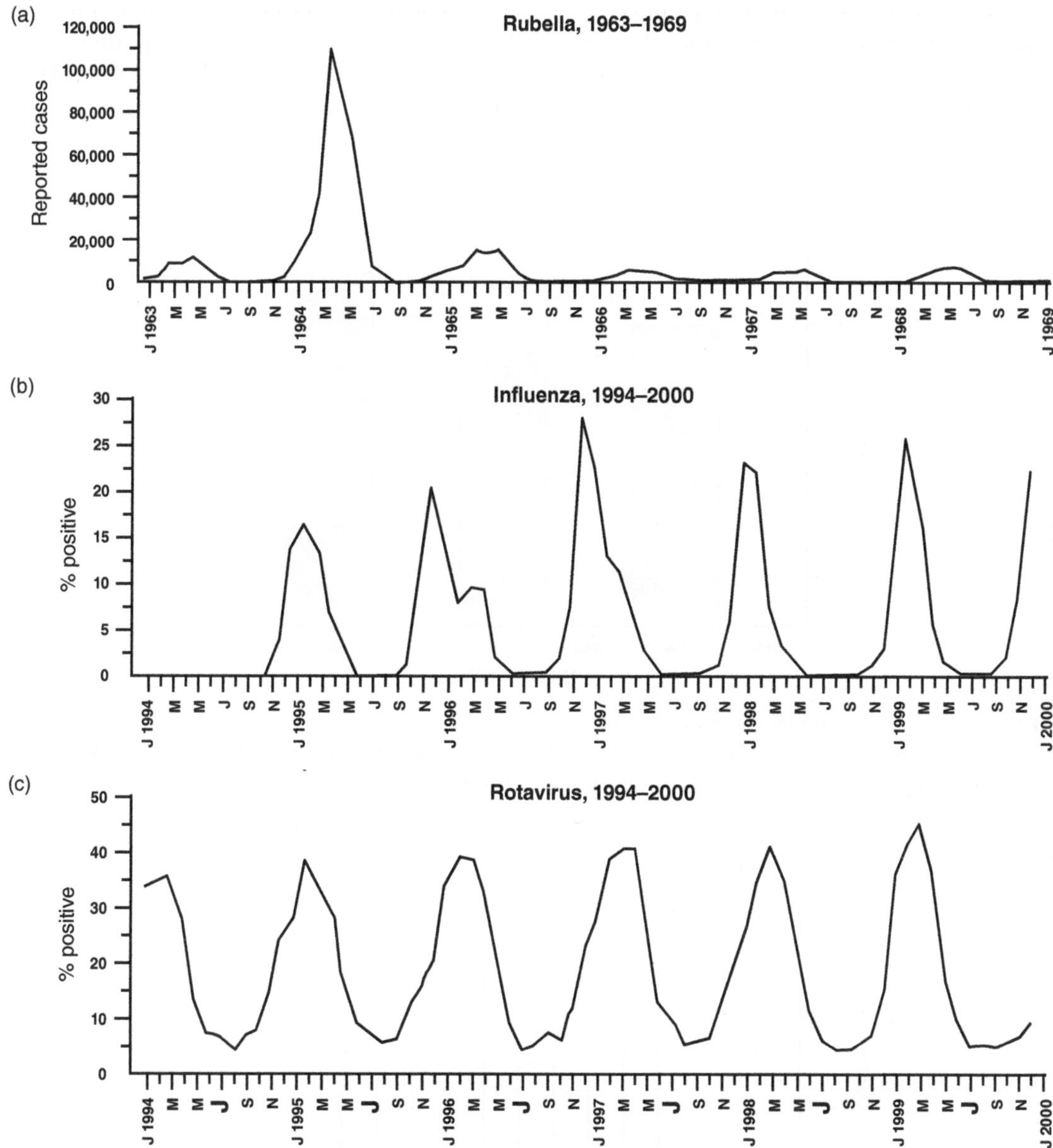

FIGURE 10.3 Seasonal Pattern of Rubella, Influenza and Rotavirus.

Source: S. F. Dowell. "Seasonal Variation in Host Susceptibility and Cycles of Certain Infectious Diseases." *Emerging Infectious Diseases*, 2001, 5: 369–74.

Day of week and time of day. For some conditions, displaying data by day of the week or time of day may be informative. Analysis at these shorter time periods is particularly appropriate for conditions related to occupational or environmental exposures that tend to occur at regularly scheduled intervals. In Figure 10.4, farm tractor fatalities are displayed by days of the week. Note that the number of farm tractor fatalities on Sundays was about half the number on the other days. The pattern of farm tractor injuries by hour, as displayed in Figure 10.5 peaked at 11:00 a.m., dipped at noon, and peaked again at 4:00 p.m. These patterns may suggest hypotheses and possible explanations that could be evaluated with further study.

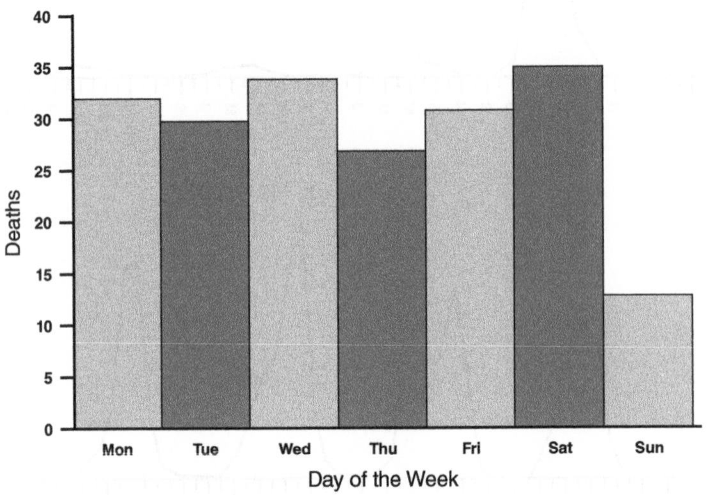

FIGURE 10.4 Farm Tractor Injuries by Day of Week.

Source: R. A. Goodman, Smith, J. D., Sikes, R. K., Rogers, D. L., and Mickey, J. L. "Fatalities Associated with Farm Tractor Injuries: An Epidemiologic Study." *Public Health Reports,* 1985, 100: 329–333.

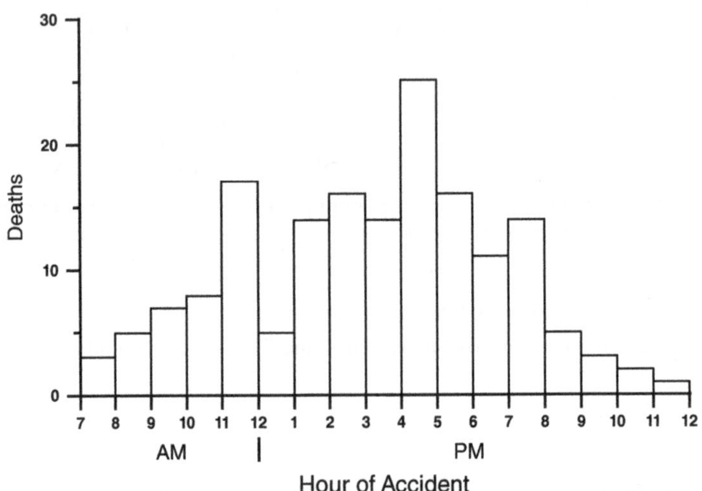

FIGURE 10.5 Farm Tractor Injuries by Hour of Day.

Source: R. A. Goodman, Smith, J. D., Sikes, R. K., Rogers, D. L., and Mickey, J. L. "Fatalities Associated with Farm Tractor Injuries: An Epidemiologic Study." *Public Health Reports,* 1985, 100: 329–333.

Epidemic period. To show the time course of a disease outbreak or epidemic, epidemiologists use a graph called an epidemic curve. As with the other graphs presented so far, an epidemic curve's y-axis shows the number of cases, while the x-axis shows time as either date of symptom onset or date of diagnosis. Depending on the incubation period (the length of time between exposure and onset of symptoms) and routes of transmission, the scale on the x-axis can be as broad as weeks (for a very prolonged epidemic) or as narrow as minutes (e.g., for food poisoning by chemicals that cause symptoms within minutes). Conventionally, the data are displayed as a histogram (which is similar to a bar chart but has no gaps between adjacent columns). Sometimes each case is displayed as a square, as in Figure 10.6. The shape and other features of an epidemic curve can suggest hypotheses about the time and source of exposure, the mode of transmission, and the causative agent.

Place

Describing the occurrence of disease by place provides insight into the geographic extent of the problem and its geographic variation. Characterization by place refers not only to place of residence but to any geographic location relevant to disease occurrence. Such locations include place of diagnosis or report, birthplace, site of employment, school district, hospital unit, or recent travel destinations. The unit may be as large as a continent or country or as small as a street address, hospital wing, or operating room. Sometimes place refers not to a specific location at all but to a place category such as urban or rural, domestic or foreign, and institutional or noninstitutional.

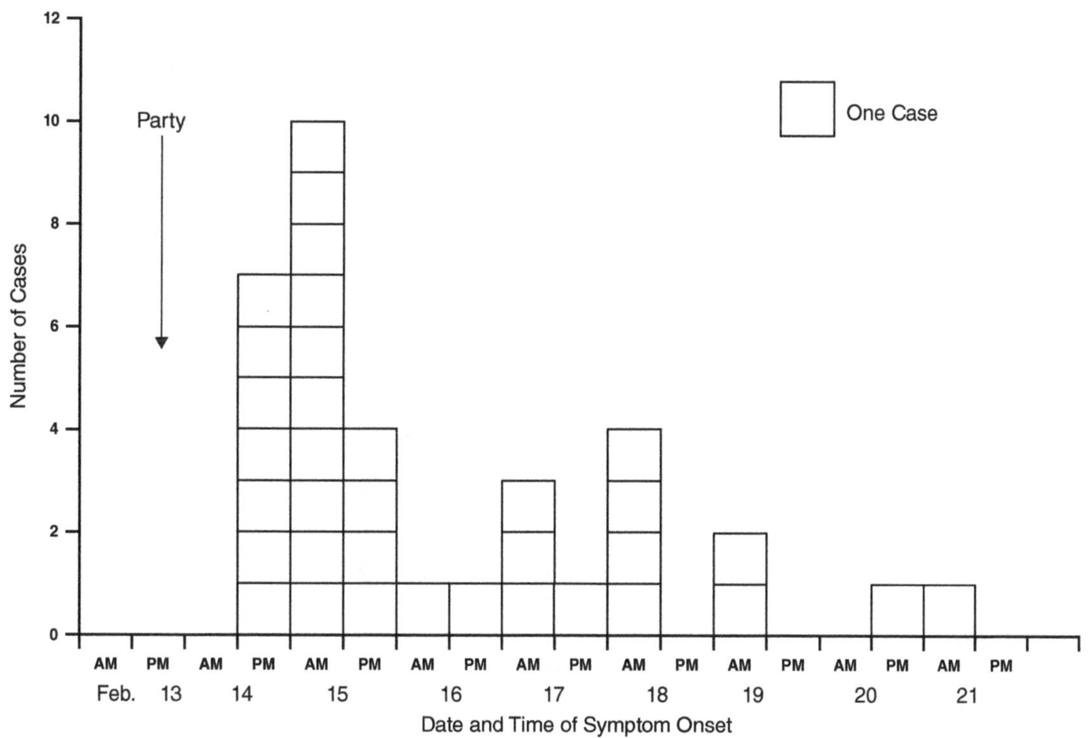

FIGURE 10.6 Cases of *Salmonella* Enteriditis in Chicago, February 13–21, by Date and Time of Symptom Onset.

Source: M. Cortese, Gerber, S., Jones, E., and Fernandez, J. A. (2003). *Salmonella enteriditis outbreak in Chicago.* Presented at the Eastern Regional Epidemic Intelligence Service Conference, March, Boston.

Consider the data in Tables 10.1 and 10.2. Table 10.1 displays SARS data by source of report, and reflects where a person with possible SARS is likely to be quarantined and treated. In contrast, Table 10.2 displays the same data by where the possible SARS patients had traveled, and reflects where transmission may have occurred.

TABLE 10.1 Reported Cases of SARS through November 3, 2004–United States, by Case Definition Category and State of Residence.

Location	Total Cases Reported	Total Suspect Cases Reported	Total Probable Cases Reported	Total Confirmed Cases Reported
Alaska	1	1	0	0
California	29	22	5	2
Colorado	2	2	0	0
Florida	8	6	2	0
Georgia	3	3	0	0
Hawaii	1	1	0	0
Illinois	8	7	1	0
Kansas	1	1	0	0
Kentucky	6	4	2	0
Maryland	2	2	0	0
Massachusetts	8	8	0	0
Minnesota	1	1	0	0
Mississippi	1	0	1	0
Missouri	3	3	0	0
Nevada	3	3	0	0
New Jersey	2	1	0	1
New Mexico	1	0	0	1
New York	29	23	6	0
North Carolina	4	3	0	1
Ohio	2	2	0	0
Pennsylvania	6	5	0	1
Rhode Island	1	1	0	0
South Carolina	3	3	0	0
Tennessee	1	1	0	0
Texas	5	5	0	0
Utah	7	6	0	1
Vermont	1	1	0	0
Virginia	3	2	0	1
Washington	12	11	1	0
West Virginia	1	1	0	0
Wisconsin	2	1	1	0
Puerto Rico	1	1	0	0
Total	**158**	**131**	**19**	**8**

Source: Adapted from Centers for Disease Control. *Severe Acute Respiratory Syndrome (SARS) Report of Cases in the United States*, http://www.cdc.gov/od/oc/media/presskits/sars/cases.htm.

TABLE 10.2 Reported Cases of SARS through November 3, 2004–United States, by High-Risk Area Visited.

Area	Count*	Percent
Hong Kong City, China	45	28
Toronto, Canada	35	22
Guangdong Province, China	34	22
Beijing City, China	25	16
Shanghai City, China	23	15
Singapore	15	9
China, mainland	15	9
Taiwan	10	6
Anhui Province, China	4	3
Hanoi, Vietnam	4	3
Chongqing City, China	3	2
Guizhou Province, China	2	1
Macoa City, China	2	1
Tianjin City, China	2	1
Jilin Province, China	2	1
Xinjiang Province	1	1
Zhejiang Province, China	1	1
Guangxi Province, China	1	1
Shanxi Province, China	1	1
Liaoning Province, China	1	1
Hunan Province, China	1	1
Sichuan Province, China	1	1
Hubei Province, China	1	1
Jiangxi Province, China	1	1
Fujian Province, China	1	1
Jiangsu Province, China	1	1
Yunnan Province, China	0	0
Hebei Province, China	0	0
Qinghai Province, China	0	0
Tibet (Xizang) Province, China	0	0
Hainan Province	0	0
Henan Province, China	0	0
Gansu Province, China	0	0
Shandong Province, China	0	0

** 158 reported case-patients visited 232 areas*

Data Source: D. L. Heymann, and Rodier, G. "Global Surveillance, National Surveillance, and SARS." *Emerging Infectious Diseases*, 2004, 10: 173–175.

Although place data can be shown in a table such as Table 10.1 or Table 10.2, a map provides a more striking visual display of place data. On a map, different numbers or rates of disease can be depicted using different shadings, colors, or line patterns, as in Figure 10.7.

Another type of map for place data is a spot map. Spot maps generally are used for clusters or outbreaks with a limited number of cases. A dot or X is placed on the location that is most relevant to the disease of interest, usually where each victim lived or worked, just as John Snow did in his spot map of the Golden Square area of London. If known, sites that are relevant, such as probable locations of exposure, are usually noted on the map.

Analyzing data by place can identify communities at increased risk of disease. Even if the data cannot reveal why these people have an increased risk, it can help generate hypotheses to test with additional studies. For example, is a community at increased risk because of characteristics of the people in the community such as genetic susceptibility, lack of immunity, risky behaviors, or exposure to local toxins or contaminated food? Can the increased risk, particularly of a communicable disease, be attributed to characteristics of the causative agent such as a particularly virulent strain, hospitable breeding sites, or availability of the vector that transmits the organism to humans? Or can the increased risk be attributed to the environment that brings the agent and the host together, such as crowding in urban areas that increases the risk of disease transmission from person to person, or more homes being built in wooded areas close to deer that carry ticks infected with the organism that causes Lyme disease?

Person

Because personal characteristics may affect illness, organization and analysis of data by "person" may use inherent characteristics of people (for example, age, sex, race), biologic characteristics (immune status), acquired characteristics (marital status), activities (occupation, leisure activities, use of medications/tobacco/drugs), or the conditions under which they live (socioeconomic status, access to medical care). Age and sex are included in almost all data sets and are the two most commonly analyzed "person" characteristics. However, depending on the disease and the data available, analyses of other person variables are usually necessary. Usually epidemiologists begin the analysis of person data by looking at each variable separately. Sometimes, two variables such as age and sex can be examined

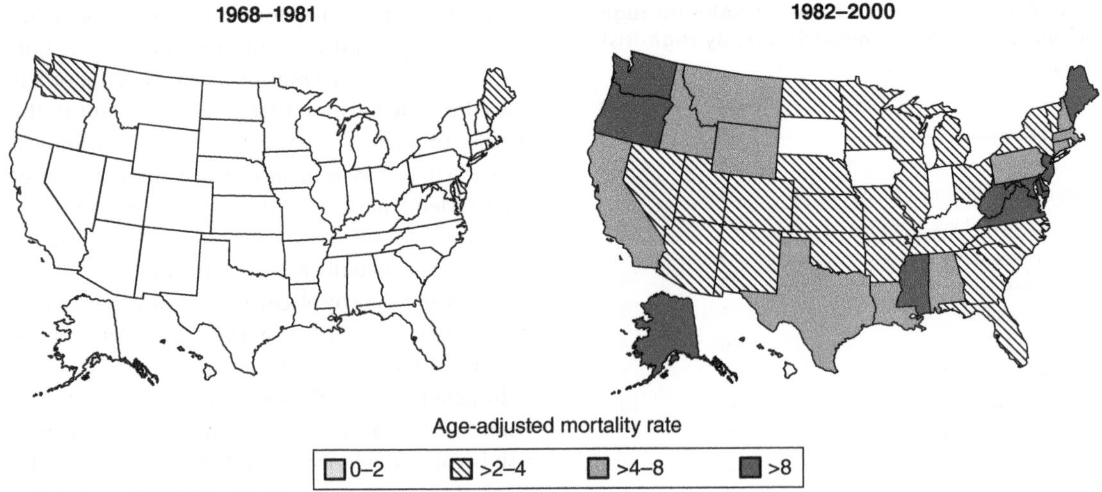

FIGURE 10.7 Mortality Rates for Asbestosis, by State, United States, 1968–1981 and 1982–2000.
Source: Centers for Disease Control and Prevention. "Changing Patterns of Pseumoconiosis Mortality—United States, 1968–2000." *MMWR,* 2004, 53: 627–632.

simultaneously. Person data are usually displayed in tables or graphs.

Age. Age is probably the single most important "person" attribute, because almost every health-related event varies with age. A number of factors that also vary with age include: susceptibility, opportunity for exposure, latency or incubation period of the disease, and physiologic response (which affects, among other things, disease development).

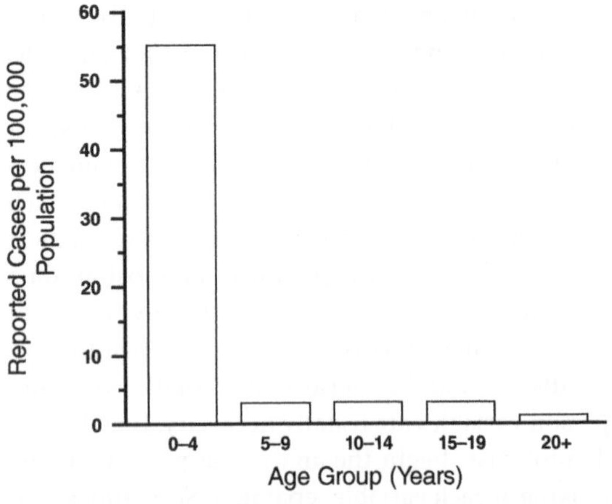

FIGURE 10.8A Pertussis by Five-Year Age Groups.

When analyzing data by age, epidemiologists try to use age groups that are narrow enough to detect any age-related patterns that may be present in the data. For some diseases, particularly chronic diseases, 10-year age groups may be adequate. For other diseases, 10-year and even 5-year age groups conceal important variations in disease occurrence by age. Consider the graph of pertussis occurrence by standard 5-year age groups shown in Figure 10.8a. The highest rate is clearly among children 4 years old

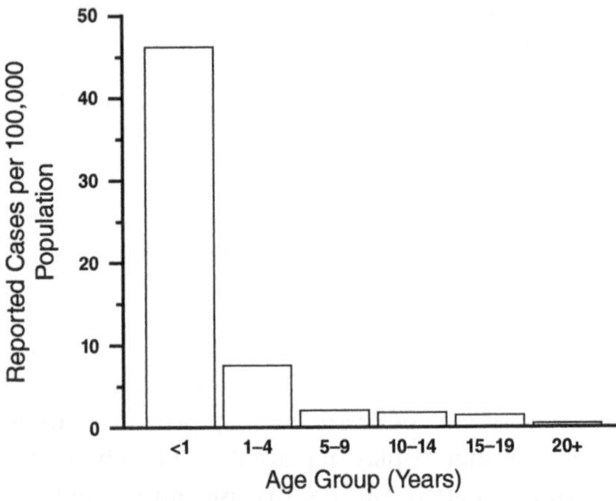

FIGURE 10.8B Pertussis by Less Than One, Four-Year, Then Five-Year Age Groups.

and younger. But is the rate equally high in all children within that age group, or do some children have higher rates than others?

To answer this question, different age groups are needed. Examine Figure 10.8b, which shows the same data but displays the rate of pertussis for children under 1 year of age separately. Clearly, infants account for most of the high rate among 0–4 year olds. Public health efforts should thus be focused on children less than 1 year of age, rather than on the entire 5-year age group.

Sex. Males have higher rates of illness and death than do females for many diseases. For some diseases, this sex-related difference is because of genetic, hormonal, anatomic, or other inherent differences between the sexes. These inherent differences affect susceptibility or physiologic responses. For example, premenopausal women have a lower risk of heart disease than men of the same age. This difference has been attributed to higher estrogen levels in women. On the other hand, the sex-related differences in the occurrence of many diseases reflect differences in opportunity or levels of exposure. For example, Figure 10.9 shows the differences in lung cancer rates over time among men and women. The difference noted in earlier years has been attributed to the higher prevalence of smoking among men in the past. Unfortunately, prevalence of smoking among women now equals that among men, and lung cancer rates in women have been climbing as a result.

Ethnic and racial groups. Sometimes epidemiologists are interested in analyzing person data by biologic, cultural or social groupings such as race, nationality, religion, or social groups such as tribes and other geographically or socially isolated groups. Differences in racial, ethnic, or other group variables may reflect differences in susceptibility or exposure, or differences in other factors that influence the risk of disease, such as socioeconomic status and access to

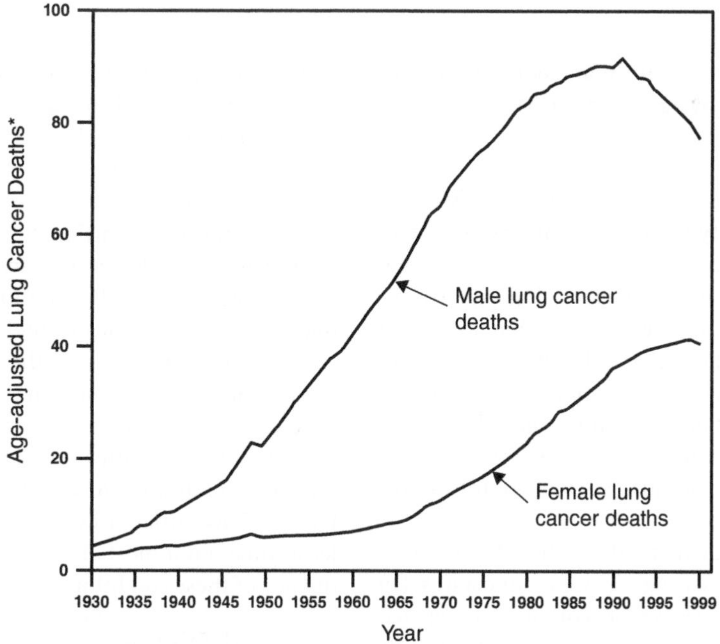

FIGURE 10.9 Lung Cancer Rates in the United States, 1930–1999.

Data Source: American Cancer Society. Available from http://www.cancer.org/docroot/PRO/content/PRO_1_1_Cancer_Statistics_2005_Presentation.asp.

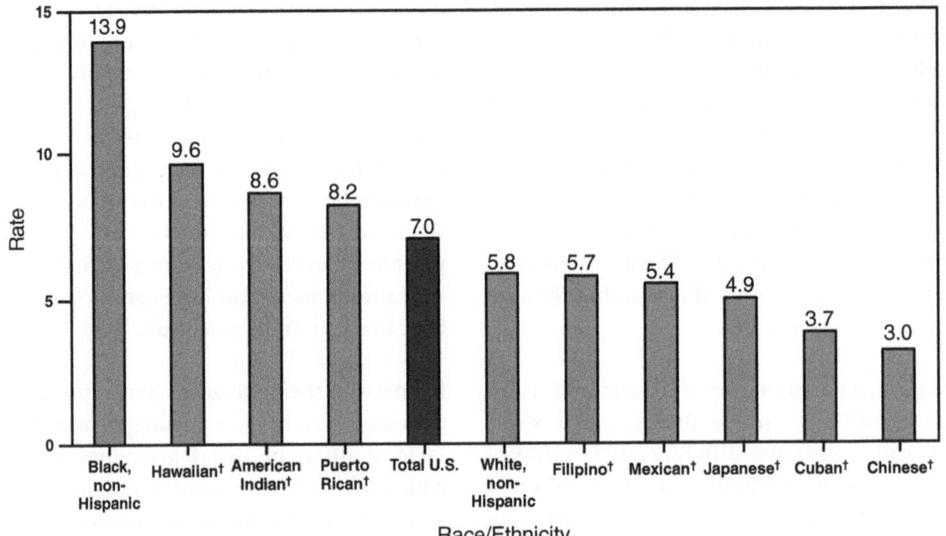

FIGURE 10.10 Infant Mortality Rates for 2002, by Race and Ethnicity of Mother.

Source: Centers for Disease Control and Prevention. "QuickStats: Infant Mortality Rates, by Selected Racial/Ethnic Populations—United States, 2002." *MMWR*, 2005, 54(5): 126.

health care. In Figure 10.10, infant mortality rates for 2002 are shown by race and Hispanic origin of the mother.

Socioeconomic status. Socioeconomic status is difficult to quantify. It is made up of many variables such as occupation, family income, educational achievement or census track, living conditions, and social standing. The variables that are easiest to measure may not accurately reflect the overall concept. Nevertheless, epidemiologists commonly use occupation, family income, and educational achievement, while recognizing that these variables do not measure socioeconomic status precisely.

The frequency of many adverse health conditions increases with decreasing socioeconomic status. For example, tuberculosis is more common among persons in lower socioeconomic strata. Infant mortality and time lost from work due to disability are both associated with lower income. These patterns may reflect more harmful exposures, lower resistance, and less access to health care. Or they may in part reflect an interdependent relationship that is impossible to untangle: Does low socioeconomic status contribute to disability, or does disability contribute to lower socioeconomic status, or both? What accounts for the disproportionate prevalence of diabetes and asthma in lower socioeconomic areas?

A few adverse health conditions occur more frequently among persons of higher socioeconomic status. Gout was known as the "disease of kings" because of its association with consumption of rich foods. Other conditions associated with higher socioeconomic status include breast cancer, Kawasaki syndrome, chronic fatigue syndrome, and tennis elbow. Differences in exposure account for at least some if not most of the differences in the frequency of these conditions.

Level of Disease

The amount of a particular disease that is usually present in a community is referred to as the baseline or **endemic** level of the disease. This level is not necessarily the desired level, which may in fact be zero, but rather is the observed level. In the absence of intervention and assuming that the level is not high enough to deplete the pool of susceptible persons, the disease may continue to occur at this level indefinitely. Thus, the baseline level is often regarded as the expected level of the disease.

Endemic refers to the constant presence and/or usual prevalence of a disease or infectious agent in a population within a geographic area.

Occasionally, the amount of disease in a community rises above the expected level. **Epidemic** refers to an increase, often sudden, in the number of cases of a disease above what is normally expected in that population in that area. **Outbreak** carries the same definition of epidemic, but is often used for a more limited geographic area. **Cluster** refers to an aggregation of cases grouped in place and time that are suspected to be greater than the number expected, even though the expected number may not be known. **Pandemic** refers to an epidemic that has spread over several countries or continents, usually affecting a large number of people.

Measures of Risk

Incidence, prevalence, and mortality rates are three frequency measures that are used to characterize the occurrence of health events in a population.

Morbidity has been defined as any departure, subjective or objective, from a state of physiological or psychological well-being. In practice, morbidity encompasses disease, injury, and disability. In addition, although for this lesson the term refers to the number of persons who are ill, it can also be used to describe the periods of illness that these persons experienced, or the duration of these illnesses.

Incidence refers to the occurrence of new cases of disease or injury in a population over a specified period of time. Although some epidemiologists use incidence to mean the number of new cases in a community, others use incidence to mean the number of new cases per unit of population.

Prevalence, sometimes referred to as prevalence rate, is the proportion of persons in a population who have a particular disease or attribute at a specified point in time or over a specified period of time. Prevalence differs from incidence in that prevalence includes all cases, both new and preexisting, in the population at the specified time, whereas incidence is limited to new cases only.

- Prevalence and incidence are frequently confused. Prevalence refers to proportion of persons who have a condition at or during a particular time period, whereas incidence refers to the proportion or rate of persons who develop a condition during a particular time period. So prevalence and incidence are similar, but prevalence includes new and preexisting cases whereas incidence includes new cases only.

A **mortality rate** is a measure of the frequency of occurrence of death in a defined population during a specified interval. Morbidity and mortality measures are often the same mathematically; it's just a matter of what you choose to measure, illness or death.

TABLE 10.3 Frequently Used Measures of Mortality.

Measure	Numerator	Denominator	10^n
Crude death rate	Total number of deaths during a given time interval	Mid-interval population	1,000 or 100,000 100,000
Infant mortality rate	Number of deaths among children < 1 year of age during a given time interval	Number of live births during the same time interval	1,000
Maternal mortality rate	Number of deaths assigned to pregnancy-related causes during a given time interval	Number of live births during the same time interval	100,000

Analytic Epidemiology

As noted earlier, descriptive epidemiology can identify patterns among cases and in populations by time, place and person. From these observations, epidemiologists develop hypotheses about the causes of these patterns and about the factors that increase risk of disease. In other words, epidemiologists can use descriptive epidemiology to generate hypotheses, but only rarely to test those hypotheses. For that, epidemiologists must turn to analytic epidemiology.

The key feature of analytic epidemiology is a comparison group. Consider a large outbreak of hepatitis A that occurred in Pennsylvania in 2003. Investigators found almost all of the case-patients had eaten at a particular restaurant during the 2–6 weeks (i.e., the typical incubation period for hepatitis A) before onset of illness. While the investigators were able to narrow down their hypotheses to the restaurant and were able to exclude the food preparers and servers as the source, they did not know which particular food may have been contaminated. The investigators asked the case-patients which restaurant foods they had eaten, but that only indicated which foods were popular. The investigators, therefore, also enrolled and interviewed a comparison or control group—a group of persons who had eaten at the restaurant during the same period but who did not get sick. Of 133 items on the restaurant's menu, the most striking difference between the case and control groups was in the proportion that ate salsa (94% of case-patients ate, compared with 39% of controls). Further investigation of the ingredients in the salsa implicated green onions as the source of infection. Shortly thereafter, the Food and Drug Administration issued an advisory to the public about green onions and risk of hepatitis A. This action was in direct response to the convincing results of the analytic epidemiology, which compared the exposure history of case-patients with that of an appropriate comparison group.

When investigators find that persons with a particular characteristic are more likely than those without the characteristic to contract a disease, the characteristic is said to be associated with the disease. The characteristic may be a:

- Demographic factor such as age, race, or sex;
- Constitutional factor such as blood group or immune status;
- Behavior or act such as smoking or having eaten salsa; or
- Circumstance such as living near a toxic waste site.

Identifying factors associated with disease help health officials appropriately target public health prevention and control activities. It also guides additional research into the causes of disease.

Thus, analytic epidemiology is concerned with the search for causes and effects, or the why and the how. Epidemiologists use analytic epidemiology to quantify the association between exposures and outcomes and to test hypotheses about causal relationships. It has been said that epidemiology by itself can never prove that a particular exposure caused a particular outcome. Often, however, epidemiology provides sufficient evidence to take appropriate control and prevention measures.

Epidemiologic studies fall into two categories: **experimental** and **observational**.

Experimental studies

In an experimental study, the investigator determines through a controlled process the exposure for each individual (clinical trial) or community (community trial), and then tracks the individuals or communities over time to detect the effects of the exposure. For example, in a clinical trial of a new vaccine, the investigator may randomly assign some of the participants to receive the new vaccine, while others receive a placebo shot. The investigator then tracks all participants, observes who gets the disease that the new vaccine is intended to prevent, and compares the two groups (new vaccine vs. placebo) to see whether the vaccine group has a lower rate of disease. Similarly, in a trial to prevent onset of diabetes among high-risk individuals, investigators randomly assigned enrollees to one of three groups—placebo, an anti-diabetes drug, or lifestyle intervention. At the end of the follow-up period, investigators found the lowest incidence of diabetes in the lifestyle intervention group, the next lowest in the anti-diabetic drug group, and the highest in the placebo group.

Observational studies

In an observational study, the epidemiologist simply observes the exposure and disease status of each study participant. John Snow's studies of cholera in London were observational studies. The two most common types of observational studies are cohort studies and case-control studies; a third type is cross-sectional studies.

Cohort study. A cohort study is similar in concept to the experimental study. In a cohort study the epidemiologist records whether each study participant is exposed or not, and then tracks the participants to see if they develop the disease of interest. Note that this differs from an experimental study because, in a cohort study, the investigator observes rather than determines the participants' exposure status. After a period of time, the investigator compares the disease rate in the exposed group with the disease rate in the unexposed group. The unexposed group serves as the comparison group, providing an estimate of the baseline or expected amount of disease occurrence in the community. If the disease rate is substantively different in the exposed group compared to the unexposed group, the exposure is said to be associated with illness.

The length of follow-up varies considerably. In an attempt to respond quickly to a public health concern such as an outbreak, public health departments tend to conduct relatively brief studies. On the other hand, research and academic organizations are more likely to conduct studies of cancer, cardiovascular disease, and other chronic diseases which may last for years and even decades. The Framingham study is a well-known cohort study that has followed over 5,000 residents of Framingham, Massachusetts, since the early 1950s to establish the rates and risk factors for heart disease. The Nurses Health Study and the Nurses Health Study II are cohort studies established in 1976 and 1989, respectively, that have followed over 100,000 nurses each and have provided useful information on oral contraceptives, diet, and lifestyle risk factors. These studies are sometimes called **follow-up** or **prospective** cohort studies, because participants are enrolled as the study begins and are then followed prospectively over time to identify occurrence of the outcomes of interest.

An alternative type of cohort study is a **retrospective** cohort study. In this type of study both the exposure and the outcomes have already occurred. Just as in a prospective cohort study, the investigator calculates and compares rates of disease in the exposed and unexposed groups. Retrospective cohort studies are commonly used in investigations of disease in groups of easily identified people such as workers at a particular factory or attendees at a wedding. For example, a retrospective cohort study was used to determine the source of infection of cyclosporiasis, a parasitic disease that caused an outbreak among members of a residential facility in Pennsylvania in 2004. The investigation indicated that consumption of snow peas was implicated as the vehicle of the cyclosporiasis outbreak.

Case-control study. In a case-control study, investigators start by enrolling a group of people with disease (at CDC such persons are called case-patients rather than cases, because case refers to occurrence of disease, not a person). As a comparison group, the investigator then enrolls a group of people without disease (controls). Investigators then compare previous exposures between the two groups. The control group provides an estimate of the baseline or expected amount of exposure in that population. If the amount of exposure among the case group is substantially higher than the amount you would expect based on the control group, then illness is said to be associated with that exposure. The study of hepatitis A traced to green onions, described above, is an example of a case-control study. The key in a case-control study is to identify an appropriate control group, comparable to the case group in most respects, in order to provide a reasonable estimate of the baseline or expected exposure.

Cross-sectional study. In this third type of observational study, a sample of persons from a population is enrolled and their exposures and health outcomes are measured simultaneously. The cross-sectional study tends to assess the presence (prevalence) of the health outcome at that point of time without regard to duration. For example, in a cross-sectional study of diabetes, some of the enrollees with diabetes may have lived with their diabetes for many years, while others may have been recently diagnosed.

From an analytic viewpoint the cross-sectional study is weaker than either a cohort or a case-control study because a cross-sectional study usually cannot disentangle risk factors for occurrence of disease (incidence) from risk factors for survival with the disease. On the other hand, a cross-sectional study is a perfectly fine tool for descriptive epidemiology purposes. Cross-sectional studies are used routinely to document the prevalence in a community of health behaviors (prevalence of smoking), health states (prevalence of vaccination against measles), and health outcomes, particularly chronic conditions (hypertension, diabetes).

In summary, the purpose of an analytic study in epidemiology is to identify and quantify the relationship between an exposure and a health outcome. The hallmark of such a study is the presence of at least two groups, one of which serves as a comparison group. In an experimental study, the investigator determines the exposure for the study subjects; in an observational study, the subjects are exposed under more natural conditions. In an observational cohort study, subjects are enrolled or grouped on the basis of their exposure, then are followed to document occurrence of disease. Differences in disease rates between the exposed and unexposed groups lead investigators to conclude that exposure is associated with disease. In an observational case-control study, subjects are enrolled according to whether they have the disease or not, then are questioned or tested to determine their prior exposure. Differences in exposure prevalence between the case and control groups allow investigators to conclude that the exposure is associated with the disease. Cross-sectional studies measure exposure and disease status at the same time, and are better suited to descriptive epidemiology than causation.

Measures of Association

The key to epidemiologic analysis is comparison. Occasionally you might observe an incidence rate among a population that seems high and wonder whether it is actually higher than what should be expected based on, say, the incidence rates in other communities. Or, you might observe that, among a group of case-patients in an outbreak, several report having eaten at a particular restaurant. Is the restaurant just a popular one, or have more case-patients eaten there than would be expected? The way to address that concern is by comparing the observed group with another group that represents the expected level. Examples of measures of association include risk ratio (relative risk), rate ratio, odds ratio, and proportionate mortality ratio.

A **risk ratio** (RR), also called relative risk, compares the risk of a health event (disease, injury, risk factor, or death) among one group with the risk among another group. It does so by dividing the risk (incidence proportion, attack rate) in group 1 by the risk (incidence proportion, attack rate) in group 2. The two groups are typically differentiated by such demographic factors as sex (e.g., males versus females) or by exposure to a suspected risk factor (e.g., did or did not eat potato salad). Often, the group of primary interest is labeled the exposed group, and the comparison group is labeled the unexposed group.

METHOD FOR CALCULATING RISK RATIO.

The formula for risk ratio (RR) is:

$$\frac{\textit{Risk of disease (incidence proportion, attack rate) in group of primary interest}}{\textit{Risk of disease (incidence proportion, attack rate) in comparison group}}$$

A risk ratio of 1.0 indicates identical risk among the two groups. A risk ratio greater than 1.0 indicates an increased risk for the group in the numerator, usually the exposed group. A risk ratio less than 1.0 indicates a decreased risk for the exposed group, indicating that perhaps exposure actually protects against disease occurrence.

BOX 10.1 Examples: Calculating Risk Ratios

Example A: In an outbreak of tuberculosis among prison inmates in South Carolina in 1999, 28 of 157 inmates residing on the East wing of the dormitory developed tuberculosis, compared with 4 of 137 inmates residing on the West wing.[11] These data are summarized in the two-by-two table so called because it has two rows for the exposure and two columns for the outcome. Here is the general format and notation.

TABLE 10.4A General Format and Notation for a 2×2 Table.

	Ill	Well	Total
Exposed	a	b	$a + b = H_1$
Unexposed	c	d	$c + d = H_0$
Total	$a + c = V_1$	$b + d = V_0$	T

In this example, the exposure is the dormitory wing and the outcome is tuberculosis) illustrated in Table 3.12B. Calculate the risk ratio.

TABLE 10.4B Incidence of Mycobacterium Tuberculosis Infection Among Congregated, HIV-Infected Prison Inmates by Dormitory Wing, South Carolina, 1999.

	Yes	No	Total
East wing	a = 28	b = 129	$H_1 = 157$
West wing	c = 4	d = 133	$H_0 = 137$
Total	32	262	T = 294

Data source: S. I. McLaughlin, Spradling, P., Drociuk, D., et al. "Extensive Transmission of Mycobacterium Tuberculosis among Congregated, HIV-Infected Prison Inmates in South Carolina, United States." *International Journal of Tuberculosis and Lung Disease*, 2003, 7: 665–672.

To calculate the risk ratio, first calculate the risk or attack rate for each group. Here are the formulas:

Attack Rate (Risk)

Attack rate for exposed = a/a + b

Attack rate for unexposed = c/c + d

For this example:

Risk of tuberculosis among east wing residents
= 28/157
= 0.178
= 17.8%

Risk of tuberculosis among west wing residents
= 4/137
= 0.029
= 2.9%

The risk ratio is simply the ratio of these two risks:

Risk ratio = 17.8/2.9 = 6.1

Thus, inmates who resided in the East wing of the dormitory were 6.1 times as likely to develop tuberculosis as those who resided in the West wing.

BOX 10.2 Examples: Calculating Risk Ratios

Example B: *In an outbreak of varicella (chickenpox) in Oregon in 2002, varicella was diagnosed in 18 of 152 vaccinated children compared with 3 of 7 unvaccinated children. Calculate the risk ratio.*

TABLE 10.5 Incidence of Varicella Among Schoolchildren in Nine Affected Classrooms, Oregon, 2002.

	Varicella	Non-case	Total
Vaccinated	a = 18	b = 134	152
Unvaccinated	c = 3	d = 4	7
Total	21	138	159

Data Source: B. D. Tugwell, Lee, L. E., Gillette, et al. "Chickenpox Outbreak in a Highly Vaccinated School Population." *Pediatrics*, 2004, 113(3 Pt 1): 455–459.

Risk of varicella among vaccinated children = 18/152 = 0.118 = 11.8%

Risk of varicella among unvaccinated children = 3/7 = 0.429 = 42.9%

Risk ratio = 0.118/0.429 = 0.28

The risk ratio is less than 1.0, indicating a decreased risk or protective effect for the exposed (vaccinated) children. The risk ratio of 0.28 indicates that vaccinated children were only approximately one-fourth as likely (28%, actually) to develop varicella as were unvaccinated children.

SECTION 2 CASES FOR TEACHING AND LEARNING

Many of the cases here were prepared by the Centers for Disease Control and Prevention (CDC) to train the Epidemic Intelligence Service officers described in Mark Pendergrast's chapter (9). Instructor's guides for many of the CDC cases are available to teachers or students who register at https://aptr.site-ym.com/store/default.aspx.

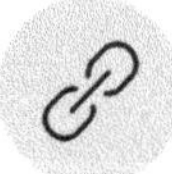

Visit our companion website, **www.oup.com/us/brown-closser**, for direct links to these featured online resources.

CDC, *An Epidemic Disease in South Carolina*

This case, written by Alexander Langmuir, founder of the Epidemic Intelligence Service, brings students through data collection and analysis in Joseph and Mary Goldberger's landmark historical investigation of a mysterious disease in South Carolina. This case requires students to use analytic and descriptive epidemiology. It also introduces pellagra, a disease that illustrates the importance of the social determinants of health.

CDC, *An Outbreak of Enteritis during a Pilgrimage to Mecca*

In this outbreak investigation case, students apply epidemiology to determine the cause of a gastrointestinal illness outbreak that occurred during the Hajj.

CDC, *Oswego – An Outbreak of Gastrointestinal Illness Following a Church Supper*

In this classic "church supper case," students must use epidemiology to determine which food served at a church supper made everyone sick.

CDC, *An Outbreak Investigation of a Neurologic Syndrome among Factory Workers in Taiwan*

In this outbreak investigation case, students use epidemiological methods (including a 2×2 table) to determine the cause of an outbreak of botulism.

CDC, *Paralytic Illness in Ababo*

In this case, students must design a surveillance system for polio and apply epidemiological concepts such as incidence, prevalence, morbidity, and mortality.

CDC, *Surveillance for E. Coli 0157:H7 – Information for Action*

Students investigate data from *E. Coli* infections in Oregon to learn about surveillance, including applying the concepts of epidemic, expected versus observed cases, and person/place/time.

Cynthia Morrow et al., *Outbreak of Tuberculosis in a Homeless Men's Shelter*

Through an investigation of a tuberculosis outbreak in a homeless shelter in upstate New York, students apply basic epidemiological concepts including incidence, prevalence, agent/host/environment, surveillance, and prevention. The case also introduces tuberculosis and directly observed therapy (DOT).

SECTION 2 VIDEOS AND WEB RESOURCES

Visit the companion website, www.oup.com/us/brown-closser, for direct links to the online resources featured below.

FRED Measles Epidemic Simulator

This website simulates measles epidemics in various cities in the United States at different levels of vaccination coverage.

MMWR QuickStats

This website provides a range of recent Centers for Disease Control (CDC) releases about the epidemiology of a variety of diseases and risk factors in the United States. It usefully introduces students to the range of epidemiological work that the CDC does.

EPIDEMIOLOGICAL METHODS

The following freely available resources are available for those who want to engage in self-study of the field of epidemiology.

Public Health 101 – CDC

Sections of this course are included in this book (Chapter 10). The entire course is freely available online, and it provides an excellent introduction to epidemiology.

Supercourse: Epidemiology, the Internet and Global Health – WHO Collaborating Center, University of Pittsburgh

This is a repository of over 200,000 lecture slides in epidemiology and global health. Many complex topics and methodologies are presented with clear animations.

Activepi Web – David Kleinbaum

This is a free online interactive multimedia textbook covering the basics of epidemiology.

SECTION

3

Metrics and the Burden of Disease

This section of the book continues the themes of the last section about epidemiological methods. Studying the **burden of disease** involves counting the numbers of people affected by different health issues. On the surface, this is a pretty dry enterprise. But what this work has the power to reveal is not dry at all: the story of how human health, disease, and death is patterned across the world is fascinating and often disturbing. The fact, for example, that a preventable and treatable illness like diarrhea kills an estimated 2,000 children *every day* reveals a great deal about global inequality.

Reducing those people into "cases" for quantitative analysis certainly makes it difficult to see people's suffering. However, when people in global health discuss infant mortality, it is important to remember the parents of each child, and the terrible emotional pain of losing a child—even when it might be relatively common in some contexts. Perhaps epidemiology might seem like accounting or financial analysis, but the "things" being counted are human lives.

Quantitative analysis is extremely important for making wise decisions about where time and money can best be invested to improve health. The burden of different health problems varies between nations and social contexts. It is important to measure the burden of disease in a way that takes into account both **morbidity** and **mortality**. One of the articles in this section involves the question of determining the most **cost-effective** ways to spend money in global health projects. The results about "best buys" might be surprising to you.

Yet making decisions in global health primarily based on "best buys" and cost effectiveness is controversial. As the selection about the work of Paul Farmer illustrates, sometimes it is right to do things that are not necessarily cost-effective. The film and website *The Life Equation* in the Web Resources for this section explore this controversy in depth.

Counting is complicated—and all the numbers used in epidemiology and global health might not be exactly accurate, particularly in low resource settings. The article by Adeola Oni-Orisan might be considered a warning about the impossibility of quantitative data being exactly correct. The challenge is often about the methods—*how* things are measured.

Metrics are important tools for decision making. Yet understanding the nitty-gritty details of how global health data are collected and created is also important for understanding the human side of global health issues, and the limitations of the data we have. Both numbers and an understanding of the humanity they reflect are important in setting priorities going forward.

» CONCEPTUAL TOOLS «

Measuring the Burden of Disease

Epidemiologists measure both **morbidity** and **mortality** when evaluating the **burden of disease**. Many types of health issues contribute to morbidity and mortality.

- **Infectious diseases** such as HIV, tuberculosis, **malaria**, and diarrhea are caused by pathogens like viruses or bacteria and are transmitted from person to person. Today, morbidity and mortality resulting from infectious disease is primarily concentrated in settings of poverty.
- **Chronic diseases** like cancer and heart disease are major causes of morbidity and mortality across the globe. These diseases are generally not spread by person-to-person contact. Rather, risk for these diseases is structured by factors like diet and environment.
- **Injuries** are also a major cause of morbidity and mortality worldwide. These include accidents well as intentional injuries (like murder and suicide). In many parts of the world, **road traffic accidents** are a major contributor to morbidity and mortality.
- **Mental health** issues are another big contributor to morbidity and mortality. Although often neglected, mental health issues are a major cause of illness and death globally. Mental illnesses vary widely across cultures, but at least two categories of mental illness—depression and schizophrenia—seem to be present worldwide.

Epidemiologists use a number of measures, including years of life lost (**YLLs**) and disability-adjusted life years (**DALYs**), to measure the burden of disease in populations.

- The YLL tells you how many years of life were lost due to a given health issue. It is calculated using standard life expectancies, and the ages of death of people killed by a disease or health issue. Therefore, the YLL weights diseases that tend to kill people in childhood more heavily than those that kill people in old age. The YLL can be useful because we might think that diseases that kill people in their youth are more urgent issues than those that kill people in old age. (Obviously, this is a value judgement.)
- The DALY tells you how many years of *healthy* life were lost due to a given health issue. The DALY takes into consideration both years of life lost due to death (mortality), *and* the burden of living with a disability (morbidity). The DALY is useful because many health issues cause disability but not death. For example, the parasitic disease onchocerciasis causes nearly a million cases of blindness every year. These health issues do not show up at all in YLL calculations, but nonetheless may cause a lot of human suffering.

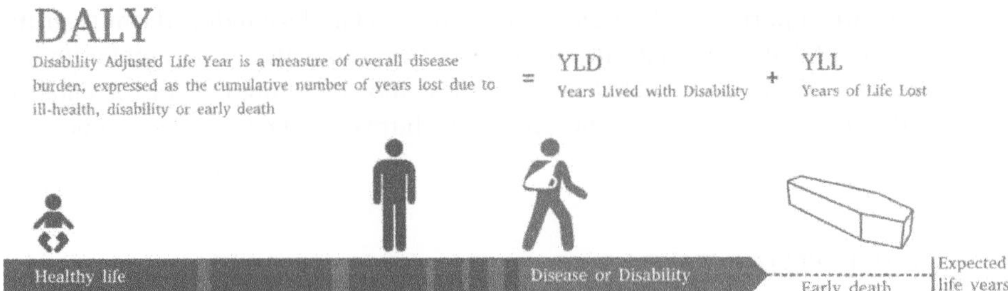

FIGURE CT3.1 The Disability Adjusted Life Year, or DALY

Source: Artwork by Planemad, vectorized by Radio89, licensed under the Creative Commons Attribution-Share Alike 3.0 Unported license.

In calculating a DALY, years lived with a disability are discounted considered "lost" or "damaged" based on how severe experts think the disability is. This is, of course, a value judgment, and not everyone agrees with how DALYs are calculated.

Measures of the burden of disease also play a role in **cost-effectiveness analysis.**

- These analyses compare the costs of a given health intervention to the impacts of that intervention on a health outcome. For example, cost-effectiveness analyses often report the effectiveness of different health interventions in terms of cost per DALY averted. Drawing on this kind of analysis, Chapter 11 describes some of the "best buys in global health." It can be very useful for health officials with a limited budget to know how they can use their budgets to achieve the most impact. If there are several potential population-level interventions to choose from for a given health issue, it's helpful to know which one will be able to save the most lives with a given amount of money.
- While cost-effectiveness analyses can sometimes be very useful, they can also be used in problematic ways. For example, Paul Farmer and Jim Kim (the authors of Chapter 8) found that in the early days of advocating for anti-retroviral therapy treatment for HIV/AIDS globally, many global health officials objected that providing this life-saving medication was not cost-effective in Africa (see Reading #8). In this case, the logic of cost effectiveness was used to deny treatment to poor people (even though that same treatment was considered essential for rich people). Careful attention must be paid during cost-effectiveness analysis to ensure that a determination of the relative value of health interventions does not become a determination of the relative value of human lives.

EPIDEMIOLOGICAL AND DEMOGRAPHIC TRANSITIONS

- **There have been three epidemiological transitions in human history.** The first occurred at the time of the Neolithic Revolution, when humans learned how to domesticate plants and animals, a process that began about 10,000 years ago.

Agriculture meant that there was a fundamentally different relationship between humans and their environment than was the case with hunter-gatherers. A denser population, less diverse diet, more social stratification, and close contact with animals all led to negative impacts on health overall, particularly increases in infectious disease.

- The second epidemiological transition happed in Europe in the 19th century. In this transition, infectious disease declined, life expectancy increased, and chronic disease increased. **This decline in mortality and increase in population growth is primarily the result of socioeconomic changes (affecting hygiene, nutrition, etc.) and not because of therapeutic inventions of biomedicine.** As later chapters of this book will explore in detail, the **determinants of health** are much more about our environments and our access to resources than our clinical care.
- Demographic historians have made significant progress in understanding the role of breast-feeding and birth-spacing patterns on total fertility that also play an important role in population change—most strikingly in the **demographic transition** from large completed families to small completed families. It is often represented graphically like in Figure CT3.2.

As this graph shows, in the demographic transition, first death rates fall, followed by birth rates. Thus, the demographic transition is tied to the second epidemiological transition. The idea here is that once death rates decline due to the second

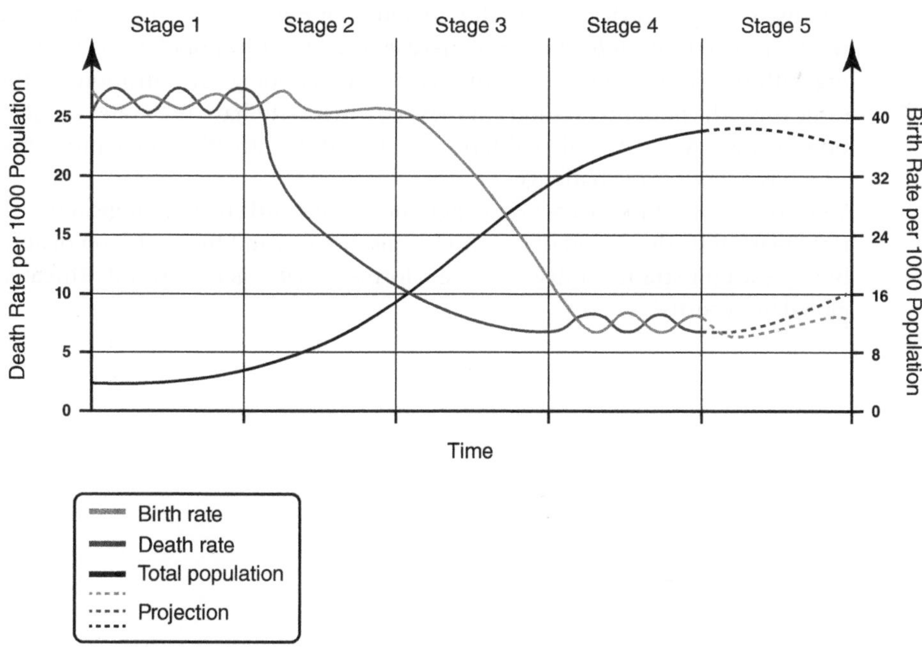

FIGURE CT3.2 The Demographic Transition.

epidemiological transition, birth rates decline too, a bit later. The result is a rapid rise in population that then levels off.

- Not everywhere in the world experienced the second epidemiological transition or the demographic transition. It happened in rich countries, and among rich people in poor countries. But for poor people in poor countries, it didn't happen, and they continue to experience both high birth rates and high death rates.
- **High income, middle income, and low income countries have substantially different epidemiological profiles and different burdens of disease.** Poor countries are mostly likely to have heavy burdens of infectious disease, including so-called tropical diseases. The main problem with the term "tropical diseases" is that it implies that the prevalence of diseases is somehow rooted in the climate and geography of a region. In fact, many so-called tropical diseases like malaria used to be common in the American Midwest and southern England. In modern world history, most of the industrialized countries that became colonial powers were located in temperate climates, and most of the colonies were located in warmer tropical environments. The two kinds of countries had, and continue to have, substantially different epidemiological profiles. But these differences are not just the result of temperature and humidity. Rather, there is clear evidence that the primary factor involved in the transmission of so-called tropical diseases is poverty. Many have suggested that scientists rename these diseases "diseases of poverty." A history of colonialism and, more importantly, postcolonial patterns of economic inequity play a central role in the creation of poverty and therefore the continuation of "tropical" disease.
- Because many countries have both rich and poor populations, they experience what is called the **double burden of disease**. Their wealthy populations are dealing with the chronic diseases of the second epidemiological transition. At the same time, the poor populations in these countries still have high rates of infectious disease. Any national health policy has to deal with all of these problems, which is a significant challenge.
- Some observers think we are now experiencing the third epidemiological transition, marked by the spread of new infectious diseases and the evolution of antibiotic resistant strains of disease. New forms of pathogens certainly threaten global biosecurity.

BOX 3.1 The Institute for Health Metrics and Evaluation: Years of Life Lost and Disability Adjusted Life Years Lost

The Institute for Health Metrics and Evaluation (IHME) is an organization based in Seattle that does a global burden of disease evaluation every few years.

Leading Causes of Death Worldwide—Years of Life Lost

According to the IHME study, the leading causes (years of life lost; YLLs) globally in 2015 were

1. Ischemic heart disease (coronary artery disease, including heart attacks)
2. Cerebrovascular disease (strokes)
3. Lower respiratory infections (lung infections, including pneumonia)
4. Neonatal preterm birth complications
5. Diarrheal diseases
6. Neonatal encephalopathy (usually caused by the baby not getting enough oxygen during birth)
7. HIV/AIDS
8. Road injuries
9. Malaria
10. Chronic obstructive pulmonary diseases (chronic lung diseases, including emphysema)

You may find some of the diseases on this list surprising. Many of them are easily preventable and easily treatable. Treatment of diarrheal disease, for example, is discussed in Chapter 5.

DALYs

IHME also evaluated DALYs. Here are the top 10 causes of global DALYs lost in 2015:

1. Cardiovascular diseases
2. Diarrhea, lower respiratory infections, and other common infectious diseases
3. Neoplasms
4. Neonatal disorders
5. Other noncommunicable diseases
6. Mental and substance use disorders
7. Musculoskeletal disorders
8. Diabetes, urogenital, blood, and endocrine diseases
9. Unintentional injuries
10. HIV/AIDS and tuberculosis

Comparing this list with the YLL list can help you understand the differences between the YLL and DALY measures. Make sure you understand why some health issues rank high for DALYs but not for YLLs.

Health and Wealth

Figure CT3.3 from IHME shows countries in 2015 according to the Socio-Demographic Index, a measure that includes the wealth, education, and fertility of the country (lower fertility contributes to a higher Socio-Demographic Index score). You can learn more about this index on the Lancet's YouTube video, "Causes of Death: Global Burden of Disease Study," https://www.youtube.com/watch?v=ERvFgjBHizo.

The IHME then listed the diseases that cause the most YLLs in these different categories of countries (Table CT3.1). Look at this list carefully, looking for patterns across different income groups. Consider which countries are most affected by infectious disease, and by injuries.

As discussed in Chapter 10, data on health conditions are often not very good. Therefore, these lists should be considered the best estimates we have rather than hard and fast truth.

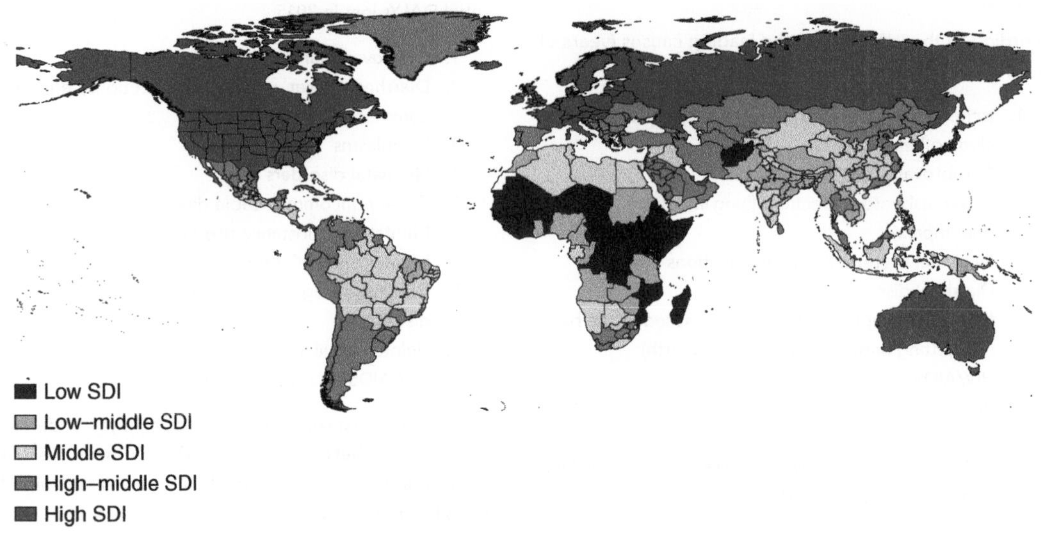

FIGURE CT3.3 SDI Quintiles by GBD Subnational Level 1 Geography, 2015.

Source: : Based on W. Haidong, Naghavi, M., Allen, C., et al. "Global, Regional and National Life Expectancy, All-Cause Mortality, and Cause-Specific Mortality for 249 Causes of Death, 1980–2015." *Lancet*, 2105, 388(100053): 1459–1544.

TABLE CT3.1 Diseases That Cause the Most YLLs by SDI Category.

	High SDI	High-middle SDI	Middle SDI	Low-middle SDI	Low SDI
1	Ischaemic heart disease	Ischaemic heart disease	Ischaemic heart disease	Lower respiratory infection	Lower respiratory infection
2	Stroke	Stroke	Stroke	Neonatal encephalitis	Malaria
3	Lung cancer	Road injuries	Road injuries	Diarrhea	Diarrhea
4	Self harm	Lung cancer	Chronic obstructive pulmonary disease	Neonatal preterm	HIV
5	Alzheimer's	Lower respiratory infection	Lower respiratory infection	Ischaemic heart disease	Neonatal preterm
6	Lower respiratory infection	HIV	Neonatal preterm	HIV	Neonatal encephalitis
7	Colorectal cancer	Chronic obstructive pulmonary disease	Congenital disorders	Malaria	Congenital disorders
8	Chronic obstructive pulmonary disease	Congenital	Neonatal encephalitis	Stroke	Neonatal sepsis
9	Road injuries	Self-harm	Diabetes	Congenital disorders	Meningitis
10	Breast cancer	Diabetes	Tuberculosis	Chronic obstructive pulmonary disease	Protein-energy malnutrition

Source: W. Haidong, Naghavi, M., Allen, C., et al. "Global, Regional and National Life Expectancy, All-Cause Mortality, and Cause-Specific Mortality for 249 Causes of Death, 1980–2015." *Lancet*, 2105, 388(100053): 1459–1544.

11 USING EVIDENCE ABOUT "BEST BUYS" TO ADVANCE GLOBAL HEALTH

There are so many health problems in today's world, especially in low- and middle-income countries, and there are limits on the amount of money that can be spent. Which health problems are the most important? How should countries or nongovernmental organizations decide on where to invest resources and time? Answering these questions is difficult. Some students feel overwhelmed when they learn about the number, scope, and complexity of health challenges. Moreover, given the scope of the problems and all the confusing data that exists, it can be difficult to know how to go about answering those questions.

Should a donor, nongovernmental organization, or community group decide on what problems to address simply because they feel passionately about an issue? Some projects, like Operation Smile, emphasize health care for particular individual patients like with the surgical repair for children born with a cleft palate. Other projects might aim at the global eradication of a disease like polio or Guinea worm. All of this global health work is important, but they all have different price tags and effect different populations.

However, some people think that decisions about priorities should not be made based on how passionately some people feel about a particular problem but rather decided rationality based on data. They argue that epidemiological and economic evidence should be the basis for deliberate decision-making about how to improve world health at the most efficient price. This is a cost-effectiveness approach; it can also be called "getting the most bang for the buck." This type of decision-making requires two things: good data and some agreement about what the goals of global health are (i.e., prevention or cure). When you start to learn more about the history of international and global health programs, it seems that some past decisions were not made in this rational way.

This article concerns the Disease Control Priority Project in its second edition (DCP2). The project involved more than 500 experts, and they produced a huge volume. The DCP2 is related to the larger effort to provide evidence about the global burden of disease. As you have seen in the box about Institute for Health Metrics and Evaluation in the Conceptual Tools for this section, the Global Burden of Disease project developed new metrics for determining the negative health impact of different diseases and health problems on a particular population. One important measure was a unit called the disability-adjusted life year lost(DALY). This article shows how to use epidemiological and economic data comparing the costs and gains in DALYs for particular countries and particular types of global health programs. This is what the authors call "best buys." The rule of thumb is that an intervention is cost-effective cost per DALY averted is less that the per capita GDP in a particular country.

There are three issues to note in this article. First, there can be no single list of "best buys" in disease control because priorities must be determined in relation to the particular ecological, epidemiological, and economic context of a country or region. A disease control project may be cost efficient, but if the disease is relatively rare, it may not be the best choice for a country. Second, remember that there are always problems with the best available data even though they are better than ever before.[1] Third, the DCP2 only considers priorities in terms of disease control and, therefore, other types of nonmedical interventions, like education or improved nutrition, are not considered. There is a similar project about the "best buys" in economic development, called the Copenhagen Consensus (http://www.copenhagenconsensus.com). Its list of the cost effectiveness of different world economic development

[1] Some skeptics say that the acronym for "best available data" is BAD.

Ramanan Laxminarayan and Lori Ashford, "Using Evidence about 'Best Buys' to Advance Global Health," Disease Control Priorities Project, 2006.

goals is regularly updated by a panel of Nobel laureates in Economics.

This article is in the form of a technical brief for policymakers; some students think it is a bit dry. However, pay attention to the examples because there are some surprises.

As you read this article, consider the following questions:

- In your opinion, is cost effectiveness the best way to set priorities? What other factors do you think need to be considered in deciding on strategies?
- How much is a life worth? What should society pay for an extra year of your life? What do you think of the morality of asking such questions?
- Is it best to do the easiest things first (i.e., the "low-hanging fruit")? Or is it smarter to tackle the biggest problems first?
- There is clear evidence that health is related to wealth and income inequality—but is solving the problem of poverty the responsibility of the health sector? Why or why not?
- Which of the "best buys" did you find most surprising? Why?

CONTEXT

Ramanan Laxminarayan directs the Center for Disease Dynamics, Economics and Policy. He is also a senior research scholar and lecturer at Princeton University. His research deals with the integration of epidemiological models of infectious diseases and drug resistance into the economic analysis of public health problems. He has worked for the World Health Organizaiton, World Bank, Centers for Disease Control and Prevention, DCP2, and the Institute of Medicine. He has a particular interest in understanding drug resistance as a problem of managing a shared global resource. Lori Ashford is the Technical Director for Policy Information at the Population Reference Bureau. She has a particular interest in reproductive health in policy and practice. This article was published on the Internet by DCP2 (http://www.dcp-3.org/dcp2/).

How much should it cost to save a life? If you had a million dollars for health, what would be the best way to spend it? How can we change incentives for health systems to adopt cost-effective interventions? These are some of the questions addressed by the Disease Control Priorities Project (DCPP), an international partnership launched earlier this decade to help policymakers decide how best to allocate their scarce health resources. The questions are pertinent today because the vast improvements in health over the last 50 years have not been shared equally across the globe. While life expectancy has risen dramatically worldwide—six years per decade just between 1960 and 1990—wide differences remain between developed and developing countries.

Low-income countries do not have to wait to become wealthy to become healthier, however. Experience has shown that, even in the absence of income growth, using existing knowledge and technologies can reduce deaths and illnesses even in the poorest countries. These health improvements, in turn, will help countries achieve their development goals.

DCPP provides the latest evidence on "best health buys" in developing countries, based on studies that have identified successful and cost-effective interventions. Evidence about what works, however, is only a starting point. Planning strategically about where and how much to invest, delivering health services more efficiently, and ultimately increasing the total resources available for health will be key to advancing global health.

The Disease Control Priorities Project

DCPP was launched in 2001 to help policymakers in developing countries identify the most pressing health problems and most effective strategies to address them. A joint effort of the Fogarty Center of the U.S. National Institutes of Health, the World Health Organization, and the World Bank, the project received major support from the Bill & Melinda Gates Foundation. Its main product is the 2nd edition of *Disease Control Priorities in Developing Countries (DCP2)*—an expansion and update of the 1st edition published in 1993, whose findings were incorporated in the World Bank's widely disseminated 1993 *World Development Report: Investing in Health.*

More than 500 health experts contributed to *DCP2*, which contains 73 chapters with wide-ranging information on the diseases and health conditions that afflict people worldwide. In addition to examining the disease burden (deaths and disabilities) resulting from specific health conditions, the chapters highlight cost-effective interventions based on careful analysis of prevention and treatment alternatives in different health care settings. A companion volume, *Priorities in Health*, available in seven languages, synthesizes *DCP2's* main messages into a plain-language reference guide for policymakers. Another major volume, *Global Burden of Disease and Risk Factors*, serves as a single source of data on health conditions worldwide as of the early 2000s, and gives details on the underlying methods for the cost-effectiveness calculations and conclusions presented in *DCP2*.

DCPP's resources are primarily aimed at public-sector health administrators, but they also provide an abundance of information for donor and technical assistance agencies, health professionals in the public and private sectors, and educators and advocates concerned with global health.

A Focus on Cost-Effectiveness

DCPP identified cost-effective opportunities that policymakers often ignore or underfund, as well as current investments that consume unnecessary resources. The project compared the cost-effectiveness of diverse health interventions using disability-adjusted life years (DALYs), a metric developed in the early 1990s to express health gains or losses in a common unit. DALYs measure the extent to which premature death and disability lower people's health status, and allow analysts to compare the value of health interventions that have multiple or different health outcomes, occurring at different ages.[1]

DCPP researchers aimed to identify the health services and strategies that would avert the most DALYs at the lowest cost. For example, heart disease is a major killer in rich countries and increasingly so in poorer ones. But the average cost of a coronary artery bypass is $37,000 per DALY averted, well beyond the per capita income of most countries. In contrast, a polypill—several medications for preventing heart disease combined in a single pill—costs only $409, on average, per DALY averted. While there is no "best" level of cost-effectiveness, governments should ideally choose to invest more in the lower-priced intervention and less in the higher-priced one—with all other things being equal.

DALYs and other measures of cost-effectiveness have limitations, however. The reliability of the estimates depends on the quality of available data, which is weak in many developing countries. Other factors also enter into policy decisions, such as the capacity of health systems, financial constraints, and cultural and ethical considerations. Equity is also a consideration, because it may be more cost-effective to serve people living in urban areas than those living in widely dispersed, rural areas—who tend to be poorer. Governments may intentionally direct more resources for serving vulnerable, hard-to-reach populations, thereby increasing the cost per person or cost per health outcome.

Best Buys in Health

DCPP examined the burden of hundreds of health conditions in developing countries and the cost-effectiveness of hundreds of interventions to address them. The findings are catalogued in the main *DCP2* volume and its companion materials. Some of the best health buys proved surprisingly simple—and often overlooked.

The most cost-effective health care solutions can be as simple and inexpensive as advising people at risk of heart disease to take an aspirin a day, and teaching mothers to keep their newborns clean and warm. Among the many surprising findings: A newborn can be resuscitated with a self-inflating bag that costs as little as $5 in developing countries, and the bag can be reused an infinite number of times.

The project identified 10 best health buys—based on cost per DALY averted—that have proven effective in developing countries:

1. Vaccinate children against major childhood diseases, including tuberculosis, diphtheria, whooping cough, tetanus, polio, and measles (the traditional expanded program of immunization).
2. Monitor children's health to prevent or, if necessary, treat childhood pneumonia, diarrhea, and malaria.

3. Tax tobacco products to increase consumers' costs by at least one-third and reduce cases of cardiovascular disease, cancer, and respiratory disease (see Box 11.1).
4. Prevent the spread of HIV through a coordinated approach that includes: promoting 100 percent condom use among populations at high risk of infection; treating other sexually transmitted infections; providing antiretroviral medications to pregnant women; and offering voluntary HIV counseling and testing.
5. Give children and pregnant women essential nutrients, including vitamin A, iron, and iodine, to prevent maternal anemia, infant deaths, and long-term health problems.
6. Provide insecticide-treated bed nets, household spraying of insecticides, and preventive treatment for pregnant women to drastically reduce malaria in areas where it is endemic.
7. Enforce traffic regulations and install speed bumps at dangerous intersections to reduce traffic-related injuries.
8. Treat tuberculosis patients with short-course chemotherapy to cure infected people and prevent new infections. (see Box 11.2).
9. Teach mothers and train birth attendants to keep newborns warm and clean to reduce illness and death.
10. Promote the use of aspirin and other inexpensive drugs to prevent and treat heart attack and stroke.

Other critical health measures—such as emergency surgery to treat injuries, childbirth complications, and abdominal conditions like appendicitis—can be more expensive in some places but worth the investment because they treat serious conditions that would otherwise be fatal or severely disabling. DCPP found emergency surgery to be most cost-effective in South Asia and Sub-Saharan Africa, where the cost of health services is relatively low and the burden of disease due to conditions requiring surgery is high (see Box 11.3).[2] This finding was surprising, because health experts had long considered surgery an unaffordable luxury in the poorest countries.

Putting Cost-Effectiveness in Context

To guide policies more precisely, data on cost-effectiveness must be viewed alongside information about the larger context, such as the prevailing burden of disease, existing health interventions, and the capacity of the health system. The burden caused by a particular disease is key because policymakers will want to direct health spending to interventions that are likely to have the greatest impact on the nation's health. In developed countries, for example, a large share of health resources is devoted to addressing noncommunicable diseases, such as heart disease and stroke, cancer, diabetes, and other illnesses associated with comfortable lifestyles (overeating, smoking) and greater longevity.

Many developing countries face a "double burden" of disease. They are still grappling with diseases related to poverty—communicable diseases such as malaria and tuberculosis; poor maternal and newborn health; and undernutrition—while also seeing a rise in the diseases that typically affect more affluent populations. By 2001, noncommunicable diseases accounted for nearly half of the disease burden of developing countries (see Figure 11.1). In

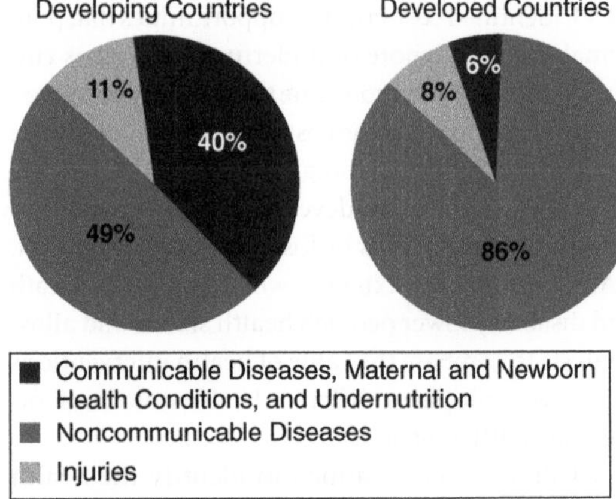

Note: The burden of disease is measured in disability-adjusted life years (DALYs) lost due to specific health conditions.

FIGURE 11.1 Burden of Disease, 2001.

Source: R. Laxminarayan, Mills A. J., Breman, J. G., et al. "Advancement of Global Health: Key Messages from the Disease Control Priorities Project." The Lancet, 2006, 367: 1193–2008.

addition, injuries, most of which are preventable, account for a higher burden of disease in developing countries compared with developed countries.

Health interventions that address a large disease burden (in terms of DALYs) and are cost-effective (in terms of cost per DALY averted) provide good value. Tables 11.1 and 11.2 show the best health buys that DCPP identified for South Asia and Sub-Saharan Africa, along with the total burden of disease addressed by the interventions. In both regions, the best buys include immunizing children against the major childhood diseases, providing emergency surgery for injuries and other urgent health complications, supporting an essential package of maternal and newborn care, and undertaking a coordinated approach to prevent HIV/AIDS.

Other interventions, such as improving the safety of blood supply to prevent new HIV infections, may be highly cost-effective but affect only a small number of people or provide a small improvement in health. Whether to invest in these interventions is a matter of judgment and availability of funds. These are only a few examples of the myriad options that policymakers must weigh. The more information about costs and burden of disease that policymakers have, the better they will be able to decide among alternative investments.

TABLE 11.1 Best Buys in South Asia.

Health Intervention	Cost (in us $) per DALY Averted*	Burden of Targeted Diseases (Millions of DALYs)*
Childhood immunization	$8	28
HIV/AIDS prevention	$9–126	7
Surgical services and emergency care	$6–212	48–146
Tuberculosis (prevention and treatment)	$8–263	14
Management of acute respiratory illnesses (under age 5)	$28–264	10–26
Cardiovascular diseases (prevention and management)	$9–304	26–39
Tobacco use and addiction	$14–374	16
Maternal and neonatal care	$127–394	38–48

TABLE 11.2 Best Buys in Sub-Saharan Africa.

Health Intervention	Cost (in US $) per DALY Averted*	Burden of Targeted Diseases (Millions of DALYs)*
Childhood immunization	$1–5	14–31
Prevention of traffic crashes	$2–12	6
Malaria prevention	$2–24	35
Surgical services and emergency care	$7–215	25–134
Management of childhood illnesses	$9–218	10–45
Cardiovascular diseases (prevention and management)	$9–273	5
HIV/AIDS prevention	$6–377	57
Maternal and neonatal care	$82–409	30–38

* Ranges in cost per DALY averted reflect variation in costs across interventions and locations. Ranges in burden of targeted disease arise from differences in estimates provided by different sources.

Note: A DALY is a composite unit that measures the amount of health lost due to a particular disease or condition. The components of the interventions listed in the table are described in the text referring to the 10 "best buys" in health.

Source: Laxminarayan, R., J. Chow, and S.A. Shahid-Salles. 2006. "Intervention Cost-Effectiveness: Overview of Main Messages," in *Disease Control Priorities in Developing Countries*, 2d edition, ed. D.T. Jamison et al.: 54–55.

Planning Strategically within Countries

The pattern of disease can vary greatly from one country to another and also within countries; thus, policymakers should not study and address diseases in isolation. They should use all of the available evidence about the disease burden in their country and develop packages of interventions that provide the greatest value for money—thereby attaining the greatest health improvements for the most people at the lowest cost. This approach should result in allocating substantial resources for the poor, who typically suffer the greatest disease burden and would benefit most.

Cost-effectiveness must be considered not just for specific interventions, but also for different levels of care, such as community health centers, district hospitals, and second- and third-level (referral) hospitals. The evidence from *DCP2* suggests that governments should focus on ensuring that primary health care systems work well, with local district hospitals as a focal point. Such systems could address up to 90 percent of health care needs in developing countries.

DCP2 showed that basic health care in district hospitals can be highly cost-effective, at $13 to $104 per DALY averted. In addition, the project found that training lay first-responders to emergencies and volunteer paramedics costs between $5 and $11 per DALY averted, depending on the region. Equipping ambulances with trained paramedics costs $46 to $137 per DALY averted in urban areas, and two to four times as much in rural areas. These are relatively inexpensive, but often overlooked, strategies for saving people's lives.

Planning strategically requires reliable evidence, however, which depends on well-functioning reporting systems. In most developing countries, reporting systems from the community and district level to higher levels are still weak and not well coordinated. Strong health information systems, including surveillance for early detection of outbreaks of disease, will be critical for planning and investing in the most appropriate health interventions.

Strengthening Health Systems

The cost-effective interventions described in *DCP2* will not reach their full potential as long as skilled health personnel and physical infrastructure are lacking in many developing countries. In addition to choosing the most cost-effective and high-impact interventions, policymakers and planners must ensure that health systems are strong enough to carry them out.

Strengthening health systems is a wide ranging subject, requiring action on many fronts. Some areas of health system reform include: strengthening human resources; improving oversight and regulation of public and private health services; reforming organizational structures; and targeting public

BOX 11.1 Curbing Tobacco Use

Cigarette smoking and other forms of tobacco use impose a large and increasing public health burden worldwide. Today, more than 1.1 billion people smoke, with about 83 percent living in developing countries. Tobacco use is linked to an estimated 5 million deaths annually, from cardiovascular disease, lung and other cancers, and respiratory diseases. Interventions to curb tobacco use reduce a large burden of deaths and are highly cost-effective. They include:

- Raising tobacco taxes by up to 70 percent;
- Providing universal access to therapies that help people quit smoking;
- Restricting smoking in public places and workplaces;
- Educating the public about the risks of tobacco addiction; and Banning tobacco advertising and promotion.

Tobacco taxes discourage people from starting smoking and encourage smokers to quit; they also can increase governments' tax revenues. The cost-effectiveness of raising cigarette prices by 33 percent ranges from $3 to $42 per DALY averted in low-income countries. Nicotine replacement therapy (costing from $55 to $751 per DALY averted) and other non-tax interventions listed above are relatively less cost-effective, but still belong in any tobacco control program.

See fact sheet, "Tobacco Addiction," April 2006, at www.dcp2.org/file/52/DCPP-Tobacco.pdf, and Chapter 46 of *DCP2*.

BOX 11.2 Preventing and Controlling Tuberculosis

Tuberculosis is the second largest cause of death from an infectious agent worldwide—killing about 1.7 million people in 2003. Despite declines in cases in some countries, the number of cases is growing worldwide (an estimated 8.8 million cases in 2005), in part driven by the spread of HIV in Africa.

Treating all forms of active TB with short-course chemotherapy is among the most cost-effective of all health interventions, because it cures infected individuals and prevents the spread of the disease. An internationally recommended strategy, DOTS (directly observed treatment short-course) costs $5 to $35 per DALY averted in developing countries. Successfully implementing it requires:

- Political commitment;
- Correctly diagnosing cases;
- Administering the standard course of drugs under observation;
- Ensuring regular drug supplies; and Maintaining a standard surveillance and reporting system.

The BCG (Bacille Calmett-Guerin) vaccination for children is also cost-effective ($40 to $170 per DALY averted), in reducing the burden of TB associated with meningitis in children. But because BCG hardly affects the huge burden of pulmonary TB in adults, the development of a new vaccine targeting adults is highly desirable.

The management of TB in people infected with HIV requires higher investment than is needed for DOTS alone. Nevertheless, the cost is still typically less than $1 per day of healthy life gained—a strong argument for integrating treatment for HIV patients into an enhanced TB control strategy.

See fact sheet, "Tuberculosis," April 2006, at www.dcp2.org/file/3/DCPP-TB.pdf, and Chapter 16 of *DCP2.*

health spending to ensure that the neediest people receive services.

A lack of trained health personnel, from nurses and doctors to higher-level managers, is severely affecting health services in the poorest countries. Because these personnel support the entire health system, many health system reforms may not succeed until the shortage of human resources is overcome. Health managers at the district level, in particular, need information, tools, and training to adapt their services to the local disease burden.

Progress Following the Launch of DCPP

Since the early 2000s, the global health community has made progress in several critical areas, boosted in part by the greater visibility that major health problems received after the launch of DCPP and related health initiatives. Examples include worldwide progress in controlling tobacco use; advances in newborn survival; promoting essential surgery in Sub-Saharan Africa (see Box 3), and new approaches to curb the spread of HIV.

Tobacco Control

The WHO Framework Convention on Tobacco Control is a 21st century achievement in global health: It is the first international treaty that WHO has negotiated. The treaty is based on scientific evidence from around the world on the harmful effects of tobacco on health, and on what is known about the most effective ways to curb the demand for and supply of tobacco products (see Box 11.1).

To reduce the demand for tobacco, the treaty calls for increasing taxes and prices, protecting people from exposure to tobacco smoke, regulating the content and labeling of tobacco products, banning certain types of advertising and promotion, and helping addicted people reduce their dependence on tobacco. To curb supply, the treaty calls on countries to end illegal trade in tobacco products and sales of tobacco to minors, and support economically viable alternatives to the tobacco industry.

As of June 2008, 168 countries and territories signed the treaty, and 157 ratified it nationally. Such an achievement demonstrates that the world's governments understand the evidence on tobacco's harmful effects and agree that the solutions are both necessary and feasible. As with any solutions that require changing behavior, however, implementation will be both challenging and complex.

Saving Newborn Babies

The problem of newborn deaths has been on policymakers' back-burner for decades, in spite of the fact that 38 percent of all deaths of children under age 5 occur in the first month of life. The lack of attention has been partly due to a belief that high technology care would be needed to save newborn lives.

Contrary to this belief, DCPP found that about 40 percent of newborn deaths could be averted with simple solutions carried out in the home and community. These solutions include keeping a newborn warm and clean, breastfeeding early and exclusively, protecting against infection through proper hygiene, and treating infections with antibiotics. Incorporating this package into standard maternal and child health care has proven highly cost-effective. In India, the newborn care package can cost as little as $24 per DALY averted, and in Sub-Saharan Africa as low as $46 per DALY averted.[3]

Around the time that *DCP2* went to press, newborn survival made headlines in a series of articles that appeared in the journal, *The Lancet*, and in WHO's *2005 World Health Report*. Several international partnerships devoted to maternal and child health also called for expanding available solutions in countries with unacceptably high newborn death rates.[4]

These global efforts helped put newborn babies on governments' health policy agendas—in many countries for the first time. As a result, progress has been seen in major policy statements, budget commitments, and new or revitalized initiatives in South Asia and Sub-Saharan Africa—the regions with the highest burden of newborn deaths. For example, in Africa, at least 20 countries have requested technical assistance to develop or strengthen newborn health programs. The African Union adopted a "Roadmap for Maternal Health" that called for increased emphasis on newborn survival.

Examples of actions in specific countries include:

- India is training 300,000 village workers whose primary responsibility will be newborn care.
- Pakistan is adding that responsibility to its successful Lady Health Workers program, which employs 100,000 workers.
- Tanzania's Ministry of Health is integrating newborn survival into local health planning. A district planning tool that ties the local burden of disease to the district health budget has been adapted to show the large number of newborn deaths, increasing the districts' interest in investing in newborn health.

New Approaches to Curb the Spread of HIV

Medical and behavioral research has provided many of the breakthroughs that have helped curb the global AIDS pandemic. Successful prevention programs rely on many well-tested components: 100 percent condom use among populations most at risk of contracting HIV; voluntary testing and counseling to allow people to learn their status and receive support; and preventing mother-to-child transmission of HIV through antiretroviral therapy, among other behavior-change measures. Health experts have long called for research into other prevention measures, particularly because prospects for an AIDS vaccine are dim in the near future.

An additional prevention measure, male circumcision (MC), came to light following clinical trials in South Africa, Kenya, and Uganda in the mid-2000s. *DCP2* had noted that the evidence suggesting that MC decreases the risk of acquiring HIV was strong. By 2007, the evidence from additional studies was irrefutable, leading WHO to recommend that countries add MC to national HIV prevention programs, particularly in countries in Sub-Saharan Africa where large percentages of men are uncircumcised. MC is cost-effective because the procedure is inexpensive, requiring only an outpatient facility and local anesthesia (it is even more cost-effective when performed on infants). In terms of saving lives, one simulation showed that in the next 20 years, MC could prevent 5.7 million people of both sexes in Africa from contracting HIV and 3 million from dying—at least as effective as the long-hoped-for AIDS vaccine.[5]

Global Health Challenges Ahead

Despite continued progress in controlling the world's major diseases, four important global health challenges remain:

- The rapid growth of noncommunicable diseases in developing countries, while their public health systems are still grappling with the conventional diseases of poverty.

- The HIV/AIDS pandemic, which continues to spread unchecked in some countries.
- The possibility of an outbreak of another pandemic, such as SARS, avian flu, or dengue fever.
- The high prevalence of malaria, tuberculosis, diarrhea, and pneumonia that persists in the poorest countries.

To address these challenges, interventions that are known to be cost-effective should be adopted on a wider scale. For example, developing countries that are now facing a rise in noncommunicable diseases can apply many interventions that were first developed in industrialized countries, such as tobacco control programs, at a reasonable cost.

But policymakers need to recognize the importance of these health threats and respond to them. To develop appropriate responses, health information systems must be strengthened to monitor and report on new and existing cases of diseases and other health conditions, and to identify the populations that are most vulnerable and in need of services.

Recommended Actions

Policymakers and health program planners in developing countries have a wealth of information to draw from on the burden of disease and on interventions that have proven successful and affordable. To put this knowledge into practice, actions are needed on the part of both national governments and the international health community:

BOX 11.3 Expanding Access to Surgery in the Poorest Countries

Surgical services have typically not been a priority in many developing countries because they are considered unaffordable in places where doctors and well-equipped facilities are scarce. Yet DCPP researchers found that surgery need not be provided in expensive, high-technology hospitals and that it can be highly cost-effective—even on par with widely accepted preventive health care such as child immunizations.

Four types of surgery are most critical for saving lives and reducing disabilities in developing countries:

- Emergency care to injury victims, to avoid preventable deaths and reduce disabilities that burden families and communities;
- Addressing the complications of pregnancy and childbirth, such as obstructed labor;
- Managing a variety of abdominal conditions, such as appendicitis, ulcers, intestinal obstructions, and other conditions that can be life-threatening; and
- Elective surgery for relatively simple conditions such as cataracts, hernias, clubfoot, and middle ear infections.

DCPP found the highest burden of surgical conditions (in terms of DALYs lost relative to the size of the population) to be in Sub-Saharan Africa. Most of the health conditions requiring surgery are treatable, and many simple surgical procedures can be performed by trained clinicians without medical degrees. The costs attributable to surgical patients in district hospitals in Sub-Saharan Africa translate to only $33 per DALY gained, making emergency surgical care among the most cost-effective interventions in the region.

Following the release of *DCP2*, the Rockefeller Foundation brought together leaders in surgery and related fields along with health policymakers and economists at a conference on expanding access to surgical services in Sub-Saharan Africa. The meeting, held in Bellagio in June 2007, took stock of evidence about the cost-effectiveness of surgical services in the poorest countries; assessed constraints to integrating surgery into district health services in Sub-Saharan Africa; and prepared a roadmap to improve access to surgical services in that region.

DCPP thus expanded an effort that had started in Sub-Saharan Africa several decades ago. In Mozambique and other East African countries, thousands of clinical officers (not doctors) have been trained and are performing essential surgery as competently as doctors. Programs have been carefully evaluated in at least three countries, showing that thousands of lives have been saved. DCPP promises to spread this knowledge much more widely.

See fact sheet, "Promoting Essential Surgery in Low-Income Countries: A Hidden Cost-Effective Treasure," June 2008, at www.dcp2.org/file/158/dcpp-surgery.pdf, and Chapter 67 of *DCP2*; and "Experts Develop Roadmap to Promote Essential Surgery at the District Level," June 2007, at www.dcp2.org/news/57.

National Governments

- Use the results of cost-effectiveness analysis to invest limited resources more wisely.
- Plan strategically to invest in those cost-effective interventions that address the largest disease burden in a country.
- Identify the health problems shared by industrialized and developing countries and opportunities for transferring knowledge.
- Expand the use of successful public-private partnerships for developing products and providing services.
- Increase the efficiency of health systems by introducing the latest health information technology and training health personnel to use it.
- Conduct operational research to determine how best to adapt important, long-term health interventions to a local setting.

"For prevention and treatment programs to work, policymakers must have access to the best possible research and analysis to ensure that their health investments save as many lives as possible."

– Ramanan Laxminarayan in *The Lancet* (Vol. 367), April 8, 2006.

International Health Community

- Increase support for global health research to attract and keep scientists in the developing world.
- Create a global health network that allocates a larger share of development assistance for research on neglected health conditions in developing countries.

While priority-setting can make limited resources go further, accomplishing all of these actions will not be possible without additional resources. The information provided by DCPP helps fill important gaps in knowledge, but the knowledge cannot be put into practice if health systems remain severely underfunded and understaffed. Increasing the flow of resources to health, drawing on both donor support and national spending, will be essential to implement the cost-effective interventions that DCPP has identified.

For More Information

DCPP publications and resources can be found at www.dcp2.org. The entire *DCP2* volume is available and can be downloaded by chapter. Other tools and resources, such as fact sheets (highlighting the major findings of *DCP2* by topic area), graphics, maps, and feature stories are also available on the website.

Acknowledgments

This policy brief is adapted from an article appearing in *The Lancet* in April 2006, written by Ramanan Laxminarayan and the editors of *DCP2*. Ramanan Laxminarayan is a senior fellow at Resources for the Future and Lori Ashford is program director for policy communications at the Population Reference Bureau. The authors would like to thank Fariyal Fikree, Anthony Measham, and Richard Skolnik for their contributions to this brief.

REFERENCES

1. See fact sheet, "Using Cost-Effectiveness Analysis for Setting Health Priorities," March 2008, at www.dcp2.org/file/150/DCPP-CostEffectiveness.pdf, and Chapter 2 of *DCP2*. A DALY (loss) that is averted is the same as a DALY gained.
2. See fact sheet, "Promoting Essential Surgery in Low-Income Countries," June 2008, at www.dcp2.org/file/158/dcpp-surgery.pdf, and Chapter 67 of *DCP2*.
3. See fact sheet, "Newborn Health," April 2006, at www.dcp2.org/file/11/DCPP-NewbornHealth.pdf, and Chapter 27 of *DCP2*.
4. Lawn J. 2007. *Newborn Survival: A Snapshot of Progress Since 2005*, accessed online June 23, 2008 at www.dcp2.org/features/48.
5. Williams, B. et al. 2006. "The Potential Impact of Male Circumcision on HIV in Sub-Saharan Africa." *PLoS Medicine* 3(7): e262; Klausner, J. et al. 2008. "Is Male Circumcision as Good as the HIV Vaccine We've Been Waiting For?" *Future HIV Therapy* 2(1); and Benderly, B.L. 2008. *The Kindest Cut: Proof that Male Circumcision Is Cost-Effective Against Transmission of HIV Brings New Hope for Sub-Saharan Africa*, accessed online July 15, 2008 at www.dcp2.org/features/60.

TRACY KIDDER

12 THE LONG DEFEAT

This reading is an excerpt from a famous book called Mountains Beyond Mountains *with the subtitle* The Quest of Dr. Paul Farmer, a Man Who Would Cure the World. *Every student of global health should read the book, not because Paul Farmer should be everyone's role model, but because the author does such a good job describing rural Haiti and a project called* Zanmi Lasante*–Partners in Health (PIH) (www.pih.org). Paul Farmer is definitely an inspirational figure, and PIH is an exceptional institution that delivers quality health care to the poorest of the poor in places like Haiti, Peru, and Rwanda. This nongovernmental organization was started by Farmer and his fellow physician-anthropologist Jim Kim (now the president of the World Bank) and Ophelia Dahl using funds from the philanthropist Tom White.*

This chapter is about the "preferential option for the poor" that guides PIH's work. This is a radical philosophical and ethical notion because it means that the poor should go to the front of the line when it comes to health care and related services. This notion has its roots in liberation theology from Latin America, which states that it is a central task of Christians (and their institutions) to address problems of poverty and social injustice. A preferential option for the poor is far more than "equal opportunity." As the beginning of the reading explains, it is a type of triage where no one is denied treatment and where the sickest and most needy people get the best and quickest services. There are ethical and practical issues at stake here.

This selection provides a very interesting discussion of the moral dilemmas involved in deciding where to invest funds in global health. Chapter 11 discussed "best buys," but sometimes making life and death choices should not be a question of metrics or measurement. Since wealthy people usually have access to expensive lifesaving treatments, the focus on measurement and cost effectiveness in global health could be considered to be based on an assumption that some peoples' lives are worth more than others. Sometimes the right thing to do is expensive. This issue is also explored in the website The Life Equation, *listed in the Web Resources for this section.*

There is another assumption hidden in the emphasis on measurement and cost-effectiveness in global health. It is the assumption that there simply is not enough money to fix everything—that there is a limit of the amount that can be spent on disease prevention and health care. Paul Farmer argues that there has never been so much wealth in the world, yet there has also never been such economic inequality. When some of the richest individuals in the world have decided to give most of their money to institutions promoting global health, the funds for both programs and research have increased enormously. There is enough wealth in the world to supply basic health for all. The challenges are to redistribute money from the world's richest to the poorest and to have governments spend more on the health of their citizens and global well-being and less on their military or comforts of the "1 percent."

It is easy to criticize Farmer's approach as being inefficient or economically irrational. Health problems in low-income countries represent emergencies that ethically demand immediate attention. While PIH does important prevention work, if we think back at the cartoon depicting public health as opposed to health care (Reading 1), the PIH doctors are knee-deep in human suffering. One can easily argue that PIH's model is unsustainable or that it fits the "medical missionary" model in the history of international/global health (Reading 35).

This is why Farmer can describe his career as "the long defeat." But the in-the-trenches work of PIH has led to broad public health impacts. There have been two important global health issues in which PIH's research and example have made huge changes in global health policy. In the 1990s, some people said that it would be impossible to deliver complex and expensive anti-retroviral therapy treatment for people who had HIV/AIDS and were the poorest of the poor. One infamous excuse for the failure to expand treatment was that poor people could not tell time and thus wouldn't take their drugs correctly. PIH demonstrated that such assumptions were patently wrong, and the World Health Organization (WHO) and UNAIDS policies changed.

The second global health policy to be reversed through the efforts of PIH concerned the treatment of multiple-drug-resistant tuberculosis (MDR-TB). Prior to PIH's actions, the WHO policy was to provide directly observed therapy (DOTS) only to patients without drug-resistant TB; there was no alternate plan in the case of drug-resistant infection. Some people argued that MDR-TB was too complicated and not cost-effective to treat in low-resource settings, so the answer, in essence, was to "let them die." But PIH, particularly Jim Kim, showed that MDR-TB patients could be effectively treated in low-resource settings, and the WHO policy changed to one called DOTS+, which includes systems for treating MDR-TB.

"Quest" is a good word to describe the work of Paul Farmer and PIH. When faced with the huge burden of global health problems and the sheer amount of human suffering, the idea of "health for all" might seem quixotic and idealistic. But from a moral and ethical point of view, what else is there to do but try?

As you read this chapter, consider the following questions:

- **Farmer argues that "the idea that some lives matter less than others is the root of all that is wrong with the world." In your opinion, is this correct? Why or why not? Are all lives of equal value?**
- **Why is this reading placed in the section of this book about the burden of disease and the problems of measurement?**
- **In your opinion, is the "preferential option for the poor" in health care a realistic idea? What would Paul Farmer say to the word "realistic" in the previous sentence?**
- **Farmer strongly objects to the widespread assumption that there is not enough money in the world to provide quality health for all people, and he objects to criticisms that his approach is not economically or strategically rational. How might you paraphrase his viewpoint? Do you agree?**
- **At the beginning of this book (Reading 1), we argued that one does not need to be a doctor to be involved in Global Health. After reading this article, does this seem to be true? What are advantages and disadvantages of being a physician in this field?**

CONTEXT

Tracy Kidder is a well-known author who has ten nonfiction books on a very wide range of topics, from this biography of Paul Farmer to a memoir of the renovation of his house. He has won the Pulitzer Prize twice: once for an early work on computer engineers and again for his latest book entitled, *A Truck Full of Money: One Man's Quest to Recover from Great Success* (2016). Tracy Kidder is a master storyteller.

Some months back, a boy named Alcante arrived at Zanmi La-sante's Children's Pavilion. He had lumps on his neck, symptomatic of scrofula. First-line drugs wiped out the infection. The swellings disappeared, leaving only a few small scars, and Alcante gained eight pounds, about 10 percent of his total weight. The boy was thirteen, and seemed younger because he was so small and trusting. He was the kind of child who takes strangers by the hand, and he was very beautiful looking—a perfect little body, shiny dark eyes, dimples. He changed the atmosphere in the Children's Pavilion and lessened the tightening Farmer felt in his chest as he climbed the stairs to that wing. For Farmer, the children's ward contained Zanmi Lasante's most harrowing sights and painful ghosts, and I think Alcante came to seem like the guardian angel of the place, or like Farmer's. He kept the boy in Cange several weeks longer than necessary. He called him "a P.O.P."—a prisoner of Paul. Finally, he sent him home.

As a rule, a child with scrofula gets it from a close contact, usually the mother or father. So one of Zanmi Lasante's community health workers brought the rest of Alcante's family to Cange—they were "trolled in," as Farmer puts it. Several had TB, including Alcante's father, who is still in therapy. Now Farmer wants to see for himself what home means to Alcante. He plans to hike to their homestead. "The family is so afflicted," he explains, then adds, "Some people would say this is a scattershot approach. We would answer, 'Not at all. It's through journeys to the sick that we identify needs and problems.'"

Alcante lives in a town called Casse. The hike is longer than the first long one I took with Farmer to Morne Michel, but the trails aren't as steep. This is what he told me last night. So I have only a vague idea of how many hours the trip will take, until we're walking out the front gate and Ti Jean, who is coming with us, asks if I have brought my flashlight.

I haven't. I offer to go back for it. Farmer doesn't think I should. Inevitably, some emergency will have cropped up, and going back will get him entangled in it. Delay now will mean further delay. Farmer is wearing a baseball cap, which looks a few sizes too large, and for a moment I imagine him a gawky teenager on the way to a ball game with his dad. His thin frame and the shininess of his face make this possible, and also a quality of innocence that surfaces at times—he's apt, for example, in the midst of an erudite discourse on the economic distribution of infectious disease, to startle you by interjecting, eagerly, "Ask me a question about *Lord of the Rings.*" He's reread those books again and again over the years since he was eleven. But now he's leading the way out of Zanmi Lasante, in every sense the man in charge, and I realize I'm not worried about the flashlight. This strikes me as unusual. I've never found it easy to trust another person to lead me anywhere, but I trust Farmer.

We head off along dirt paths etched into the sides of the hills beside the Péligre Reservoir, and soon I'm scrambling up the eroded face of a cliff. I'm drenched with sweat by the time we get to the top, where Farmer is waiting for me. I'm reminded of the epic hike to Morne Michel. As we go on, Farmer calls back over his shoulder—his voice makes it plain he's joking—that if I have chest pains, I should tell him right away. I take a long swig of water as we stride across a ridge through yellow grass, Farmer pointing out "the peculiarly steep and conical hill" on which he sat in solitude years ago, writing *AIDS and Accusation.*

Ti Jean is carrying a large water jug, filled from a tap at the medical complex. It's potable water. Farmer and Ti Jean have immunity to whatever microorganisms it contains, but American visitors who drink it often come down with bowel troubles, not dangerously but uncomfortably. So I've brought my own jug of filtered water, but it isn't very large. By the time we make our first stop, I've drunk half, and Ti Jean and Farmer and Zanmi Lasante's pharmacist, who is also coming along, haven't even opened their jug.

Farmer has planned an intermediate house call on the way to Alcante's home in Casse. Somewhere in the mountains, we stop at a hut—two tiny rooms, dirt floors, a roof of banana fronds, pro-Aristide posters on the walls, and an elderly-looking couple sitting together on a straw mat. Farmer has brought along the man's medical records. He sits down on a chair near the doorway and reads aloud from them. "Since 1989 he's been coming to ZL and he's been getting antihypertensives. I saw him last in 1997 and he had malaria and then it says, 'Come back Thursday for a follow-up.' He didn't come back. And oops, here we go, it says here, 'Trouble standing up.' And his son had come for medicine for his blood pressure." Farmer kneels on the dirt floor and takes the man's pulse and blood pressure, then puts on a stethoscope and listens to his chest for a while. Cocks crow outside. The air inside is still and hot, vibrating with flies. The old man says he felt a little pain at the center of his chest and afterward weakness in his legs. Farmer says to me, "I know what I'm going to do. Get his blood pressure down to normal, then get him two Canadian crutches. I think he probably had a stroke, but he should be able to recover is what I'm saying. His deficit is *minimal.* So I have to get somebody to help me get the Canadian crutches here. To get his blood pressure just right would be easy at the Brigham. It's not easy here, and how do we check and make sure he's doing his physical therapy?"

The old man's wife says she wants her blood pressure checked, too. Kneeling beside her, Farmer says in English, "She's sixty-two. Going on a hundred," adding, as if to himself, "We are far from the Brigham, my friend." The woman's pressure is high, too, he says. I, meanwhile, am trying to think of what Farmer said to me a year ago about the profound difference between being bedridden in a nice house outside Boston and mat-ridden in a hut like this, but I can't stop thinking at the same time about the little pain that has been flitting around behind my left nipple, on and off ever since that first cliff climb.

Finally, I tell Farmer about the pain. Then I apologize, and he says, "Don't be silly. Tell me more about it." He asks me a dozen questions, and says he thinks I just have heartburn. "But if it gets worse, you have to tell me. You don't want to see Alcante that bad. Promise?"

Several small children have come to the doorway. They stand there, peering in. Farmer says to them, speaking of the sad-looking woman of the house, "You love her a lot? Do you tell her? Don't lie to me now." The children giggle. The old woman smiles. Farmer nods toward a naked toddler in the doorway. "Look at his toy."

The child is sucking the thumb of one hand. In the other, he holds a piece of coarse hemp string. A rock is tied to the end of it.

"Rocks 'R' Us," says Farmer, and I laugh. I can't stop. Farmer starts laughing, too, saying, "Now *I'm* going to have chest pain. God is going to strike me dead." He says that he's going to give me half a beta-blocker just in case, and still I can't stop laughing.

"God is going to strike me dead," he says again. "For drinking more than my share of water, for not living humbly, for my *bad* sense of humor. It's your fault. I'm playing to my audience."

But, I think, he hasn't drunk any water yet.

He gives the couple their pills and instructions. Good-byes are always long in Haiti. When we get outside, Farmer says, "This was a *bel kout nas*, a good cast of the net. We came to see Papa and got Grandma, too. Just in time. Before she got run over by a reindeer."

I've heard him use the fishing metaphor many times. When a sick person is discovered by accident, he usually says he's made a lucky catch. As if Zanmi Lasante didn't have enough patients already.

"Is there a long way still to go?" I ask, as we walk on.

"Oh, yeah! This is a quarter of the way there."

"A quarter?"

Since the death of the boy John, I've been trying to form my question for Farmer about that case. I remember a remark he made to me a year ago in these hills: "You *should* compare suffering. Which suffering is worse. It's called triage."

The term comes from the fourteenth-century French *trier*, "to pick or cull," and was first used to describe the sorting of wool according to its quality. In modern medical usage, *triage* has two different meanings, nearly opposite. In situations where doctors and nurses and tools are limited, on battlefields, for instance, one performs triage by attending first to the severely wounded who have the best chance of survival. The aim is to save as many as possible; the others may have to die unattended. In the peacetime case, however, in well-staffed and well-stocked American emergency rooms, for example, *triage* isn't supposed to imply withholding care from anyone; rather, it's identifying the patients in gravest danger and giving them priority.

Farmer has constructed his life around this second kind of triage. What else is a "preferential option for the poor" in medicine? But Haiti more nearly resembles a battlefield than a place at peace. Walking behind him, I say there must always be situations here where the choice to do one necessary thing also means the choice not to do another—not just to defer the other but not to do it.

"All the time," he says.

"Throughout your whole career you've had to face this, right?"

"Yes. I do it every day. Do this instead of that. Every day all day long, that's all I do. Is not do things."

So, I ask, what about the case of John? What about the twenty thousand dollars that PIH spent on the medevac flight to get him out of Haiti? Not long after John died, a PIH-er, a relatively new one, said to me that she couldn't help thinking of all the things they could have done with that twenty thousand dollars. What is his response to that? "I don't mean this at all critically," I add, hurrying along behind him.

"Come on," he says over his shoulder. "I'm not hypersensitive. But we've already discussed this, so many times. I'm just failing to do a good job or you're not convinced. Maybe I'll never convince you that the choices we make are good ones."

I don't want to nettle him. For one thing, he's both my guide and my doctor for today. But I recognize his tone of voice. He's not really irritated. He's just delivering a preamble, warming up his argument.

He continues, talking over his shoulder to me as we walk on. "Let me say a couple of things about this particular case, if you like. One is, remember of course that John was referred to Boston as dying of a treatable tumor, a very rare tumor. He wasn't referred to Mass General before we knew what he had. So when he was referred, it was for free care because he had such a rare thing and it was treatable, and the predicted cure rate was sixty to seventy percent. All right. Good enough. That was what the decision was made on. And there was no way for us to find out that John didn't have locally invasive disease without metastases, because it required a diagnostic test that we can't do here. So the other thing is, the bottom line is, why do we intervene as aggressively as we can with that kid and not with another? Because his mother brought him to us and that's where he was, in our clinic."

"I wondered when Serena and Carole came to get him, if you'd have decided to bring him after all, if you'd been there. He was so emaciated."

"The emaciation wouldn't have stopped me. If I'd seen him and seen how far he'd gone downhill, I wouldn't have stopped the process. Why? On what grounds? We didn't know until he got to Boston that the cancer had invaded his vertebrae."

We climb another cliff, and I am breathing too hard to speak. After a short pause, he says, "I have to tell you, though, I'm a little troubled by these comments from the new PIH-er. Because I have to *work* with these people. The last thing I want to do is expend my energy trying to convince my own coworkers. Now I have to, of course. But I don't like it. The Haitians have a lot to say about inviting the wrong people into your midst, you know."

"I don't want to misrepresent it," I say. "Your PIH-er wasn't saying you shouldn't have brought John to Boston. Only that it was a shame you had to spend so much, given what else you could do with twenty grand."

"Yeah, but there are so many ways of saying that," he replies. "For example, why didn't the airplane company that makes money, the mercenaries, why didn't they pay for his flight? That's a way of saying it. Or how about this way? How about if I say, I have fought for *my whole life* a long defeat. How about that? How about if I said, That's all it adds up to is defeat?"

"A long defeat."

"I have fought the long defeat and brought other people on to fight the long defeat, and I'm not going to stop because we keep losing. Now I actually think sometimes we may *win*. I don't dislike victory. You and I have discussed this so many times."

"Sorry."

"No, no, I'm not complaining," he says. "You know, people from our background—like you, like most PIH-ers, like me—we're used to being on a victory team, and actually what we're really trying to do in PIH is to make common cause with the *losers*. Those are two very different things. We *want* to be on the winning team, but at the *risk* of turning our backs on the losers, no, it's not worth it. So you fight the long defeat." He pauses. "How you feelin'? Is that chest pain gone?"

I am overheated, but that little flitting pain hasn't come again.

Farmer continues, "And most of the time when people ask about triage, most of the time they're asking not with open hostility but deep distrust of our answer. They already have the answer. And that of course is the energy-draining process, because you understand that a substantial proportion of the questions are asked in a, you know, in a very, what's the word?"

"With an animus?"

"Yeah."

He's silent as we scrabble down a hilly section of the trail. At the bottom, he resumes. "The salary of a first-world doctor. How about that? Talk about all the money that could have been spent on other things, what about a doctor's salary?"

I laugh. "I hadn't thought of that."

"Well, of course. See, the truly humble think of that before they say the other. I'm not truly humble. I'm trying to be humble. So let me ask you another question. What is it that makes people not think that? Why doesn't a young American doctor say, 'Gee, my salary is five times what John's airplane ride cost. And I'm twenty-nine or thirty-some years old.' If you say that stuff out loud, you sound like an asshole. Whereas if you say the other stuff, you just sound thoughtful. Now what's wrong with that? What's wrong with this picture? If you say, Well, I just think how much could have been done with twenty thousand dollars, you sound thoughtful, sensible, you know, reasonable, rational, someone you really want on your side. However, if you were to point out, *But* a young attending physician makes *one hundred thousand* dollars, not twenty, and that's *five* times what it cost to try to save a boy's life—that just makes you sound like an asshole. Same world, same numbers, same figures, same currency. It's just, you know, I never have been able to figure it out. I mean, I've figured it out, but I realize now it takes *so much time* to get to that point, to explain it, without offending someone. So what are you thinkin'?"

"I like the line about the long defeat," I tell him.

"I would regard that as the basic stance of O for the P," he replies. "I don't care if we lose, I'm gonna try to do the right thing."

"But you're going to try to win."

"Of course! We're not, you know, masochistic. And then all the victories are gravy, you know? The other option is to be jaded because you've been fighting a defeat for eighteen years, and trying to stop it, at least save the elbow joint for Kenol, you know." He's referring to a current patient, a boy back in Cange whose hand got caught in a sugarcane press—a "low medieval device," Farmer called it—and ended up with gangrene. In the end, his arm had to be amputated above the elbow joint. (After the operation, he said he wanted a radio. Farmer bought him one on his latest Miami day. Zanmi Lasante will send him to school.)

"How's your chest?" Farmer asks.

It feels all right, in fact. But there is only one mouthful of water left in my jug, and Farmer has said he'd prefer that I not drink the unfiltered water Ti Jean is carrying. So, for the moment, I think I'd rather be thirsty.

Farmer goes on, "If we could identify losers like John, and not waste our time and energy on them, then we'd be all good, as they say in the States. Right? But the point of O for the P is that you never do that. You never risk that. Because before you turn your back on someone like John you have to be really really sure, and the more you learn about John's family the more you realize that the whole family, their whole—I mean, they're basically extinct, right? He was the last kid. They're extinct. His mother's bloodline is just gone. It sounds Darwinian, but you know what I mean. Shit, man, how can you be an O for the P doc and be willing to take that risk without all the data you can get? Every patient is a sign. Every patient is a test. Like this guy we just saw. The guy's living in dirt, the guy who needs Canadian crutches? You realize how much shit I'd get for that, Canadian crutches in rural Haiti?"

"Because they're not appropriate technology?"

"Yeah. Now you can see the critiques revealed for what they are. But I have to limit the amount of time I put into explaining all that or it just sucks your soul dry. If I spent all my time arguing, No, this man needs Canadian crutches *and* a roof *and* a floor. I mean, if you're only defensive. If you say, Fuck you, man, I already *built* a thousand houses in this country, how many have you built? That doesn't go anywhere either. But that's the very doctor they'd be criticizing, one who's already done his housing fellowship and his practicum in blah blah blah. If you spend all your time arguing about that stuff, defending yourself, you don't get your work done. It must mean *something* that Ti Jean doesn't talk about things like appropriate technology."

We are walking, Farmer has said, through what used to be rebel territory, during both Haiti's slave days and the years when the U.S. Marines occupied the country. It seems different from the areas near Cange. The farmyards and even the hilltops look a little more fertile, a little less bereft of soil and trees. But the land is just as crowded. We have been trudging through deep country, far from anything that could even be called a road, and yet there's hardly been a moment when other people haven't been in sight or just around the next turn in the trail.

We've forded one big river—pigs rooting in the banks, chunks of earth falling into the water, and irrationally, I felt as though I should catch the soil in my arms and put it back. I'm not sure how many hours we've been walking. It must be at least four. We've crossed ridge after ridge, and we're still encountering the works of PIH. Some are inanimate—a school that Zanmi Lasante built out here in the mountains—but mostly they're patients. I've lost count of their numbers, and we're still running into them. There are the fairly healthy-looking ones who say to Farmer in Creole, "Hi, my Doc," or "How's my Doc's little body today?" And patients who are works in progress. The most memorable for me is a girl whose neck and chest were burned some time ago. It looks as if the flesh on the lower part of her face had melted and then hardened into a beard of skin, the strands of the beard attaching her jaw and chin to her chest and shoulders more and more tightly as she's grown. Never mind the grotesque scarring, in another year or so, her mouth will be pulled permanently open. Unless she gets to a plastic surgeon. Farmer has been trying to arrange the necessary operations in the United States. "It's a *bwat*," he says.

"We getting close to Casse?" I ask.

"Well, you don't want to know just yet." He smiles. He stops and points to a hilltop in the distance. "Wait'll we get over that ridge. Then I'll break it to you. Khyber Pass. Ruby Ridge. I'm sorry. *Lord of the Rings*, Redhorn Pass. Smell this. It's campêche."

I drank my last sip of water some time ago, and I'm feeling slightly dizzy as we continue on. My mouth has grown so dry that I croak when I try to speak.

Farmer has noticed. He starts calling out, "Do you have oranges?" at every farmyard we pass. I end up sitting with my back against a tree, devouring six oranges, one right after the other. And when we finally reach Casse, a brown and dusty, dirt-street market town, constructed of wood and corrugated metal, Farmer feeds me Cokes.

"I can't tell you how much better I feel."

"Hydration," he says.

Zanmi Lasante's local health worker—a barefoot woman in a dress—shows us the way to Alcante's house. (Farmer waited for her to find us. He didn't ask the strangers in Casse for directions. "Because they're Hats, there would be no shortage of wrong answers. You learn that in year three or four.") Another half hour's walk and we arrive at the farm, which consists of a stand of millet, a cook shack with a three-rocks fireplace, and a hut made of what is known as wattle and daub—that is, dried mud and sticks. The roof is old banana bark, patched all over with rags.

"Alcante!" says Farmer. "I'm happy to see you."

"And I'm delighted to see you!" says the shiny little boy. He calls to his sisters, emerging from the hut, "Are there any more chairs here? We need more chairs."

"The little social director," Farmer says to me. "He's just so . . ." His voice trails off. He grins.

Alcante's father was shaving when we arrived—with a painted shard of glass for a mirror and a razor blade and no soap or water. He finishes the job: Gradually, the rest of the family emerges from the hut, and I am reminded of the routine at the circus in which an apparently endless stream of people comes out of a tiny car. I estimate the hut to be about ten feet by twenty, and I count ten souls who live in it. Farmer gazes at the hut. "Well, I guess I don't need to do a house inspection." He stares at it some more. "On a scale of one to ten, this is a one."

A long chat ensues. From it Farmer draws a variety of lessons for me. Of the several cases of TB in this family, only the father's was detectable by sputum smear. That is, his was the only case that involved the lungs and was contagious, the only epidemiologically significant case, the only kind of case that DOTS addresses. "So here's a house full of TB, where you only have one case according to the DOTS system," says Farmer. "The rest had extrapulmonary disease, which doesn't count. It can kill ya but it doesn't count." He adds, and for a moment he is back in Peru, "We never wanted to get rid of *las normas*, we just wanted to extend them, and add some flexibility."

There's also a sociopolitical lesson to draw, of course: "Look at Alcante's family. It's intact, the kids are bright and clever, and the father can't walk. And they just can't make it. It's fucking unfair. The woman who said to me years ago, Are you incapable of complexity? That was an epiphany for me. Are you going to punish people for thinking TB comes from sorcery? It's like the guy on our own team, a nice guy, who said he would help with a water project in a town here, but only if the people really showed they wanted it. What if that standard had been applied to me when I was a kid, before I knew that water could carry organisms that made people sick?"

He concludes the dismount, saying, "I'm glad we came, because now we know how grim it is and we can intervene aggressively."

I know what this means: a new house with a concrete floor and metal roof, further arrangements for improving the family's nutrition, school tuition for the kids. Here's a good deed in progress, and a perfect example of the Farmer method. First, you perform what he calls "the distal intervention" and cure the family of TB. Then you start changing the conditions that made them especially vulnerable to TB in the first place.

I am aware of other voices that would praise a trip like this for its good intentions, and yet describe it as an example of what is wrong with Farmer's approach. Here's an influential anthropologist, medical diplomat, public health administrator, epidemiologist, who has helped to bring new resolve and hope to some of the world's most dreadful problems, and he's just spent seven hours making house calls. How many desperate families live in Haiti? He's made this trip to visit two.

I think of the wealthy friend of Howard Hiatt's who balked at contributing to PIH because, while he knew about Farmer's work in Haiti and considered it impressive, he doubted anyone could reproduce it. I've heard variations on that theme. Farmer and Kim do things that no one else can do. Zanmi Lasante won't survive Farmer. Partners In Health is an organization that relies too much on a genius. All the serious, sympathetic critiques come down to these two arguments: Hiking into the hills to see just one patient or two is a dumb way for Farmer to spend his time, and even if it weren't, not many other people will follow his example, not enough to make much difference in the world.

But standard notions of efficiency, notions about cost-effectiveness, about big people performing big jobs, haven't worked so well themselves. Long ago in North Carolina, Farmer watched the nuns doing menial chores on behalf of migrant laborers, and in the years since he's come to think that a willingness to do what he calls "unglamorous scut work" is the secret to successful projects in places like Cange and Carabayllo. "And," he says, "another secret: a reluctance to do scut work is why a lot of my peers don't stick with this kind of work." In public health projects in difficult locales, theory often outruns practice. Individual patients get forgotten, and what seems like a small problem gets ignored, until it grows large, like MDR. "If you focus on individual patients," Jim Kim says, "you can't get sloppy."

That approach has worked for PIH. And I can imagine Farmer saying he doesn't care if no one else is willing to follow their example. He's still going to make these hikes, he'd insist, because if you say that seven hours is too long to walk for two families of patients, you're saying that their lives matter less than some others', and the idea that some lives matter less is the root of all that's wrong with the world. I think he undertakes what, earlier today, he called "journeys to the sick" in part because he has to, in order to keep going. "That's when I feel most alive," he told me once on an airplane, "when I'm helping people." He makes these house calls regularly and usually without *blan* witnesses, at times when no one from Harvard or WHO can see him kneeling on mud floors with his stethoscope plugged in. This matters to him, I think—to feel, at least occasionally, that he doctors in obscurity, so that he knows he doctors first of all because he believes it's the right thing to do.

If you do the right thing well, you avoid futility. His patients tend to get better. They all get comforted. And he carries off, among other things, images of them and their medieval huts. These refresh his passion and authority, so that he can travel a quarter of a million miles a year and scheme and write about the health of populations. Doctoring is the ultimate source of his power, I think. His basic message is simple: This person is sick, and I am a doctor. Everyone, potentially, can understand and sympathize, since everyone knows or imagines sickness personally. And it can't be hard for most people to imagine what it would be like to have no doctor, no hope of medicine. I think Farmer taps into a universal anxiety and also into a fundamental place in some troubled consciences, into what he calls "ambivalence," the often unacknowledged uneasiness that some of the fortunate feel about their place in the world, the thing he once told me he designed his life to avoid.

"The best thing about Paul is those hikes," Ophelia says. "You have to believe that small gestures matter, that they do add up." Earlier today Farmer said that he'd brought on others to fight "the long defeat." The numbers are impressive. They include priests and nuns and professors and secretaries and businessmen and church ladies and peasants like Ti Jean and also dozens of medical students and doctors, who have enlisted to work in places such as Cange and Siberia and the slums of Lima. Some of the students and doctors work for nothing, some earn much less than they could elsewhere, some raise their own salaries through grants. I once heard Farmer say that he hoped a day would come when he could do a good job just by showing up. It seems to me that time has already arrived. A great deal of what he's started goes on without him now, in Roxbury and Tomsk and Peru and, some of the year, in Haiti. Meanwhile, other definitions than the usual, of what can be done and what is reasonable to do in medicine and public health, have spread from him. They're still spreading, like ripples in a pond.

How does one person with great talents come to exert a force on the world? I think in Farmer's case the answer lies somewhere in the apparent craziness, the sheer impracticality, of half of everything he does, including the hike to Casse.

ADEOLA ONI-ORISAN

13 COUNTING IS COMPLICATED

The first section of this book described the fundamental challenges facing global health and emphasized the epidemiological methods used to understand those problems and better design solutions. As you see when you look at the websites of institutions like the World Health Organization, quantitative information is at the core of global public health. Surveillance data are useful for monitoring new health problems and evaluating progress in meeting global health goals.

However, it is critical to always remember that there are real human beings represented in those sterile-looking numbers, tables, and graphs. Disease rates and statistics on unnecessary premature mortality sometimes distract us from remembering the terrible suffering they represent: these statistics represent real human lives and deaths. This article represents a qualitative ethnographic study based upon on-the-ground observations; it provides narrative evidence (i.e., it tells a story) about how quantitative data are collected.

Global health data are valuable but are never exact. Medical anthropologists argue that data are "socially constructed." In other words, data are created by human beings, molded by biases in sampling, changed by operational definitions, inflected by competing priorities, and swayed by the fact that people do not always tell the truth. For example, health problems might be exaggerated to attract funding, while the success of an intervention might be exaggerated to make a program, an organization, or certain people look good.

Donors and international aid agencies demand "metrics" from their partners and employees. Constantly collecting these numbers represents a significant burden on some health-care workers, especially nurses and community health workers. Accountability may be important, but it also reflects differences in power. In this article, Adeola Oni-Orisan describes how, on a small scale, maternal mortality data in Nigeria were influenced by politics on multiple levels. On the international level, decreasing maternal mortality was a significant focus of the United Nation's **Millennium Development Goals.**

Improvement of maternal mortality statistics, the topic of this article, requires more than improvement in health care. Maternal mortality is unnecessary and preventable, but its causes are complex, and, as this article shows, data about these deaths may be unreliable.

As you read this article, consider the following questions:

- **Why was Blessing's death not counted? Consider both the technical reasons given and the political reasons behind the decision.**
- **How might the failure to count cases like Blessing's affect the overall assessment of Nigeria's campaign to reduce maternal mortality?**
- **How are global health agendas linked to monetary resources and the local acceptance of externally designed programs? What does this say about political power?**
- **How did the obligation to count impede clinical care? Why might counting be more important in public health than in clinical medicine?**

CONTEXT

Adeola Oni-Orisan is a PhD candidate in medical anthropology at the University of California, San Francisco, and is also completing her MD degree at the Harvard Medical School. She is interested in sub-Saharan Africa (specifically Nigeria) and a wide variety of research topics including gender, maternal health, the politics of international aid, and the intersection of ritual and **health behaviors**. A previous version of this article appeared in the volume *Metrics: What Counts in Global Health*, edited by Vincanne Adams (Durham, NC: Duke University Press, 2016). Many of the ethnographic studies in that volume describe the ways in which global health data are "constructed" and interpreted.

"The hospital is politically motivated," Dr. Oloke informed me amid the morning bustle of activity at the Hospital for Mothers and Children (HMC). Women were lining up along the hospital's concrete walls, waiting for registration to open. Some carried babies tied to their backs with printed fabrics while others with rounded bellies shifted uncomfortably in place. Meanwhile the staff was setting up for what would be yet another day of caring for hundreds of women and children. Fresh-faced nurses in pastel-colored scrubs were taking over for their weary night-shift colleagues, and the doctors, including Dr. Oloke, were collecting in small groups according to rank, swapping stories about the previous night.

On this morning there was troubling news to be shared. A woman had died overnight. Blessing, a forty-one-year-old mother of three, had delivered her fourth healthy baby at a police clinic nearby, but difficulty arose during the delivery of the placenta. The clinicians could not remove it entirely, and Blessing started to bleed uncontrollably likely from where the torn placenta remained attached to her uterus. She was referred to the Hospital for Mothers and Children, but according to Dr. Oloke, she didn't arrive there until three hours later. When she finally arrived in a personal car, she was accompanied by her husband, some relatives, and a unit of blood meant to be transfused into her at the hospital. Dr. Oloke was waiting in the emergency room when Blessing was carried in. He recounted to me that just as he approached her he saw that she was "white, cold, gasped, and stopped breathing." He could do nothing more than declare her deceased.

The following morning, Dr. Oloke had been called into the hospital chief medical director's office. "[Dr. Adetunde] read my documentation [and] concluded [Blessing] was dead even before she came in even though her last breath was in my presence," he told me as he walked out of the director's office. I asked him why the director would come to this conclusion, and it was then that he declared, "The hospital is politically motivated. She would have been an *unnecessary* mortality."

It was the beginning of the month and the hospital was preparing for its monthly mortality and morbidity review. This was a meeting that all the hospital employees, from doctors to gardeners, were expected to attend in order to review the hospital's performance and present the total number of mortalities for the previous month. These numbers would be used to tabulate the local government area's in-hospital maternal mortality rates. Since the hospital had only had one other death that month, adding Blessing's death would have doubled the maternal mortality rate. But because she had left the police clinic still breathing, she would not be added to their death toll either. Thus her death would not be counted. As far as the official health facility records and state government reports were concerned, Blessing did not count.

The story of the death of Blessing is all too familiar. Similar anecdotes of maternal mortality are told in global health classrooms and conferences all over the world. Stories like these, with anonymized victims and struggling health care providers, have a way of emotionally priming listeners for the devastating numbers that will follow, the astounding rates at which women die giving birth in lower-income countries. Listeners are meant to multiply the story they have heard by the regional mortality rates that usually follow to arrive at the appropriate level of dismay, gaining a feeling of urgency in the process. Along the way from anecdotal cases to national statistics to global health textbooks, the sometimes staggering, sometimes subtle differences in the circumstances of each particular person who dies, each woman who does not make it through childbirth alive, are lost.

Dr. Oloke's story gives us a little more to think about. His story and that of Blessing suggest that the numbers do much more than account for death. They even do more than simply obscure the experiences of women in childbirth. His story tells us that as a result of the power that they are invested with, these numbers can become political instruments. Put another way, at times these numbers do a better job of reflecting a government's political goals than the facts of the situation they purport to tell us about.

The global health industry's dependence on specific kinds of quantitative knowledge—particularly numerical data in maternal health—influences both healing and local governance. This article is about the Healthy Mothers Healthy Babies (HMHB) program in a southwestern state in Nigeria. My discussion is based on research interviews with doctors, nurses, patients, and government officials in HMHB health facilities, where I also engaged in ethnographic fieldwork.

By exploring both local political decision-making and everyday clinical encounters, I draw attention to the ways counting is complicated. That is to say, the numerical metrics required by global health funders today not only have the power to determine which interventions are successes and which are failures, which will be funded and which will not, but they also carry the political authority to determine who will get reelected to office, who will be promoted to chief medical director of a hospital, and who will win a government contract. Metrics, in other words, carry a political efficacy that comes to bear on how health care is delivered.

Politics and metrics are thus entangled in the push for numerical evidence of effectiveness. Demands for accountability in global maternal health encourage states to organize themselves as recipient nations in and around problems concerning not health per se, but numbers meant to represent health. When local sovereignty—local political authority grounded in territory—is tethered to the numbers games that arrive with global health grant-giving organizations, practices of accountability, cost efficiency, and translatability can create perverse incentives for local politicians.

Linking Numbers and Dollars

The previous governor of this state in southwestern Nigeria, a physician and a former state commissioner for health, began making good on his campaign promises to improve the state's health system almost as soon as he took office in early 2009. Since then, the state has in many ways organized itself around agendas set by the United Nations, the World Health Organization (WHO), and other leading international health organizations. One of the administration's first initiatives, the HMHB program, was the governor's specific response to a World Bank study, the 2008 Nigeria Demographic and Health Survey (NDHS). The NDHS study found that this Nigerian state was one of the furthest from reaching the United Nation's Millennium Development Goal 5, which aimed to improve maternal health by achieving universal access to reproductive health and reducing maternal deaths to three quarters of the rate in 1990 by 2015. HMHB revamped the state's provision of maternal and child health care, by offering free biomedical services to all pregnant women and children under five.

But the HMHB program represents more than a reaction by health planners to health concerns. HMHB also represents the outcome of a new alliance in the structures of funding for global health. While government programs have long been dominated by global health agendas that link monetary resources to acceptance of externally designed plans, it is worth exploring how this process continues today through various forms of counting.

Less than two years after the launch of HMHB, the state became the recipient of a $60 million health investment loan from the World Bank. This is not entirely surprising since it was the World Bank that sponsored the NDHS, the study that motivated the creation of HMHB in the first place. At this point, the state began gathering its own data. They found that the maternal mortality rate, originally estimated at 545 deaths per 100,000 live births in the 2008 NDHS, had been reduced to 253, a more than 50 percent reduction. With this quantitative evidence, the program gained international recognition and has since received additional grants from the Ford Foundation and the Bill and Melinda Gates Foundation.

With the links between health statistics and international agency financial support established, the government naturally sought to keep the grant money flowing in by continuing to supply the data needed to affirm the impact of this money. On a Fall 2011 visit to Nigeria, Bill Gates met with President Goodluck Jonathan to launch the Governor's Immunization Leadership Challenge. The initiative was aimed at eradicating new cases of polio from Nigeria by the end of 2012, and an award for the states that immunized the most babies was set at $500,000, with the promise of an additional $250,000 if the government of the winning states made a matching contribution. The funds, potentially $1 million in total, were to be put toward further improving health care and delivery in the winning states. Of the six states that emerged as winners in early 2013, the state that had recently launched the HMHB initiative came in first with the highest recorded rates of polio vaccination in Nigeria. The achievement was highly publicized in a year in which the governor was up for reelection. Several local news organizations reported on the state's success, applauding its governor as the best performing governor in the country.

These patterns of funding and accountability seen in the race to stop polio spilled over into other maternal and child health efforts. In a meeting between high-level state government officials and representatives from Family Health Organization, a Nigerian nongovernmental organization chosen by the Gates Foundation to ensure proper usage of the contest winnings, attendees deliberated over how the contest winnings should be used. While the principal problem discussed was the fact that women still choose to deliver at church-based birthing centers and with traditional birth attendants (TBAs), the meeting attendees agreed that money should go to scaling up the HMHB program. One high-level state government official explained, "If we improve facilities, we can improve facility deliveries by 20 to 30 percent, . . . [and] TBAs will naturally phase out." Caught up in the fervor of success that was mapped out in the polio contest, they sought to align themselves with more easily quantifiable goals (number of births in facilities) rather than orient themselves toward the particularities of a pressing local problem (for example, by improving TBA training or supporting care at church-based birthing centers).

What is interesting about this case is how the numbers, once produced, became instruments for political mobility. The Gates Foundation Immunization Leadership Challenge and the subsequent events in this state tied successful health statistics to the problem of securing resources to do any health work at all. The numbers here represented more than simple metrics to help decide which interventions worked and which did not; they became indices of successful governance and were the conduit for securing more aid. Let us not forget that the official name of the contest was the Governor's Immunization Leadership Challenge. The statistics generated in the polio campaign became quickly visible not just in Millennium Development Goals status reports and Gates Foundation annual letters but also in the local state's election campaigns, helping voters to discern good leaders from bad ones. The problem with the increasing reliance on numbers, however, is that once they circulate in this political way, it becomes difficult to question them. Their power multiplies.

With so many international dollars at stake, it is no wonder that maintaining and managing "the numbers" is seen as a primary task of politicians. The specifics of how this is accomplished are important to track, as the consequences for the health of those who are not counted are potentially devastating.

The Stakes beyond Health

International donor reliance on quantitative metrics for accountability creates perverse incentives for individuals in recipient countries to produce numbers in specific ways—often in ways that are more about political than health goals. Those who stand to gain politically if they can produce evidence of a successful intervention have an incentive to provide numbers that demonstrate success. HMHB has brought millions of dollars into the state, boosting the economy and creating jobs. While there is positive value in these changes, the fact that where the money goes is assessed exclusively with numbers can also be problematic. Everyone, from patients to doctors and government officials, becomes complicit in the push to produce good data, that is, data that show improvement. Bad data, data that might show weakness in the system, are frequently discounted or kept invisible. The business of global health creates pressure for "death data to 'go missing,'" (cf. Erikson 2012: 379) as seen in Blessing's story.

Some Nigerians are able to capitalize on incoming sources of funding, while others do not share in the spoils. The fates and fortunes of many individuals are tied to the success of the program. One of those people is the previous governor of the state, mentioned above. He ran on a platform that featured his state health achievements and is the first governor to win a second term in this state. Along with the commissioner of health, he travels across the globe, presenting lectures on the success of HMHB at conferences in places ranging from Washington, DC to Beijing. Citizens of this state refer to HMC and the HMHB program as "the governor's brainchild." Patients associate the care they receive at the hospital with the governor and the state's prosperity, and many enthusiastically support the hospital, rejoicing in its reported successes. The governor and his wife were wildly popular, drawing considerable attention at even the sight of their motorcade.

Many of the doctors I spoke to at HMC also associate the HMHB program and health care with the potential for political achievement. When asked what specialty they wanted to go into after finishing their intern year, the most common answer was, "Politics." Doctors aspire to complete a residency, which is not actually a requirement to practice in Nigeria, or a master's degree in business administration or public health from an overseas university as a means of rising up the medical ladder and, subsequently, the political ladder. The current commissioner of health was previously the chief medical director of a hospital before obtaining a foreign degree and being appointed to office.

Hopes of benefiting from the success of the HMHB program did not end with doctors. Over lunch, the commissioner of health's driver, Taiwo, told me he had been working for the ministry for ten years, but, he assured me, the present commissioner had been his "best boss." Taiwo said he had learned so much from the commissioner and that the commissioner made it a point of taking care of his employees. "We are all praying for them to nominate him to the federal office. Maybe Goodluck Jonathan will just pick him [to be the nation's minister of health], and we will all just go with him to Abuja!"

Individuals and private companies that previously had little to do with health care have begun to shift their focus to health in order to win government contracts and profit from the HMHB program rollout. I spent one afternoon with the commissioner of health as he sifted through a foot-high stack of mail. There were dozens of proposals from both NGOs and private companies. One man wrote to request more money for the gas station that the state had acquired from him in order to have the land to build a second HMC. Other companies wrote proposals to provide the new hospitals with everything from flat screen TVs to continuing education seminars for staff. The careers of many individuals are contingent on the continued success of the program; they rely on the production of specific kinds of data to show that the program has done what it set out to do. And this is what the quantitative data collected are effective at doing. With so much relying on the state's maternal mortality rates, it is not surprising that everyone becomes complicit in projecting a successful HMHB program.

The chief medical director of HMC, Dr. Adetunde, is not alone in wanting to discount Blessing's death. Erikson (2012: 373) reminds us that in the global health business, "whether statistics are accurate enough to improve health is less important than whether statistics are performed and work to enable economic systems." Statistics "enable other things of value, like gainful employment and profit-making" (373). This leads to systems of data production that do not always align with local needs. If numbers that show positive outcomes become compulsory in the eyes of the donors who keep programs in nations like Nigeria alive, little room is left for questioning the numbers or how they are collected. Yet, when numbers become essential to local political and economic success—as I illustrated with the governor's popularity, several doctors' aspirations, and private business contract winners—it becomes important to ask how the numbers must change, how they must be produced, and what purposes they must serve far beyond the problems of women like Blessing.

Limiting Possibilities for Care

Aid industry mandates to collect data as "proof of success" force individuals to collect, analyze, and make decisions based on numerical data in ways that can constrain doctors and hurt patients. Even the very act of gathering data can affect the ways data collectors are oriented toward and interact with patients. The possibilities for caregiving, a supposed primary goal of global health, are undermined by the need to provide data that pleases both overseas funding sources and local political agendas. As Adams (2013: 55) notes, the turn in global health communities toward an insistence on numerical data leads to a "shift in priorities in caregiving practices in public health such that 'people [no longer] come first.'"

The demand for data that can be used to prove the success of HMHB has not only changed the way women receive care (in ways that are not always beneficial to the patients); it has also constrained the way doctors are allowed to practice. The day after Eid, the feast at the end of the Muslim holy month of Ramadan and a federal holiday in Nigeria, a man named Sunday approached Dr. Olamide, the chief medical director of the newly built HMC in his town. Sunday explained that his wife, Funmi, needed to be seen urgently. That morning she had started coughing, and the sutures from the cesarean section she had the week before had opened up. He claimed that nobody would attend to her in the emergency department. Dr. Olamide told Sunday to go back to the emergency department and that the nurses there would help him. When, a few minutes later, Dr. Olamide noticed that Funmi was still not being helped, he charged down the hall to see what was the delay. He stormed into the emergency room, flinging reprimands at the nurse, "Why was this patient not seen? This is an emergency!"

Dr. Olamide lead Funmi into a makeshift examination "room" in the corner of the emergency room, surrounded the bed with blue cloth dividers, and asked her to lie down. Pulling up her top, we were all shocked to see a loop of Funmi's bowels protruding from the incision in her abdomen. Dr. Olamide yelled for other doctors to come help place an IV, start her on antibiotics, draw blood to be cross-matched in preparation for surgery, and cover the exposed intestines with sterile gauze. Funmi lay on the bed, becoming more terrified with every exclamation from Dr. Olamide.

In the aftermath, I talked to everyone involved in the incident. When I asked Funmi what happened, she explained that in the morning when she was coughing, her belly had burst open. She said she hadn't told anyone in the emergency room that her insides had broken through her skin because no one had asked. She told them only that she wanted to see a doctor. Both the nurse and the intern said they hadn't know that Funmi had a burst abdomen and that they were just following protocol. Before being seen by a nurse, a patient is normally expected to go to hospital registration to get a registration card and casebook. The casebook contains the patient's medical history, and she cannot be seen without it. Detailed records must be taken at the start of every patient encounter. Once the casebook is obtained, a nurse can see the patient, followed by a doctor.

While these expectations for record-keeping protocol might seem commonplace and even reassuring to the outsider, demands for accountability can structure and shape how medicine gets practiced in hospitals. One might find oversight like this in any emergency ward in any country. However, in this state the overwhelming presence of the HMHB program (and its need to prove its success in order to ensure continued funding) became a particularly strong structuring force in determining how clinical care was carried out, how triage was determined, and how patients were made visible or invisible. The dedication to record-keeping outweighed a dedication to the patient so that there was no room for improvising on behalf of the patient even in her pressing medical circumstances. The worry is that for hospitals like those in the HMHB program, where staff are trained to consider the urgency of recording data on patients to be just as important as attending to their health needs, these record-keeping operations can sometimes get in the way of appropriate care. Possibilities for successful clinical care are sometimes impeded by the compulsion to produce data. At the same time, it is this compulsion to produce data for the HMHB program that is vital to the survival of not only hospitals but also careers like that of Dr. Olamide.

Younger doctors, not yet caught up in HMHB propaganda, were particularly vocal about the conflicts of interest inherent in the program. They expressed discontent with their supervisors' political pandering at the expense of patient well-being. They considered such pandering a form of "politics" in the sense that they suspected their supervisors were depending on the success of HMHB for personal gain and thus to become potential candidates for promotion. Many also recognized that these successes depended on a process of data collection that was at odds with the notion of best practices that they had been taught in medical school. Contestation between caregivers was often aroused by the explicit perception that decisions were being made on the basis of the need for certain kinds of numbers and certain kinds of outcomes.

These same doctors often talked about how the relationship between the hospital, the HMHB initiative, and the government's office was constraining their medical decisions in ways that were not necessarily medically justifiable. Recognizing that the numbers that HMHB strives to produce are not neutral, caregivers felt constrained in the care they give by a political vision and global processes that are beyond their control.

Conclusion

The story of the HMHB program in southwestern Nigeria is one where the state gains economic power through interactions with global health agencies. The regional government works with multilateral development agencies and not-for-profit private grant-making foundations to ensure its own survival. Local health actors aspire to become ministers, politicians, and leaders who will govern by way of the demands set by the agendas of international donors.

Because of the way development aid is tied to productivity and success, the work of health development increasingly relies on numbers to not only guide but also to give support to specific health activities. The demand for certain kinds of success-showing numbers forms a sort of governance over both clinical practices and political processes. That is, on their way to affecting health outcomes, the numbers have a way of producing political effects that exceed the mere production of numerical facts. This is not simply a case of neutral numbers falling into the wrong hands. The numbers themselves are produced and performed in ways that imbue them with political efficacy. The work they do—a result of the work done to produce them—can have real consequences for both how patients are treated and who wins elections.

I am not suggesting that the call for accountability underlying the steadily growing push for a universal metrics in global health is necessarily a bad thing. However, when the numbers go unquestioned, when they are allowed to stand for much more than they were originally intended to measure and become instruments of political aggrandizement, we should be wary. Numbers are seductive in their seamless utility. They turn complicated, messy local realities into manageable, translatable, comparable figures. However, these same qualities give the increasing primacy of numbers in global health an ominous power that can elide clinical realities, compromise care, and hide some kinds of death.

Relying only on numbers to create global health agendas has the potential for detrimental effects. The HMHB program demonstrates that numbers are not only hard to collect in an unbiased manner but may not accurately describe a situation, as was the case for Blessing. At every level of data production, efforts to direct flows of money and political power weaken claims to objectivity. The point is this: there is no such thing as objectivity in this sort of situation. There are only numbers and politics. Recognizing how these work as well as when and how they don't is more important than ever. When doing global health means doing global health *research*, certain health solutions and health practices that cannot be measured numerically are left out. Blessing was uncounted because she was marked as dying in transit and her death would have marred the hospital's claim to success. Money is spent on building more government health facilities rather than negotiating solutions with traditional birth attendants or church-based facilities because the numbers of women who attend government health facilities can be more easily counted and monitored. Meanwhile up to 80 percent of women in much of Nigeria still deliver outside of a hospital or clinic.

The care they get is unquantifiable by global health standards and thus remains unaccounted for.

My hope in presenting cases like this is that questions about how we produce numbers and demonstrate accountability will be more carefully considered, particularly as the global health industry continues to mandate that we use numbers-based ways of knowing the world in relation to a diverse and complex set of health problems and situations. Rather paradoxically numerical standards for effectiveness can sometimes create incentives for recipient countries and organizations to "perform good data" in ways that limit potentially productive possibilities for health care.

REFERENCES

Adams, V. 2013 "Evidence Based Global Public Health: Subjects, Profits, Erasures" in J. Beihl and A. Petryna, eds. *When people come first: Critical studies in global health.* Princeton University Press.

Erikson, Susan. L. (2012). Global Health Business: The Production and Performativity of Statistics in Sierra Leone and Germany. *Medical Anthropology,* 31(4), 367–384.

SECTION 3 CASES FOR TEACHING AND LEARNING

Visit the companion website, www.oup.com/us/brown-closser, for direct links to the featured online resources.

Mary Applegate and Debra Blog, *Maternal Mortality*

In this case, students must classify maternal deaths in the United States. The system described here is interesting to compare with what is happening in Adeola Oni-Orisan's description of counting maternal mortality in Nigeria.

Brooks et al., *The Global Trachoma Mapping Project*

This case describes the process of developing a surveillance and mapping system for trachoma cases globally.

Centers for Disease Control and Prevention, *Establishing an Injury Surveillance System*

In this case, students must design a surveillance system for injury surveillance in children in Massachusetts and then use data to determine what public health priorities should be. Students practice calculating years of Life Lost, which can also be helpful in understanding the Disability Adjusted Life Years concept. Students can learn about sources of current health data by being asked to update the information on page 4.

Cibula et al., *Community Health Assessment: Onandaga County, New York and Pitt County, North Carolina*

In these two cases (similar except for the setting), students go through the process of deciding how to carry out a community health assessment in New York or North Carolina, including determining what indicators to use and figuring out how to collect data.

Madore et al., *Electronic Medical Records at the ISS Clinic in Mbarra, Uganda*

In this case, students learn about keeping electronic records for HIV/AIDS cases in Uganda. It addresses the political and funding aspects of sustaining disease surveillance programs.

SECTION 3 VIDEOS AND WEB RESOURCES

Visit the companion website, **www.oup.com/us/brown-closser**, for direct links to the featured online resources.

Gapminder

This site is home to a wealth of resources about historical and current disease distribution and health inequalities. The interactive data in the "Gapminder Tools" feature are great to explore; the "Dollar Street" feature is a compelling way to investigate global inequality; and a variety of videos make demographics accessible and fascinating.

The Life Equation

This feature-length film follows a woman with cervical cancer in Guatemala and a physician in Nepal to explore the logic and the moral dilemmas of cost-effectiveness reasoning. The film's website also has a wealth of video and material that walks students through the main ideas of the film, from information on how DALYs are calculated to poignant vignettes that illustrate key dilemmas in cost-effectiveness reasoning.

Data Visualizations – Institute for Health Metrics and Evaluation

The Institute for Health Metrics and Evaluation (IHME) has a number of fascinating data visualizations: for example, exploring health in the United States at the county level and looking at global trends in tobacco use.

Our World in Data – Max Roser

A source for interactive maps based on IHME's burden of disease estimates.

If It Were My Home

This website allows students to calculate demographic and other characteristics of one country in comparison to another. For example, "if Italy were your home instead of the United States you would be 69.86% more likely to be unemployed; make 43.94% less money; be 87.54% less likely to be in prison; spend 65.91% less money on health care; be 78.95% less likely to be murdered; be 46.35% less likely to die in infancy; live 2.47 years longer."

Worldometers

This website tracks estimated deaths by many major causes in real time. It can be used to quickly illustrate the scale of major issues like HIV and smoking.

Health Map – Boston Children's Hospital

An interactive website that visualizes locations of outbreaks of disease around the world. Since this site mostly pulls information from Internet sources, it is not comprehensive but it is an interesting tool for students to discuss as part of a larger conversation about surveillance methods.

Global Health Estimates – PLOS Collections

The PLOS Medicine Collection of papers debating the uses of global health estimates is an excellent academic resource for more advanced students interested in the debate around the uses of data in Global Health. For a more broadly accessible introduction to these issues, see *The Life Equation*.

PART

2

Ecological Determinants of Health

SECTION

4

Water

This section considers one of the fundamental requirements for human life: water. The other fundamental requirements for life —air and food—are the subjects of the next sections. There is a saying in medicine about the "rule of threes" for survival: in general, a person can live for three minutes without air, three days without water, and three weeks without food.

Going without water is, of course, lethal. More than half of your body weight is water. Humans must maintain a balance of fluids, so the amount of liquid one needs depends on how much that person is losing because of factors like temperature and physical activity. In extreme conditions, a body can lose more than one liter of fluid in a single hour. As we saw in the reading on infant diarrhea dehydration deaths (Reading 5), the replacement of body fluids (with the correct mineral balance) is a key aspect of medical care for diarrheal illness both in the hospital and at home.

Many people live in areas where there is not enough water for either drinking or hygiene. Living with water insecurity is terrible and unhealthy—including for mental health—as explored in Reading 15.

It is also severely detrimental to health when the water one has access to is contaminated. Contaminated water, especially when drinking water is contaminated by sewage or human feces, is a major cause of disease and death throughout the world. In Reading 2, we discussed how fecal material infected the water supply in a neighborhood in 19th-century London, but this kind of contamination is continually recurring, like in an outbreak of cholera in Haiti in 2010. Chapter 14 discusses these issues.

Water contamination is not just about infectious disease. Chapter 16 describes the case of Flint, Michigan, where disadvantaged minority populations were exposed to the dangerous heavy metal of lead, which can cause damage to the nervous system, learning disabilities, shorter stature, impaired hearing, and problems in red blood cells. This is the kind of water contamination that would be less likely to occur in a white majority, wealthy, and politically important place. What happened in Flint reminds us that it is difficult to separate health, economics, and politics.

» CONCEPTUAL TOOLS «

- The World Health Organization defines "**environmental health**" as "those aspects of human health, including quality of life, that are determined by physical, chemical, biological, social, and psychosocial factors in the environment." The field of environmental health aims to evaluate and prevent these health problems.
- The burdens of environmental issues do not fall equally on all populations. As events like the Flint water crisis (described in this section of the book) illustrate, disadvantaged populations often bear the brunt of environmental issues. **Environmental justice** is the effort to ensure that all populations are equally protected from environmental health risks.

WATER

- **Clean water, quality sanitation, and good hygiene can dramatically improve health. Water, sanitation, and hygiene (WASH)** is a field within global health that works to improve water and sanitation quality and access to achieve health impacts. While the sector has branched out into addressing other problems, at the core of the WASH sector is the prevention of the spread of diseases that are transmitted through the fecal–oral route by maintaining clean water, containing feces (sanitation), and promoting hygienic practices.
- **Humans live in a world of microbes.** These microorganisms are affected by ecology. For example, *Vibrio cholerae*, the bacteria that causes **cholera**, can live in brackish or marine waters in many parts of the world; depending on the ecology of the area, it may be plentiful or absent entirely. While people may get cholera from natural sources (like eating poorly cooked shellfish), because cholera is transmitted fecal–orally from person to person, it most commonly spread in areas with poor WASH.
- **Many waterborne diseases have fecal–oral transmission.** This means that a disease-causing agent like a virus or bacteria is transmitted from person to person by getting excreted in the feces of one person and then by a second person ingesting a tiny amount of those feces into their mouths. That second person then gets infected. This happens more often than we like to think about. You have probably experienced a disease with fecal–oral transmission in the recent past; most diarrheas, whether they are viral, bacterial, or protozoal, are transmitted via the fecal–oral route. Many other diseases, including polio, cholera, *E. Coli*, and *Salmonella*, are transmitted this way too.
- How do those feces get into people's mouths? There are lots of ways: for example, in the United States, undetected diaper leaks are one way this happens. But the major culprits globally are the **Four Fs: fluids, fields, flies, and fingers**. Examine Figure CT4.1. If you were in a rural village in Nigeria, can you think of how fecal–oral transmission for each of the four Fs could occur? What about in the place you live now? Can you think of ways the transmission could be stopped?

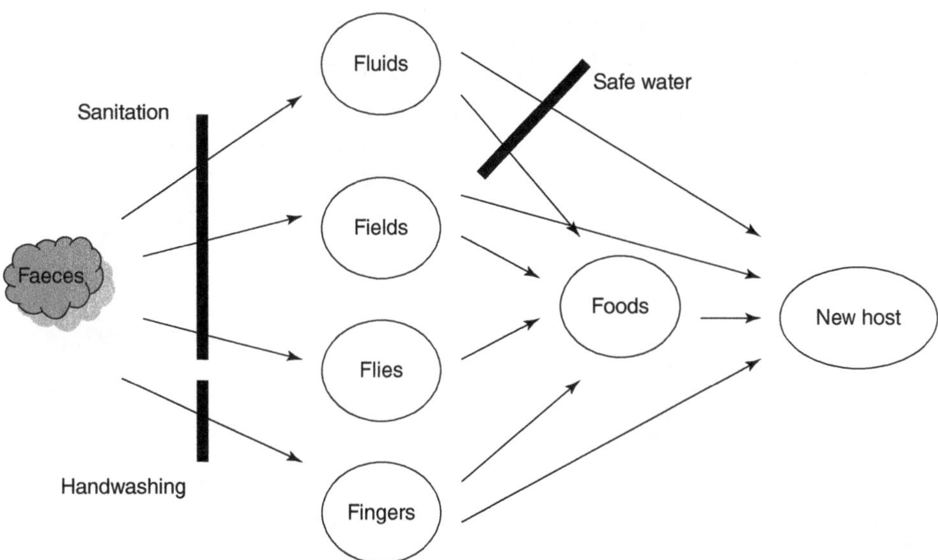

FIGURE CT4.1 Fecal–Oral Disease Transmission Pathways and Interventions to Break Them.
Source: © 2010 Mara D, Lane J, Scott B, Trouba D (2010) Sanitation and Health. PLoS Med 7(11): e1000363. This is an open-access article distributed under the terms of the Creative Commons Attribution License, which permits unrestricted use, distribution, and reproduction in any medium, provided the original author and source are credited.

- **Without good sanitation facilities in an area, fecal–oral transmission happens much more frequently.** While "sanitation" can have a lot of meanings (e.g., in the United States, people who pick up garbage can be called "sanitation workers"), in global health, sanitation generally refers to the safe disposal of human fecal matter. For example, if people defecate in the open—in spaces like fields, forests, or clearings between buildings—fecal run-off can end up in drinking water. Also, flies will probably land on those feces, and those same flies may also land on food. Even simple latrines with a slab or platform over a hole in the ground can significantly reduce fecal–oral disease transmission. (Toilets attached to sewage systems, septic tanks, or other safe disposal systems are, of course, much better, since buried feces can seep into the groundwater, infecting it.)
- **Open defecation is very common in many rural areas globally**. Part of the reason for this is that the basic hole-in-the-ground type latrines that very poor people can afford to build are sometimes very unpleasant to use: they can smell awful, be swarming with flies, and afford little or no privacy. The people who use them often are responsible for emptying out tanks or storage systems; they often cannot afford to hire someone else and understandably do not want to do so themselves. Going in the open air may be a much more pleasant alternative. Unfortunately, such open defecation contributes to the fecal–oral transmission of disease. In urban areas, the problem is more likely to be **open sewers/drains** that don't keep fecal matter away from flies or from water sources, or insufficiently treated sewage being dumped directly into water sources.

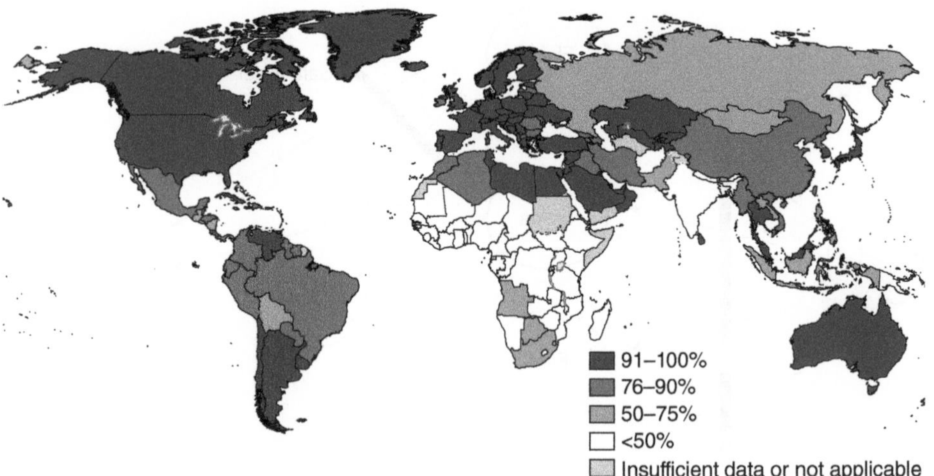

FIGURE CT4.2 Proportion of the Population Using Improved Sanitation Facilities in 2015.
In forty-seven countries, areas or territories, less than half the population uses improved sanitation in 2015.

Image source: UNICEF and World Health Organization. *25 Years: Progress on Sanitation and Drinking Water: 2015 Update and MDG Assessment,* http://apps.who.int/iris/bitstream/10665/177752/1/9789241509145_eng.pdf?ua=1.

- As Figure CT4.2 shows, many people worldwide do not have access to improved sanitation. In fact, nearly two and a half *billion* people worldwide do not have access to improved sanitation facilities (meaning, e.g., they have only a hole in the ground for a latrine, or they go outside). And, as you might expect, these are the poorest people in the world's poorest countries.
- Globally, access to sanitation is better in urban than in rural areas. About a quarter of people who live in rural areas defecate in the open. But this number is a lot lower than it was 25 years ago.
- In addition to good sanitation, getting drinking water from a clean and protected source is another way to stop fecal–oral transmission. In many areas of poor countries, the infrastructure to provide such water does not exist (Figure CT4.3).
- **There has been enormous progress on this front in the last 25 years.** In fact, more than a third of the world has gotten access to clean drinking water in that time period. More work remains to be done, but a huge amount of progress has been made.
- The result of subpar water and sanitation coverage is dramatic. The IHME estimates that substandard WASH was responsible for almost 2 million deaths in 2015. Improved WASH can eliminate this problem.
- **Water insecurity, when people do not have access to enough water, is a serious problem worldwide. Water-washed diseases** are diseases that occur because people do not have enough water to thoroughly clean their hands and faces

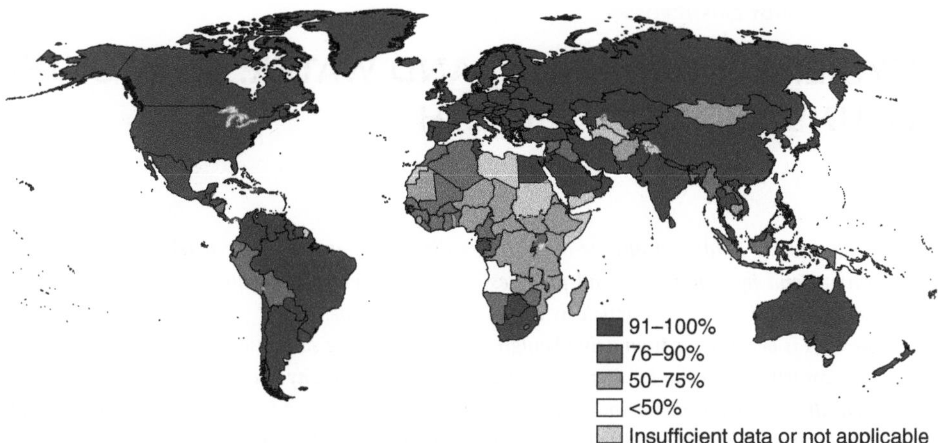

FIGURE CT4.3 Proportion of the Population Using Improved Drinking Water Sources in 2015.

Countries in which less than 50 percent of the population uses improved drinking water sources are all located in sub-Saharan Africa and Oceania.

Image source: UNICEF and World Health Organization. *25 Years: Progress on Sanitation and Drinking Water: 2015 Update and MDG Assessment,* http://apps.who.int/iris/bitstream/10665/177752/1/9789241509145_eng.pdf?ua=1

regularly. This means that both water quality and water quantity are important health issues. One important water-washed disease is trachoma, an eye infection that is common when people do not have enough water to wash their faces. Repeated trachoma infections can end in blindness. Nearly 2 million people globally have vision impairment or blindness as a result of trachoma.

JAMIE BARTRAM AND SANDY CAIRNCROSS

14 HYGIENE, SANITATION, AND WATER: FORGOTTEN FOUNDATIONS OF HEALTH

This article evaluates the burden of disease owing to water, sanitation, and hygiene issues, and proposes some potential solutions. Much of this article is about diarrheal disease. This is because far from being benign, diarrhea is a huge contributor to the burden of disease globally. Diarrheal disease is estimated to be the fifth biggest contributor to years of life lost (YLL). This means that of all the diseases in the world, diarrhea is number five in terms of its global contribution to loss of life. Diarrhea kills mostly very young children and infants, particularly those who are malnourished.

Diarrhea is really your body's response to infection—it happens because your body is doing its best to flush an invading pathogen out of your gut. Children die not from their infections per se, but from dehydration resulting from diarrhea. As is discussed in Chapter 5, oral rehydration therapy (ORT) is a lifesaving and inexpensive strategy that can save the lives of infants and children with diarrhea. But, particularly since diarrhea can exacerbate problems of malnutrition, it would be better if they did not get the infections that cause diarrhea in the first place.

Diarrhea is caused by a range of pathogens, from bacteria to viruses to protozoa. What all of these agents have in common is ***fecal–oral transmission****. The life-threatening dehydration that diarrhea causes can be treated with ORT (Reading 5), but that solution does nothing about the ultimate cause of the problem. Fecal–oral transmission of infectious disease is a question of water and sanitation infrastructure and the obligation of nations to provide clean water to their citizens.*

As this article argues, improving sanitation and water supply can prevent a range of diseases beyond diarrhea. This includes ***waterborne*** *diseases with fecal–oral transmission like polio and hepatitis A, E, and F (other kinds of hepatitis have other kinds of transmission—many are bloodborne). Improving water supply can also prevent diseases that are* ***water-washed****—that is, they rely on people having an adequate supply of water to maintain good hygiene.*

Improving sanitation can also break the transmission pattern of many parasitic worms. Hookworm is one common example; it relies mainly on ***open defecation*** *to maintain its life cycle. Its eggs are in the stool of infected people. If those people go to the bathroom outside, the larvae will grow in the soil. If someone walks through that soil barefoot, the larvae can infect that person through their feet, later developing into worms in the small intestine, beginning the cycle again. Basic sanitation improvements in rural areas can prevent these parasitic infections.*

Beyond infrastructure improvements, the article also mentions handwashing. The importance of handwashing is a central public health tenet because it prevents the spread of many different disease organisms. This is the reason that departments of public health across the country post signs in bathrooms reminding food preparation employees about the importance of handwashing. But, getting people to wash their hands consistently is extremely challenging. Even health-care workers like doctors, who know how important it is, often don't do it.

As you read this selection, consider the following questions:

- **Why do the authors say that water, sanitation, and hygiene (WASH) issues are the "forgotten" foundations of health?**
- **One very important part of this article is the table showing how many people across the world have (and do not have) improved sanitation and water supply. Take a look at the definitions used for "improved" sanitation and water supply in the table. Do the figures here surprise you?**

- **Why do you think it is the case that, as the article states, "water and sanitation are the top priority for the poor"?**
- **Do you think governments should prioritize investing in preventative measures like sanitation and water improvements or providing health care to people who are already sick? Why?**

CONTEXT

Jamie Bartram is the director of the Water Institute at the UNC Gillings School of Global Public Health. He has written extensively on issues of water quality and on evaluating the burden of disease from poor water, sanitation, and hygiene. Sandy Cairncross is a public health engineer who has worked on water and sanitation engineering projects for the governments of Lesotho and Mozambique. He has also worked extensively on WASH-related diseases. He is professor of environmental health at the London School of Hygiene and Tropical Medicine.

Globally, around 2.4 million deaths (4.2% of all deaths)[1] could be prevented annually if everyone practised appropriate hygiene and had good, reliable sanitation and drinking water. These deaths are mostly of children in developing countries from diarrhoea and subsequent malnutrition, and from other diseases attributable to malnutrition.

A Massive Disease Burden Is Associated with Deficient Hygiene, Sanitation, and Water Supply

While rarely discussed alongside the "big three" attention-seekers of the international public health community—HIV/AIDS, tuberculosis, and malaria—one disease alone kills more young children each year than all three combined. It is diarrhoea,[2] and the key to its control is hygiene, sanitation, and water (HSW).

Figure 14.1 breaks down the preventable HSW-associated disease burden. It is dominatedby mortality from infectious diarrhoea, nearly 90% of which is borne by children under five years old and 73% of which occurs in only 15 developing countries.[1] Moreover, mortality from diarrhoea is only part of the disease burden. Even using the most conservative scenarios, the long-term sequelae due to diarrhoea in early childhood contribute more DALYs than do the deaths.[3]

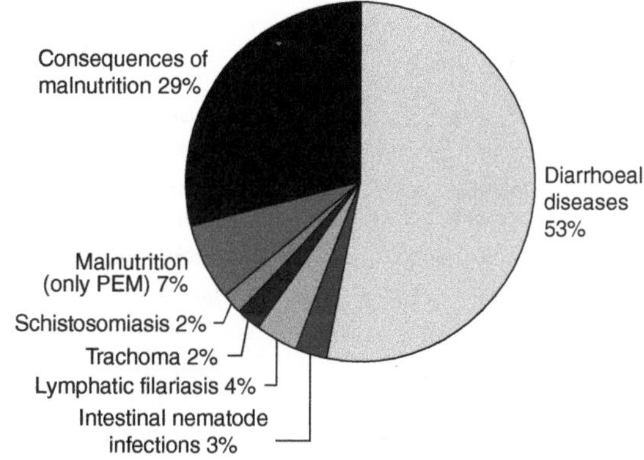

FIGURE 14.1 Contributions in DALYs of Individual Diseases to the Total Burden of Ill-Health Preventable by Improvements in HSW.

PEM = protein-energy malnutrition.

Source: A. Prüss-Üstün, Bos, R., Gore, F., and Bartram, J. (2008). *Safer Water, Better Health: Costs, Benefits and Sustainability of Interventions to Protect and Promote Health.* Geneva: World Health Organization.

Regrettably, it is no surprise that much ill health is attributable to a lack of HSW. Globally, nearly one in five people (1.1 billion individuals) habitually defecates in the open. Conversely, 61% of the world's population (4.1 billion people) has some form of improved sanitation at home—a basic hygienic latrine or a flush toilet. Between these two extremes, many households rely on dirty, unsafe latrines or shared toilet facilities.[4] Not only can it prevent endemic diarrhoea, adequate sanitation can help to prevent intestinal helminthiases, giardiasis, schistosomiasis, trachoma, and numerous other globally important infections (Table 14.1).

TABLE 14.1 Environmental classification of water - and excreta-related infections.

Category	Examples	Control Strategies
A. Feco-oral (Potentially water-borne or water-washed)	*Viral* Hepatitis A, E, and F Poliomyelitis Viral diarrhoeas *Bacterial* Campylobacteriosis Cholera Pathogenic *E. coli* Salmonellosis Typhoid, paratyphoid *Protozoal* Amoebiasis Cryptosporidiosis Giardiasis	Improve water quality (to prevent water-borne transmission), improve water availability, hygiene promotion (to prevent water-washed transmission)
B. Purely water-washed	*Skin and eye infections* Scabies Conjunctivitis Trachoma *Louse-borne infections* Relapsing fever	Improve water availability, hygiene promotion
C. Soil helminths	Ascariasis Trichuriasis Hookworm infection	Sanitation, hygiene promotion, treatment of excreta before re-use
D. Tapeworms	*Taenia solium* infection *Taenia saginata* infection	As C above, plus meat inspection and cooking
E. Water-based diseases	*Bacterial* Cholera Legionellosis Leptospirosis *Helminthic* Schistosomiasis Clonorchiasis Dracunculiasis	Reduce contact with/consumption of infected water, sanitation, treatment of excreta before re-use
F. Insect vector diseases	*Water-related* Dengue Yellow fever Malaria West African trypanosomiasis *Excreta-related* Bancroftian filariasis Trachoma Fly- and cockroach-borne excreted infections[a]	Reduce number of potential breeding sites and need to pass near them, improve surface water drainage, use repellent/insecticide where appropriate
G. Rodent-borne diseases	Rodent-borne excreted infections Leptospirosis Tularaemia	Rodent control, hygiene promotion, reduce contact with infected water

[a]Excreted infections comprise all those in Categories A, C, and D plus helminthic diseases in Category E. doi:10.1371/journal.pmed.1000367.t001

Source: Adapted from D. D. Mara, and Feachem, R. G. A. "Unitary Environmental Classification of Water- and Excreta-Related Diseases." *Journal of Environmental Engineering*, 1999, 125(4): 334–339.

The situation for drinking water appears better than that for sanitation. Although around 13% of the world's population (884 million people) lives in households where water is collected from distant, unprotected sources, 54% (3.6 billion) receives piped water at home. However, many piped water systems in developing and middle income countries work for only a few hours per day and/or are unsafe. In larger Asian cities, for example, more than one in five water supplies fails to meet national water quality standards.[5] Reliable safe water at home prevents not only diarrhoea but guinea worm, waterborne arsenicosis, and waterborne outbreaks of diseases such as typhoid, cholera, and cryptosporidiosis.

Much of the impact of water supply on health is mediated through increased use of water in hygiene. For example, hand washing with soap reduces the risk of endemic diarrhoea, and of respiratory and skin infections, while face washing prevents trachoma and other eye infections. A recent systematic review of the literature[6] confirmed that hygiene, particularly hand washing at delivery and postpartum, also helps to reduce neonatal mortality. It might be argued that water supplies also make flush toilets feasible, but this does not necessarily add to their health benefits, as we have seen no credible evidence that the health benefits of sanitation cannot be achieved by dry latrines, if they are properly built and maintained.[7]

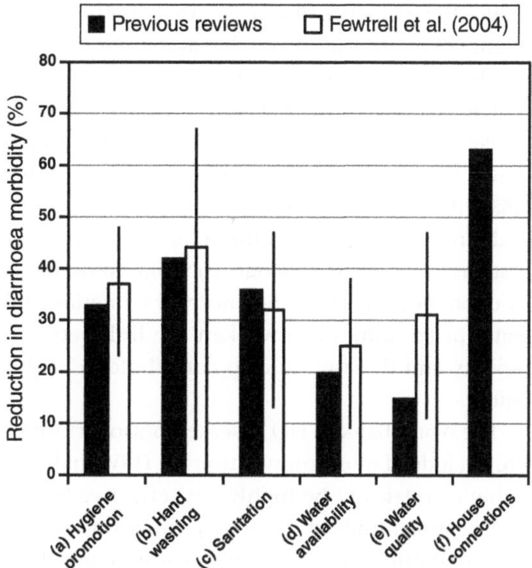

FIGURE 14.2 Results of Reviews of the Effect on Diarrhea of HSW Interventions.

Results of the previous reviews are for the better-quality studies. The reduction for household drinking water connections is in addition to reductions for water quality and availability of public sources.

Source: L. Fewtrell, Kaufmann, R. B., Kay, D., et al. "Water, Sanitation, and Hygiene Interventions to Reduce Diarrhoea in Less Developed Countries: A Systematic Review and Metaanalysis." *Lancet Infectious Diseases*, 2005, 5: 42–52.

This Disease Burden Is Largely Preventable with Proven, Cost-Effective Interventions

Figure 14.2 shows the average reductions in diarrhoea incidence found to be associated with HSW interventions in several literature reviews. The impact of "real world" interventions varies widely in response to local factors such as which pathogens are contributing to disease and the relative contribution of different transmission routes.

A balanced interpretation of the available evidence suggests that a reasonably well-implemented intervention in one or more of hygiene, sanitation, water supply or water quality, where preexisting conditions are poor, is likely to reduce diarrhoeal disease prevalence by up to a third. Still greater reductions (up to 63%) are associated with water piped to one or more taps on a property.[8] Such a major impact merits far more attention from health professionals and health systems than has been common in recent decades.

We now know that frequent bouts of diarrhoea and intestinal parasitosis are important causes of malnutrition, which renders children more susceptible to other diseases. For example, when malnourished children are recovering from an episode of diarrhoea, they are unusually susceptible to pneumonia; this diarrhoea-induced susceptibility may be associated with as much as 26% of all childhood pneumonia episodes.[18] Similarly, while 7% of the HSW-associated disease burden is directly associated with malnutrition, reductions in diarrhoea also reduce the incidence of diseases that are the consequence of malnutrition and that account for 29% of the disease burden (Figure 14.1).

The disease burden weighs heavily on both households and health systems. It has been estimated that the health costs alone amount to some US$340 million for households lacking water supply and sanitation and US$7 billion for national health systems.[19] The household burden weighs most heavily upon the poor, but well-conceived sanitation and water programmes can weaken the link between poverty and disease[20] and so contribute to health equity.

The World Bank/WHO Disease Control Priorities Project judged most interventions in HSW in developing countries to be highly cost-effective health interventions. Indeed, hygiene promotion was the most cost-effective of all major disease control interventions at US$5 per DALY averted, with sanitation promotion also in the top ten at just over US$10 per DALY.[21]

The Benefits of These Interventions Are Greater than the Health Benefits Alone

Environmentally caused mortality and malnutrition have substantial economic costs. In Ghana and Pakistan, for example, the indirect effect on child mortality of environmental risk factors mediated by malnutrition adds more than 40% to the cost of directly caused child mortality.[22] If one takes into account the effect of such malnutrition on impaired school performance and delayed entry into the labour market, the cost doubles to 9% of gross domestic product (GDP). With the possible exceptions of malaria and HIV/AIDS in Africa, it is hard to think of another health problem so prejudicial to household and national economic development.

Lack of sanitation also leads to intestinal helminth infections, which cause stunting, late entry to school, and impaired cognitive function.[23,24] Furthermore, inadequate sanitation and water supply are associated with much loss of time spent on water collection or seeking a place to defecate. An analysis of survey data from 39 African countries showed that for 160 million people (many of them women), collection of each container of water took substantially more than 30 minutes.[4,25] A World Bank study[26] found that, even ignoring the effect of water supplies on health, the value of time saved from water collection alone was sufficient to justify investments in rural water supply in most settings. Finally, a WHO report suggests that the time lost in collecting water and seeking somewhere to defecate could be valued at US$63 billion annually.[27]

When all these benefits are accounted for, many HSW investments yield a net benefit in the range US$3–46 per dollar invested.[19,27]

HSW Continues to Have Health Implications in the Developed World

The impacts of poor HSW are not restricted to the developing world. Take the example of hand washing, which reveals an inappropriate level of complacency concerning hygiene in developed nations. Two intervention studies of hand washing with soap conducted in child-care centres in the US[34] and Australia[35] found reductions in diarrhoea of roughly 50%, similar to the reductions found in developing countries.[11]

TABLE 14.2 Proportion of the Population of Developing Countries with Access at Each Level, in 1990 and 2008, to Sanitation and Water Supply.

	Proportion with Access (%)	
Level of Access	1990	2008
Excreta disposal		
Open defecation	32	21
Unimproved	18	14
Shared	9	13
Improved	41	52
Water supply		
Unimproved	29	16
Other improved	32	35
House connection	39	49

Notes: "Unimproved" sanitation facilities are those with no hygienic separation of faeces from human contact; e.g. open pit, platform or bucket latrines. "Improved public" water sources include public taps or standpipes, tube wells or boreholes, protected dug wells and rainwater collection. "Piped water at home" means inside the user's dwelling, plot or yard.

Source: World Health Organization and UNICEF. (2010). *Progress on Sanitation and Drinking Water;* 2010 Update, https://www.unicef.org/eapro/JMP-2010Final.pdf.

In another study, carers of young children in the UK washed their hands with soap after changing nappies on only 42% of occasions.[36]

The idea that sanitation continues to have health implications in the developed world is a surprise to many. It should not be, given that flush toilets transport excreta but do not render it innocuous. Sewage treatment even in the most developed nations is not universal or fully effective, and effluent discharged into rivers and coastal areas constitutes a health risk to bathers, among others. The costs of dealing with such effluent are considerable.[37,38]

The Overlooked Foundation

Health evidence confirms that the burden of disease associated with inadequate HSW is overwhelmingly (although not exclusively) carried by the poor and disadvantaged in the developing world and is a major contributor to the cycle of poverty. Stated this way, HSW are *problems*.

Dealing effectively with HSW has the potential to reduce child mortality, one of the more recalcitrant health statistics, by a third. Investment in HSW in developing countries contributes to practically all of the MDGs, yields benefits that can be valued at many times their costs, and can reach even the poorest. Stated this way, HSW are *solutions*.

How well are national governments and donors responding to the challenge of providing HSW for all? Three statistics are especially telling. First, water and sanitation are the top priority for the poor. In participatory poverty assessments such as those carried out for national Poverty Reduction Strategic Plans (PRSPs), water appears among the top two priorities, even in apparently water-rich countries such as Papua New Guinea[49] and Uganda.[50] Second, despite the "Water for Life" decade, the International Year of Sanitation, and numerous regional interministerial conferences, sanitation is still accorded low priority. If sanitation appears at all in a national PRSP, it is usually with a zero budget allocation. Drinking water fares little better; in four out of five African countries studied, funds allocated in PRSP action plans (or related documents) did not match the importance of water issues noted in earlier descriptive parts of the same PRSPs.[51] Finally, despite commitments to target aid and to the "Paris Principles" of Aid Effectiveness,[52] six of the ten countries in which more than half of the population live on less than a dollar a day receive less than the median aid per capita for sanitation and drinking water.[53]

There is clearly much room for health professionals and health systems to do more for HSW, and an urgent need for them to do so. One of the really important things they can do is to engage more with other sector professionals with whom they share many goals such as the prevention of faecal-oral disease transmission. Moreover, health sector professionals are well placed to champion the massive changes in attitudes and practices required to progress HSW up the political ladder and out to everyone without good HSW services.

REFERENCES

1. Prüss-Üstün A, Bos R, Gore F, Bartram J (2008) Safer water, better health: costs, benefits and sustainability of interventions to protect and promote health. Geneva: World Health Organization.
2. Boschi-Pinto C, Velebit L, Shibuya K (2008) Estimating child mortality due to diarrhoea in developing countries. Bull World Health Organ 86: 710–717.
3. Guerrant RL, Kosek M, Lima AA, Lorntz B, Guyatt HL (2002) Updating the DALYs for diarrhoeal disease. Trends Parasitol 18: 191–193.
4. WHO and UNICEF (2010) Progress on Sanitation and Drinking Water; 2010 update. Joint Monitoring Programme for Water Supply and Sanitation.
5. WHO and UNICEF (2000) Water Supply and Sanitation Global Assessment Year 2000 Report. Joint Monitoring Programme for Water Supply and Sanitation.
6. Chant R (2008) The role of water, hygiene and sanitation in neonatal mortality [MSc dissertation]. London: London School of Hygiene & Tropical Medicine.
7. Cairncross S, Kolsky PJ (1997) Letter: water, waste and well-being. American J Epidemiol 146: 359–360.
8. Esrey SA, Potash JB, Roberts L, Schiff C (1991) Effects of Improved Water Supply and Sanitation on Ascariasis, Diarrhoea, Dracunculiasis, Hookworm Infection, Schistosomiasis and Trachoma. Bull World Health Organ 69: 609–621.

11. Curtis V, Cairncross S (2003) Effect of washing hands with soap on diarrhoea risk in the community: a systematic review. Lancet Inf Dis 3: 275–281.
18. Schmidt WP, Cairncross S, Barreto ML, Clasen T, Genser B (2009) Recent diarrhoeal illness and risk of lower respiratory infections in children under the age of 5 years. Int J Epidemiol. doi:10.1093/ije/dyp159.
19. Hutton G, Haller L (2004) Evaluation of the costs and benefits of water and sanitation improvements at the global level. Geneva: World Health Organization, WHO/SDE/WSH/04.04.
20. Genser B, Strina A, dos Santos LA, Teles CA, Prado MS, Cairncross S, Barreto ML (2008) Impact of a city-wide sanitation intervention in a large urban centre on social, environmental and behavioural determinants of childhood diarrhoea: analysis of two cohort studies. Int J Epidemiol 37: 831–840.
21. Laxminarayan R, Chow J, Shahid-Salles SA (2006) Intervention Cost-Effectiveness: Overview of Main Messages. In: Jamison DT, Breman JG, Measham AR, et al. (2006) Disease Control Priorities in Developing Countries. [2]nd edition. Washington DC: The World Bank. pp 35–86.
22. Acharya A, Paunio M (2008) Environmental Health and Child Survival; Epidemiology, Economics, Experiences. Washington DC: The World Bank (Environment Department).
23. Nokes C, Grantham-McGregor SM, Sawyer AW, Cooper ES, Bundy DA (1992) Parasitic helminth infection and cognitive function in school children. Proc Biol Sci 247: 77–81.
24. Sakti H, Nokes C, Hertanto WS, Hendratno S, Hall A, et al. (1999) Evidence for an association between hookworm infection and cognitive function in Indonesian school children. Trop Med Int Health 4: 322–334.
25. Fry RK (2008) Incorporating water quantity into the water access indicator: the effect on estimates of 'adequate' access to water for health in Sub-Saharan Africa. [MSc dissertation]. London School of Hygiene & Tropical Medicine.
26. Churchill AA, de Ferranti D, Roche R, Tager C, Walters AA, et al. (1987) Rural water supply & sanitation; time for a change. World Bank Discussion Paper No. 18. Washington DC: The World Bank.
27. Hutton G, Haller L, Bartram J (2007) Global Cost-Benefit Analysis of Water Supply and Sanitation Interventions. J Water Health 5: 481–502.
34. Black RE, Dykes AC, Anderson KE, Wells JG, Sinclair SP, et al. (1981) Handwashing to prevent diarrhea in day-care centers. Am J Epidemiol 113: 445–451.
35. Roberts L, Jorm L, Patel M, Smith W, Douglas RM, et al. (2000) Effect of infection control measures on the frequency of diarrheal episodes in child care: a randomized, controlled trial. Pediatrics 105: 743–746.
36. Curtis V, Biran A, Deverell K, Hughes C, Bellamy K, et al. (2003) Hygiene in the home: relating bugs and behaviour. Soc Sci Med 57: 657–672.
37. Georgiou S, Bateman IJ (2005) Revision of the EU Bathing Water Directive: economic costs and benefits. Mar Pollut Bull 50: 430–438.
38. [No authors listed] (1994) Address by Lord Clinton-Davis at Institution's Annual Dinner on 23rd February 1994. Water Environment J 8: 335–339.
49. ADB (2002) Priorities of the Poor in Papua New Guinea. Manila: Asian Development Bank.
50. Williamson T, Slaymaker T, Newborne P (2004) Towards better integration of water and sanitation in PRSPs in Sub-Saharan Africa: Lessons from Uganda, Malawi and Zambia. Water Policy Programme Briefing 5. London: Overseas Development Institute.
51. Newborne P, Slaymaker T, Calaguas B (2002) Poverty Reduction and Water: 'Watsan and PRSPs' in sub-Saharan Africa Water Policy Programme Briefing 3. London: Overseas Development Institute.
52. OECD (2005) Paris Declaration on Aid Effectiveness, Ownership, Harmonisation, Alignment, Results and Mutual Accountability. Paris: Development Assistance Committee, Organization for Economic Cooperation and Development, available: http://www.oecd.org/dataoecd/11/41/34428351.pdf. Accessed 30 September 2010.
53. WHO (2008) Towards a Global Annual Assessment of Drinking-water and Sanitation. Geneva: WHO.

AMBER WUTICH AND ALEXANDRA BREWIS

15 WATER, WORRY, AND MENTAL HEALTH

Recently, many people in the United States have been asked to think about and cut back on their water use. Most people affected by such shortages live in California. Although estimates vary somewhat, the average person in California uses between 100 and 300 gallons of water every day. (This is just water they use at home and doesn't include the water needed to grow the food they eat and produce the clothes they wear.)

Many populations globally, however, have access to only a tiny fraction of that amount of water for all of their drinking, cooking, bathing, landscaping, and cleaning needs. Table 15.1 from the World Health Organization shows levels of water access (l/c/d refers to liters per person per day) and their implications for hygiene and health. Keeping in mind that there are about four liters per gallon, you can see that even in a drought situation, Californians' water access would still be considered "optimal" by global standards.

As the chart shows, maintaining basic hygiene with limited water availability can be extremely difficult.

Water access can also have health effects beyond the direct ones described in the previous selection (Chapter 14). This article is about a way in which water quality and availability may contribute to health outcomes that may not be immediately obvious: through impacts on mental health.

Mental health, which is discussed in more detail in Chapter 43, is very complicated. It includes psychoses like schizophrenia, as well as more common disorders like depression, anxiety, and alcohol or drug dependency. Many mental illnesses manifest themselves in culturally specific ways. However, symptoms of psychosis and depression, for example, are common across the world.

In studies across the world, symptoms of mental illness (including hearing voices, feeling worthless or anxious, and a number of other symptoms) are correlated with low social status, particularly to lower levels of education. Mental health symptoms don't seem to be directly related to income per se but are more likely to be related

TABLE 15.1 Levels of Water Access and Their Implications for Hygiene and Health.

Service Level	Access Measure	Needs Met	Level of Health Concern
No access (quantity collected often below 5 l/c/d)	More than 1000m or 30 minutes total collection time	Consumption – cannot be assured Hygiene – not possible (unless practised at source)	Very high
Basic access (average quantity unlikely to exceed 20 l/c/d)	Between 100 and 1000m or 5 to 30 minutes total collection time	Consumption – should be assured Hygiene – handwashing and basic food hygiene possible; laundry/ bathing difficult to assure unless carried out at source	High
Intermediate access (average quantity about 50 l/c/d)	Water delivered through one tap on-plot (or within 100m or 5 minutes total collection time)	Consumption – assured Hygiene – all basic personal and food hygiene assured; laundry and bathing should also be assured	Low
Optimal access (average quantity 100 l/c/d and above)	Water supplied through multiple taps continuously	Consumption – all needs met Hygiene – all needs should be met	Very low

Source: World Health Organization.

Revised from A. Wutich, Brewis, J. B. R. Chavez, and C. L. Jaiswal. "Water, Worry, and Dona Paloma: Why Water Security Is Fundamental to Global Mental Health." *Global Mental Health: Anthropological Perspectives*, edited by Brandon A. Kohrt and Emily Mendenhall, 57–72. London: Routledge, 2016.

to insecurity, threats of extreme scarcity, or threats of violence (which can have a relationship with income).

Although research on the topic is in its infancy, ***water insecurity*** *is correlated with mental health outcomes in several contexts. Amber Wutich, one of the authors of this article, did groundbreaking work in Bolivia, showing that water insecurity was significantly associated with symptoms of psychosocial distress, including anger and anxiety. She also found that women—who in Bolivia, like in most of the world, do most of the work of water collection—scored higher on water insecurity measures than men.*

Following that work, others (including one of the co-editors of this textbook) have done survey research on the same topic in Ethiopia and found similar results: in Ethiopia, too, water insecurity is associated with symptoms of psychosocial distress.

Understanding why this would be the case requires different methods than survey research—it necessitates qualitative methods like interviews to understand people's experiences of water insecurity. This article is an example of this work. By going in-depth into one woman's life, it examines the pathways that may link water insecurity with mental health outcomes.

As you read this selection, consider the following questions:

- **Why would water insecurity lead to stigma?**
- **Which of the authors' potential solutions do you think is the most effective? The most likely to be implemented?**
- **In your opinion, why is there a connection between mental health and insecurities (water, food, safety)?**
- **What do the authors mean in saying that we need to remove shame from global health?**

CONTEXT

Amber Wutich and Alexandra Brewis are both medical anthropologists and professors at Arizona State University. They both work extensively on resource scarcity, with a focus on water insecurity. Dr. Wutich directs the Global Ethnohydrology Study, a multiyear study of water knowledge and management in ten countries. Dr. Brewis's research has been concerned with how culture shapes human biology—she has worked extensively on stigma, particularly related to obesity.

The World Health Organization estimates that half of everyone globally will struggle with a psychological disorder in their lifetime, such as depression, anxiety, or addictive disorders. Depression is now recognized as the leading cause of disability, and women are significantly more affected than men. Much of this is due to women's lower social status and the burdens of gender-based expectations, including their unrelenting responsibilities for caring for others.

At the same time, poor water quality is a threat to global health because it can harbor and transmit infectious disease or toxins. But for millions worldwide, inadequate water *quantity* is also a major global health challenge. In rural areas, where people are vulnerable to drought and often lack adequate water infrastructure, water scarcity poses an enormous threat to farming lifeways and food security. Even in cities, the urban poor can experience water shortages due to decaying infrastructure, under-serviced neighborhoods, and the rising price of water. And, when water is scarce, the struggle to get enough water to drink, cook, and bathe often falls to women in the household.

Our story about how women's lives, water, and mental health collide starts with Doña Paloma. Amber first met her in 2004 in Villa Israel, a squatter settlement at the extreme southern end of the city of Cochabamba, Bolivia.[1] Four years before, Cochabambans had launched protests against their government's privatization of water. So powerful was their political action that it led to a new government and a new constitution that enshrined water rights. Yet, in 2004 nearly half the city's population still lacked good access to municipal water. As Doña Paloma said at that time, "Without water, we have absolutely nothing. I worry about water all the time."

[1] Names and some minor details have been changed to protect informants.

Doña Paloma was 29 years old, doing a double-shift—working to make money and to care for her husband, four children, mother-in-law, and brother-in-law. Funny and frank, Doña Paloma was well known in the community, and active in the squatter settlement's struggle to obtain basic public services like schools, clinics, streets, and stormwater channels. She had spent months with the other women of Villa Israel digging out those stormwater channels, hauling, and stacking boulders to create barriers against flash floods. But their top priority, a regular, safe water supply, continued to elude them.

Both geography and politics were stacked against the residents of Villa Israel. Most of the municipal water infrastructure in the Cochabamba Valley is located in the north. The squatter settlements are in the south of the city where groundwater is scarce. Rain comes only in short bursts in the summer, so each household's rainwater tanks sit empty much of the year. Family garden plots often died before ripening.

After years of struggling to dig their own groundwater well, Dona Paloma's community finally managed to build a small tapstand system. These tapstands are public outdoor faucets, which are commonly owned, maintained, and administered by the community. Only home owners in Villa Israel are eligible to use the tapstands, and then at best their quota is four buckets of water per family. Renters, new homeowners, and households too poor to pay the required monthly tapstand fee are excluded, and this adds up to nearly three-quarters of residents.

Doña Paloma's family were one of the lucky few with the rights and income to access the tapstand. But with 8 people in the family, four buckets of water added up to just a bit more than drinking water. There was still not enough for basic cooking, bathing, and other household chores.

The only real alternative at that time was to buy water from vending trucks. Vendors dislike driving to Villa Israel. Selling water in the city's outskirts meant high gas costs and the risk that rough, unpaved roads would damage their trucks. On most days, just one or two trucks made the trip, on other days none at all. With so little water to buy, the struggle for water was often humiliating. Doña Paloma and her neighbors were often forced to chase the water vendors up the street, pleading with them to sell water. When the vendors refused, people had the added humiliation of begging their neighbors to lend them just enough water for their family to drink.

Over the next two years, Doña Paloma told many other stories about her struggle to make ends meet. While they had enough to drink, her greatest anguish for her family was always about water: getting enough to cook, wash their bodies and clothes, flush the toilet, and clean their home. Doña Paloma reminisced about the early days of the squatter settlement, when "there was enough to plant corn and potatoes". As she talked, Doña Paloma showed many of the signs of depression and anxiety; she worried constantly, complained of fatigue, and was socially withdrawn. She said "I don't really have any friends. I say hello to my neighbors, but I don't like to talk to people," and preferred to sleep when she had the time. Water worries also spilled into conflicts with neighbors that turned to hate.

"One day the water ran out and I could not cook anything," Doña Paloma stated when Amber visited her again in the height of the dry season. Doña Paloma's husband was out of town, trying to find a better paying job. Doña Paloma was working 15 hour days, leaving little time for her to wait at the tapstand or chase down the water vendor—and only if they could afford it. Her youngest son had diarrhea "because of the water," and her household seethed with anger and resentment. Doña Paloma summed up: "There is nothing I like about living here anymore. I am sick of not having any water. I want to sell my house and move away."

Amber visited Doña Paloma again as that dry season neared its end, to find her family was moving to another less-established squatter settlement. Selling the old home yielded cash for a move. But in doing so, her family lost access to Villa Israel's tapstands. They were now completely dependent on the water vendors. She remained constantly worried about money and water. The construction of the new house was completely stalled because there was not enough water to mix the concrete. With no hope of access to piped water in her new community, Doña Paloma found that move had not helped solve the water problem at all. Things were even worse, and she was more worried than ever.

Water Scarcity, Emotions, and Mental Health

While there is widespread appreciation that poverty worsens mental health, exactly *how* that happens is not well understood. A puzzling question is: does water scarcity cause mental health conditions like depression, or is the issue how people experience and understand water shortages? Based on our anthropological analysis of the case of Villa Israel and other similarly water-scarce communities, we propose that the *social processes* that create scarcity—rather than scarcity itself—are most harmful to mental health. And we suggest there are three key factors involved in how this works: uncertainty, injustice, and stigma.

Uncertainty

In the squatter settlements in south-side Cochabamba, people anxiously awaited the arrival of the summer rainy season. Drought years were the worst of years. Gardens withered, wells and water reservoirs stayed empty, and many families were forced to move. Studies from across the globe show droughts trigger anxiety, depression, and other mental health issues, because they threaten people's ability not only to thrive but in many cases to survive. Even in Australia, where there is good water infrastructure, the drought in 2000–2012 devastated people. Farmers' crops died; their incomes and savings were lost; and their long-term ability to farm was threatened. As a result, people felt financial strain, loss, and fears for the future. Farmers, in particular, experienced more stress, anxiety, depression, and suicides.

For farmers and squatters alike, uncertainty about water availability will come in non-drought years too. In Cochabamba, water vending was not part of an organized municipal delivery system; it was unpredictable. Unlike municipal transport or trash removal, water vendors are not providing a public service. They act as independent or unionized entrepreneurs who are free to choose where they pursue profits. They strongly prefer clients who bought in bulk, as this cuts their delivery costs. We found in interviews that in more central, better established, and more economically stable squatter settlements, water vending services were more predictable and thus less stressful. When there were many bulk buyers, however, it was almost impossible for Doña Paloma and other small-scale buyers to convince the water vendors to deliver to their homes. Unpredictability around when water would be available and when severe shortages might strike a family next were a major source of worry for Doña Paloma and others like her.

Injustice

Just before she decided to move away from the community, Doña Paloma told us "We don't participate in community governance anymore. It's just for suckers." Doña Paloma's stories of life in Villa Israel conveyed her sense that community leaders had mismanaged residents' contributions to solving the water problem. She described all of Villa Israel's efforts to truly solve its water problems, including getting a groundwater well with enough output to support the community and installing taps in each home, as failed projects. Furthermore, Doña Paloma felt that corruption and incompetence in Villa Israel's community governance was at the root of these failures. Her sense of injustice led her to disengage from local action and, ultimately, to leave the community itself. Doña Paloma's take on the community water system was unusual for Villa Israel. While many people expressed frustration with the tapstand system—the shortages, exclusion of renters, timing of water distribution, or squabbling of neighbors—most agreed that the rules about who had access themselves were fair and equitable.

In other Cochabamba squatter settlements, however, this was not the case. There was anger around community-owned and administered water systems. "The leaders are . . . just swindling us" said a resident of another squatter settlement. Other frequently cited injustices included being cut off from the municipal water system and the water price gouging. When we analyzed reports of anxiety and depression symptoms of standard scales from across 23 squatter settlements in Cochabamba, we found this sense of injustice predicted worse symptoms of anxiety and depression. Women were most affected.

Around the world, new research suggests this is a wider pattern. We suspect that the association between water insecurity and mental ill-health is worst where power inequities abound. In South Africa, for instance, apartheid produced long-standing inequities and exclusions in water distribution. For blacks, this exclusion has been a source of profound shame, which has further hampered their participation in reforming the water sector and thus put them at greater risk for water insecurity (Goldin 2011). In an anthropological study of a Mexican town, *sufriendo del agua* (suffering from water) was found to be common, and lead to feelings of frustration, anguish, bother, worry, and anger. Those who suffered most were residents who depended on the community water system, experienced water shortages, and felt that new and wealthy residents had taken advantage of the system (Ennis-McMillan 2006). In all cases, psychosocial distress seems to emerge between the twin stresses of water shortages and injustices in water distribution.

Stigma

Doña Paloma once exclaimed in frustration, "I feel dirty because there is not enough water with more water I could clean the rooms, the bathroom, grow plants, *everything*!"

As she explained it, water helped Doña Paloma live what she defined as a life of dignity—being able to be proud of well-groomed children, a tidy home, and a green garden. Accordingly, lack of water was a source of shame, and her feelings are echoed in studies from around the world. In Madagascar, for instance, it is shameful to be dirty in front of your friends, and Tanzania, a person who is not clean is "like a mad person people avoid him but feel sorry for him" (Curtis et al. 2009).

Infectious diseases borne of water insecurity, ranging from skin infections to diarrheal illnesses, can be profoundly stigmatizing. This stigma intensified if the disease is also seen as a marker of poverty, filthiness, and contamination. In Brazil's cholera-stricken urban neighborhoods, for instance, the urban poor came to feel that "We ARE the cholera!"—a powerful statement conveying their feelings of culpability, stigma, and social exclusion (Nations and Monte 1996).

There are local variations in what is shameful, and hence what hurts emotionally. In Cochabamba's squatter settlements, for example, many families relied on kin, neighbors, and friends for gifts and loans of water. In some cases, people formed long-standing bonds of mutual assistance. Others, like Doña Paloma, preferred to pay neighbors for any water they were able to give. But many people we interviewed across Cochabamba's squatter settlements were not able to reliably get water in these ways. As recent migrants, they lacked the deep community connections, social acumen, and financial resources to navigate the social complexities of water loans and purchases as successfully as Doña Paloma. In such cases, people saw water loans as a stigmatized source of last resort. When families were forced to beg their neighbors for water, the experience was deeply degrading—if refused, it was utterly humiliating. In Cochabamba, people who begged for water were also more likely to experience anxiety and depression, as were women who were more reliant on neighbors as a source.

Similar patterns have also been seen in studies in the wake of famine and other food shortages. People who resort to socially-stigmatized forms of eating and food acquisition (like eating "famine foods", borrowing, and begging) are more likely to feel shame, anxiety, and depression.

What to Do?

There are several ways we can break the connection between insecurity and mental ill-health around the world. All have their own limits and challenges.

Change the System

One of the most powerful ways to address the negative health impacts of poverty is to change the system that produces it. This approach can have many positive downstream effects, including increasing incomes, improving physical health, and improving educational outcomes. There is encouraging evidence that some interventions, such as conditional cash transfer programs (Lund 2011), can make a difference to household wealth, opening more economic options as ways of coping with shortage.

Another promising, but as-yet unexplored approach, would be to improve water systems. Water insecurity produces a range of negative health and economic outcomes—including mental ill-health—in many parts of the world. For example, in Cochabamba, the most direct way to address mental distress and illness related to water insecurity might be to extend the municipal water system to the city's squatter settlements.

People living in Cochabamba's squatter settlements (and their political allies) have made many efforts to achieve this. After the end of Cochabamba's Water War, the municipal water authority, SEMAPA, regained control of water distribution. The protesters demanded that they be given a larger voice in water decision-making, and won a place at the table for community organizations that represented south-side communities. In 2004, SEMAPA expanded its service area to include the south-side squatter settlements. With funding from the Inter-American Development Bank and others, SEMAPA committed to expand the municipal water grid to the south-side.

Unfortunately, it is much easier to promise such changes on paper than to make them a reality in the poorest neighborhoods. Historical inequities, power imbalances, and corruption—all problems that existed long before the Water War and continue to persist—have derailed these plans to extend SEMAPA infrastructure. In 2007 alone, for example, external reviews of SEMAPA found 51 "irregularities" representing misuses or losses of between $600,000 and $1,000,000 USD of funds meant for managing and improving the water system (Driessen 2008). And so, even in Cochabamba—a global symbol of the triumph of common people against private water interests—the poor remain excluded from municipal water service, left only with hope.

The activists empowered by the Water War have found other, smaller ways to make an impact. After the local mayor's office reneged on its promise to build a major subterranean tank, one group negotiated directly with the European Union for a large grant. Stable, predictable water is now delivered to 20,000 residents by five community-owned water tanker trucks.

Other Cochabamba communities have devised their own affordable, small-scale solutions. Villa Israel had already built its own local tapstand system. When it did not yield enough water to support a growing population, community leaders bought land nearby so they could drill a new well. But, unfortunately for them, that adjacent community caught wind of the plan and legally blocked it. So Villa Israel built a major subterranean water tank, holding the amount of water that two tanker trucks could deliver in one day. While this is not enough to support the community permanently, it provides an important buffer—one step toward secure and affordable water provision. As these examples demonstrate, there are rarely easy solutions for the poor, but targeted interventions can at least shift things in the right direction.

Treat Mental Health

Fear, anxiety, and hopelessness are normal emotional responses to living in an unfair system where one's survival and dignity are constantly under siege. Over time, however, chronic distress can become a more serious mental health disorder, such as anxiety or depression. Untreated depression or anxiety disorders can interfere with people's productivity or income-earning ability, pushing them further into poverty. In such cases, appropriate, high-quality mental health treatment may help people break the cycle of mental illness and poverty.

In this sense, Doña Paloma's unfinished story represents that of millions of people in poor neighborhoods all over the world, where the stresses of resource insecurity and the inaccessibility of mental health care intersect. Doña Paloma showed several symptoms of anxiety and depression—including feeling nervous, anxious, fearful, unhappy, tired, socially disengaged, and hopeless—every time we interviewed her.

Professional mental health care providers would ideally provide treatment for anxiety, depression, and other common mental disorders, but there are simply not enough providers and clinics available to help everyone who needs treatment, especially in communities like Villa Israel. Perhaps 90% of people in low income communities are left without any options for treatment (Patel and Thornicroft 2009).

But it is unlikely that Doña Paloma would seek out formal mental health care, even if it were available. Her 3 am–8 pm workdays left little time for self-care and her financial situation made it difficult to pay for doctors. And, perhaps most important of all, few in south-side Cochabamba saw these feelings as indicative of illness; rather, they were seen as a common and normal (though lamentable) result of being unable to safeguard their survival and dignity.

The main question here is: if building more mental healthcare infrastructure still isn't enough to meet people's needs to cope with these types of profound stresses, what other approaches might work? One promising approach is called *task-sharing*. In this approach, community members are trained and guided to serve as the first line of assessment and intervention for people showing symptoms of common mental disorders. A single psychiatrist working with a legion of community-based workers is considered to be cost-effective because the only ongoing investment is the continuous training of volunteers (Beaglehole 2008).

One further point: even if treatment with a legion of volunteers is cost effective, that does not mean it is socially just. Community members who provide community-based social support, through task-sharing psychotherapy or other mental health programs, should be adequately compensated. If such treatments rely on the unpaid labor of community volunteers, the treatment system adds a burden to community non-professionals—who are often urgently in need of a path out of poverty (Maes et al. 2010).

Treatment for mental illness related to resource insecurity needs to be very carefully designed for a much larger reason. Connecting resource insecurity to mental illness runs a very real risk of contributing to the "medicalization of poverty" (Moreira 2003). This is when we recast normal emotional and physiological responses to poverty as pathologies, and can lead to interventions that focus on treating the symptoms of poverty rather than the root of the problem. For example, weakness, shaking, and irritability symptoms in Brazilian urban poor were treated with psychiatric medication, even though the real cause was outright hunger (Scheper-Hughes 1992). As Moreira explains, "The poor are thus transformed into patients. Poverty becomes a mental illness. A problem that is principally social and political is treated like a psychiatric symptom" (2003: 70). When poverty is medicalized, the purses of the poor are also emptied—to pay for costly medicines and treatments like anti-depressants.

Advance Women's Rights and Empowerment

Women in Villa Israel had more worries than men because household water provision is socially defined, for the most part, as their problem to solve. Were these burdens shared more broadly, the effects on women might be more muted. But, when households were in true crisis, men and women shared the burden of worry and the responsibility for finding water. And Doña Paloma and the women of Villa Israel had some autonomy to act politically to address social problems, such as organizing together to build stormwater drains. The situation is far worse elsewhere.

In many other parts of the world, women's opportunities to find solutions are further undermined by their lack of autonomy to decide and act. Reminders of women's low social and political power exacerbates the likelihood of depression, because the sense of frustration and unfairness is further compounded. For example, in Soviet era Uzbekistan, women made many gains through greater access to education and employment. During the Post-Soviet years, when religious fundamentalism resurged, women found themselves blocked from even visiting a doctor's office or supermarket alone. Women that thought they should have rights were even more likely to be depressed (and suffered other stress-related health effects like high blood pressure). Women whose husbands' supported the idea of women's empowerment, however, had less depression.

In this way, the World Health Organization's approach to addressing global mental health has identified three primary factors for improving mental health for women globally, especially depression, and these focus on addressing women's lower social rank and advancing women's empowerment. These are: (1) ensuring women having sufficient autonomy to exercise some control in response to severe events,

(2) providing women, in particular, access to some material resources that allow the possibility of making choices in the face of severe events, and (3) encouraging family, friends, or health providers to give women better emotional support. Underlying all of these is the need for women and girls to be treated as valued and equal members of society, a grand social project that is limping forward too slowly in many places.

Remove Shame from Global Health

The potential mental health implications of shame deserve greater attention within in the global health community. A regularly deployed tactic to encourage hand-washing and improved sanitation are "shaming interventions" designed to stigmatize "dirty" people in order to make people want to wash more. Given that people in places like Villa Israel do not have enough water to wash regularly, and these interventions are designed to make people who don't wash feel bad about themselves, such interventions could worsen the mental health of people who are already quite vulnerable. The potential impacts of these types of shame-based global health interventions clearly need to very carefully considered.

Final Words

Even as diarrheal and other water-borne diseases continue to threaten millions globally, the health implications of water are not just about water quality. They are also tied up in issues of scarcity and uncertainty. As water becomes increasingly scarce and commoditized, worries over water are likely to be a continually rising global health challenge.

Unless real structural solutions are implemented that meet the human need for stable and safe water supplies, there is every reason to anticipate even more damaging mental health effects in the years ahead. And the brunt of this likely will fall to women living in the poorest communities. Since water appears to be a key part of the relationship between poverty and mental health, direct interventions to improve water provision and accessibility may offer a way to break the cycle of poverty and mental illness.

From the perspective of mental health provision to the world's poor, this reminds us that all mental health policies ultimately start with delivering the very basics. These include the most fundamental material matter of all: water. And the most basic social principle: equity.

REFERENCES

Beaglehole, R., Epping-Jordan, J., Patel, V., Chopra, M., Ebrahim, S., Kidd, M., & Haines, A. 2008. Improving the prevention and management of chronic disease in low income and middle-income countries: a priority for primary health care. *Lancet* 372, 940–949.

Curtis, Valerie, Lisa Danquah, and Robert Aunger. 2009. Planned, motivated and habitual hygiene behaviour: an eleven country review. *Health Education Research* 24(4): 655–673.

Driessen, T. 2008. Collective management strategies and elite resistance in Cochabamba, Bolivia. *Development*, 51(1), 89–95.

Lund, Crick, Mary De Silva, Sophie Plagerson, Sara Cooper, Dan Chisholm, Jishnu Das, Martin Knapp, and Vikram Patel. 2011. Poverty and mental disorders: breaking the cycle in low-income and middle-income countries. *The Lancet* 378(9801): 1502–1514.

Maes, K. C., Kohrt, B. A., & Closser, S. 2010. Culture, status and context in community health worker pay: Pitfalls and opportunities for policy research. A commentary on Glenton et al. 2010. *Social Science & Medicine* 71(8): 1375–1378.

Moreira, Virginia. 2003. Poverty and Psychopathology. In *Poverty and Psychology: From Global Perspective to Local Practice*. Eds, S. Carr and T. Sloan. New York: Kluwer Academic. Pp. 69–86.

Nations, M.K. and C.M.G. Monte. 1996. "I'm not a dog, no!": cries of resistance against cholera control campaigns. *Social Science and Medicine* 43(6):1007–1024.

Patel, V., & Thornicroft, G. 2009. Packages of care for mental, neurological, and substance use disorders in low- and middle-income countries. *PLoS Medicine*, 6(10), e1000160.

Reddy, B. and M. Snehalatha. 2011. Sanitation and Personal Hygiene: What Does it Mean to Poor and Vulnerable Women? *Indian Journal of Gender Studies* 18(3):381–404.

Scheper-Hughes, Nancy. 1992. *Death Without Weeping: The Violence of Everyday Life in Brazil*. Berkeley: University of California Press.

ANNA MARIA BARRY-JESTER

16 WHAT WENT WRONG IN FLINT

This article is about a very rich but very unequal country. In 2015 in Flint, Michigan, government officials changed the source of the community's water intake. Local citizens noticed right away—the water looked dirty, tasted bad, and started causing a variety of health problems. But the governmental response was extremely slow. To get the government's attention, "citizen scientists" had to go to extreme efforts, and their volunteer work demonstrated that the water was heavily contaminated with lead and other chemicals that had leached into the water from old pipes.

The serious effects of lead poisoning—even from exposure to tiny amounts—has been known for a long time. Lead causes poor cognitive development in children, and like undernutrition (Reading 21), it can affect the overall economic productivity of a society.

In the 1970s, in a major public health achievement, leaded gasoline was banned in the United States because the lead from the gasoline got into the air and into people's bodies. (Lead had been added to gasoline starting in the 1920s as a way to make engines less noisy.) Lead paint was also banned in the 1970s, although it still exists in almost every house built prior to that time.

In the case of Flint, the public health system responsible for ensuring water safety did not work. And, when citizens raised questions, authorities failed to listen citizens' concerns and became defensive. The question is why. Why was there was a political decision to change the source of the city's water from Lake Huron to the polluted Flint River? Why was the response of government institutions so slow?

Section 7 of this book—on the social determinants of health—may help explain the situation. Flint has a majority poor African-American population, and the city has suffered incredible losses of industrial production in the past 30 years. Cleaning up environmental pollution from unregulated industrial production in the past continues to be a challenge. The cost of pollution—whether by bacteria, heavy metals, or greenhouse gases—ends up being paid in poor health.

As you read the following article, consider the following questions:

- **In your opinion, was what happened in Flint simply the result of a poor decision made by a government official who was not from the community? Or is the entire episode an example of unconscious racism in an overall society?**
- **Why do you think there were disagreements about the water tests? What did the "citizen scientists" have to do to get new tests of water quality?**
- **In the 1980s, the Food and Drug Administration forbade the use of artificial sweeteners (cyclamates) in drinks because of rat studies that showed risk of bladder cancer. The dosage of the chemical that the rats were subjected to was the equivalent of a person drinking more than 500 cans of cyclamate-sweetened soda a day for years. In your opinion, how should people determine what is the appropriate level of risk the government to use? Are the Public Health authorities being too protective?**
- **In the London cholera outbreaks of the 19th century, (Reading #2) a landlord drank the water from a pump that his tenants had complained looked and smelled bad. He did this to show the people that the water was safe to drink, but he contracted cholera and died. In the case of Flint, the effects of lead poisoning in water are less dramatic; they require time and mostly affect children's cognitive development. In your opinion, how are the two examples of water pollution different?**

CONTEXT

This article appeared in the online publication FiveThirtyEight in January 2016. This website is associated with the quantitatively oriented public intellectual Nate Silver. Anna Maria Barry-Jester is a journalist who publishes regularly on public health, food, and culture for the website.

1. An Unnatural Disaster

FLINT, Mich.—As I walked into Jackie Pemberton's petite white house in the southeast corner of Flint, she apologized for the mess (there wasn't one) and offered me a cup of coffee. "River water all right?" her husband, John, asked without a hint of irony. Jackie burst into laughter.

Jackie has lived in Flint for much of the past 48 years, and for many of those, she owned a drain-cleaning business that counted several industrial factories as clients. "I saw what they put down those drains," she told me, shaking her shoulder-length salt-and-pepper hair in disgust. So when the city switched its water source from Lake Huron to the murky waters that ran through Flint in April of 2014, she refused to drink it. The idea of it made her ill, she said, thinking about all the industrial chemicals, sewage and road salt that had made their way into the river over the years. John, however, keeps an old soda bottle filled with water by his side whenever he's home, and he filled it with tap water frequently. Mindful of her limited budget as a retiree, Jackie gave in after six or eight weeks and started drinking the water as well.

By late summer, they both started having stomach problems, losing hair and developing rashes, as did several of their children and grandchildren who either lived elsewhere in the city or periodically came to stay with them. In August (2014), *E. coli* was found in the city's water, forcing Flint to issue multiple advisories to residents to boil the water before use. By October, the Pembertons had become regulars at City Council meetings along with a group of other residents concerned about water that smelled of sulfur and chlorine, often came out of the tap tinted the color of urine or rust, and appeared to be causing a long list of health concerns.

"I drank the water for eight or nine months," John said. "In the poor parts of town, those people drank it for one and a half years. Some still are."

Today, we know that those health concerns include poisoning from a well-understood neurotoxin: lead. That realization has led to international outrage, protests from Flint residents, and the resignation of several federal, state and local employees, though not as many as some Flint residents would like. More than a year after residents started sounding alarm bells, it's now clear that employees at the state's Department of Environmental Quality collected insufficient data and ignored the warning signs visible in what they did collect. In the process, they allowed the residents of Flint to be poisoned.

Officials at the Michigan Department of Environmental Quality, the agency in charge of making sure water is safe in the state, made a series of decisions that had disastrous consequences:

- Against federal guidelines, they chose not to require the Flint water plant to use optimized corrosion control, despite telling the Environmental Protection Agency they were doing so in an email on Feb. 27, 2015.
- They took few samples and took them from the wrong places, using a protocol known to miss important sources of lead, which some say didn't comply with a 25-year-old law meant to prevent lead exposure in residential water.
- They threw out two samples whose inclusion would have put more than 10 percent of the tests above what's known as the "actionable level" of lead, 15 parts per billion. Had the DEQ not done so, the city would have been required to warn residents that there was a

If the DEQ had **included all of the water samples it took,** federal law would have demanded further steps ...

... but the **exclusion of two high-lead samples** put the city's water supply below the threshold for mandatory action.

LEAD LEVELS IN WATER SAMPLES

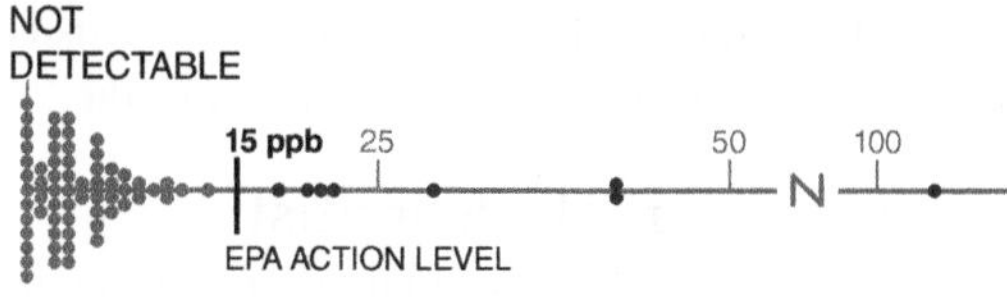

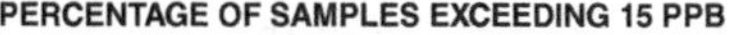

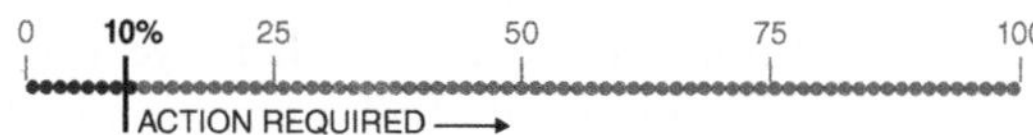

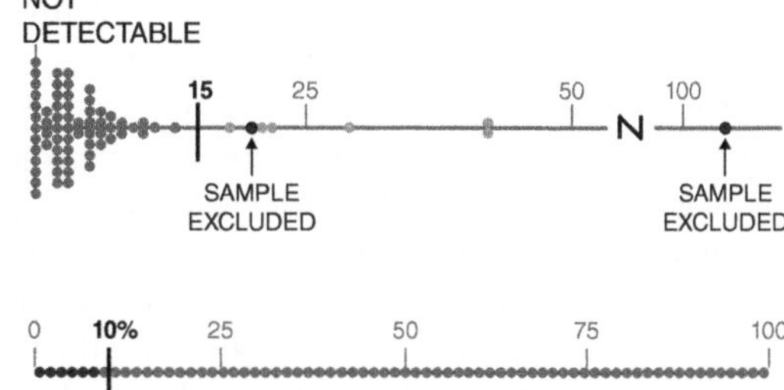

FIGURE 16.1 The Difference Two Data Points Make: The Michigan Department of Environmental Quality's Analysis of Flint's Water Supply.

Source: Michigan Department of Environmental Quality (http://www.flintwaterstudy.org).

problem with lead in the water back in the summer of 2015, or possibly earlier.[1]

Because of those transgressions, the Flint River's corrosive water ate through the protective film inside the city's old pipes, allowing odorless, tasteless lead to leach into the water. They are also what has featured in most of the news coverage of Flint: important questions about which officials knew what, and when. Gov. Rick Snyder has said the failures here had nothing to do with the fact that Flint's residents are largely poor and majority black, but that didn't assuage many who feel this wouldn't have happened in a wealthier, whiter city.

Also worthy of examination is how a wealth of other data and information, gathered by the city's residents, was largely ignored. When the county declared a public health emergency on Oct. 1, 2015, it was not a revelation for many residents. They had been fighting for months to convince officials that something was wrong. Instead of heeding those reports, priority was given to the official data—data that was flawed and shortsighted. As a result, the percentage of children with elevated blood lead levels in Flint doubled.

If it weren't for a few dozen residents and a handful of crusading experts who pushed back against the official narrative, we still wouldn't know the truth.

2. Flint River

The Flint River enters the city at its northeast corner through wooded park land. It winds past the city's water treatment plant, with its giant cartoon-spaceship-shaped water tower, and then runs along an industrial stretch that was home to Buick City, a sprawling 400-acre complex that employed more than 26,000 people at its peak. Most of the buildings have been torn down since the complex shuttered in 1999, its demise part of Flint's transition from a working-class city of nearly 200,000 in 1960 to one of about 99,000. As of 2013, the median household income was $24,834, half the statewide median, and 42 percent of residents lived below the federal poverty level. From the old Buick City footprint, the river crosses the city center, running through the

[1] The DEQ has said one sample was removed because it had a whole house filter (samples are supposed to be taken from the most high-risk homes, which ostensibly shouldn't include homes with filters, though in this case the home had some of the highest lead levels). The other was thrown out because it was from a business. The DEQ maintains that it was following federal law, while some experts say samples are not to be thrown out even if they don't meet requirements. The EPA is reviewing the issue.

University of Michigan's Flint campus and underneath Chevrolet Avenue, where workers marched in victory in 1937 after a sit-down strike that transformed the newly formed United Automobile Workers into a powerful union.

The person who decided to use the river as a water source was one of a succession of emergency managers in Flint, Darnell Earley. Earley was appointed by Snyder under a controversial law that allows the governor to install managers whose power trumps that of elected officials. Over the last five years, more than 50 percent of Michigan's black population has, at some point, lived in a city with a state-installed manager.

For nearly 50 years, the city bought its water from Detroit, which pumped it out of Lake Huron. But in 2013, the city voted to join a new pipeline being built to the lake, prompting Detroit to cancel its agreement. Rather than agree to a new short-term contract with Detroit, Earley decided[2] to use the river that runs through the heart of the cash-strapped city. The state treasurer signed off on the move.

The switch has been described as an effort to save money, but Flint's water system hadn't been a drain on the budget. In fact, the water paid for itself and then some, paying out about $1.5 million annually to the city's general fund in the years leading up to the switch, according to Dayne Walling, who was mayor in 2009–15.[3]

Walling toasted the new source on April 25, 2014, the day of the switch. When residents started to complain of foul odors and strange tastes that summer, Walling told a local newspaper that they were "wasting their precious money buying bottled water." But last week, sitting in a cafe just a couple of blocks from the river, he expressed regret that he hadn't challenged state and federal officials throughout the last year and a half who repeatedly told him everything was OK. "Even though we disagreed on many things," he said of Earley, "I fundamentally trusted that it would be done right. That was a mistake."

3. The Self-Taught Scientist

LeeAnne Walters, a 37-year-old mother of four with a self-described "Jersey girl" persistence, started losing her eyelashes sometime in the summer of 2014. She also noticed that one of her 3-year-old twins, Gavin, who already had a compromised immune system, was constantly ill and had stopped growing, in addition to the rashes the rest of her kids were developing. In January she received a notice that there were TTHMs[4] in the water, a byproduct of the chlorine that was being used to clear up the E. coli that had been found in the city's water on multiple occasions over the summer. She joined other residents at public forums with the emergency manager, bringing along a jug of brown water that came from her tap. State and city officials repeated the familiar phrase that it met federal standards—even after a local General Motors plant had been allowed to switch back to Detroit's water in October because the river water was corroding machine parts.

But research told Walters she was getting half-truths. She stayed up late into the night after the kids were in bed, learning everything she could about what might be happening to her family and friends. "I decided, I guess I got to figure the science part of this, because you can't argue with the science," she told me over the phone from her new home in Virginia. "If you don't know what you're talking about, they can say whatever they want. But if you know what you're talking about, then they have to listen."

In the last decade or so, researchers have learned a lot about how to gather water samples that will accurately measure risk, and Walters now understands the science of water testing better than many experts. She explained to me in great detail the many ways the city's testing protocol underestimated the risk:

- The city's original target was 100 samples, the federally required number for a city with more

[2] Earley has written that the switch to Flint River water was based on a Flint City Council vote. There is no evidence to suggest the City Council voted on the temporary water switch, though it did vote to join the pipeline, and two City Council members and then-Mayor Dayne Walling told me they did not make the decision to switch to river water. Either way, Earley was the one who could ultimately make that decision, and he signed the request to the state treasurer to do so.

[3] Walling lost a re-election campaign in 2015 to Karen Weaver. Water concerns were a key issue during the campaign.

[4] Total trihalomethanes.

than 100,000 people and the number that DEQ agreed to with the city. But after city workers had trouble collecting that many samples, the DEQ dropped the requirement to 60, saying Flint's population of just more than 99,000 was under the six-figure mark. Scientific experiments aren't supposed to change protocol partway through.

- Residents were asked to test water after it had been sitting for more than six hours, as required by federal law, but were also asked to flush the systems the night before. This "pre-flush" is known to lower detection in samples.
- Samples were collected in bottles with a small neck, which requires filling with a small stream, rather than opening the tap as you would when you fill a glass of water. The slower the stream, the less likely lead is to corrode from the pipe into the sample.
- The law requires that the city test the most at-risk homes, but it didn't have a record of where its lead service pipes were (lead is often introduced in corroded pipes as it travels to homes), or which homes were likely to have lead pipes.

In February, Walters asked the city to test her home's water, and says she got a panicked phone call telling her the water samples found lead levels of 104 and 397 parts per billion, far above the threshold of 15 ppb that puts a federally mandated response plan into motion. (The amount of iron in the water exceeded measurement capabilities.) The DEQ would later tell the EPA the lead was coming from her indoor plumbing, which was rather unlikely since the house had been plumbed with plastic pipes when the Walters family bought it a few years ago, before the city started using river water. She also had Gavin's blood lead levels tested again, and the results were disturbing. They had gone from 2 micrograms per deciliter (µg/dL) before the switch to the Flint River to 6.5 µg/dL after. Although no lead exposure is considered safe, anything above 5 µg/dL triggers a public health response in the United States.

Lead is an extensively studied neurotoxin, and decades of research show that there is no safe level of exposure. Although most elevated blood lead levels today are not high enough to cause immediate problems, there are many long-term effects of lead exposure, even for small doses. While it's impossible to say what effect a low exposure will have on an individual child, research is fairly clear on what it does to a population. It causes miscarriages and low birth weight for babies, and it shifts the entire IQ of a population down a few points. It's also believed to cause decreases in impulse control and increases the incidence of attention deficit hyperactivity disorder, learning disabilities and potentially violent behavior. Newer research suggests that exposure can also affect DNA, carrying damage on to the children and grandchildren of those exposed. The effects of low exposure on adults haven't been studied as closely, but they include an increased risk of hypertension and decrease in cognitive function. In a city like Flint, rife with poverty, high violent crime rates and low high school graduation rates, lead exposure is yet another layer of trauma.

Walters says when she brought her concerns to city officials, they told her that they were following the law, and if she had a problem, she could take it up with the EPA. So she did.

She wrote to several people at the regional EPA office, including Miguel Del Toral, who happens to be a national expert on the Lead and Copper Rule (LCR). He was familiar with how sampling protocol in the LCR often misses the highest lead levels and had published a study about it in Chicago. In one of many conversations, Del Toral told Walters that he didn't understand how the lead in her water could be so high when the city was using corrosion control. Walters told him that was easy—they weren't using corrosion control.

4. The Self-Funded Whistleblower

Marc Edwards was in his lab at Virginia Tech when Del Toral let him know that a woman whose child had lead poisoning would be calling about a water test. The youthful 52-year-old civil engineer is a national expert on corrosion control and has spent much of his career proving that water can be a significant source of lead if not treated properly. In 2007, he was awarded a MacArthur genius grant, largely for work he'd done exposing dangerous levels of lead in Washington, D.C., drinking water, a scandal that ultimately forced the Centers for Disease Control and Prevention to admit that it had misled the public on the risks.

When Walters shared her samples with Edwards, Edwards saw the highest lead levels he'd seen in 25 years of this research. The amount, 13,200 ppb, qualified the water as toxic waste.

By the time Edwards had completed his testing, Del Toral had already written a memo detailing the high lead levels at the Walterses' home; the city's lack of compliance with federally required corrosion control; and substandard testing procedures that "could provide a false sense of security to the residents of Flint."

Del Toral gave a copy of the report to Walters, who eventually shared it with an investigative reporter at the Michigan American Civil Liberties Union named Curt Guyette. In July, Guyette published the first news report warning of a potential lead crisis. Guyette says this crisis is the most egregious betrayal of public trust that he's seen in his decades of investigative reporting on Detroit.

Still, Walters says she got nowhere with the DEQ. "When Miguel gave me that report, I did not make that public to get him in trouble; I made that public because I felt people had a right to know," Walters told me recently. "I hoped that [DEQ employees] would do their jobs, that they would finally listen." Instead, Del Toral's supervisor, Susan Hedman, who recently said she would resign over her role in Flint, apologized to the state for his sharing the drafted memo, and Walters says DEQ staff bragged that he'd "been handled" and called him a "rogue employee" to the press.

Edwards thought his role was done after testing Walters's water, but when he heard what was happening to Del Toral, he was furious. "You can't stand by when a city is not following a federal law," he said. "You've got one child lead poisoned already and one house that's the worst you've ever seen. You've just got to find out what the hell is going on."

MICHIGAN
Flint

WATER SAMPLES
■ BELOW EPS ACTION LEVEL (15 PPB) ■ ABOVE ACTION LEVEL

Michigan Department of Environmental Quality

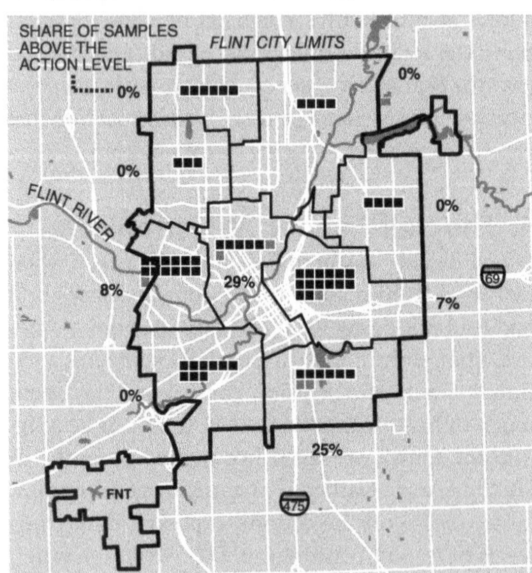

Flint Water Study's Analysis

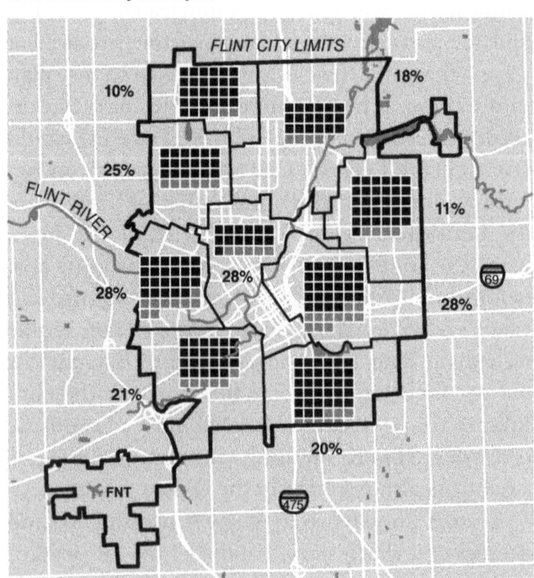

FIGURE 16.2 Water Sampling in Two Separate Studies: How the Sampling and Results from City and State Testing and the Flint Water Study Compare, by Ward.

Source: Michigan Department of Environmental Quality (http://www.flintwaterstudy.org).

His team, Flint Water Study, bought 300 testing kits, mostly with his own funds,[5] and sent them to a church in Flint. Walters and dozens of other residents fanned out across the city, ending up with 271 samples from homes in each of the city's ZIP codes.

The water sample results were startling—and very different from what the city had found in its testing. That was in part because the new samples were more thorough—they tested the water three times under different conditions instead of just once, and they took a larger number of samples from every ward in the city. In Ward 9, where the Walterses and Pembertons lived, 51 percent of water samples showed lead higher than 5 ppb, and 20 percent were above 15 ppb. Under federal law, when 10 percent of samples are above 15 ppb, it should trigger public warnings. And the numbers were high all over the city.

5. The Relentless Pediatrician

While Edwards showed that there was lead in Flint's water, it was a pediatrician in the city's public health system who realized just how grave an effect it was having. As the Virginia Tech testing was going on in August, Mona Hanna-Attisha, a pediatrician who runs the pediatric medical residency program at Flint's Hurley Medical Center, heard from a friend who worked for the EPA in Washington during the earlier lead crisis that Flint wasn't using corrosion control. Hanna-Attisha's friend, Elin Betanzo, implored her: "Can't you look into that?"

She could. Hanna-Attisha pulled up the results of all the lead tests from her clinic, which sits atop the city's sprawling and elaborate farmers market. The levels looked higher than normal, but the sample size was small and didn't represent the whole city. She tried to get data from the state, which keeps detailed records on lead levels, but they wouldn't give it to her in a time frame that she considered acceptable given the level of potential danger. Then a light bulb went off with one of her colleagues. Her clinic is part of Hurley Medical Center, the city's public health system, which is the biggest show in town when it comes to pediatrics; she estimates that 60 percent to 70 percent of lead lab tests are processed through the medical center. So she applied for permission to research all the center's lead labs. Then she and another doctor spent several mostly sleepless nights poring over the data.[6] "Our mantra was no eating and no going to the bathroom until we get this done," she told me. "Only coffee and wine." They double- and triple-checked their findings. And then they held a news conference.

"Research isn't supposed to be released in press conferences; it's supposed to be released in journals," Hanna-Attisha said recently in an office sprinkled with her children's art, pushing horn-rimmed glasses up her nose. "But in this case, the risk to the public was just too great."[7]

After the Sept. 24 news conference, where Hanna-Attisha announced that the percentage of children with elevated blood lead levels had gone from 2.4 percent to 4.9 percent citywide, the governor's spokeswoman said that Hanna-Attisha had "spliced and diced" the data to get those numbers. Hanna-Attisha says a DEQ spokesperson called her comments "unfortunate." A week later, the county declared a public health emergency.

On Oct. 16, 2015, the city switched back to water from Detroit. It's not clear how long it will take for the protective film to redevelop inside the pipes. Until it does, the water won't be safe to drink.

6. What Now?

At the beginning of this year, three months after the state acknowledged that there was lead in the water in Flint, Gov. Snyder declared a state of emergency,

[5] Although Edwards got a National Science Foundation grant to do the work, more than three-quarters of the more than $180,000 cost of testing came out of Edwards's discretionary research funds and personal bank account. Guyette, who was involved in gathering the water samples, said Edwards never said anything about the money. "I had no idea until the beginning of January that he was paying for this with his own funds," Guyette told me.

[6] Hanna-Attisha used data from the study Edwards organized, Flint Water Study, to hypothesize where a higher percentage of children might have elevated blood lead levels after the water switch. For her study, she used data available as of Sept. 26, 2015, which did not include all of the samples in the final Flint Water Study data set. You'll see some slight discrepancies in our charts as a result.

[7] She later published the study in the American Journal of Public Health.

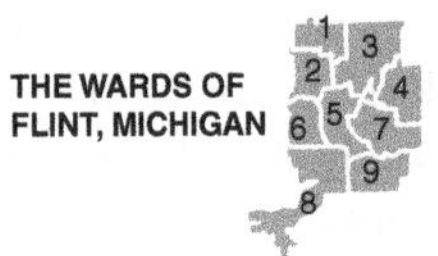

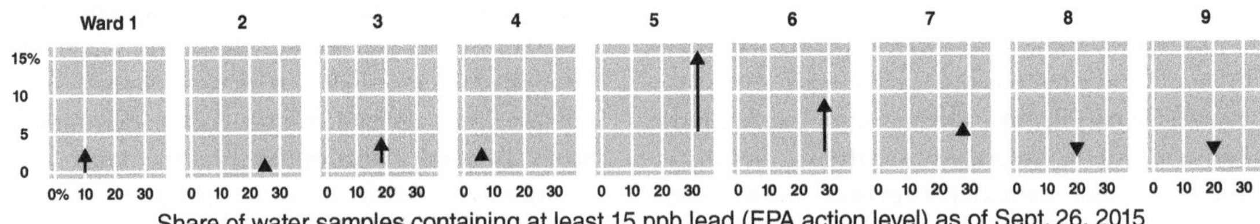

FIGURE 16.3 How Blood Lead Levels Changed in Flint's Children: Before and After the City's Water Source Was Switched to the Flint River in April 2014.

Source: Hanna-Attisha, Mona et al. "Elevated Blood Lead Levels in Children Associated With the Flint Drinking Water Crisis." *American Journal of Public Health* 106, no. 2 (February 1, 2016): pp. 283–290.

sending state police door to door to deliver supplies to residents and opening several sites for water and filter pickup. On Jan. 22, the EPA declared "imminent and substantial endangerment" and took responsibility for the water from the DEQ.

Walters is now coordinating with Yanna Lambrinidou, a medical ethnographer who got involved with a similar D.C. lead crisis as a concerned parent, to push the EPA to improve the Lead and Copper Rule, the law that's supposed to regulate lead in drinking water. Lambrinidou was asked to be on an advisory council that proposed revisions to the law late last year and says that the group's recommendations, currently being reviewed by the EPA, could actually make the law weaker. She wrote a dissent to the report, which along with the proposal is currently with the EPA; the agency says it will make proposed changes available for public comment in 2017.

Lambrinidou says her experience in Washington has made trust a complicated topic. "You know that the people you are supposed to trust are putting you in harm's way, and there's really very little that you can do about it. It's really a complete betrayal of the most basic assumptions that you have, that you rely on to live your day-to-day life," she said.

Walters's husband, who was in the naval reserve, went back into active duty so the family could move out of Flint. Even in their new home in Virginia, she says, they continue to drink bottled water and have a five-minute limit on showers.

Hanna-Attisha is working on several programs she hopes can mitigate the effects of the lead exposure in children. These include getting healthy food to kids (one of the best ways to counteract lead exposure), improving early education options, bringing in mental health specialists and making sure kids can visit their doctors regularly. "We need to throw every single thing we can at these kids now," Hanna-Attisha said. "They are owed this."

Edwards says this has been one of the most amazing experiences of his life, to watch the residents of Flint become citizen scientists. "Half the water industry does not understand what these people learned on their own to protect their children," he said. Siddhartha Roy, a graduate student at Virginia Tech who has worked with Edwards throughout the Flint research, made some of the calls to residents whose water had tested high for lead. Although some expressed shock and concern over how they would pay for bottled water or a filter, he says many expressed relief at having the concerns they'd been expressing for months validated. "One woman said to us, 'You mean that's the results for my tap? That's empowering.' She actually used the word 'empowering,'" Roy said.

Like Roy, I was shocked when I first heard that. How could finding poison in your water be empowering? But when you've spent nearly a year being told by public officials that your own experience isn't what you think it is, even grave news can be rewarding.

Dozens of Flint's residents who had been gathering data and information for nearly a year knew something wasn't right. While state and federal agencies almost obsessively focused on proving that they were meeting federal regulations, rather than taking a deeper look at whether Flint's drinking water was safe, residents begged them to pay attention to the valuable data they'd collected through their bodies and research. There was power in finally having irrefutable proof, and finally having someone listen.

Still, they'd gladly trade that power for clean water.

SECTION 4 CASES FOR TEACHING AND LEARNING

Visit the companion website, www.oup.com/us/brown-closser, for direct links to the featured online resources.

Addy et al., *When Work Makes You Sick: A Farmworker's Experience in the Field*
This case uses the Center for Disease Control and Prevention's pesticides database to explore associations between pesticide use and illness. It provides the basis of a possible student debate over whether the pesticide Mevinphos should be banned.

Susan Holman and Leila Shayegan, *Toilets and Sanitation and the Khumb Mela*
Students learn about the substantial challenges in providing sanitation for the Khumb Mela festival in Allahabad, India. This case is told from the perspective of undergraduate student observers. Instructors may want to develop questions for students to answer as they read the case.

LeBlanc et al., *Get the Lead Out! An Interdisciplinary Case Study for Science Students*
In this case, suitable for courses with access to a chemistry lab, students investigate lead concentrations in groundwater samples.

The Camel Challenge
Limiting water use can be an effective way to reflect on and understand the impact of water scarcity. This exercise requires participants to only use water that they have carried on foot a significant distance. Guidelines for the challenge are on the companion website.

SECTION 4 VIDEOS AND WEB RESOURCES

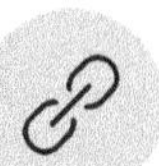

Visit the companion website, www.oup.com/us/brown-closser, for direct links to the featured online resources.

Baseball in the Time of Cholera
This documentary describes the 2010 Haitian cholera epidemic from the perspective of a young baseball player and delves into the controversy surrounding the source of the epidemic (likely United Nations peacekeeping troops). (30 min)

Foul Water Fiery Serpent
This documentary follows the Carter Center's dracunculiasis (Guinea worm) eradication program in sub-Saharan Africa. It explains the epidemiology of the disease and describes

the effort to eradicate it, focusing particularly on the young Americans involved in the eradication effort. Short excerpts can easily be used as part of classroom lectures. (60 min)

Trachoma: Defeating a Blinding Curse
A second documentary following a Carter Center program, this film follows the Trachoma Control Program in rural Amhara, Ethiopia. Trachoma is a water-washed disease. Again focusing primarily on American staff, this documentary describes the strategy of latrine building, face-washing, treatment, and surgery. (60 min)

***Bad Data and Worse Decisions Poisoned Flint* – What's the Point? Five Thirty Eight podcast**
This podcast features the author of Chapter 16 discussing the Flint water crisis, covering many of the issues in that reading. (30 min)

The Warriors of Qiugang
This documentary follows a conflict between a Chinese village and a chemical company over water contamination. (39 min)

Flow: For Love of Water
This feature-length documentary explores the impact of water privatization worldwide.

Aqueduct – World Resources Institute
This website contains maps and predictions of global water supply and shortage. Students can use these maps along with the maps in the Conceptual Tools in this section for a fuller understanding of the areas of the world most affected by water and sanitation issues. The future predictions can also be used in discussions of the impact of increased water scarcity globally with population growth and climate change.

SECTION

5

Air

Like water, air is necessary for life, and, as is the case for water, contaminated air is a major cause of disease and death. This section of the book discusses four major ways in which air quality affects our health: (i) indoor and outdoor air pollution, (ii) cigarette smoking, (iii) person-to-person transmission of air-borne pathogens, and (iv) climate change (an issue that includes, but goes far beyond, air quality).

Indoor and outdoor air pollution have far-reaching and often quite surprising health effects. People seldom have a choice about whether or not they breathe in pollutants. Many rapidly industrializing urban centers in middle income nations across the globe have severe problems with air pollution. And globally, many air pollutants are found inside the home—particularly in rural areas. As explored in Chapter 17, indoor air pollution from wood fires for cooking and heating are a major cause of sickness, particularly for women and children.

Cigarette smoking contributes to indoor air pollution, as well as killing directly. Smokers willingly inhale carcinogens and the additive chemical nicotine with every puff that they enjoy. As described in Chapter 6, it was not until the midcentury that the causal relationship between cigarettes and lung cancer was proven though epidemiological studies. Cigarettes are very profitable for companies, but if used as intended, they are are likely to kill their consumers. Chapter 18 explores how the variety of multinational corporations sometimes called "Big Tobacco" has profound negative effects on public health globally.

The fact that we share the air we breathe means that diseases can be spread through the air. This is why we are taught to cover our nose when we sneeze. Ecology is hugely important in health—humans and many of the diseases that affect us are part of ecological systems. These ecological systems affect infectious diseases, including airborne diseases like tuberculosis (TB), the insect vectors that carry many infectious diseases, and a wide variety of other factors.

The far-reaching impacts of ecology on health can be clearly seen in the case of climate change. Climate change is about air (extreme temperatures) and water (drought, floods, and storms) that endanger people's health. However, the effects of climate change on health are much multifaceted and complex, as seen in Chapter 19.

»CONCEPTUAL TOOLS«

Air Pollution

- **Air pollution** is a major cause of poor health worldwide. Air pollutants directly not only cause chronic health problems like asthma but also worsen or cause infectious diseases like lower-respiratory infections and chronic respiratory-related conditions like cardiovascular disease and chronic respiratory diseases.
- **Outdoor air pollution** causes a wide variety of health problems, although not all are well understood. As just one surprising example, studies have shown that deaths from sudden infant death syndrome happen more frequently in the United States when outdoor air pollution levels are high.

  A classic example of the striking effects of outdoor air pollution is the "killer" London smog of 1952. Weather conditions made coal plant emissions combine with fog (smog), and the thick cloud hung over the city for 4 days. Epidemiological analyses show that between 5,000 and 12,000 people died as a result of this 4-day smog event.
- **Indoor air pollution**, primarily from burning wood for cooking or heat, is also a major health issue. This issue is discussed in depth in Chapter 17. Indoor air pollution contributes to a variety of health problems, from pneumonia and TB to strokes and cataracts.

Smoking

- **Smoking** is a major cause of death globally, and secondhand smoke is a major contributor to indoor air pollution. With increased tobacco regulation in rich countries, "Big Tobacco" has turned its attention to getting people in poor countries hooked on cigarette smoking. The problem is difficult for those in public health to address effectively, because some governments acquire significant tax revenue from the production and consumption of cigarettes.
- The absolute number of smokers in low- and middle-income countries is astounding—in China alone, there are approximately 300 million smokers who consume around twenty cigarettes a day. Worldwide, cigarettes smoking is more of a problem for men than women, although in rich countries, rates are more equal.
- Smoking can be considered a type of intentional air pollution.

Ecology and Infectious Disease

- The importance of ecology in health goes far beyond air. Ecological factors heavily influence water, food, and social factors influencing health.
- One clear example of the importance of ecology in global health is vector-borne disease. **Vectors** are arthropods (insects) that transmit disease from person to person. Many diseases are vector-borne, from Zika (transmitted by mosquitoes) to Lyme disease (transmitted by ticks). Arthropod vectors are cold-blooded, and so ecological change (including climate change) can affect the transmission of vector-borne diseases.

- **Malaria** is a vector-borne disease that is a major health issue globally—the World Health Organization estimates that there were over 200 million cases of malaria in 2015, including over 400,000 deaths, mostly in children. Malaria is caused by a parasite that is transmitted by *Anopheles* mosquitoes (there are many different species of mosquitoes globally). Drugs to treat and cure malaria exist. Because the parasite evolves drug resistance extremely quickly, the World Health Organization recommends a combination of drugs called artemisinin-based combination therapy. Many people who get malaria, however, do not get the right drugs in time. Prevention of transmission through interventions like bed nets treated with long-lasting insecticides can also be helpful.
- Humans have ecological systems within our own bodies. Living within us, there are a multitude of microorganisms, many of which are beneficial. Biologists call this internal ecology the "microbiome."
- One microbe that many humans harbor is the bacteria that causes TB. In fact, around 30% of the world's population is infected with TB. But this doesn't mean that a third of the world is sick from TB. In the vast majority of those infected people, the bacteria stay inactive in the lungs (this is called "latent" TB). But in some cases, people's immune system can't keep the bacteria in this inactive state (this is particularly likely to happen if the person is also infected with HIV). In these cases, the person develops active TB. People with active TB can spread it to others through the air by coughing or talking. TB is a major cause of death worldwide, killing almost 2 million people a year, most of them poor people in the prime of life.

  Effective treatment for TB exists—drug therapy that must be taken for several months on a daily basis. Since these drugs have serious side effects, global recommendations are that a health worker watches the patient take their drugs—something called **directly observed therapy (DOT)**. When DOT is not done, people often do not finish their medicine, leading to antibiotic-resistant bacteria. Drug-resistant TB is a growing global problem. About 500,000 people developed active multidrug-resistant tuberculosis (MDR-TB) in 2015—a version of the disease resistant to the most commonly used drugs. And there are some cases, called XDR-TB, that are completely untreatable by any drug we have.
- **TB is transmitted through the air, which again shows the importance of indoor air quality for health.** The statement by the Canadian Tuberculosis Committee (see box) describes how TB is transmitted and specifically why it is an issue in certain populations in Canada.

Climate Change

- **We live in the Anthropocene, the age of humans, in which humans are causing enormous changes to ecological systems globally.** One of the most striking examples of this is climate change. Figure CT5.1 shows the impacts that climate change is already having on the ecology of the United States.
- Climate change will have multiple and far-reaching health effects. Table CT5.1 shows a few of the most important.

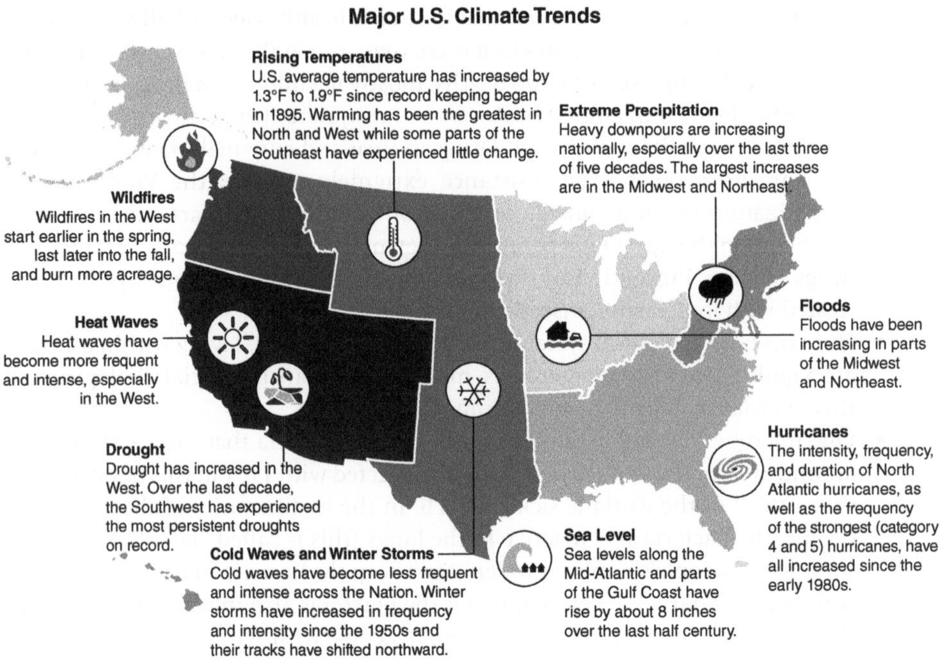

Major U.S. Climate Trends
Rising Temperatures
U.S. average temperature has increased by 1.3°F to 1.9°F since record keeping began in 1895. Warming has been the greatest in North and West while some parts of the Southeast have experienced little change.
Extreme Precipitation
Heavy downpours are increasing nationally, especially over the last three of five decades. The largest increases are in the Midwest and Northeast.
Wildfires
Wildfires in the West start earlier in the spring, last later into the fall, and burn more acreage.
Heat Waves
Heat waves have become more frequent and intense, especially in the West.
Floods
Floods have been increasing in parts of the Midwest and Northeast.
Hurricanes
The intensity, frequency, and duration of North Atlantic hurricanes, as well as the frequency of the strongest (category 4 and 5) hurricanes, have all increased since the early 1980s.
Drought
Drought has increased in the West. Over the last decade, the Southwest has experienced the most persistent droughts on record.
Sea Level
Sea levels along the Mid-Atlantic and parts of the Gulf Coast have rise by about 8 inches over the last half century.
Cold Waves and Winter Storms
Cold waves have become less frequent and intense across the Nation. Winter storms have increased in frequency and intensity since the 1950s and their tracks have shifted northward.

FIGURE CT5.1. Major U.S. Climate Trends.

Image source: US Global Change Research Program Climate and Health Assessment, https://health2016.globalchange.gov/climate-change-and-human-health.

TABLE CT 5.1 Health Effects of Climate Change.

	Climate Driver	Exposure	Health Outcome	Impact
Extreme Heat	More frequent, severe, prolonged heat events	Elevated temperatures	Heat-related death and illness	Rising temperatures will lead to an increase in heat-related deaths and illnesses.
Outdoor Air Quality	Increasing temperatures and changing precipitation patterns	Worsened air quality (ozone, particulate matter, and higher pollen counts)	Premature death, acute and chronic cardiovascular and respiratory illnesses	Rising temperatures and wildfires and decreasing precipitation will lead to increases in ozone and particulate matter, elevating the risks of cardiovascular and respiratory illnesses and death.
Flooding	Rising sea level and more frequent or intense extreme precipitation, hurricanes, and storm surge events	Contaminated water, debris, and disruptions to essential infrastructure	Drowning, injuries, mental health consequences, gastrointestinal and other illness	Increased coastal and inland flooding exposes populations to a range of negative health impacts before, during, and after events.

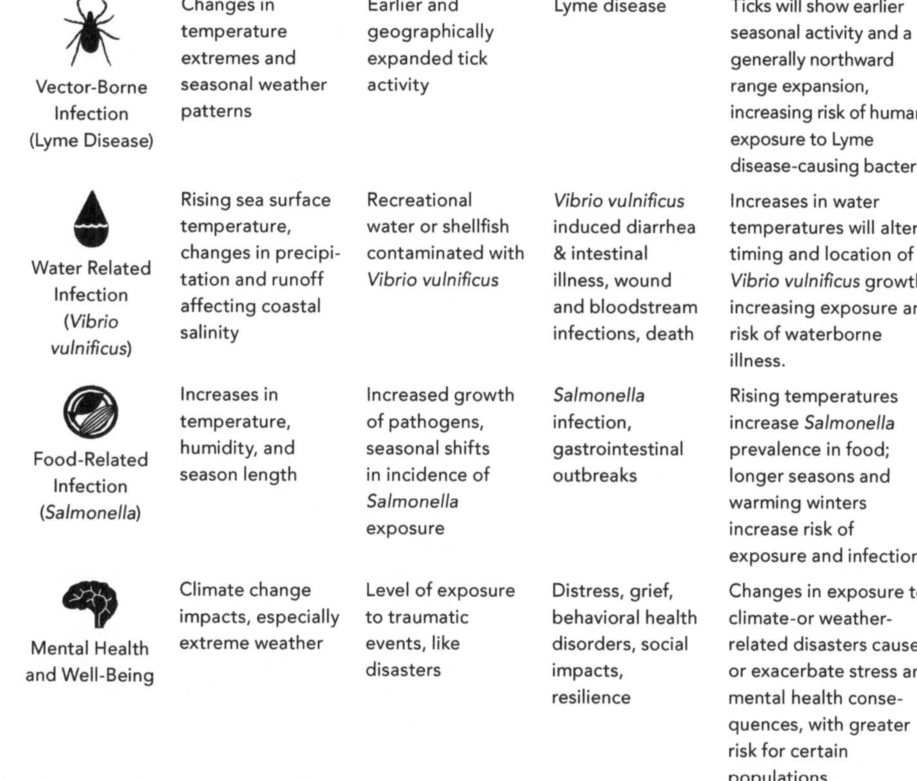

Vector-Borne Infection (Lyme Disease)	Changes in temperature extremes and seasonal weather patterns	Earlier and geographically expanded tick activity	Lyme disease	Ticks will show earlier seasonal activity and a generally northward range expansion, increasing risk of human exposure to Lyme disease-causing bacteria.
Water Related Infection (*Vibrio vulnificus*)	Rising sea surface temperature, changes in precipitation and runoff affecting coastal salinity	Recreational water or shellfish contaminated with *Vibrio vulnificus*	*Vibrio vulnificus* induced diarrhea & intestinal illness, wound and bloodstream infections, death	Increases in water temperatures will alter timing and location of *Vibrio vulnificus* growth, increasing exposure and risk of waterborne illness.
Food-Related Infection (*Salmonella*)	Increases in temperature, humidity, and season length	Increased growth of pathogens, seasonal shifts in incidence of *Salmonella* exposure	*Salmonella* infection, gastrointestinal outbreaks	Rising temperatures increase *Salmonella* prevalence in food; longer seasons and warming winters increase risk of exposure and infection.
Mental Health and Well-Being	Climate change impacts, especially extreme weather	Level of exposure to traumatic events, like disasters	Distress, grief, behavioral health disorders, social impacts, resilience	Changes in exposure to climate-or weather-related disasters cause or exacerbate stress and mental health consequences, with greater risk for certain populations.

Source: US Global Change Research Program Climate and Health Assessment, https://health2016.globalchange.gov/climate-change-and-human-health.

BOX 5.1 An Advisory Committee Statement (ACS): Canadian Tuberculosis Committee

Housing conditions are used as socio-economic indicators of health and well-being. Poor housing quality and overcrowding are associated with poverty, specific ethnic groups and increased susceptibility to disease. Crowding, poor air quality within homes as a result of inadequate ventilation, and the presence of mold and smoke contribute to poor respiratory health in general and have been implicated in the spread and/or outcome of tuberculosis (TB).

According to the 2001 Canadian Census, First Nations, Inuit and recent immigrants (foreign-born) have a disproportionately higher share of housing needs than other Canadians. They have the highest risk of living in houses that are overcrowded and in disrepair, and/or they live in houses that cost more than 30% of their before-tax household income.

TB in First Nations Populations On and Off Reserve

TB rates continue to be a major public health problem in Canada in First Nations, Métis, Inuit and foreign-born populations. First Nations people living on reserves have an 8–10 times higher TB notification rate than do non-Aboriginal Canadians; they also have a higher than average household occupancy density and a poorer quality of housing than other Canadians. It is not surprising, therefore, that TB rates are higher in Canada's First Nations populations than among Canadian-born, non-Aboriginal people. Factors contributing to the high rates of TB among First Nations are the prevalence of latent infection, co-morbidities (including diabetes), substance abuse, genetic factors and socio-economic factors. Socio-economic factors that have been implicated in health outcome include ethnicity, income, employment

continued

status, education, poverty and housing conditions. Overcrowded houses and poor ventilation increase both the likelihood of exposure to the TB mycobacterium and progression to disease.

TB TRANSMISSION

TB infection is spread when an individual with active respiratory TB coughs or sneezes *M. tuberculosis* bacilli that become aerosolized droplets of less than 5 µm diameter. An increased density of droplet nuclei in the air leads to an increased risk of infection. As the number of inhaled bacilli increases, so too does the risk that disease will develop in individuals after they have become infected. An individual with active pulmonary TB (smear-positive) who is sneezing or coughing vigorously and frequently will exhale 10^6 contaminated droplets. Some, but not all, of the droplets will contain the *M. tuberculosis bacilli.* The aerosolized droplets settle very slowly and can remain suspended in the air for many hours. Therefore, TB transmission occurs with greater prevalence in poorly ventilated and crowded spaces.

Environmental factors related to housing that may enhance the likelihood of TB transmission include the following:

1. exposure of susceptible individuals to an infectious person in a relatively small, enclosed space;
2. inadequate ventilation that results in either insufficient dilution or removal of infectious droplet nuclei;
3. recirculation of air containing infectious droplet nuclei;
4. duration of exposure; and
5. the susceptibility of the exposed person.

What Housing Factors Might Contribute to TB Transmission?

CROWDING

Crowding has been identified as both a risk factor for TB transmission and a characteristic of First Nations housing both on and off reserve. In communities where persons with TB disease live, crowded housing leads to an increased risk in terms of exposure to *M. tuberculosis.* The risk of exposure is also increased if there is limited air movement in an enclosed space.

The overall average number of persons per room for First Nations people is 20% higher than for the rest of the Canadian population. People in on-reserve houses were more than twice as likely to live in crowded conditions as those in non-reserve First Nations households.

INADEQUATE VENTILATION

Transmission of *M. tuberculosis* bacteria to a non-infected person is more likely if there is poor ventilation. Occupancy density, room volume and air change rate are all directly correlated with the number of new TB infections among persons who share airspace.

MOLD AND TOBACCO SMOKE

Homes that have inadequate ventilation (either mechanical or natural) are often damp or have mold growth resulting from high humidity and condensation. The absence of adequate central heating and insulation is an important factor in the growth of mold in a house.

Dampness and mold have not been directly linked with the acquisition of TB infection. However, they have been implicated in increased susceptibility to respiratory infection, asthma and allergies among Canadian children.

It has also been found that the presence of mold and fungi in homes is associated with suppressed T-cell production, which has been linked to slower recovery from TB.

A higher incidence of TB transmission to children has been associated with exposure to environmental tobacco smoke.

DURATION OF EXPOSURE

The extent and persistence of contact with an infected person are the main environmental factors for the transmission of TB. Thus, transmission of TB occurs most frequently as a result of prolonged contact in enclosed environments with an infectious person. Persons who are at the greatest risk of exposure to TB are those who live and sleep in the same household as an infected person. The amount of shared air space for occupants of a small house is significantly higher than one would find in a larger house occupied by the same number of people.

NIGEL BRUCE, ROGELIO PEREZ-PADILLA, AND RACHEL ALBALAK

17 INDOOR AIR POLLUTION IN DEVELOPING COUNTRIES

The air we breathe is usually not under our control. One might inhale tuberculosis (TB) bacteria while sleeping in a crowded family bedroom. You might live in a heavily polluted city like Beijing, and the constant inhalation of pollutants damage would damage your lungs. Or, the air inside your home might be contaminated with smoke from cooking fires. **Indoor air pollution** *is a major global health burden. Many women in low-income countries are exposed to indoor air pollution on a daily basis because of what they burn for cooking for their families. While we think of lung cancer as being associated with smoking, about two-thirds of the women who have lung cancer in India, China, and Mexico have never smoked cigarettes.*

Smoke from burning wood, dung, or coal affects women and children the most. In adults, it can increase risk for a wide variety of health problems such as pulmonary TB, chronic obstructive pulmonary disease, lung cancer, and cataracts. In children, the health problems are also severe. Babies born from mothers exposed to indoor air pollution are more likely to have a low birth weight—a serious risk factor for mortality. They are also more likely to have acute respiratory infections, ear infections, and asthma. The families who burn wood or dung for cooking and heating are the poorest of the poor. They might prefer to use a cleaner fuel source, but that can be an expensive luxury.

There have been many projects worldwide aimed at providing cleaner burning stoves as a solution. Engineers have regular competitions for clean stove designs. Supplying cleaner and more comfortable stoves is a great thing, and they are much appreciated by recipients when designed to meet the needs of the cook. However, as this article suggests, they may not be the solution in regard to health risks. Even if the stoves are cleaner, they may still emit too many toxic particles. It appears that as severe poverty declines, families may begin to utilize cleaner but more expensive fuel. As such, the solution to the health problem is ultimately economic, that is, poverty reduction. Nevertheless, the pediatric health challenges of respiratory infections must be addressed immediately with basic medical care.

As you read the following article, consider the following questions:

- **Outdoor air pollution caused by automobiles and industries might be addressed by governmental laws of environmental protection. In your opinion, who or what should be responsible for improving indoor air pollution?**
- **In some parts of India, dried cow dung is a typical cooking fuel for the rural poor, and it has a surprisingly nice scent and adds flavor to the cooked food. Do you find that idea disgusting? If so, why?**
- **Passive cigarette smoke is a type of indoor air pollution. What are some factors that might contribute to passive cigarette smoke or smoking cooking fires being a long-term health risk?**
- **Almost 50 percent of world's population rely on simple stoves that have incomplete combustion and pollute the inside of the house. In your opinion, is this an important problem? Is it more important than diarrhea dehydration deaths or polio? How did you decide that?**
- **According to the article, how do the epidemiological costs of indoor air pollution compare with those of cigarette smoking?**

N. Bruce, R. Perez-Padilla, and R. Albalak. "Indoor Air Pollution." *Bulletin of the World Health Organization*, 2000, 78(9): 1078–1092. The photos included here are not original to the article. They are included for illustrative purposes.

CONTEXT

This article was published in the official journal of the World Health Organization. Nigel Bruce teaches public health at the University of Liverpool; Rogelio Perez-Padilla is the head of Medicine at National Institute of Respiratory Diseases, Mexico; and Rachel Albalak works in the Caribbean regional office of the Centers for Disease Control and Prevention.

Introduction

Indoor air pollution can be traced to prehistoric times when humans first moved to temperate climates and it became necessary to construct shelters and use fire inside them for cooking, warmth and light. Fire led to exposure to high levels of pollution, as evidenced by the soot found in prehistoric caves.[1] Approximately half the world's population and up to 90% of rural households in developing countries still rely on unprocessed biomass fuels in the form of wood, dung and crop residues.[2] These are typically burnt indoors in open fires or poorly functioning stoves. As a result there are high levels of air pollution, to which women, especially those responsible for cooking, and their young children, are most heavily exposed (Fig. 17.1).

In developed countries, modernization has been accompanied by a shift from biomass fuels such as wood to petroleum products and electricity. In developing countries, however, even where cleaner and more sophisticated fuels are available, households often continue to use simple biomass fuels.[3] Although the proportion of global energy derived from biomass fuels fell from 50% in 1900 to around 13% in 2000, there is evidence that their use is now increasing among the poor.[1] Poverty is one of the main barriers to the adoption of cleaner fuels. The slow pace of development in many countries suggests that biomass fuels will continue to be used by the poor for many decades.

Notwithstanding the significance of exposure to indoor air pollution and the increased risk of acute respiratory infections in childhood, chronic obstructive pulmonary disease and lung cancer,[3,4] the health effects have been somewhat neglected by the research community, donors and policy-makers. We present new and emerging evidence for such effects, including the public health impact. We consider the prospects for interventions to reduce exposure, and identify priority issues for researchers and policy-makers.

Biomass fuel is any material derived from plants or animals which is deliberately burnt by humans. Wood is the most common example, but the use of animal dung and crop residues is also widespread.[5] China, South Africa and some other countries also use coal extensively for domestic needs.

In general the types of fuel used become cleaner and more convenient, efficient and costly as people move up the energy ladder.[6] Animal dung, on the lowest rung of this ladder, is succeeded by crop residues, wood, charcoal, kerosene, gas and electricity. People tend to move up the ladder as socio-economic conditions improve. Other sources of indoor air pollution in developing countries include smoke from nearby houses,[6] the burning of forests, agricultural land and household waste, the use of kerosene lamps,[7] and industrial and vehicle emissions. Indoor air pollution in the form of environmental tobacco smoke can be expected to increase in developing countries. It is worth noting that fires in open hearths and the smoke associated with them often have considerable practical value, for instance in insect control, lighting, the drying of food and fuel, and the flavouring of foods.[3]

Many of the substances in biomass smoke can damage human health. The most important are particles, carbon monoxide, nitrous oxides, sulphur oxides (principally from coal), formaldehyde, and polycyclic organic matter, including carcinogens such as benzo[*a*]pyrene.[5] Particles with diameters below 10 microns (PM_{10}), and particularly those less than 2.5 microns in diameter ($PM_{2.5}$), can penetrate deeply into the lungs and appear to have the greatest potential for damaging health.[8]

The majority of households in developing countries burn biomass fuels in open fireplaces, consisting of such simple arrangements as three rocks, a

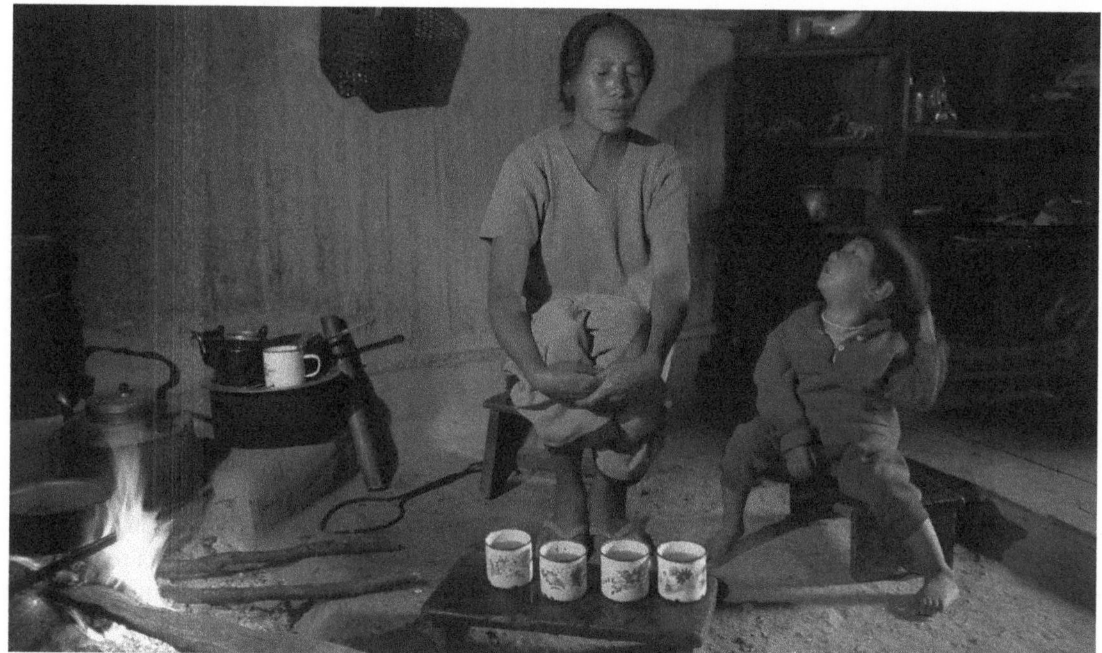

FIGURE 17.1 A Woman in Nagaland, India Cooks over an Open Wood Fire in her Home.
Source: Photo by Jerry Redfern/LightRocket via Getty Images

U-shaped hole in a block of clay, or a pit in the ground, or in poorly functioning earth or metal stoves[3] (Fig. 17.2). Combustion is very incomplete in most of these stoves, resulting in substantial emissions which, in the presence of poor ventilation, produce very high levels of indoor pollution.[9] Indoor concentrations of particles usually exceed guideline levels by a large margin: 24-hour mean PM_{10} levels are typically in the range 300–3000 μg/m^3 and may reach 30 000 μg/m^3 or more during periods of cooking.[6,7,9–20]

The United States Environmental Protection Agency's standards for 24-hour average PM_{10} and $PM_{2.5}$ concentrations are 150 μg/m^3 and 65 μg/m^3 respectively.[8] The mean 24-hour levels of carbon monoxide in homes using biomass fuels in developing countries are in the range 2–50 ppm; during cooking, values of 10–500 ppm have been reported. The United States Environmental Protection Agency's 8-hour average carbon monoxide standard is 9 ppm or 10 mg/m^3.[8]

A health effect is determined not just by the pollution level but also, and more importantly, by the time people spend breathing polluted air, i.e. the exposure level.[1] Exposure refers to the concentration of pollution in the immediate breathing environment during a specified period of time. This can be measured either directly through personal monitoring or indirectly by combining information on pollutant concentrations in each microenvironment where people spend time with information on activity patterns.[21] Information on such patterns is very important for understanding the dynamic relationship between levels of pollution and behaviour. As pollution levels are reduced it is possible that people will spend more time indoors or nearer the sources of pollution. If this happens a reduction in ambient pollution will not necessarily result in a proportionate decrease in exposure, and there will be important implications for interventions.

People in developing countries are commonly exposed to very high levels of pollution for 3–7 hours daily over many years.[22] During winter in cold and mountainous areas, exposure may occur over a

[1] Strictly, the dose that determines the health effect. In practice this is a complex issue that is difficult to assess. It is not considered further in this review.

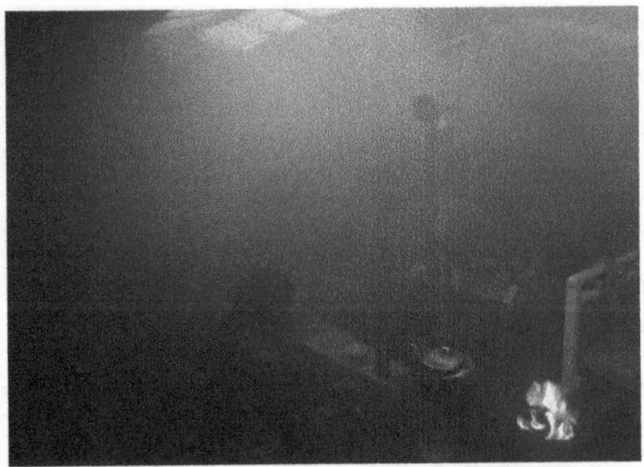

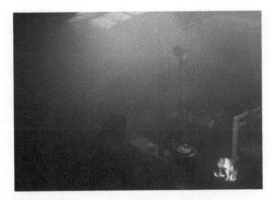

FIGURE 17.2 Indoor Air Pollution in a Yak Hair Tent in Tibet.

Photo credit: Steve Sclar

substantial portion of each 24-hour period.[13] Because of their customary involvement in cooking, women's exposure is much higher than men's.[23] Young children are often carried on their mothers' backs while cooking is in progress and therefore spend many hours breathing smoke.[1]

TABLE 17.1 Mechanisms by Which Some Key Pollutants in Smoke from Domestic Sources May Increase the Risk of Respiratory and Other Health Problems.

Pollutant	Potential Health Effects
Particules (small particles less than 10 microns, and particularly less than 2.5 microns aerodynamic diameter)	• Wheezing, exacerbation of asthma • Respiratory infections • Chronic bronchitis and chronic obstructive pulmonary disease • Exacerbation of chronic obstructive pulmonary disease
Carbon monoxide	• Low birth weight (fetal carboxyhaemoglobin 2–10% or higher) • Increase in perinatal deaths
Polycyclic aromatic hydrocarbons, e.g. benzo[a]pyrene	• Lung cancer • Cancer of mouth, nasopharynx and larynx
Nitrogen dioxide	• Wheezing and exacerbation of asthma • Respiratory infections • Reduced lung function in children
Sulphur dioxide	• Wheezing and exacerbation of asthma • Exacerbation of chronic obstructive pulmonary disease, cardiovascular disease
Biomass smoke condensates including polycyclic aromatics and metal ions	• Cataract

Source: N. Bruce, Perez-Padilla, R., and Albalak, R. "Indoor Air Pollution in Developing Countries." *Bulletin of the World Health Organization*, 2000, 78(9): 1078–1092.

Prospects for Interventions

The goal of interventions should be to reduce exposure to indoor air pollution, while meeting domestic energy and cultural needs and improving safety, fuel efficiency and environmental protection. Interventions should be affordable, perhaps requiring income generation and credit arrangements, and they should be sustainable. The evaluation of interventions should take into consideration all these criteria in addition to emphasizing the importance of reducing exposure to indoor air pollution.

Exposure can be reduced by means of improved stoves, better housing, cleaner fuels and behavioural changes. Cleaner fuels, especially liquefied petroleum gas, probably offer the best long-term option in terms of reducing pollution and protecting the environment, but most poor communities using biomass are unlikely to be able to make the transition to such fuels for many years.

The use of improved biomass stoves has given varying results and has often been unsuccessful. However, evaluation has been very limited and has not considered the range of criteria outlined above. Indeed, until recently, the main emphasis of stove programmes has been to reduce the use of wood, and consequently there has been relatively little evaluation of reductions in exposure.[129] Nevertheless, there are examples of large-scale rural stove programmes, for instance in China.[130] Under the Chinese programme, which began in 1980, improved stoves had been installed in over 172 million homes by the end of 1995. Smaller programmes, for example in western Kenya, have been enthusiastically adopted, mainly because of the participation of local women in construction and dissemination.[131] Although improved stoves are usually capable of reducing ambient pollution and personal exposure, the residual levels for stoves in regular use are still high, mostly in the range 500 to several thousand μg/m^3 TSP or PM_{10}).[115, 132, 133]

Relatively little information is available on the potential of other types of intervention, including the use of cleaner fuels, particularly for poor rural communities. A study of patterns of fuel use in households following electrification in a traditionally wood-burning area of South Africa showed that,

TABLE 17.2 Numbers of Deaths Attributable to Indoor Particles Air Pollution, by Setting.

Author	Total Deaths Attributable to Indoor Particles Air Pollution	Excess Mortality by Setting (Deaths and % of Total)			
		Developed Countries		Developing Countries	
		Urban	Rural	Urban	Rural
Smith	2.8 million	640,000 23%	1,800,000 67%	250,000 9%	30,000 1%
Schwela	2.7 million	363,000 13%	1,849,000 68%	511,000 19%	Not calculated

Source: N. Bruce, Perez-Padilla, R., and Albalak, R. "Indoor Air Pollution in Developing Countries." Bulletin of the World Health Organization, 2000, 78(9): 1078–1092.

while there was a shift to the use of electricity, the more polluting fuels continued to be used, particularly for cooking and heating.[134] The main reasons for not using electricity more were its cost and that of electrical appliances, although other factors, such as seasonal energy requirements and cultural beliefs, are also important in this connection.

In the field of development, household energy is important from the health, environmental and economic standpoints. This is consequently a very important field for interventions, and one in which technical and policy research needs to be closely linked to development work in a range of countries and settings.

Conclusion

Indoor air pollution is a major public health hazard for large numbers of the world's poorest, most vulnerable people and may be responsible for a similar proportion of the global burden of disease as risk factors such as tobacco and unsafe sex. The greatest contribution to this burden results from childhood acute lower respiratory infections. The evidence on which these estimates are based, however, is rather limited. It is important to extend and strengthen it, particularly for the most common and serious conditions including acute lower respiratory infections and tuberculosis, to quantify exposure, and to ensure that confounding is adequately dealt with. A few well-conducted randomized controlled studies on the health impact of reducing exposure would markedly strengthen the evidence, and should be feasible at the household level. For conditions where the evidence is very limited (e.g. low birth weight) or where a long latent period would make an intervention study impractical (e.g. tuberculosis, cataract), further observational studies are desirable.

Although work on interventions to reduce exposure has given mixed results, there is a wide range of possibilities and there has been some success in terms of both exposure reduction and uptake. The development and evaluation of interventions should take account of the many aspects of household energy supply and utilization, and should include assessment of pollution and exposure reductions, fuel efficiency and impact on the local and global environment, safety, capacity to meet household needs, affordability and sustainability. There is a need for a coordinated set of community studies to develop and evaluate interventions in a variety of settings, together with policy and macroeconomic studies on issues at the national level, such as fuel pricing incentives and other ways of increasing access by the poor to cleaner fuels. Also required is a systematic, standardized approach to monitoring levels and trends of exposure in a representative range of poor rural and urban populations.

Finally, it is necessary to keep in mind the close interrelationship between poverty and dependence on polluting fuels, and consequently the importance of socioeconomic development, which should be at the core of efforts to achieve healthier household environments.

REFERENCES

1. Albalak R. *Cultural practices and exposure to particles pollution from indoor biomass cooking: effects on respiratory health and nutrtitional status among the Aymara Indians of the Bolivian Highlands* [Doctoral dissertation]. University of Michigan, 1997.
2. World Resources Institute, UNEP, UNDP, World Bank. *1998–99 world resources: a guide to the global environment.* Oxford, Oxford University Press, 1998.
3. Smith KR. *Biomass fuels, air pollution, and health. A global review.* New York, Plenum Press, 1987.

4. Chen BH et al. Indoor air pollution in developing countries. *World Health Statistics Quarterly*, 1990, 43: 27–138.
5. De Koning HW, Smith KR, Last JM. Biomass fuel combustion and health. *Bulletin of the World Health Organization*, 1985, 63: 11–26.
6. Smith KR et al. Air pollution and the energy ladder in Asian cities. *Energy*, 1994, 19: 587–600.
7. McCracken JP, Smith KR. Emissions and efficiency of improved woodburning cookstoves in highland Guatemala. *Environment International*, 1998, 24: 739–747.
8. United States Environmental Protection Agency. Revisions to the National Ambient Air Quality Standards for Particles Matter. *Federal Register*, July 18 1997, 62: 38651–38701.
9. *Air quality guidelines for Europe*. Copenhagen, World Health Organization Regional Office for Europe, 2000 (in press).
10. Anderson HR. Respiratory abnormalities in Papua New Guinea children: the effects of locality and domestic wood smoke pollution. *International Journal of Epidemiology*, 1978, 7: 63–72.
11. Collings DA, Sithole SD, Martin KS. Indoor woodsmoke pollution causing lower respiratory disease in children. *Tropical Doctor*, 1990, 20: 151–155.
12. Martin KS. Indoor air pollution in developing countries. *Lancet*, 1991, 337: 358.
13. Norboo T et al. Domestic pollution and respiratory illness in a Himalayan village. *International Journal of Epidemiology*, 1991, 20: 749–757.
14. Saksena S et al. Patterns of daily exposure to TSP and CO in the Garhwal Himalaya. *Atmospheric Environment*, 1992, 26A: 2125–2134.
15. Ellegard A. Cooking fuel smoke and respiratory symptoms among women in low-income areas of Maputo. *Environmental Health Perspectives*, 1996, 104: 980–985.
16. Robin LF et al. Wood-burning stoves and lower respiratory illnesses in Navajo children. *Pediatric Infectious Diseases Journal*, 1996, 15: 859–865.
17. Ellegård A. Tears while cooking: an indicator of indoor air pollution and related health effects in developing countries. *Environmental Research*, 1997, 75: 12–22.
18. Albalak R, Frisancho AR, Keeler GJ. Domestic biomass fuel combustion and chronic bronchitis in two rural Bolivian villages. *Thorax*, 1999, 54 (11): 1004–1008.
19. Albalak R et al. Assessment of PM_{10} concentrations from domestic biomass fuel combustion in two rural Bolivian highland villages. *Environmental Science and Technology*, 1999, 33: 2505–2509.
20. Zhang J et al. Carbon monoxide from cookstoves in developing countries: 2. Potential chronic exposures. *Chemosphere-Global Change Science*, 1999, 1: 367–375.
21. Lioy PJ. Assessing total human exposure to contaminants: a multidisciplinary approach. *Environmental Science and Techonology*, 1990, 24 (7): 938–945.
22. Engel P, Hurtado E, Ruel M. Smoke exposure of women and young children in highland Guatemala: predictions and recall accuracy. *Human Organisation*, 1998, 54: 408–417.
23. Behera D, Dash S, Malik S. Blood carboxyhaemoglobin levels following acute exposure to smoke of biomass fuel. *Indian Journal of Medical Research*, 1988, 88: 522–542.
115. Naeher L et al. Indoor, outdoor and personal carbon monoxide and particle levels in Quetzaltenango, Guatemala: characterisation of traditional, improved and gas stoves in three test homes. Geneva, World Health Organization, 1996 (unpublished document, Acute Respiratory Infections Programme).
126. *Health and environment in sustainable development*. Geneva, World Health Organization, 1997 (unpublished document WHO/EHG/97.8).
129. Bruce N. *Lowering exposure of children to indoor air pollution to prevent ARI: the need for information* and *action*. Arlington, Environmental Health Project, 1999 (Capsule Report 3).
130. Lin D. The development and prospective of bioenergy technology in China. *Biomass and Bioenergy*, 1998, 15: 181–186.
131. *Indoor air pollution from biomass fuel*. Geneva, World Health Organization, 1992 (unpublished document WHO/PEP/92-3).
132. Reid H, Smith KR, Sherchand B. Indoor smoke exposures from traditional and improved cookstoves: comparisons among rural Nepali women. *Mountain Research and Development*, 1986, 6: 293–304.
133. Ezzati M, Mbinda MB, Kammen DM. Comparison of emissions and residential exposure from traditional and improved cookstoves in Kenya. *Environmental Science and Technology*, 2000, 34: 578–583.
134. Luvhimbi, Jawrek H. Household energy in a recently electrified rural settlement in Mpumalanga, South Africa. *Boiling Point*, 1997, 38: 30–31.

18 TOBACCO INDUSTRY INTERFERENCE: A GLOBAL BRIEF

There are real enemies to global health efforts. This article is about the international tobacco industry and how it continues to undermine the work of the World Health Organization (WHO) and national public health agencies in protecting peoples' health. Cigarette smoking is a major cause of preventable death in the world, leading to around 6 million deaths every year.

Cigarette smoking has declined in high-income countries over the past 50 years, but few young people realize how common smoking was in the United States in the 1950s and 1960s. At the peak of smoking in the United States, over two-thirds of American men smoked, and each of them smoked an average of about 4,000 cigarettes a year. The tobacco industry became so successful, in large measure, because of its effective advertising and marketing strategies; it made the cigarette cool and sexy. The industry spent more on the advertising of cigarettes than actually producing them. The profits were enormous.

As discussed in Reading 6, the biomedical reality that cigarette smoking caused cancer took a great deal of effort for public health authorities to establish. Using legal means and public education, public health advocates finally won out in the end—at least in rich countries. They did so despite the fact that the highly profitable tobacco industry was well organized for active opposition to the truth. Globally, the culmination of the WHO's antismoking efforts was the agreement called the Framework Convention on Tobacco Control, signed by over 200 nations. The framework laid out goals and plans such as antismoking regulations concerning advertising to minors, increasing health education, limiting secondhand smoke, and providing services to help current smokers quit. These are proven strategies; increasing taxes on the product and educating young people to discourage them to start smoking are effective at lowering smoking rates.

However, tobacco sales remain good business. Cigarettes have advantages over other consumer products—like the fact they are highly addictive. Smoking is an efficient way to deliver the very addictive drug of nicotine, and, therefore, the habit is extremely difficult to stop. Cigarettes are also inexpensive to make and require almost no innovation. Moreover, the future of the tobacco industry is bright because there is a growing world market. As rates of smoking have declined in rich nations, they have continued to grow in low- and middle-income countries. There are an estimated 1 billion smokers in the world today, with the greatest number in China.

This article describes how the tobacco industry continues to fight against public health and the ways they "fight dirty." The militant tone of this article is rather unusual for the WHO. But the strategies employed to influence governments throughout the world to support the tobacco industry—ranging from legal intimidation to the seduction of charities—must be frustrating when there are so many lives at stake. In the past, when global health efforts were so focused on decreasing child mortality from infectious disease, there was the criticism that Global Health was "saving the children for the tobacco industry." Given how deadly cigarettes and addictive cigarettes are, it is a good thing that the WHO is engaging in the fight against a clever and rich enemy.

As you read this article, consider the following questions:

- **Do you smoke cigarettes? Why or why not?**
- **In your opinion, why is the tobacco industry focusing on their expansion into the markets of low- and middle-income countries? What power do these companies have in regard to local governments?**

World Health Organization. *Tobacco Industry Interference: A Global Brief.* Washington, DC: WHO, 2012. http://apps.who.int/iris/bitstream/10665/70894/1/WHO_NMH_TFI_12.1_eng.pdf.

- **Of the different tactics used by the tobacco industry detailed in the article, which do you think is the most devious? Which do you think is the cleverest?**
- **The Framework Convention on Tobacco Control was a remarkable achievement for global health. After reading this article, would you defend or criticize that statement?**
- **The cover of this WHO document has a gangster in a black fedora and a black overcoat with a tiny label "Big Tobacco." He is removing a No Smoking symbol from a wall. Do you think that such a depiction is fair? Or are people working in the tobacco industry just doing their job?**

CONTEXT

This pamphlet was published by the WHO in 2012. The tobacco control section of the WHO is very small, especially when seen in comparison with the number of people working for Big Tobacco. Like many WHO documents, it does not have a specific author. Unlike many WHO documents, which usually are very diplomatic, it does not mince words.

Stop Tobacco Industry Interference in Tobacco Control

Curbing the Tobacco Epidemic

Tobacco addiction is a global epidemic that ravages entire countries and regions, wreaking the most havoc in the most vulnerable countries and creating an enormous toll of disability, disease, lost productivity and death. Tobacco use continues to be the leading global cause of preventable death. It kills nearly 6 million people every year through cancer, heart disease, respiratory diseases, childhood diseases and others. It also causes hundreds of billions of dollars of economic losses worldwide every year. If current trends continue, by 2030 tobacco will kill more than 8 million people worldwide every year, with 80% of these premature deaths occurring among people in low- and middle-income countries. Over the course of the 21st century, tobacco use could kill up to a billion people unless urgent action is taken.

We know what works to curb the tobacco epidemic. The action we need to take is laid out in the WHO Framework Convention on Tobacco Control (WHO FCTC). So far, 173 nations (plus the European Union) have pledged to work together to implement the Convention in order to protect present and future generations from the devastating health, social, environmental and economic consequences of tobacco consumption and exposure to tobacco smoke. However, these tobacco control efforts are systematically opposed by the tobacco industry. Who or what is the tobacco industry and what forms do its interference with public health efforts take?

Tobacco Industry Opposition

What Is the Tobacco Industry?

The "tobacco industry" includes manufacturers, importers and distributors of tobacco products and processors of tobacco leaf – an entire group of businesses whose only goal is to make profits, directly or indirectly, from tobacco products.

The tobacco industry has energetically promoted tobacco sales, despite knowing for decades that tobacco use and exposure to secondhand tobacco smoke damaged people's health. Despite a promise to investigate and share all research findings with the public, made in 1954,[1] the tobacco industry has hidden the facts from the public and continues to deny the full impact of tobacco products in order to maintain profits and increase sales. Dependency on tobacco is engineered, in the case of smoking, by careful, calculated formulations of more than 1000 chemical and other ingredients.[2,3] The tobacco industry sells a product that, unlike any other legal commercial good, kills up to half its regular users when consumed as directed by the manufacturer.

The Tobacco Industry Puts Profits before People

There is a fundamental and irreconcilable conflict between the tobacco industry's interests and public health policy interests. In one corner, the tobacco industry produces and promotes a product that has been scientifically proven to be highly addictive, to harm and kill many and to give rise to a variety of social ills, including increased poverty. In the opposite corner, many governments and public health workers try to increase the health of the population by implementing measures to reduce tobacco use. The tobacco industry recognizes the impact of these measures and actively fights against these efforts because of their negative effect on its sales. Time and time again, the industry has used its resources to halt these public health policies where it can, water them down when it cannot stop them altogether, and undermine their enforcement when they are adopted.

The tobacco industry has decades of experience of operating away from the public eye. Although these covert tactics continue, in recent years tobacco industry opposition has become more aggressive and overt. It increasingly includes direct counteraction against policies and strategies contained in, and promoted by, the WHO FCTC.[4] The objective is to extend the tobacco industry's sphere of influence with the aim of reaching all levels and sectors of government, as well as nongovernmental groups including the private sector and civil society, while trying to appear before politicians and the public as indispensable contributors to economic and social welfare.

Forms of Tobacco Industry Interference

In its efforts to derail or weaken strong tobacco control policies, tobacco industry interference takes many forms. These include:

- manoeuvering to hijack the political and legislative process;
- exaggerating the economic importance of the industry;
- manipulating public opinion to gain the appearance of respectability;
- fabricating support through front groups;
- discrediting proven science; and
- intimidating governments with litigation or the threat of litigation.

Manoeuvering to Hijack the Political and Legislative Process

In a presentation to the Philip Morris Board of Directors in 1995, the then Senior Vice-President of Worldwide Regulatory Affairs of the company stated: "Our goal is to help shape regulatory environments that enable our businesses to achieve their objectives . . . [fighting] aggressively with all available resources, against any attempt, from any quarter, to diminish our ability to manufacture our products efficiently, and market them effectively . . . ".[5]

The range of strategies used by the tobacco industry, then and now, to influence the political and legislative process includes conspiring with lobbyists to promote self-interested decisions in preference to those that serve the public good. Existing evidence suggests, for example, that in several countries the tobacco industry tried to undermine the country's position in the negotiation of the WHO FCTC and continues to attempt to derail the treaty's implementation.[6,7,8,9,10,11,12,13,14] The tactics used by the tobacco industry included: the inciting of controversy between financial, trade and other ministries on one side and the health ministry on the other side; the use of business associations and other "front groups" to lobby on the industry's behalf; and the securing of industry access to the WHO FCTC negotiations through its well established links with the International Organization for Standardization.[15] Other evidence shows that the industry has sought to weaken legislation in many countries in all regions of the world.

Manoeuvering to influence political and legislative decisions also involves: creating and exploiting legislative loopholes; demanding a seat at government decision-making tables; promoting voluntary regulation instead of legislation; and drafting and distributing sample legislation that is favourable to the tobacco industry. There have been cases of industry representatives actually writing the language of tobacco control and other legislation, to ensure that any regulatory measures would not be too restrictive on the industry's aggressive marketing practices.[16,17]

Another common strategy is entering into industry partnerships with different branches of government to fund joint projects, such as border patrols to prevent illicit trade, sports programmes for children, support for meetings and events and sponsoring of meetings that play on human rights concerns and condemn regulatory initiatives.[18,19,20] Other strategies include making political campaign contributions, chalking up favours by financing government initiatives on other health issues and defending trade benefits at the expense of health. All these strategies, along with the claims of wanting "reasonable" regulation that is ineffective, give the industry constant access to individuals in power and the potential to manipulate the policy-making process.

Exaggerating the Economic Importance of the Industry

The tobacco industry boosts its efforts to interfere in the political process by exaggerating its own contribution, expressed in terms of employment, tax contributions and other economic indicators, to the economy of a country, region, province or municipality. Not only is the economic information overhyped, but it also ignores the negative economic impact of tobacco use, including the drain on the public purse caused by the need to treat the millions of people afflicted by diseases caused by tobacco.

The industry claims, for example, to generate a high level of direct and indirect employment. It opposes tobacco control measures on the grounds that they would have a negative impact on employment and therefore on the country's economy. Using this argument, the industry lobbies against tobacco tax increases, predicting catastrophic consequences for its business. In reality, evidence has shown, at least to date, that job losses in the tobacco sector have little to do with stricter tobacco control measures. A recent publication[21] highlights how the tobacco industry lobbied against cigarette taxation and tariffs on the pretext that reduced production costs would preserve jobs. Despite obtaining tax advantages, the industry still reorganized and consolidated its production processes, leading to job losses in the sector. In fact, even if its demands are met, it is not uncommon for the industry to threaten to close a factory or department and move elsewhere, despite its claims to social commitment and responsibility.

Sound economic studies show that industry claims of potential job and other economic losses resulting from stricter tobacco controls are significantly overstated anyway; in fact, these losses are negligible. If consumption declines, job losses in tobacco-dependent sectors, are more than offset by increases in employment in other sectors with no negative impact on the overall economy.[22]

Manipulating Public Opinion to Gain the Appearance of Respectability

Public opinion governs the workings of our society, and the tobacco industry devotes considerable resources to trying to twist it. The industry is aware that the views of millions of people every day are influenced by the mass media. The tobacco industry uses public relations firms and other groups to concoct and spin the news to promote its lethal business. Public relations firms have often been used in an attempt to manipulate the media and public opinion about various aspects of tobacco control and to gather the support of persons who oppose government "intrusion" in business and taxation, thus instigating general antiregulatory and antigovernment views.

However, the main way of manipulating public opinion is corporate social responsibility (CSR) activity, also known as "social investment". While CSR activities in many industries reflect an honest commitment to behave ethically and contribute to economic development, while improving the quality of life of the workforce, the local community and society at large, for the tobacco industry it is a self-serving strategy. CSR activities by the tobacco industry may include ineffective youth smoking prevention campaigns which allow the industry to present itself as "caring" for the very youngsters to whom it also markets its deadly products. The industry takes pains to support social programmes for tobacco growers and their children and unrelated social causes such as programmes to combat domestic violence against women, disaster relief efforts and environmental causes and groups. Every time a group accepts funds from or works with the tobacco industry, the industry claws back some of the respectability it has lost through the social, economic, environmental and health damage caused by its products. In summary, the tobacco industry uses CSR to claim that it cares for society and the environment and to present itself as a responsible member of society.

These CSR efforts interfere with health policy by winning goodwill for the industry among politicians and the public. The industry uses CSR to seduce groups not related to tobacco – sometimes not even related to health – into becoming industry allies. In this way, when there are attempts to regulate tobacco marketing, for example, the industry can call on a host of organizations which are well disposed towards it, or in its debt, to speak on its behalf.

This phenomenon has recently been seen in countries from regions as diverse as Africa[23] and Europe,[24] where representatives of tobacco companies complained that a proposed ban on sponsorship, a recognized form of marketing, was harmful and unnecessary. A chorus of protests from charities supporting causes such as mental health and care for the elderly was then quoted in the media and presented as opposition to proposed legislation banning tobacco marketing. Media reports focused on the loss of income for the charitable organizations, and not on the health gains to be made by restricting tobacco marketing.

Fabricating Support through Front Groups

Years of deception have so isolated the tobacco industry from business and citizens that it needs to simulate support. To this end, the industry uses front groups. Front groups are organizations that purport to serve a public cause while actually serving the interests of a third party, sometimes obscuring or concealing the connection between them. The tobacco industry uses phony "grassroots" groups to give an impression of social support for its interests, typically "smokers' rights" groups, "citizens' rights" groups and business groups.

"Smokers' rights" groups are created and promoted behind the scenes to preserve the social acceptability of smoking and speak out for allowing smoking in public places. Philip Morris proposed adopting a variety of personas: "Sometimes we will need to speak as independent scientists, scientific groups and businessmen; at other times we will talk as the industry; and, finally, we will speak as the smoker".[25] Since smoke-free policies are widely supported by the general public, the "smokers' rights" groups try to maintain a "controversy" about secondhand smoke in the social arena and focus the debate on the smoker rather than the tobacco industry or the harmful effects of the smoke itself. "Smokers' rights" groups oppose clean indoor air laws and policies, and take a stand on other issues as well, such as tobacco taxes and advertising bans.[26]

Business front groups are used to argue that tobacco control policies cause economic damage to the businesses they claim to represent. The tobacco industry is known for funding tobacco growers' associations and creating or funding restaurant or bar organizations to oppose smoke-free measures in the hospitality sector. Their role is to insist that banning smoking would cost them business and to create an aggressive mentality in legitimate restaurant and bar operators against government smoke-free policies. The tobacco industry has also created front groups to oppose consumer regulation, depicting it as an attack on individual freedom. It describes these regulation efforts as part of the "nanny culture" led by a "growing fraternity" of food and anti-tobacco "cops", "health care enforcers", "anti-meat activists" and "meddling bureaucrats" who "know what's best for you".[27]

Discrediting Proven Science

The scientific evidence about the harm caused by tobacco and secondhand smoke is so strong and extensive that the industry needs to discredit it in order to get around or weaken tobacco control legislation. "Doubt is our product", a cigarette executive once observed, "since it is the best means of competing with the 'body of fact' that exists in the minds of the general public. It is also the means of establishing a controversy".[28]

The efforts of the tobacco industry to deny the lethal effects of secondhand smoke are well known. For decades the industry has known that secondhand smoke is toxic. One company, for example, privately performed extensive research on secondhand smoke in a secret laboratory and demonstrated its toxicity.[29,30] It then designed a global programme with other tobacco companies, hiring scientists and lobbyists to dispute scientific evidence about health risks. The industry hired scientists and briefed journalists, government officials and members of the scientific community in order to keep them confused about the hazards posed by tobacco and secondhand smoke. The majority of tobacco companies continue to deny that secondhand smoke kills.[31,32]

Whether it is creating confusion about the harms of secondhand smoke, the addictiveness of nicotine or the deleterious effects of smoking, the tobacco industry's duplicitous tactics have spawned a multimillion-dollar industry which dismisses research conducted by the scientific community as "junk science". Hired consultants have increasingly tried to skew the scientific literature, and have manufactured and magnified scientific uncertainty, in order to divert policy decisions to the industry's advantage. In doing so, they have not only delayed action on tobacco control, but have weakened public health safeguards and put up barriers which make it harder for lawmakers, government agencies and courts to respond to future threats.

Intimidating Governments with Litigation or the Threat of Litigation

An often-used threat, increasingly carried out, is the threat of legal retaliation against a specific policy or set of policies. This can be at any level, from global to local. The tobacco industry, employing a veritable army of lawyers, threatens legal action against governments over tobacco control policies that threaten its profits. Legal arguments often question the constitutionality of any policy measure or legislation, claim that due process was not followed in the phase that preceded the adoption of legislation and argue against any implementation or regulatory language that follows adoption.

Since the entry into force of the WHO FCTC, domestic legal challenges by the tobacco industry and its front groups have more and more frequently failed, as courts cite the treaty as the legal foundation for strong tobacco control legislation. Recently, the industry has shifted its litigation strategy, scaling up the use of international bilateral or multilateral agreements to challenge a country's tobacco control policy in the courts. For example, the tobacco industry has recently brought actions against Australia, Norway, Uruguay and other countries which have introduced tougher tobacco control measures in line with the WHO FCTC. The industry has pursued these governments through international mechanisms and using bilateral investment agreements. It seems that these intimidation tactics are deliberately designed to deter other countries from introducing similar tobacco control measures.[33]

Tobacco Industry Interference: Always and Everywhere a Threat to Public Health

Regardless of the shape or form it takes, tobacco industry interference is always designed to thwart attempts to curb the tobacco epidemic and its negative social, economic, environmental and health consequences. While there is a growing awareness of the tobacco industry's unceasing attempts to sabotage public health, it is less well known that tobacco companies often work hand in glove with their commercial competitors to keep regulation to a minimum and obtain advantageous conditions from the government to help them run their businesses.

Three things to keep in mind about tobacco industry interference:

- it is not always obvious;
- it is not always in the area of tobacco control; and
- it is not always even in the area of health.

Tobacco industry interference is a threat to public health, whether the industry is private or state-owned. So all countries need to be aware and take action against tobacco industry interference. WHO recognizes that the tobacco industry uses back-handed methods to thwart tobacco control efforts, and urges governments to remain.

WHO FRAMEWORK CONVENTION ON TOBACCO CONTROL, ARTICLE 5.3

"In setting and implementing their public health policies with respect to tobacco control, Parties shall act to protect these policies from commercial and other vested interests of the tobacco industry in accordance with national law."

How to Beat Tobacco Industry Interference

Fortunately, to address this global threat there is a global solution. A total of 173 countries plus the European Union (comprising almost 90% of the world's population) have already agreed to implement an international treaty, the WHO FCTC, that sets out policies aimed at controlling this epidemic of disease, death and suffering. Countries that are Parties to this treaty recognize the tobacco industry as a major barrier to achieving global health and have committed themselves to overcoming this barrier, as shown by Article 5.3 of the treaty.[35]

Because the industry interferes in all countries, those countries that are not yet a Party to the WHO FCTC are also urged to counteract the industry's malicious interference and refuse to provide it with a safe haven for its business and litigation.

Everyone can help. Governments, nongovernmental organizations, academia and individual citizens can all act to put an end to tobacco industry interference.

Governments Must Act to Protect Public Health from Tobacco Industry Interference

All the Parties to the WHO FCTC have agreed on ways to stop tobacco industry interference. They have adopted Guidelines for the implementation of Article 5.3 of the WHO FCTC,[36] based on four principles:

Principle 1:
There is a fundamental and irreconcilable conflict between the tobacco industry's interests and public health policy interests.

Principle 2:
Parties, when dealing with the tobacco industry or those working to further its interests, should be accountable and transparent.

Principle 3:
Parties should require the tobacco industry and those working to further its interests to operate and act in a manner that is accountable and transparent.

Principle 4:
Because their products are lethal, the tobacco industry should not be granted incentives to establish or run their businesses.

Based on these principles, governments should take action to prevent tobacco industry interference in tobacco control and public health. They should communicate information relevant to the tobacco industry to policy-makers, decision-makers and stakeholders and establish coordinated approaches involving all sectors of the government to promote full accountability and guide all interactions with the tobacco industry, ensuring that these interactions are limited to what is strictly necessary and transparently disclosed. A monitoring system for the tobacco industry, with relevant exchanges of information at regional and global level, should be considered as an important tool to implement the Article 5.3 guidelines.

More specifically, in applying the Article 5.3 guidelines, governments should:

- Raise awareness about the addictive and harmful nature of tobacco products and about tobacco industry interference with tobacco control policies.
- Establish measures to limit interactions with the tobacco industry and ensure the transparency of those interactions that do occur.
- Reject partnerships and non-binding or non-enforceable agreements with the tobacco industry. Not accept funds or help from the tobacco industry. Not support or endorse tobacco industry attempts to organize, promote, participate in or implement youth, public education or other initiatives that are directly or indirectly related to tobacco control.
- Require that information provided by the tobacco industry be transparent and accurate. Require the tobacco industry and those

working to further its interests to submit regular, truthful, complete and precise information on tobacco production, manufacture, market share, marketing expenditures, revenues or any other activity, including lobbying, philanthropy and political contributions, as well as the disclosure or registration of tobacco industry entities, affiliated organizations and individuals acting on their behalf, including lobbyists.

- Denormalize and, to the extent possible, regulate activities described as "socially responsible" by the tobacco industry, including but not limited to activities described as "corporate social responsibility".
- Avoid giving preferential treatment to the tobacco industry.
- Treat state-owned tobacco companies in the same way as the rest of the tobacco industry.
- Avoid conflicts of interest for government officials and employees. Governmental action in this area should include:
    - mandating policy on the disclosure and management of conflicts of interest, binding on all government officials, employees, consultants and contractors;
    - implementing a code of conduct for public officials which prescribes the standards with which they should comply in their dealings with the tobacco industry;
    - prohibiting contributions by the tobacco industry or any entity working to further its interests to the coffers of political parties, candidates or campaigns, or at least requiring full disclosure of such contributions.

Nongovernmental Groups and Academia Need to Monitor and Denounce Interference

Nongovernmental groups and academia have an essential role in implementing the WHO FCTC and Article 5.3 guidelines. In fact, any institution can help to counteract tobacco industry interference. Here are some possible actions:

Identify the potential allies and front groups of the tobacco industry, using legislative and regulatory processes, in addition to any legal cases.

Monitor whether the tobacco industry is complying with national regulations and laws.

- Denounce industry interference to the media, parliamentarians and government.

Individuals: Everyone Can Help

- Be aware of the ways the tobacco industry interferes. Learn its ways and be vigilant.
- Use social media to inform others of tobacco industry interference and share your opposition to it.
- Denounce tobacco industry interference when you see it.
- Join nongovernmental groups working to stop tobacco industry interference.

REFERENCES

1. Cummings KM, Morley CP, Hyland A. Failed promises of the cigarette industry and its effect on consumer misperceptions about the health risks of smoking. *Tobacco Control*, 2002, 11:i110-i117, doi:10.1136/tc.11.suppl_1.i110 (http://tobaccocontrol.bmj.com/content/11/suppl_1/i110.full, accessed 10 May 2012).
2. Hirschhorn N. *Evolution of the tobacco industry positions on addiction to nicotine.* Geneva, World Health Organization, 2008 (http://whqlibdoc.who.int/publications/2009/9789241597265_eng.pdf, accessed 10 May 2012).
3. *Tobacco: deadly in any form or disguise.* Geneva, World Health Organization, 2006:14 (http://www.who.int/tobacco/communications/events/wntd/2006/Tfi_Rapport.pdf, accessed 10 May 2012).
4. Mackay JM, Bettcher DW, Minhas R, Schotte K. Successes and new emerging challenges in tobacco control: addressing the vector. Tob Control 2012;21:77–79 doi:10.1136/tobaccocontrol-2012-050433.
5. Philip Morris. *Corporate worldwide regulatory affairs issues review, prospects and plans, 29 April 1995* (http://legacy.library.ucsf.edu/tid/jww95a00, accessed 3 May 2012).

6. Grüning T et al. Tobacco industry attempts to influence and use the German government to undermine the WHO Framework Convention on Tobacco Control. *Tobacco Control*, 2012, 21:30–38, doi:10.1136/tc.2010.042093 (http://tobaccocontrol.bmj.com/content/21/1/30.full, accessed 4 May 2012).
7. Mamudu HM, Hammond R, Glantz SA. International trade versus public health during the FCTC negotiations, 1999–2003. *Tobacco Control*, 2011, 1:e3, Epub 13 October 2010 (http://tobaccocontrol.bmj.com/content/early/2010/10/13/tc.2009.035352.abstract, accessed 10 May 2012).
8. Otañez MG, Mamudu HM, Glantz SA. Tobacco companies' use of developing countries' economic reliance on tobacco to lobby against global tobacco control: the case of Malawi. *American Journal of Public Health*, 2009, 99(10):1759–71, Epub 20 August 2009 (http://www.ncbi.nlm.nih.gov/pubmed/19696392, accessed 10 May 2012).
9. Assunta M, Chapman S. Health treaty dilution: a case study of Japan's influence on the language of the WHO Framework Convention on Tobacco Control. *Journal of Epidemiology and Community Health*, 2006, 60(9):751–756 (http://jech.bmj.com/content/60/9/751.full, accessed 10 May 2012).
10. Lee S, Ling PM, Glantz SA. The vector of the tobacco epidemic: tobacco industry practices in low and middle-income countries. *Cancer Causes and Control*, 2012, 23 (Suppl. 1):117–29, Epub 28 February 2012.
11. Jakpor P. Nigeria: how British American Tobacco undermines the WHO FCTC through agricultural initiatives: invited commentary. *Tobacco Control*, 2012, 21(2):220.
12. Wan X et al. Conflict of interest and FCTC implementation in China. *Tobacco Control*, 14 June 2011, doi:10.1136/tc.2010.041327.
13. Mejia R et al. Tobacco industry strategies to obstruct the FCTC in Argentina. *CVD Prevention and Control*, 2008, 3(4):173–179.
14. Mamudu HM, Hammond R, Glantz S. Tobacco industry attempts to counter the World Bank report Curbing the Epidemic and obstruct the WHO Framework Convention on Tobacco Control. *Social Science and Medicine*, 2008, 67(11):1690–99, Epub 2008 Oct 22.
15. Bialous SA, Yach D. Whose standard is it, anyway? How the tobacco industry determines the International Organization for Standardization (ISO) standards for tobacco and tobacco products. *Tobacco Control*, 2001;10:96–104, doi:10.1136/tc.10.2.96.
16. Crosbie E, Sebrié EM, Glantz SA. Tobacco industry success in Costa Rica: the importance of FCTC article 5.3. *Salud Pública de México*, 2012, 54(1):28–38.
17. Albuja S, Daynard RA. The Framework Convention on Tobacco Control (FCTC) and the adoption of domestic tobacco control policies: the Ecuadorian experience. *Tobacco Control*, 2009, 18(1):18–21, Epub 2008 Oct 20.
18. Imperial Tobacco (http://www.imperial-tobacco.com/files/environment/cr2006/index.asp?pageid=34, accessed 10 May 2012).
19. British American Tobacco-Nigeria (http://www.batnigeria.com/oneweb/sites/bat_58td2C.nsf/vwpagesweblive/do65gdrq/$file/medmd6k4elm.pdf?openelement).
20. AMEInfo (http://www.ameinfo.com/news/company_news/b/British_American_Tobacco_BAT_/, accessed 10 May 2012).
21. Holden C, Lee K. 'A major lobbying effort to change and unify the excise structure in six Central American countries': how British American Tobacco influenced tax and tariff rates in the Central American Common Market. *Global Health*, 2011, 7(1):15 (http://dx.doi.org/10.1186/1744-8603-7-15, accessed 5 May 2012).
22. Health and economic impact of tobacco taxation. In: *Effectiveness of tax and price policies for tobacco control (IARC Handbooks of Cancer Prevention*, Vol. 14, Chapter 9). Lyon, International Agency for Research on Cancer/WHO, 2011.
23. African Financial Markets. *Anti-smoking laws blocking firms from charity* (http://www.africanfinancialmarkets.com/front-news-detail.php?NewsID=35348, accessed 10 May 2012).
24. Amos H. Foreign tobacco faces ban on charitable donations. *Moscow Times*, 14 December 2011 (http://www.themoscowtimes.com/news/article/foreign-tobacco-faces-ban-on-charitable-donations/449868.html#ixzz1u6xQgpB7, accessed 4 May 2012).
25. Philip Morris. Newsflow Strategic Overview. January 1989. In: Smith EA, Malone RE. 'We will speak as the smoker': the tobacco industry's smokers' rights groups. *European Journal of Public Health*, 2007, 17(3):306–313, doi: 10.1093/eurpub/ckl244 (http://eurpub.oxfordjournals.org/content/17/3/306.full#ref-1, accessed 4 May 2012).
26. Smith EA, Malone RE. 'We will speak as the smoker': the tobacco industry's smokers' rights groups. *European Journal of Public Health*, 2007, 17(3):306–313, doi: 10.1093/eurpub/ckl244 (http://eurpub.oxfordjournals.org/content/17/3/306.full#ref-1, accessed 4 May 2012).

27. Daube M, Stafford J, Bond L. No need for nanny. *Tobacco Control*, 2008;17:426–427, doi:10.1136/tc.2008.027763.
28. Brown and Williamson. *Smoking and health proposal* (Brown and Williamson Document No. 680561778-1786), 1969 (http://legacy.library.ucsf.edu/tid/nvs40f00, accessed 10 May 2012).
29. Schick S, Glantz S. Philip Morris toxicological experiments with fresh sidestream smoke: more toxic than mainstream smoke. *Tobacco Control*, 2005, 14:396–404, doi:10.1136/tc.2005.011288.
30. Diethelm PA, Rielle JC, McKee M. The whole truth and nothing but the truth? The research that Philip Morris did not want you to see. Lancet. 2005 Jul 2-8;366(9479):86–92.
31. Aguinaga Bialous S, Shatenstein S. Profits over people: tobacco industry activities to market cigarettes and undermine public health in Latin America and the Caribbean. Pan American Health Organization. November 2002.
32. Tong EK, Glantz SA. Tobacco Industry Efforts Undermining Evidence Linking Secondhand Smoke With Cardiovascular Disease. Circulation. 2007; 116: 1845–1854 doi: 10.1161/Circulation AHA.107.715888
33. *The changed face of the tobacco industry: galvanizing global action towards a tobacco-free world.* Dr Margaret Chan, keynote speech, 15th World Conference on Tobacco or Health, Singapore, 20 March 2012 (http://www.who.int/dg/speeches/2012/tobacco_20120320/en/index.html, accessed 5 May 2012).
34. World Health Assembly resolution WHA54.18, 2001 (http://www.who.int/tobacco/framework/wha_eb/wha54_18/en/index.html, accessed 5 May 2012).
35. WHO Framework Convention on Tobacco Control, Article 5.3 (http://www.who.int/fctc/guidelines/article_5_3.pdf, accessed 5 May 2012).
36. Guidelines for implementation of Article 5.3 of the WHO Framework Convention on Tobacco Control. In: *WHO Framework Convention on Tobacco Control: guidelines for implementation*. Geneva, World Health Organization, 2011 (http://www.who.int/fctc/guidelines/article_5_3.pdf, accessed 10 May 2012).

GEORGE LUBER AND STASIA WIDERYNSKI

19 THE HEALTH CONSEQUENCES OF GLOBAL CLIMATE CHANGE

The geological era in which we live is called the ***Anthropocene****. This term reflects the fact that humans have changed the Earth and its atmosphere so much that we have arrived at a new stage in the history of the planet. The Anthropocene is a different environment than the one in which our ancestors evolved. Of course, the planet changed a great deal over the millions of years of the remote past, including intermittent periods of cooling during the ice ages. Geologists and paleontologists have documented five "great extinctions" in the history of the planet. Nevertheless, the Anthropocene is unique—and uniquely dangerous.*

"Global warming" was the first label given to this phenomenon, and that sounded rather innocuous. The current label is "climate change," but that does not adequately connote its dangers. **Climate change** *is a set of interconnected patterns involving increases in the frequency and severity of extreme weather events, an overall rise in average temperature and consequently a rising sea level, and a growth of seemingly contradictory events such as droughts and floods. There is a scientific consensus about the dangers of and irreversibility of climate change. However, a minority of people prefer to ignore those warnings. Some of these deniers may confuse climate with weather. There are parallels here to the "merchants of doubt" who denied for decades the fact that cigarette smoking causes cancer and other diseases (see Reading 6). Yet denying climate change is different because the stakes are so much higher.*

Climate change is primarily the result of global industrialization and air pollution from our use of fossil fuels. The rich nations of the world have contributed the most to this problem, but they were doing so long before it was widely recognized. In the future, however, people throughout the world will pay the price—particularly the poorest people. Today, droughts in East and Central Africa that are ultimately related to climate change are causing terrible food shortages.

This article, written by members of the Climate and Health Program at the Centers for Disease Control (CDC), describes what is known about the population health effects of climate change. The list is long. Besides droughts, famines, floods, sea-level rise, and "super storms," there will be an increase in a myriad of other health problems—from allergies to heat stroke to the spread of insect-borne diseases. Global climate change is happening everywhere, but some nations and some segments of society are going to fare better than others. Just like so many other issues in global health, the ultimate outcome will be linked to socioeconomic inequalities.

As you read the following report, consider the following questions:

- **How would you use the model at the beginning of this article to explain the health effects of climate change? Try this with a friend who is not in the class. Did he or she expect that there would be so many different kinds of health effects?**
- **Why do you think there are people who want to believe that climate change is a hoax? What does this tell you about society?**
- **The authors name three main pathways by which climate change will affect health (adding to existing burdens): extreme weather, complex humanitarian emergencies, and novel infectious diseases. Which pathway do you think is most important? Why? What preventive or mitigative measures can be put in place?**
- **What does "resilience of infrastructure" mean in regard to climate change and health?**

This article is original to this volume.

- **How might some of the effects of climate change have impacts on mental health? What might public health practitioners do to decrease those negative effects?**

CONTEXT

George Luber is Chief, Climate and Health Program, Division of Environmental Hazards and Health Effects in the National Center for Environmental Health at the CDC. A medical anthropologist by training, he began his career at the CDC as an Epidemic Intelligence Service officer (see Reading 9). He has taken a leading role in discussions of climate change and health focusing on the United States and has co-authored *Global Climate Change and Human Health: from Science to Practice* (San Francisco: Jossey-Bass, 2015), as well as a number important intergovernmental assessments on climate change and health. Some people say that climate change is not always a popular topic at the CDC—it is not only political but also complex with no easy solutions. In some ways, it is the opposite of a localized outbreak of an infectious disease. Stasia Widerynski is a research fellow in Climate and Health at the CDC. Her background is in environmental science with a focus on the built environment and infrastructure.

Introduction

Weather and climate have been known to affect human health long before Hippocrates identified it as a critical determinant of health. Cold can cause hypothermia; heat can cause hyperthermia; droughts can cause famine; and floods can result in injuries, displacement, and death. Hurricanes, tornadoes, and forest fires can destroy life and property.

Mounting evidence that the earth's climate is changing has led the UN Intergovernmental Panel on Climate Change (IPCC) to conclude that "warming of the climate system is unequivocal, as is now evident from observations of increases in global average air and ocean temperatures, widespread melting of snow and ice, and rising of global average sea level." The IPCC, an international group of eminent climate scientists, reports that the majority of global increases in temperatures since the mid-20th century are very likely a result of greenhouse gases like carbon dioxide caused by human activity (IPCC 2014). Warming has already brought not only temperature and precipitation increases but also modest sea-level rise and increased weather variability, both of which will continue and will likely accelerate. Weather patterns will change everywhere, but the direction and magnitude of those changes will vary. The effects of these changes on human health will vary too, and will depend largely on the resources available for adaptation.

Climate change poses a threat to human health in a variety of ways: injury and death from heat waves, extreme storms, and reduced air quality from increasing ozone, aeroallergens, and drought-related wildfire smoke; illnesses transmitted by food, water, and vectors, such as mosquitoes and ticks; and mental health impacts subsequent to disasters.

More importantly, climate change will threaten the critical systems and infrastructure we rely on to keep us safe and healthy: communication and transportation during emergencies, food and water systems during drought, and the energy grid during prolonged heat waves. As the magnitude and frequency of extreme weather events increases, the resilience of these systems will be tested, and vulnerabilities will become more exposed. It is in this sense that climate change will serve as a "risk-multiplier" by amplifying both the exposures that bring about health risks and the vulnerabilities to these exposures.

This chapter will review the major categories of climate-sensitive health outcomes and their determinants and discuss how climate change and other trends interact as major future drivers of morbidity and mortality. In doing so, we will explore three key pathways through which climate change will act to modify disease risk: (1) adding to the cumulative burden of already-existing health threats, (2) increasing extreme weather events that have the potential to increase the probability of "complex

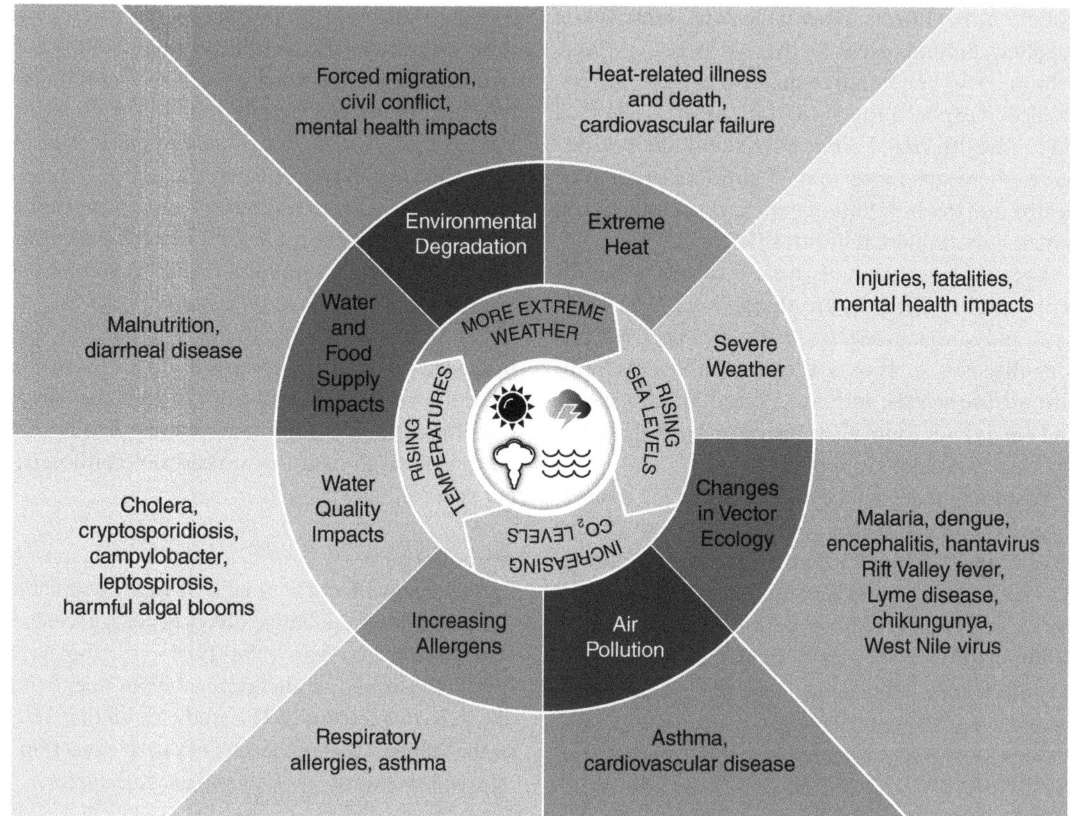

FIGURE 19.1 The Health Effects of Climate Change.
Source: George Luber, Climate and Health Program, Centers for Disease Control.

emergencies" where multiple system failures can exceed response capacity, and (3) the emergence of novel threats as a result of profound changes in disease ecology.

Climate Change Will Increase the Health Problems That Are Already Occurring

Air Pollution

Climate change is expected to impact human health by increasing air pollution in the forms of particulate matter (PM) and ground-level ozone. The increase in air pollution would make vulnerable populations and those already suffering from respiratory diseases more at risk to illnesses.

PM is a mix of microscopic solid and liquid particles, such as dirt and soot, that can be emitted from wildfires, construction sites, power plants, and fuel combustion of automobiles. PM can pose a major threat to public health because the particles can be small enough to get deep inside the lungs and even the blood stream. Those most at risk to the adverse health effects of air pollution include children, the elderly, individuals with pre-existing respiratory diseases, and those frequently exercising outside during periods of poor air quality.[1]

Ground-level ozone is a greenhouse gas that is formed naturally when chemicals that are emitted from coal-fired power plants and fuel combustion from cars, mix with sunlight. Ozone is also a key factor for creating smog, a severe and visible air pollution that affects many large cities such as Los Angeles, Beijing, New Delhi, Mexico City, and Tehran. Over one hundred major U.S. cities are periodically exposed to concentrations of ozone that exceed health based air quality standards. Worldwide, there are more than 7 million premature deaths due to air pollution exposure, making it the largest environmental health risk.[1]

Ground-level ozone is linked to many health problems, like difficulty breathing, sore throat, chest pain, and cardiac arrest. It can also aggravate respiratory diseases such as asthma, emphysema, and chronic bronchitis. Increased hospital admissions and emergency room visits have also been linked to increased levels of ground level ozone.[2,3]

Assuming there will be no future changes in environmental regulations or population growth characteristics and combined with the current air pollution health effects, scientists have estimated that there will be an additional 1,000–4,300 annual premature deaths in the United States by 2050 caused by poor air quality.[2] Global temperature rise is likely to cause decreases in air quality and increases in premature deaths because of worsened ozone and particulate matter pollution.[4]

Air pollution in India is more toxic than in any other country in the world. Although Beijing is infamous for its smog filled skies, New Delhi has surpassed it as the most polluted city in the world. According to the World Health Organization Air Pollution Database, thirteen of the top-20 most-polluted cities are in India.[5] The air in New Delhi is twenty times over the safe air limit. The pollution is caused by vehicle emission, burning solid waste, and construction sites. Weather patterns can trap the air pollution close to the ground for days, causing extreme health problems and deaths. Studies have shown that air pollution in India causes approximately half a million premature deaths annually and costs the country around $640 billion USD per year.[5]

Aeroallergens

Aeroallergens affect a large amount of the population. A nationally representative survey of allergy sensitization spanning the years 1988–1994 found that 54.3% of Americans had an allergic reaction to one or more allergens in a test study. The study found that 26.2% of the subjects had some sort of allergic reaction to ragweed, a common pollen and aero allergen.[6]

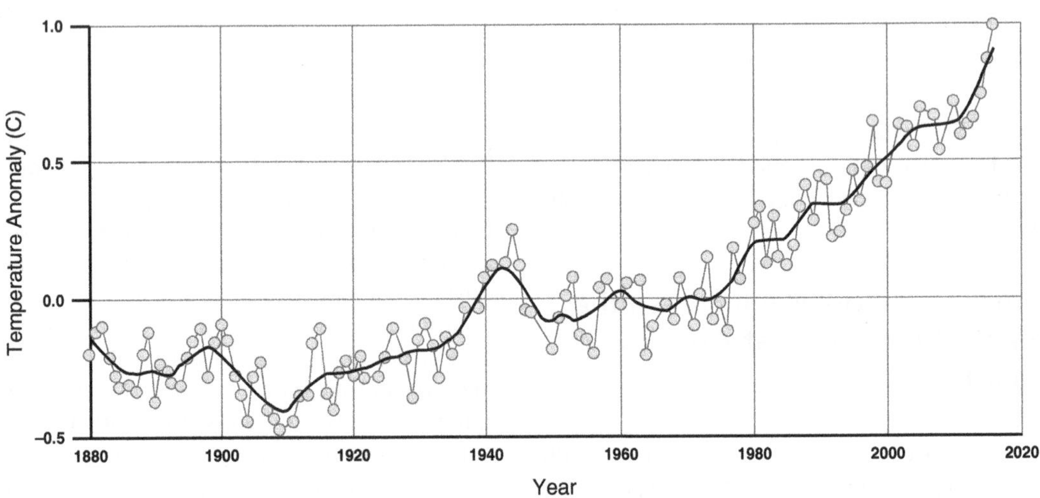

FIGURE 19.2 Change in Global Surface Temperature Compared to Average Temperatures from 1951–1980.

Temperature anomaly is a change from the average temperature.

Source: http://www.climate.nasa.gov.

Climate change has already caused longer, warmer seasons and more frost-free days. The changes in season temperature, as well as other climatic factors, have helped allergenic plant species produce pollen earlier and for a longer amount of time. The increase of carbon dioxide (CO2) gas in the atmosphere can produce a higher level of plant-based allergens because these plants use CO2 to grow and survive through photosynthesis. Higher pollen concentrations in the air and longer pollen seasons can adversely impact respiratory conditions; increase allergic sensitizations, asthma episodes, and rhinitis; and cause more visits to health care providers and emergency departments. There has also been an increase in the use of over-the-counter medications as a method to cope with the allergic reactions, rhinitis, and asthma. Other pollen-induced effects include loss of school and workdays because of allergies.[2,7,8]

Europe has been studying the trend in pollen for the past three decades and has an extensive international network that provides up to date pollen and hay-fever forecasts. Europe is a geographically complex continent with a widely diverse climate and varied types of vegetation, resulting in pollen calendars that differ widely by region. Some of the most common pollen species in Europe are birch trees, olive trees, and grasses. Urban areas seem to be more at risk for the adverse health effects of pollen than rural areas are. Studies have noted an increase in the amount of pollen in the air across Europe, as well as a shift in some pollen seasons. There has also been an increase in incidence rates of allergic illnesses, including respiratory diseases, allergic rhinitis, and asthma, which can be linked to the increase in airborne quantities of allergenic pollen.[9,10] Studies have shown that simultaneous exposure to air pollution and aeroallergens can work together to make allergy symptoms worse and create more severe health problems.[2]

Food and Waterborne Illness

Food and waterborne illnesses can be influenced by climate change through a sudden change in air and water temperature, severe precipitation patterns, or rising sea level. Extreme weather events have also been linked to foodborne illnesses. Flooding, drought, and wildfires can contaminate crops and fisheries and release metals and toxins into the environment polluting the food supply.[11,12]

Foodborne illnesses can result from eating food spoiled or contaminated by microbes, chemicals, or toxic substances. There has been an increase of food poisoning in the United Kingdom, and diarrheal diseases in Peru and Fiji, that have followed a short-term increase in temperature. There has also been a strong connection in European countries between a change in temperature and reports of salmonellosis (the foodborne illness caused by salmonella bacteria).[13,14]

Waterborne illnesses are caused by a variety of bacteria often occurring after an extreme weather event and can cause a variety of diarrheal diseases. Diarrheal diseases are a major public health issue in the developing world and affect those who consume or use untreated groundwater containing bacteria. The most vulnerable to these diseases are the young, elderly, and sick. These diseases become more common when temperatures are higher and have been found to occur with unusually low or high precipitation.[2] These diseases cause approximately 1.7 million deaths annually due to poor water sanitation.[15] The World Health Organization estimates that diarrheal diseases account for 3.7% of environmental health mortality worldwide.[16]

Outbreaks have also followed increases in stream-flow rates, rapid snowmelt, and changes in water treatment. Waterborne illnesses can also occur from exposure to ocean water after large rainstorms or when a lake or still body of water has experienced an increase in temperature. In addition, rising sea level may have an effect on the growth and spread of bacteria that causes cholera and other intestinal diseases.[2,17]

Food Security

Food security is the state of having an available, accessible, and nutritional food supply. Climate change is expected to threaten food production worldwide, increase food prices, diminish quality, and impede the distribution system, all of which decreases food security.[2] Changes in rainfall patterns, more severe weather events, and increasing competition from weeds and pests may alter crop yields, causing them to decline. The price of food is expected to rise in response. The change in seasonal patterns may also create an abundance of pests and diseases, which can affect pesticide use.[18,19]

As a developed nation, the United States will be less affected than other countries, but it won't be immune. We are already seeing food shortages in states like Alaska, where natives rely on a specific dietary pattern to meet their needs. Athabascan, Eskimo, and Aleut indigenous groups subsist on sea mammals, saltwater fish, and migratory birds. This lifestyle has connected the tribes to the land and created their culture, but as the land changes, so will their diet.[20,21]

The nutritional value of some foods is also estimated to decline. High levels of CO2 in soil is linked to decreased protein in crops, including barley, sorghum, and soy, which are highly prevalent foods in many cultures.[22,23]

Farmers are likely to use stronger pesticides to combat the increased growth of insects, weeds, and other pests. These chemicals can be toxic and will be used more frequently, increasing pests' resistance to them while making them less effective in turn. As pests become more immune or tolerant to some pesticides, farmers will have to continue to look for stronger alternatives. Farmers, workers, and consumers will all be exposed to these chemicals and substances, which can be toxic at different points of the foods system.[2]

Climate variability is not new to some of the world's main agricultural areas like the Midwestern United States, Northeastern Argentina, Southern Africa, or Southeast Australia. These areas have weather fluctuations on record over the last 100 years. But climate variability as a whole is likely to spread across all regions, and temperatures are expected to grow. If climate variability becomes more prevalent, droughts and floods may become more severe and more frequent, which is the dominant cause of short-term shortages in food production. Some of the poorest and most undernourished countries will be open to the highest levels of food insecurity. It is estimated that climate change could increase the number of undernourished people worldwide by 5–26%, depending on climate projections.[12]

The challenge of agriculture in the next century will be integrating environmental, economic, and social capital, to meet the needs of the current generation without sacrificing food security for the future.

Climate Change Will Make Extremes Weather Events More Extreme, Exceeding Our Capacity to Cope with Them

Temperature Extremes

One of the more certain impacts of future climate change will be an increase in intense heat waves. Projections show that extreme heat events will occur more frequently and become more intense in the future. Scientists are predicting that future conditions in regions that currently experience summers over 100 degrees may become uninhabitable. In 2016, India set a new all-time record for temperature at 125 degrees Fahrenheit. On the other hand, populations living in regions where extremely hot weather is relatively infrequent are vulnerable because of their inability to adapt to hot temperatures. They can have the most increased mortality during an uncommon extreme heat.[24]

High temperatures can have significant detrimental health effects. Heat waves can cause deaths from heat stroke and other heat illnesses, or exacerbate chronic conditions, including cardiovascular and respiratory diseases. Heat waves are associated with higher hospital admissions and emergency department visits for cardiovascular, kidney, and respiratory disorders.

Vulnerable populations during extreme heat events include children, low-income, and the elderly. An aging population will put severe pressure on health systems in a rapidly warming world. Elderly populations are extremely susceptible to heat waves because they are not able to regulate their body temperature as efficiently, so they are less adaptable to heat events. This population is more likely to likely to live alone and have reduced social contacts, which can increase their vulnerability to large scale heat events. As the populations of developed countries continue to age, their vulnerabilities to extreme heat will increase.[2,24,25]

Urban areas are known to be much hotter than rural areas. On average, the annual mean air temperature of a city with 1 million people or more can be 1.8–5.4°F warmer than the surrounding more rural areas.[26] This idea is known as urban heat island effect and is caused by roof tiles and pavement absorbing more heat than parks and greenery. This creates a hotter urban environment and can increase the amount of heat-related illnesses that occur in metropolitan areas. Many cities have created a Heat Health Warning System in response to the high temperatures so that their county can be quickly warned during a heat wave.

Extreme heat events have been a public health threat for decades around the world. In 1995 Chicago experienced 514 heat-related deaths and 696 excess deaths from chronic diseases being exacerbated by heat.[26] In 2003, Europe experienced a heat wave causing an excess mortality of about 30,000 deaths. France experienced a heat wave that caused 14,802 deaths in a 20-day period. The heat exacerbated chronic conditions such as cardiovascular, respiratory, and cerebrovascular disease and caused heat stroke and other heat-related illnesses.[18]

More recently, the risks of heat-related sickness and death have decreased worldwide. This could be due to better forecasting, heat health warning systems, heat action plans, or access to air conditioning for more developed countries. Despite all the progress that has been made, extreme heat events continue to be a cause of preventable mortality.[18]

Conversely, milder and shorter winters resulting from a warming climate can reduce cold-weather death and injuries. However, although future winters may see a reduction in cold mortality and injury, it will not make up for the increase in heat-related deaths that are projected to occur.[2]

Precipitation Extremes: Heavy Rainfall, Flooding, Droughts

Heavy precipitation events are expected to increase in frequency in the future. The intensification in extreme precipitation and total precipitation has led to an increase in the severity of floods, landslides, debris and mud flows in some regions. Worldwide, floods caused more than 500,000 deaths from 1980 to 2009 and are the second deadliest weather hazard in the United States.[2]

Although major precipitation and flooding can cause major health risks, other hazards often occur once a heavy precipitation event has passed. Standing water and heavy rainfall can cause an increase in waterborne disease outbreaks. Outbreaks such as pneumonia and Respiratory Syncytial Virus have been reported following a heavy rainstorm, although it is known that other variables can also affect these associations.[2, 27, 28]

Areas in South Asia, such as India, Bangladesh, the Maldives, and Sri Lanka, are facing adverse health effects as a result of more severe monsoons. During the years 1976–2005, there were 332 flood events in South Asia, the most prevalent natural disaster in the region. In 1998, a flood caused by monsoon rains killed over 2,000 people and displaced more than 20 million people in Bangladesh, India, and Nepal. Many people died from being carried away in the storm or drowning, but the floodwaters after the storms had passed were also a health concern. After the flood, an outbreak of diarrhea resulted in over 276 deaths in West Bengal.[29] Studies have also associated this and previous floods in Bangladesh and India with outbreaks of cholera, rotavirus, leptospirosis, and respiratory infections.[30, 31, 32] A study by the United Nations estimated that floods cost the Asian economy $136 billion (US dollars) annually.[33]

Flooding caused by heavy storms can also contribute to vector-borne diseases. The collection of still water provides breeding grounds for mosquitos, potentially aiding in the spread of malaria.[2]

Water can enter into building structures and cause mold contamination that grows without notice. This can lead to indoor air-quality problems and respiratory illnesses. Buildings damaged during hurricanes are especially vulnerable to this type of water intrusion. Individuals living in these buildings, and damp indoor environments are more likely to experience an increased prevalence of asthma, coughing, wheezing, and pneumonia.[2]

Drought can also damage a population's health. Drought conditions may increase exposure to a varied set of health hazards, including wildfires, dust storms, extreme heat events, flash flooding, reduced water quality, and food insecurity. Arizona and California, both dry climates, have seen severe droughts that may be linked to dust storms. These dust storms caused degraded air quality and an increased count of fungal pathogen Valley fever.[2]

Tropical Storms

Hurricanes are low-pressure weather systems that form over warm-water oceans around the world. They can be extremely destructive and have been increasing in frequency since the early 1980s, when more accurate satellite data became readily available.[2] They are referred to different names depending on where they develop. For instance, they are called typhoons if they develop in the Pacific Ocean, cyclones in the south Pacific or Indian Ocean, or hurricanes in the Atlantic or northeastern Pacific Ocean.

Rising sea surface temperatures are expected to increase tropical cyclone intensity and the height of storm surges. Over the last 35 years, there has been a large increase in the proportion of hurricanes reaching the highest hurricane categories 4 and 5. More hurricanes have been seen in the North Pacific, Indian, and Southwest Pacific Oceans.[2]

Although cyclones originating in the Bay of Bengal and the Arabian Sea have decreased in frequency, they have increased in intensity since 1970, causing significant damage in India and Bangladesh. South Asia is particularly vulnerable to cyclones; among the world's thirty-five most deadly cyclones (from the years 1584–1991), cyclones in India and Bangladesh accounted for 76% of all deaths. In the past two centuries, tropical cyclones have caused 1.9 million deaths.[34,35,36]

Storm surge is the unusually high ocean level along coastlines before a hurricane makes landfall. Without early warning and evacuation measures, drowning from a storm surge can cause 90% of cyclone-attributed mortality. While storm surge deaths have dropped significantly in developed nations because of the implementation of preparedness measures, such as early warning, evacuation, and shelter systems, drowning from a storm surge remains the primary cause of death in developing nations.[35]

Rising sea levels resulting from climate change contribute to higher storm surges, and lead to infrastructure damage, shoreline erosion, and changes in water quality and quantity, all of which can impact human health. In South Asia, sea level rise will be of particular concern to the Maldives, Bangladesh, and other countries that lie at very low elevations. Coastal populations will bear the burden of the increasing intensity of tropical cyclones, as well as the impacts on human life and property.[37]

Injury resulting from wind-strewn debris and structural collapse is a major cause of morbidity and mortality from hurricanes. There have also been reports of increased animal and insect bites in the aftermath of tropical cyclones. These bites have been associated with an increase in vector-borne diseases. Chronic diseases are exacerbated after tropical storms owing to their possible exposure to mold during clean up and recovery.[38] In low-income countries, both waterborne and vector-borne diseases have been reported following a tropical cyclone.[28]

Hurricanes also cause extremely large economic losses. Insurance companies have noted a fourfold increase in disasters since the 1960s, with a "one billion dollar storm" event occurring every year from 1987 to 1993. In 2016, there were fifteen weather and climate disaster events, with losses exceeding $1 billion each across the United States.[39,40]

Wildfires

Due to periods of drought and record high temperatures in some regions, climate change is increasing the vulnerability of forests to larger and more extreme wildfires. Many forests are currently situated in extremely dry climates. These conditions make it much easier for fires to start, and can make them much harder to control.

Wildfire smoke can be very harmful to human health. It contains air pollutants and chemicals including particulate matter, carbon monoxide, nitrogen oxides, and other toxic substances that can reduce air quality. The smoke can cause individuals to become ill, both in the direct area of the fire and to a much larger range when there is a strong wind.[2]

Exposure to smoke can cause respiratory and cardiovascular illnesses including asthma, chronic obstructive pulmonary disease, and respiratory infections. This can result in increased trips to the hospital and emergency department visit, and an increase in medication dispensations for people suffering from lung illness. A study linked wildfire smoke to an average of 339,000 deaths annually worldwide, with the most deaths being seen in sub-Saharan Africa and Southeast Asia.[41] The risk of occurrence of wildfires, exacerbated by climate change, is expected to increase in the future. The smoke emissions associated with the increase will likely cause harmful impacts on respiratory health.[2]

Climate Change Will Modify Disease Ecology Profoundly, Causing New Health Threats to Emerge

Climate change is expected to cause new and emerging threats globally, such as infectious diseases in areas that previously were uninhabitable to the viruses. Many infectious bacteria and vectors are responsive to climatic conditions and will move to areas that better suit their needs. Salmonella and cholera both flourish more rapidly at higher temperature. Mild temperate areas with low rainfall are becoming warmer in some regions. Climate change can make these areas more susceptible to disease-carrying vectors, which could trigger epidemics that areas are unprepared for and were previously unseen. Epidemics can also result from a migration of reservoir hosts or human population to a new area, for instance, during extreme weather and refugee situations.[2]

The area for many vectors to live suitably is growing because of longer periods of warm weather. In Sweden, a country with a normally mild climate, tick-borne diseases are increasing because of the warmer winters over the past few decades. Tick-borne encephalitis, Lyme disease, and other illnesses that have been practically unseen previously in this region are now moving and extending northward in Europe. This extension has been linked to the recent warming trends and the geographic range of these ticks may continue to project north and into new regions in the future.[14]

Recently, several scientists have shown an increase in highland malaria in Kenya's Western Highlands in relation to local warming trends. Research is being done to estimate how much climate change will affect future outbreaks of malaria. Several models show minimal expansion of malaria in the region over the next few decades, while other studies project a 16–28% increase in exposure by 2100.[14]

There have been more studies recently on the link between short-term climatic change events like the ENSO cycles of El Nino and La Nina and the occurrence of infectious vector-borne diseases. South Asia and South America have experienced an increase in malaria outbreaks with El Niño and La Niña weather events, while in the Asia Pacific regions, ENSO has been linked to dengue fever outbreaks shortly after. Australia has had outbreaks of Ross River virus disease that coincide with the ENSO cycles.[14]

Conclusions

The expected health effects of climate change present a novel public health problem with an unprecedented scope, timeline, and complexity. It is important to recognize, however, that specific exposures resulting from climate change are not new. Instead, familiar exposures will shift and widen in distribution, increase in frequency, and intensify in magnitude. Currently, rare events may become common, and anomalous events usual. These changes will unfold over decades. Therefore, climate change will act as a general stressor on the public health infrastructure, and gaps and weaknesses in our ability to respond to health threats must be identified and addressed.

An effective public health response will require a new, synergistic approach that can accommodate the complexity of the exposure interactions and engage a variety of stakeholder groups in efforts to develop adaptation measures. A framework for prioritizing the key public health responses to climate change can be found in the "10 Essential Services of Public Health," developed in 1994 by the American Public Health Association and its partners (Public Health Functions Steering Committee 1994). An adaptation of these essential services provides a starting point for the engagement of climate change from a public health standpoint.[1] These "Essential Services" include:

1. Monitor health outcomes to identify changing disease patterns and geographies.

Climate change will require a new approach to public health surveillance that will allow for the integration and monitoring of multiple data streams, including climate trends, meteorological data, ecological data, and changing indicators of population vulnerability. Enhanced surveillance programs, incorporating meteorological and climate data, can provide the framework for the operationalization of such a set of "climate change indicators" and help health authorities to understand the associations among long-term climate changes, weather events, ecological changes, and health outcomes.

2. Diagnose and investigate health problems and hazards in the community.

Classic public health responsibilities include identifying, investigating, and explaining health patterns at the community level. In a future climate, with altered disease ecologies, public health laboratories will need the capacity and to make rapid diagnoses and reports of altered geographic distribution and frequency of diseases.

3. Inform, educate, and empower people about health issues.

In an effort to re-frame climate change as a basic human health and welfare issue, health communicators can inform the public and policymakers about the health risks of a changing change and actions that may reduce this risk. To build effective health communication strategies, we must target specific groups with specific attention to accounting for varying levels of education as well as cultural and ethnic differences.

4. Mobilize community partnerships to identify and solve health problems.

We will need to strengthen relationships among traditional partners, such as government agencies and academia, and develop new partners, such as faith-based groups and city planning departments. Many of these relationships will develop at the local and state levels, where services are delivered. As we identify vulnerable populations and implement a response, we must integrate community expectations, beliefs, and cultural values into adaptation efforts.

5. Develop policies and plans that support individual and community health efforts.

Although the responsibility for policies to reduce greenhouse gas emissions lies outside the scope of public health, health professionals can provide compelling evidence to support climate policies that have the additional co-benefit of reducing morbidity and mortality. Public health tools such as health impact assessments can provide evidence for positive and negative effects of various approaches to climate change adaptation and mitigation and allow health departments to collaborate across policy sectors and highlight key points for public health engagement.

Preparing the public health community to face the challenge of a changing climate will require a coordinated effort at several jurisdictional scales, from international, federal, regional, to local. It is perhaps through this form of active, sustained collaboration, linking the global with the local, that we can begin to address this crisis that Margaret Chan, Director General of WHO, has described as "one of the greatest challenges of our time" (2008).

REFERENCES

1. World Health Organization (WHO). (2014, March 25). 7 million premature deaths annually linked to air pollution. Retrieved from http://www.who.int/mediacentre/news/releases/2014/air-pollution/en/
2. National Climate Assessment Human Health
3. Peel, J. L., Metzger, K. B., Klein, M., Flanders, W. D., Mulholland, J. A., & Tolbert, P. E. (2007). Ambient air pollution and cardiovascular emergency department visits in potentially sensitive groups. Am J Epidemiol, 165(6), 625–633. doi:10.1093/aje/kwk051
4. Jacobson, M. Z. 2008: On the causal link between carbon dioxide and air pollution mortality. Geophysical Research Letters, 35, L03809, doi:10.1029/2007GL031101.
5. Ghude, S. D., et. al (2016). Premature mortality in India due to PM2.5 and ozone exposure. Geophysical Research Letters, 43(9), 4650–4658. Doi: 10.1002/2016GL068949
6. Arbes, S. J., Gergen, P. J., Elliot L, & Zeldin D.C., (2005). Prevalences of positive skin test responses to 10 common allergens in the US population: results from the third National Health and Nutrition Examination Survey. J Allergy Clin Immunol, 116 (2) 377–83, doi: 10.1016/j.jaci.2005.05.017
7. Ziska, L. et al. (2011). Recent warming by latitude associated with increased length of ragweed pollen season in central North America. *Proceedings of the National Academy of Sciences*, 108, 4248–4251, doi:10.1073/pnas.1014107108.
8. Sheffield, P. E., Weinberger, K. R., Ito, K., Matte,T. D., Mathes, R. W., Robinson, G. S., & Kinney, P. L. (2011). The association of tree pollen concentration peaks and allergy medication sales in New York City: 2003–2008. *ISRN Allergy*, 2011, 1–7, doi:10.5402/2011/537194.
9. Emberlin, J., Detandt, M., Gehrig, R., Jaeger, S., Nolard, N., Rantio-Lehtimaki, A. (2002). Responses

in the start of *Betula* (birch) pollen seasons to recent changes in spring temperature across Europe. International Journal of Biometeorology, 46(4) 159–170, doi: 10.1007/s00484-002-0139-x

10. Ziello, C., Sparks, T. H., Estrella, N., Belmonte, J., Bergmann, K. C., Bucher, E., . . . & Gehrig, R. (2012). Changes to airborne pollen counts across Europe. *PloS one*, *7*(4), e34076.
11. Lake, I. R., Gillespie, I. A., Bentham, G., Nichols, G. L., Lane, C., Adak, G. K., & Threlfall, E. J. (2009). A re-evaluation of the impact of temperature and climate change on foodborne illness. Epidemiology and Infection, 137(11), 1538–1547.
12. Portier, C. J., Tart, K. T., Carter, S. R., Dilworth, C. H., Grambsch, A. E., Gohlke, J., . . . & Maslak, T. (2013). A human health perspective on climate change: a report outlining the research needs on the human health effects of climate change. Journal of Current Issues in Globalization, 6(4), 621.
13. Bentham, G. & Langford, I. H. Climate change and the incidence of food poisoning in England and Wales. International Journal of Biometeorology 39: 81–86 (1995).
14. McMichael, A. J., Woodruff, R. E., & Hales, S. (2006). Climate change and human health: present and future risks. The Lancet, 367(9513), 859–869.
15. Ashbolt, Nicholas John. "Microbial contamination of drinking water and disease outcomes in developing regions." Toxicology 198.1 (2004): 229–238.
16. Mathers, C., et al. (2008) Geneva, Switzerland: World Health Organization. vii, 146 p.
17. Portier C. J., Thigpen Tart K, Carter S. R., Dilworth C. H., Grambsch A. E., Gohlke J, Hess J, Howard S. N., Luber G, Lutz J. T., Maslak T, Prudent N, Radtke M, Rosenthal J. P., Rowles T, Sandifer P. A., Scheraga J, Schramm P. J., Strickman D, Trtanj J. M., Whung P-Y. 2010. Available: www.niehs.nih.gov/climatereport.
18. Schmidhuber, J., & Tubiello, F. N. (2007). Global food security under climate change. Proceedings of the National Academy of Sciences, 104(50), 19703–19708.
19. Brown, M. E., & Funk, C. C. (2008). Food security under climate change.
20. Loring, P. A., & Gerlach, S. C. (2009). Food, culture, and human health in Alaska: an integrative health approach to food security. Environmental Science & Policy, 12(4), 466–478.
21. Brubaker, M., Berner, J., Chavan, R., & Warren, J. (2011). Climate change and health effects in Northwest Alaska. Global Health Action, 4. doi:http://dx.doi.org/10.3402/gha.v4i0.8445.
22. Intergovernmental Panel on Climate Change (2007) Climate Change: Impacts, Adaptation and Vulnerability, Contribution of Working Group II to the Fourth Assessment Report of the Intergovernmental Panel on Climate Change (Cambridge Univ Press, Cambridge, UK) in press.
23. Intergovernmental Panel on Climate Change (2001) Climate Change: Impacts, Adaptation and Vulnerability, Contribution of Working Group II to the Third Assessment Report of the Intergovernmental Panel on Climate Change (Cambridge Univ Press, Cambridge, UK).
24. Luber, G., & McGeehin, M. (2008). Climate change and extreme heat events. American journal of preventive medicine, 35(5), 429–435.
25. M. A. McGeehin, M. A. Mirabelli, M. (2001) The potential impacts of climate variability and change on temperature-related morbidity and mortality in the United States *Environ Health Perspect*, 109 (suppl 2) pp. 185–189
26. Whitman, S., Good, G., Donoghue, E. R., Benbow, N., Shou, W., & Mou, S. (1997). Mortality in Chicago attributed to the July 1995 heat wave. American Journal of public health, 87(9), 1515–1518.
27. Curriero, F. C., J. A. Patz, J. B. Rose, and S. Lele, 2001: The association between extreme precipitation and waterborne disease outbreaks in the United States, 1948–1994. American Journal of Public Health, 91, 1194–1199, doi:10.2105/AJPH.91.8.1194.
28. Haines, A., Kovats, R. S., Campbell-Lendrum, D., & Corvalán, C. (2006). Climate change and human health: impacts, vulnerability and public health. Public Health, 120(7), 585–596.
29. Sur, D., Dutta, P., Nair, G. B., & Bhattacharya, S. K. (2000). Severe cholera outbreak following floods in a northern disrict of West Bengal. Indian Journal of Medical Research, 112, 178.
30. Kunii O, Nakamura S, Abdur R, et al. (2002). The impact on health and risk factors of the diarrhoea epidemics in the 1998 Bangladesh floods. Public Health; 116:68–74.
31. Ahern, M.,. Sari Kovats, R.,l Wilkinson, P., Few, R., & Matthies, F. (2005); Global Health Impacts of Floods: Epidemiologic Evidence. Epidemiol Rev; 27 (1): 36–46. doi: 10.1093/epirev/mxi004
32. Fun, B. N., Unicomb, L, Rahim, Z, et al. 1991. Rotavirus-associated diarrhea in rural Bangladesh: two-year study of incidence and serotype distribution. J Clin Microbiol; 29:1359–63.

33. Shrestha, M. S., & Takara, K. (2008). Impacts of floods in south Asia. Journal of South Asia Disaster Study, 1(1), 85–106.
34. Marchigiani, R., Gordy, S., Cipolla, J., Adams, R. C., Evans, D. C., Stehly, C., . . . & Bhoi, S. (2013). Wind disasters: A comprehensive review of current management strategies. International Journal of Critical Illness and Injury Science, 3(2), 130.
35. James, M. Shultz, Jill Russell, Zelde Espinel. (2005). Epidemiology of Tropical Cyclones: The Dynamics of Disaster, Disease, and Development. Epidemiol Rev 2005; 27 (1): 21–35. doi: 10.1093/epirev/mxi011
36. Doocy, S., Dick, A., Daniels, A., Kirsch, T. D., 2013. The Human Impact of Tropical Cyclones: a Historical Review of Events 1980–2009 and Systematic Literature Review. PLOS Currents Disasters. Apr 16. Edition 1. doi:10.1371/currents.dis.2664354a5571512063ed29d25ffbce74.
37. Woodward, A., Hales, S., & Weinstein, P. (1998). Climate change and human health in the Asia Pacific region: who will be most vulnerable? Climate Research, 11(1), 31–38.
38. Wilson, J. F. (2006). Health and the environment after Hurricane Katrina. Annals of Internal Medicine, 144(2), 153–156.
39. NOAA National Centers for Environmental Information (NCEI) U.S. Billion-Dollar Weather and Climate Disasters (2017). https://www.ncdc.noaa.gov/billions/
40. Lott, N., and T. Ross, (2006). Tracking and evaluating U. S. billion dollar weather disasters, 1980–2005. Preprints. AMS Forum: Environmental Risk and Impacts on Society: Successes and Challenges, Atlanta, GA, Amer. Meteor. Soc., 1.2.
41. Johnston, F. H., Henderson, S. B., Chen, Y., Randerson, J. T., Marlier, M., DeFries, R.S., Kinney, P., Bowman, D. M. J. S., & Brauer, M. (2012). Estimated global mortality attributable to smoke from landscape fires. Environmental Health Perspectives, 120, 695–701, doi:10.1289/ehp.1104422.

SECTION 5 CASES FOR TEACHING AND LEARNING

Visit the companion website, www.oup.com/us/brown-closser, for direct links to the featured online resources.

Shehnaz Alidina and Jessica Paulus, *Malaria and DDT in Uganda*

This case explores the controversy over DDT use in malaria control in Uganda. DDT is a cheap and effective insecticide against malaria-transmitting mosquitoes. But it also affects the environment – especially for birds. This is a good topic for a debate.

Bitton et al., *Tobacco Control in South Africa*

Tobacco use is huge cause of premature death throughout the world. In this case, students must consider what steps the government of South Africa could or should take to curb tobacco use in a context of tobacco industry interference. There is also a follow-up case, *Tobacco Control in South Africa: Next Steps.*

Gutiérrez-Avila et al., *Air Quality and Public Health in Megacities: Has Air Quality Improved Due to Driving Restrictions in Mexico City?*

Air quality in the huge world urban centers – like Mexico City – is terrible. This case study requires students to evaluate an effort to improve air quality in Mexico City. This detailed case describes the determinants of poor air quality in Mexico City, a program aimed at addressing those issues, and the political context of air-quality interventions.

National Institutes of Health, *Climate Change and Human Health*
Students can dig into the 2016 *Climate and Health Assessment* to lay out the drivers, mediators, and impacts of climate change on human health.

SECTION 5 VIDEOS AND WEB RESOURCES

Visit the companion website, www.oup.com/us/brown-closser, for direct links to the featured online resources.

Vector-Borne Disease

***Three Reasons We Still Haven't Gotten Rid of Malaria* – Sonia Shah**
In this TED Talk, author Sonia Shah lays out the basics of malaria and, taking a historical perspective, looks at why malaria eradication failed in the 1960s and why it will be so difficult to achieve now. Shah asks the question, What if we attacked this disease according to the priorities of the people who lived with it?

Dark Forest Black Fly
This documentary follows the onchocerciasis (river blindness) control program in Uganda sponsored by The Carter Center. It discusses vector control of blackflies, as well as mass treatment with ivermectin. (60 min)

Island Fever
A short introduction to Chikungunya, focusing on control efforts in Grenada. (15 min)

Smoking

Addiction Incorporated
This feature-length muckraking documentary follows the history of the tobacco industry in the United States.

Thank You for Smoking
This a satirical feature-length film about a spokesman for tobacco companies who is also trying to be a role model for his son.

Tobacco: John Oliver from This Week Tonight
This is a hard-hitting and humorous exposé of the tactics of international tobacco companies to squelch public health campaigns in low-and middle-income countries by threatening lawsuits. (2015, 20 minutes)

Climate Change

***An Inconvenient Truth* – Davis Guggenheim and Al Gore**
This 2006 Academy Award – winning feature-length film is still a useful primer on climate change, compellingly presenting the evidence that human activities are leading to large-scale climate impacts.

SECTION

6

Food

This section of the book considers another physical requirement for sustaining life. Obviously, we all need to eat food to provide sufficient energy for our bodies and brains. Throughout the evolutionary history of humans, food shortages were common. That is one reason why humans are the fattest of land animals—we have evolved to store energy in the form of fat during times of plenty so that it can be utilized during food shortages. Adequate diet is always important for health but especially for growing infants and children. However, too much food and being overweight can also cause health problems. Therefore, nutrition is a central part of global health.

The ultimate causes of malnutrition—both undernutrition and overnutrition—are complex because they deal with the production, distribution, and consumption of food. Because access to food is usually regulated by the market, the poor are more likely to have insufficient diets. The ultimate solutions to the challenge of malnutrition are political and economic, not medical. However, in times of crisis, food is medicine. The articles in this section cover a range of topics—from the effects of undernutrition on child development, to the causes of famines, to how food availability relates to infectious disease, including tuberculosis (TB) and AIDS.

Food insecurity—living without reliable access to a sufficient quantity of affordable, nutritious food—is a central concern in global health today. But it is not the case that many people die from an absolute lack of food, or starvation. Rather, as prices rise on certain foods, it becomes impossible for the poor to maintain a healthy diet. To live with uncertainty about your family's next meal is very stressful. It may be counterintuitive, but food insecurity can be related to the growing problem of obesity, a subject discussed in last reading of this section.

» CONCEPTUAL TOOLS «

- **There are three kinds of malnutrition: undernutrition, overnutrition, and micronutrient malnutrition.** Food is necessary for all forms of life to survive. The lack of food or a diet with an improper combination of nutrients is harmful to health, especially as a child is growing. Adequate nutrition involves both adequate quantity and adequate quality of diet. Undernútrition not only retards development but also makes an individual more vulnerable to infectious diseases. Overnutrition (and inactivity) is linked to a variety of serious noncommunicable diseases like diabetes. "Micronutrient malnutrition" refers to a lack of specific vitamins or minerals and results in specific preventable diseases.

- There is enough food for everyone in the world. **Famines and undernutrition are a result of the politics of food distribution, not an absolute lack of food.** Nevertheless, food aid (the donation of food from high-income countries to areas with food shortages) has many problems associated with it. Food aid distorts local markets and creates disincentives for local farmers. The agricultural subsidies that the United States and other wealthy nations give to their farmers also distort markets and drive down prices, frequently leading to negative consequences for the poorest farmers globally.
- **The experience of food insecurity has both physical and psychological dimensions.** Many people in the world are food-insecure, meaning that they lack reliable access to a sufficient quantity of affordable, nutritious food. There are food-insecure people even in the richest countries of the world. From a physical perspective, food insecurity results in undernutrition. It is also linked to higher rates of mental distress in many parts of the world.
- **It is impossible to separate the challenges of economic development and those of global health.** To combat food insecurity, it will be necessary to improve agricultural production, particularly in sub-Saharan Africa. This region faces both food insecurity and potential future problems created by climate change. Solving these problems will require work across many fields, from improving biotechnology to strengthening markets. Many Africans are already hard at work on these problems.

Undernutrition

- **Undernutrition is a large problem globally.** According to the United Nation's Food and Agriculture Organization, nearly 800 million people worldwide are undernourished. Globally, fewer people now are undernourished compared with 20 years ago.
- **Undernutrition in children is often measured through growth measures including stunting and wasting. Wasting** is when children have a weight for their height that is far below the average for these well-nourished children. **Stunting** is when children are much shorter than the average for their age. We know what healthy weight is for children because of a large study called the Multicentre Growth Reference Study, which collected data on 8,500 well-nourished children from settings around the world. Both stunting and wasting are signs of undernutrition and/or frequent illness in children.
- **Undernutrition is particularly concentrated in resource-poor countries.** Figure CT6.1 shows the percentage of children who are stunted across the world. Compare this map with the map of the Socio-Demographic Index in Section 3 (see box in Conceptual Tools). What are the trends, and what are the exceptions to those trends? What does this tell you about undernourishment and its relationship with poverty at the country level?

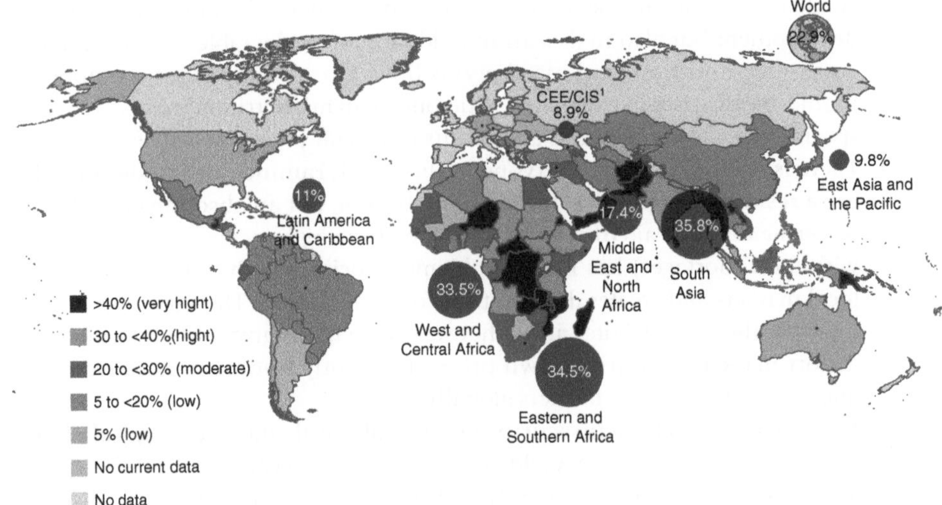

FIGURE CT6.1 Percentage of Children under Five Who Are Stunted, 2010–2016.
Image credit: UNICEF. *Undernutrition Contributes to Nearly Half of All Deaths in Children under 5 and Is Widespread in Asia and Africa,* http://data.unicef.org/topic/nutrition/malnutrition/#.

- **Undernutrition, particularly wasting, is a major risk factor for death in children.** In fact, nearly half of all deaths in children under five are a result of undernutrition. Most of these children do not directly starve; rather, they die because they are more vulnerable to other diseases. Undernourished children are much more likely to die from common killers like diarrhea, pneumonia, malaria, and measles. In fact, we can say that much of the mortality owing to these diseases is actually due to undernutrition.
- **In a vicious cycle, disease can also contribute to undernutrition.** For example, an undernourished child who gets severe diarrhea is likely to become even more undernourished, putting them at even greater risk for other health issues.
- **Undernutrition in childhood is also a risk factor for diseases later in life.** Increasingly, the study of genetics is revealing that the consequences of undernutrition in early child development may even stretch into future generations; this is called epigenetics. The Dutch famine of 1944–45, called the "hunger winter," is a particularly well-studied example. This famine had lifelong impacts on the metabolism and cognitive function of the people who were born during that period. More surprising, there are even generational effects in those people's children and grandchildren—people who never experienced the hunger winter themselves.

  Figure CT6.2 summarizes the complex causes—and effects—of undernutrition. The chart uses the term "**food insecurity**." This is a term that describes a situation when getting the quantity and quality of necessary food is not always certain. Food insecurity is usually about resources but could be about other problems, like mobility in elderly people.
- **Undernutrition is also associated with diseases like HIV and TB in adults and children.** The HIV epidemic contributes to food insecurity at a societal level in areas with high prevalence of HIV. Because so many adults are getting sick or

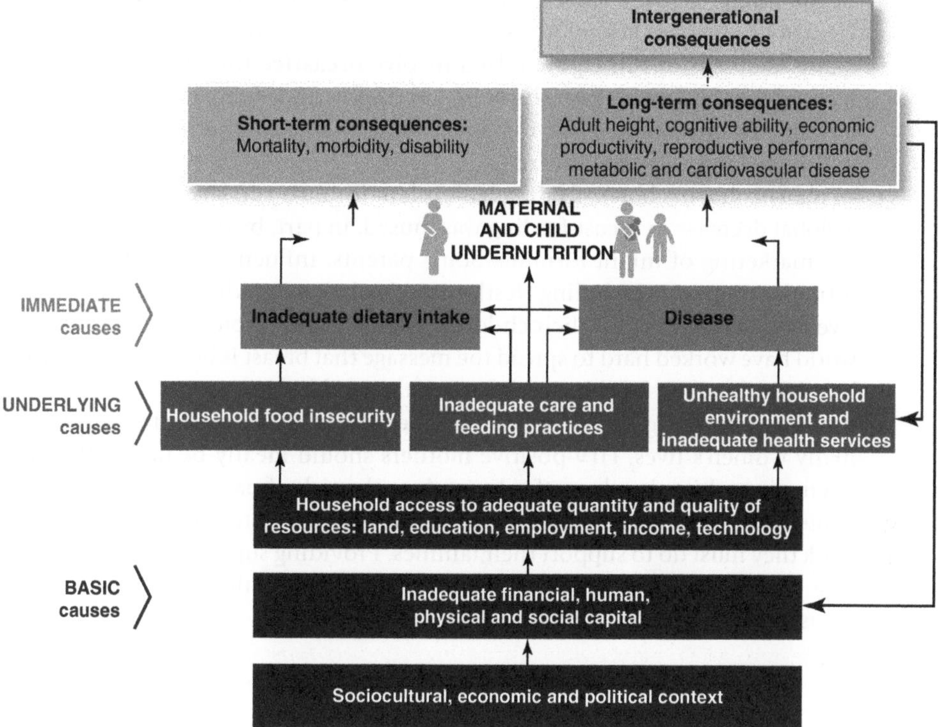

FIGURE CT6.2 Conceptual Framework of the Determinants of Child Undernutrition.
Image source: UNICEF. *Improving Child Nutrition,* https://www.unicef.org/publications/index_68661.html.

dying, there are not as many people who are able to labor to produce food. The high incidence of morbidity and mortality also means that there are often not enough healthy adults in a household to earn enough wages to secure food for the family. In addition, many families have adopted orphaned children, making more dependents per working adult.

At an individual biological level, HIV makes the problems associated with being undernourished more serious. Being infected with HIV, for example, makes children more susceptible to infectious disease like diarrhea, contributing to yet another pressure in the vicious spiral mentioned above. Severely undernourished HIV-infected children are more likely to die than those without HIV infection.

Also, food insecurity can contribute to the risk of being infected with HIV. In some contexts, for example, food insecurity may drive women into sexual relationships they would otherwise avoid. In a broad sense, then, food—or food security—can be excellent preventive medicine.

- Food can also be curative medicine. **Emergency foods can help severely wasted children and adults avoid death in the short term.** One example of a therapeutic food for severely undernourished children is Plumpy'Nut, a peanut paste packed with vitamins, proteins, and calories.

- **In the longer term, a variety of interventions can improve child nutrition.** Figure CT6.3 shows key interventions for mother and child.
- Many interventions in Figure CT6.3 involve **breastfeeding. Exclusive breastfeeding for the first six months of life, and continued breastfeeding throughout the first two years of life, is a powerful way to counter undernutrition and malnutrition in young children.**
- In many contexts, bottle-feeding with infant formula can lead to malnutrition; a global decrease in breast-feeding was caused, in part, by unethical practices in the marketing of infant formula. Some parents, influenced by advertising by formula companies including Nestlé, may think that spending money on expensive formula is better for their children. Global health professionals around the world have worked hard to spread the message that breast is best. In recent years, breastfeeding rates have increased across the world.
- Projects promoting breastfeeding must recognize the complicated realities of many women's lives. HIV-positive mothers should ideally be taking the drug nevirapine while they breastfeed to reduce the risk of passing HIV on to their babies. And some mothers may find it impossible to breastfeed alongside the work they must do to support their families. Providing support for breastfeeding in a variety of situations, without stigmatizing or shaming mothers unable to breastfeed, is an important balance.

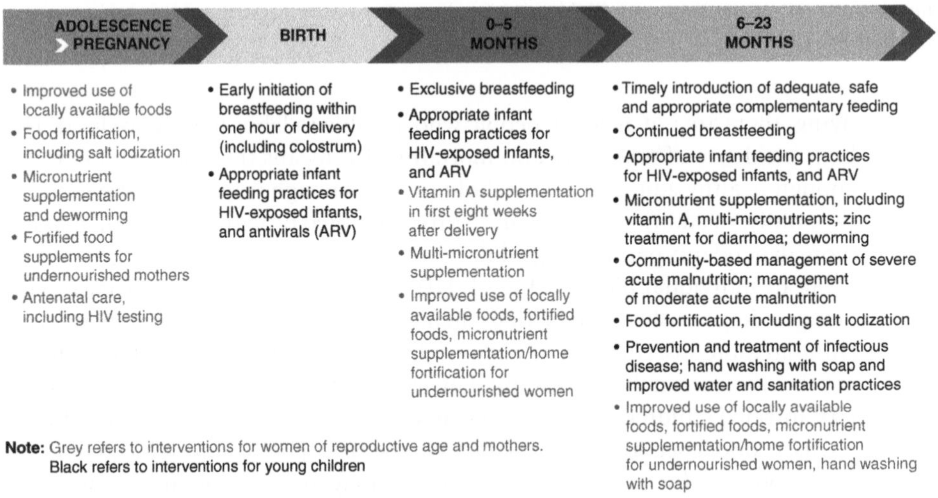

ADOLESCENCE > PREGNANCY	BIRTH	0–5 MONTHS	6–23 MONTHS
• Improved use of locally available foods • Food fortification, including salt iodization • Micronutrient supplementation and deworming • Fortified food supplements for undernourished mothers • Antenatal care, including HIV testing	• Early initiation of breastfeeding within one hour of delivery (including colostrum) • Appropriate infant feeding practices for HIV-exposed infants, and antivirals (ARV)	• Exclusive breastfeeding • Appropriate infant feeding practices for HIV-exposed infants, and ARV • Vitamin A supplementation in first eight weeks after delivery • Multi-micronutrient supplementation • Improved use of locally available foods, fortified foods, micronutrient supplementation/home fortification for undernourished women	• Timely introduction of adequate, safe and appropriate complementary feeding • Continued breastfeeding • Appropriate infant feeding practices for HIV-exposed infants, and ARV • Micronutrient supplementation, including vitamin A, multi-micronutrients; zinc treatment for diarrhoea; deworming • Community-based management of severe acute malnutrition; management of moderate acute malnutrition • Food fortification, including salt iodization • Prevention and treatment of infectious disease; hand washing with soap and improved water and sanitation practices • Improved use of locally available foods, fortified foods, micronutrient supplementation/home fortification for undernourished women, hand washing with soap

Note: Grey refers to interventions for women of reproductive age and mothers. Black refers to interventions for young children

FIGURE CT6.3 Key Proven Practices, Services, and Policy Interventions for the Prevention and Treatment of Stunting and Other Forms of Undernutrition throughout the Life Cycle.

Policy and guideline recommendations based on UNICEF, World Health Organization, and other United Nations agencies.

Source: UNICEF, Improving Child Nutrition, https://www.unicef.org/publications/index_68661.html

- The **green revolution** was the massive increase in the food produced globally throughout the 1900s as a result of new technologies, including new chemical fertilizers, varieties of crops, and systems for irrigating and harvesting food. Without the green revolution, it is likely that there would be much more undernutrition than there is today. The green revolution has led to more food being available at lower prices across the world.

  Many of us here in the United States think of organic food as inherently better for health than food produced through green revolution technologies. But the situation is complicated. When you consider the global health consequences of undernutrition, the green revolution has likely had many positive health benefits.

Micronutrient Malnutrition

- Many other interventions in the chart mention "fortified foods" or Vitamin A. These recommendations are dealing with a different kind of malnutrition—micronutrient malnutrition. It is the quality, and not just the quantity, of food that matters. Some children who are not undernourished may nonetheless be malnourished.
- A variety of diseases including pellagra and goiter are caused by micronutrient deficiencies and have been nearly eliminated in the United States through the use of food fortification. For example, fortified flour has ended pellagra as a major health issue in the United States, and iodized salt has drastically reduced rates of goiter. The use of fortified foods is increasing across the globe, but some populations, particularly poor and marginalized populations, do not have consistent access to them.
- Some micronutrients have broad and surprising health impacts. Children with enough Vitamin A are much less likely to suffer from infectious diseases including measles and diarrhea. Zinc supplementation also reduces diarrhea rates and the severity of individual episodes of diarrhea. Having enough iron in the diet increases school performance and work productivity. And eliminating iodine deficiencies can cut rates of mental impairment.

Overnutrition and Big Food

- **A third kind of malnutrition is overnutrition.** This includes the problem of energy imbalance—consuming more energy (calories) than one is using in the form of physical (and mental) activity. Overnutrition is linked to the industrialization of the food system that results in people eating more sugars and dietary fats than are optimal. Being overweight or obese is an important risk factor for noncommunicable diseases like heart disease, hypertension, diabetes, and certain cancers, which are the major cause of death in high-income countries and increasingly so in middle-income countries. While the prevalence of undernutrition is decreasing globally, the prevalence of overnutrition is a growing global problem.
- Many countries are dealing with the effects of both under- and overnutrition. This is often referred to as the **double burden of malnutrition**. Both of these problems are related to capitalist food systems: undernutrition is a result of not having enough money to purchase food, whereas overnutrition is often a result of the fact that the lowest-cost foods are often highly processed and full of added fats and sugar.

- Much of the increase in overnutrition globally is driven by the production and marketing capabilities of **Big Food**, multinational food and drink companies that produce constantly increasing amounts of what we eat across the world. Like Big Tobacco, Big Food places profits above human health. As sales have slowed in the Global North, these companies have increasingly turned their attention to the Global South, as Figure CT6.4 shows.

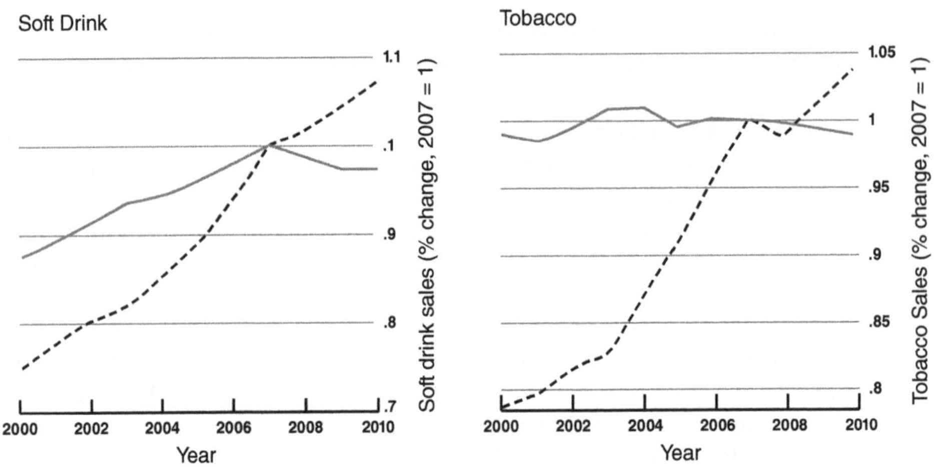

FIGURE CT6.4 Growth of Big Food and Big Tobacco Sales in Developing Countries: An Example.

Shaded gray line is developed countries, dashed black line is developing countries.

Image source: D. Stuckler, and Nestle, M. "Big Food, Food Systems, and Global Health." *PLoS Medicine,* 2012, 9(6): e1001242. doi:10.1371/journal.pmed.1001242.

THOMAS MCKEOWN

20 CLINICAL MEDICINE OR PUBLIC HEALTH? THE HISTORY OF MORTALITY DECLINE

What factors are the most important influences on population health? This is a critical question because if we know what the major causes of good (or poor) health are, then we would understand where to focus our efforts for the best results. The use of epidemiological evidence for global health decision making was covered in Section 3.

The World Health Organization says that health is not merely the absence of disease but an overall state of physical, mental, and social well-being. Describing such overall health on a global scale is not currently possible, and most scientists and scholars would agree that levels of disease in a population (morbidity) and the frequency of death at particular ages (mortality) represent essential, if gross, measures of health. In other words, most people agree that a decline in mortality in that population is a sign of improved health in that population.

As we have seen earlier, the field of global health includes both programs for the prevention of population health problems—the territory of public health—and the provision of health services to underserved populations—the domain of clinical medicine. Some undergraduate students (and most of the public) believe that clinical medicine is the most important determinant of health. That may be a reason why so many students want to become doctors.

Examining historical evidence from Europe and North America, one can see an incredible improvement in health and well-being from the mid-19th century and throughout the 20th century. There was a remarkable decline in mortality rates associated with economic improvements—an historical event that the economic historian Angus Deaton has called "the great escape" from misery. This raises a historical question: What was the role of medicine in this improvement?

If by "medicine" we mean biomedical clinical care including modern inventions such as X-rays, antibiotics, and immunizations, then it is possible to compare mortality rates before and after significant medical interventions were introduced. This is exactly the topic of Thomas McKeown's famous book The Role of Medicine: Dream, Mirage, or Nemesis? *(Oxford: Blackwell, 1979), which is summarized in this article.*

For his analysis, McKeown used the best available data source about changes in mortality during that time period: the Bills of Mortality from England and Wales, which provides statistical information on causes of death all the way back to 1870. Using this historical data, McKeown demonstrates that the greatest advancements in health occurred before specific medical interventions became available. He suggests that more significant factors determining health improvement include better sanitation, better food, and birth spacing. He concludes that preventive public health and economic development measures have a greater impact than clinical medicine and medical technology on the morbidity and mortality of a population. McKeown speculates that it is improved nutrition that had the biggest impact on health.

The field of global health must take advantage of all that is known in both prevention and biomedical health care. The historical record, however, is very clear that health is determined more by housing than hospitals. This is a classic argument that has important political and health policy implications.

As you read this selection, consider these questions:

- **Do many people actually believe the presumption that McKeown is arguing against—that**

From T. McKeown, "Determinants of Health." *Human Nature Magazine*, April 1978. *Human Nature Magazine*: Determinants of Health.

modern health improvements are caused by modern biomedicine? What do your friends think are the determinants of health?

- **Why is there connection between health and wealth?**
- **What does McKeown mean by an "engineering approach" to biomedicine?**
- **What implications does McKeown's discussion have for combating infectious diseases in low- and middle-income countries, where they are still a very significant cause of morbidity and mortality?**

CONTEXT

Thomas McKeown (1918–1988) was a medical historian at the University of Birmingham. Despite his earlier training in biochemistry and medicine, he became famous for the thesis presented in this piece. Scholars continue to debate his demographic methodology and the question of whether he focused too much on economic change, living conditions, and nutrition, while neglecting the development of basic clinical care (including nursing and sanitation within hospitals).

Modern medicine is not nearly as effective as most people believe. It has not been effective, because medical science and service are misdirected and society's investment in health is misused. At the base of this misdirection is a false assumption about human health. Physicians, biochemists, and the general public assume that the body is a machine that can be protected from disease primarily by physical and chemical intervention. This approach, rooted in 17th-century science, has led to widespread indifference to the influence of the primary determinants of human health—environment and personal behavior—and emphasizes the role of medical treatment, which is actually less important than either of the others. It has also resulted in the neglect of sick people whose ailments are not within the scope of the sort of therapy that interests the medical professions.

An appraisal of influences on health in the past suggests that the contribution of modern medicine to the increase of life expectancy has been much smaller than most people believe. Health improved, not because of steps taken when we are ill, but because we become ill less often. We remain well, less because of specific measures such as vaccination and immunization than because we enjoy a higher standard of nutrition, we live in a healthier environment, and we have fewer children.

For some 300 years an engineering approach has been dominant in biology and medicine and has provided the basis for the treatment of the sick. A mechanistic concept of nature developed in the 17th century led to the idea that a living organism, like a machine, might be taken apart and reassembled if its structure and function were sufficiently understood. Applied to medicine, this concept meant that understanding the body's response to disease would allow physicians to intervene in the course of disease. The consequences of the engineering approach to medicine are more conspicuous today than they were in the 17th century largely because the resources of the physical and chemical sciences are so much greater. Medical education begins with the study of the structure and function of the body, continues with examination of disease processes, and ends with clinical instruction on selected sick people. Medical service is dominated by the image of the hospital for the acutely ill, where technological resources are concentrated. Medical research also reflects the mechanistic approach, concerning itself with problems such as the chemical basis of inheritance and the immunological response to transplanted tissues.

No one disputes the predominance of the engineering approach in medicine, but we must now ask whether it is seriously deficient as a conceptualization of the problems of human health. To answer this question, we must examine the determinants of human health. We must first discover why health improved in the past and then go on to ascertain the important influences on health today, in the light of the change in health problems that has resulted from the decline of infectious diseases.

It is no exaggeration to say that health, especially the health of infants and young children, has been transformed since the 18th century. For the first time

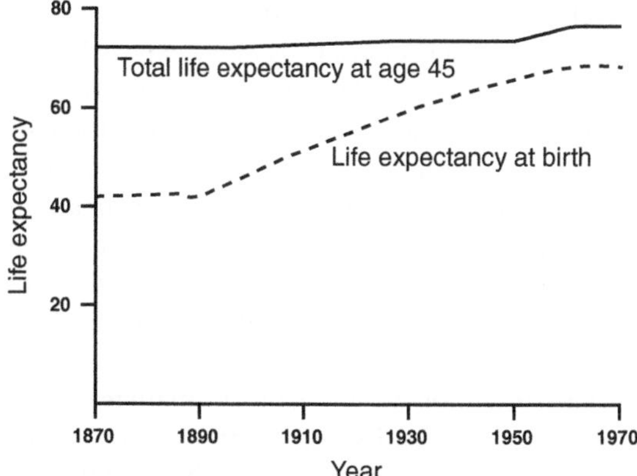

FIGURE 20.1 Life Expectancy.

Source: From *Human Nature Magazine* / McKeown. *Human Nature Magazine:* Determinants of Health. © 1978 Global Rights & Permissions, a part of Cengage Learning, Inc. Reproduced by permission. www.cengage.com/permissions.

in history, a mother knows it is likely that all her children will live to maturity. Before the 19th century, only about three out of every 10 newborn infants lived beyond the age of 25. Of the seven who died, two or three never reached their first birthday, and five or six died before they were six. Today, in developed countries fewer than one in 20 children die before they reach adulthood.

The increased life expectancy, most evident for young children, is due predominantly to a reduction of deaths from infectious diseases. Records from England and Wales (the earliest national statistics available) show that this reduction was the reason for the improvement in health before 1900, and it remains the main influence to the present day.

But when we try to account for the decline of infections, significant differences of opinion appear. The conventional view attributes the change to an increased understanding of the nature of infectious disease and to the application of that knowledge through better hygiene, immunization, and treatment. This interpretation places particular emphasis on immunization against diseases like smallpox and polio, and on the use of drugs for the treatment of other diseases, such as tuberculosis, meningitis, and pneumonia. These measures, in fact, contributed relatively little to the total reduction of mortality; the main explanation for the dramatic fall in the number of deaths lies not in medical intervention, but elsewhere.

Deaths from the common infections were declining long before effective medical intervention was possible. By 1900, the total death rate had dropped substantially, and over 90% of the reduction was due to a decrease of deaths from infectious diseases. The relative importance of the major influences can be illustrated by reference to tuberculosis. Although respiratory tuberculosis was the single largest cause of death in the mid-19th century, mortality from the disease declined continuously after 1838, when it was first registered in England and Wales as a cause of death.

Robert Koch identified the tubercle bacillus in 1882, but none of the treatments used in the 19th or early 20th centuries significantly influenced the course of the disease. The many drugs that were tried were worthless; so, too, was the practice of surgically collapsing an infected lung, a treatment introduced about 1920. Streptomycin, developed in 1947, was the first effective treatment, but by this time mortality from the disease had fallen to a small fraction of its level during 1848 to 1854. Streptomycin lowered the death rate from tuberculosis in England and Wales by about 50%, but its contribution to the decrease in the death rate since the early 19th century was only about 3%.

Deaths from bronchitis, pneumonia, and influenza also began to decline before medical science provided an effective treatment for these illnesses. Although the death rate in England and Wales

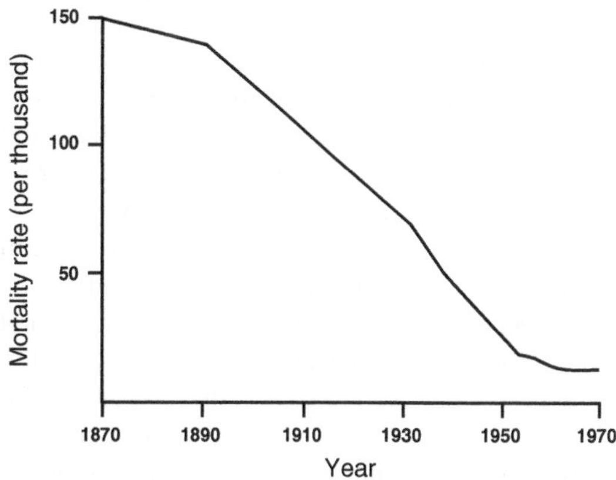

FIGURE 20.2 Infant Mortality Rate.

Source: From *Human Nature Magazine* / McKeown. *Human Nature Magazine:* Determinants of Health. © 1978 Global Rights & Permissions, a part of Cengage Learning, Inc. Reproduced by permission. www.cengage.com/permissions.

increased in the second half of the 19th century, it has fallen continuously since the beginning of the 20th. There is still no effective immunization against bronchitis or pneumonia, and influenza vaccines have had no effect on deaths.

The first successful treatment for these respiratory diseases was a sulfa drug introduced in 1938, but mortality attributed to the lung infections was declining from the beginning of the 20th century. There is no reason to doubt that the decline would have continued without effective therapeutic measures, if at a slower rate.

In the United States, the story was similar; Thomas Magill noted that "the rapid decline of pneumonia death rates began in New York State before the turn of the century and many years before the 'miracle drugs' were known." Obviously, drug therapy was not responsible for the total decrease in deaths that occurred since 1938, and it could have had no influence on the substantial reduction that occurred before then.

The histories of most other common infections, such as whooping cough, measles, and scarlet fever, are similar. In each of these diseases, mortality had fallen to a low level before effective immunization or therapy became available.

In some infections, medical intervention *was* valuable before sulfa drugs and antibiotics became available. Immunization protected people against smallpox and tetanus; antitoxin treatment limited deaths from diphtheria; appendicitis, peritonitis, and ear infections responded to surgery; Salvarsan was a long-sought "magic bullet" against syphilis; intravenous therapy saved people with severe diarrheas; and improved obstetric care prevented childbed fever.

But even if such medical measures had been responsible for the whole decline of mortality from these particular conditions after 1900 (and clearly they were not), they would account for only a small part of the decrease in deaths attributed to all infectious diseases before 1935. From that time, powerful drugs came into use and they were supplemented by improved vaccines. But mortality would have continued to fall even without the presence of these agents; and over the whole period since cause of death was first recorded, immunization and treatment have contributed much less than other influences.

The substantial fall in mortality was due in part to reduced contact with microorganisms. In developed countries an individual no longer encounters the cholera bacillus, he is rarely exposed to the typhoid organism, and his contact with the tubercle bacillus is infrequent. The death rate from these infections fell continuously from the second half of the 19th century, when basic hygienic measures were introduced: purification of water; efficient sewage disposal; and improved food hygiene, particularly the pasteurization of milk, the item in the diet most likely to spread disease.

Pasteurization was probably the main reason for the decrease in deaths from gastroenteritis and for the decline in infant mortality from about 1900. In the 20th century, these essential hygienic measures were supported by improved conditions in the home, the work place, and the general environment. Over the entire period for which records exist, better hygiene accounts for approximately a fifth of the total reduction of mortality.

But the decline of mortality caused by infections began long before the introduction of sanitary measures. It had already begun in England and Wales by 1838, and statistics from Scandinavia suggest that the death rate had been decreasing there since the first half of the 18th century.

A review of English experience makes it unlikely that reduced exposure to microorganisms contributed significantly to the falling death rate in this earlier period. In England and Wales that was the time of industrialization, characterized by rapid population growth and shifts of people from farms into towns, where living and working conditions were uncontrolled. The crowding and poor hygiene that resulted provided ideal conditions for the multiplication and spread of microorganisms, and the situation improved little before sanitary measures were introduced in the last third of the century.

Another possible explanation for the fall in mortality is that the character of infectious diseases changed because the virulence of microorganisms decreased. This change has been suggested in diseases as different as typhus, tuberculosis, and measles. There is no infection of which it can be said confidently that the relationship between host and parasite has not varied over a specified period. But for the decline of all infections, this explanation is obviously inadequate, because it implies that the modern improvement in health was due essentially to a fortuitous change in

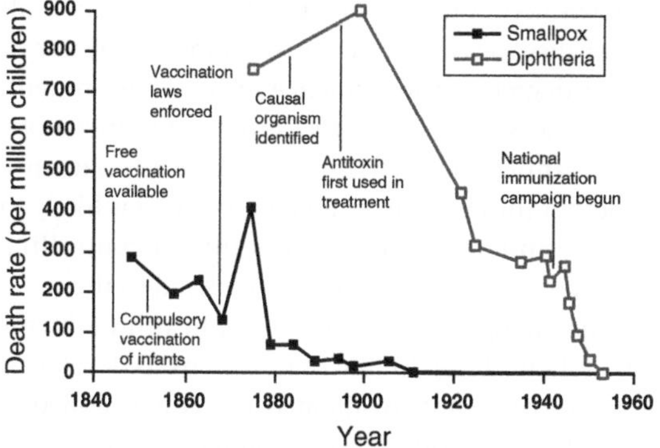

FIGURE 20.3 Child Death Rates Reduced by Medicine.

Source: From *Human Nature Magazine* / McKeown. *Human Nature Magazine:* Determinants of Health. © 1978 Global Rights & Permissions, a part of Cengage Learning, Inc. Reproduced by permission. www.cengage.com/permissions.

the nature of the infections, independent of medical and other identifiable influences.

A further explanation for the falling death rate is that an improvement in nutrition led to an increase in resistance to infectious diseases. This is, I believe, the most credible reason for the decline of the infections, at least until the late 19th century, and also explains why deaths from airborne diseases like scarlet fever and measles have decreased even when exposure to the organisms that cause them remains almost unchanged. The evidence demonstrating the impact of improved nutrition is indirect, but it is still impressive.

Lack of food, and the resulting malnutrition were largely responsible for the predominance of the infectious diseases, from the time when men first aggregated in large population groups about 10,000 years ago. In these conditions an improvement in nutrition was necessary for a substantial and prolonged decline in mortality.

Experience in developing countries today leaves no doubt that nutritional state is a critical factor in a person's response to infectious disease, particularly in young children. Malnourished people contract infections more often than those who are well fed and they suffer more when they become infected. According to a recent World Health Organization report on nutrition in developing countries, the best vaccine against common infectious diseases is an adequate diet.

In the 18th and 19th centuries, food production increased greatly throughout the Western world. The number of people in England and Wales tripled between 1700 and 1850, and they were fed on home-grown food.

In summary: The death rate from infectious diseases fell because an increase in food supplies led to better nutrition. From the second half of the 19th century this advance was strongly supported by improved hygiene and safer food and water, which reduced exposure to infection. With the exception of smallpox vaccination, which played a small part in the total decline of mortality, medical procedures such as immunization and therapy had little impact on human health until the 20th century.

One other influence needs to be considered: a change in reproductive behavior, which caused the birth rate to decline. The significance of this change can hardly be exaggerated, for without it the other advances would soon have been overtaken by the increasing population. We can attribute the modern improvement in health to food, hygiene, and medical intervention—in that order of time and importance—but we must recognize that it is to a modification of behavior that we owe the permanence of this improvement.

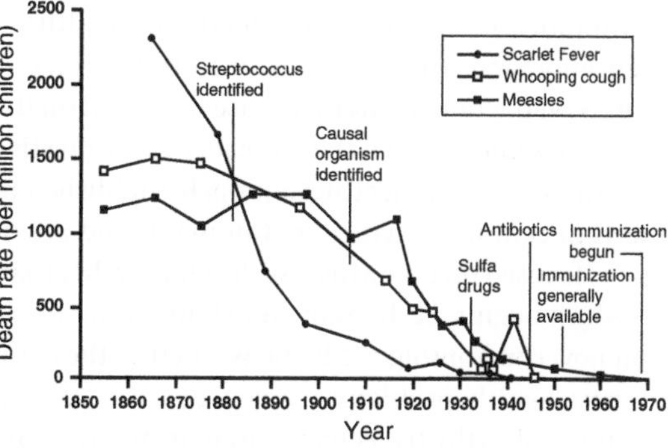

FIGURE 20.4 Other Childhood Diseases.

Source: From *Human Nature Magazine* / McKeown. *Human Nature Magazine:* Determinants of Health. © 1978 Global Rights & Permissions, a part of Cengage Learning, Inc. Reproduced by permission. www.cengage.com/permissions.

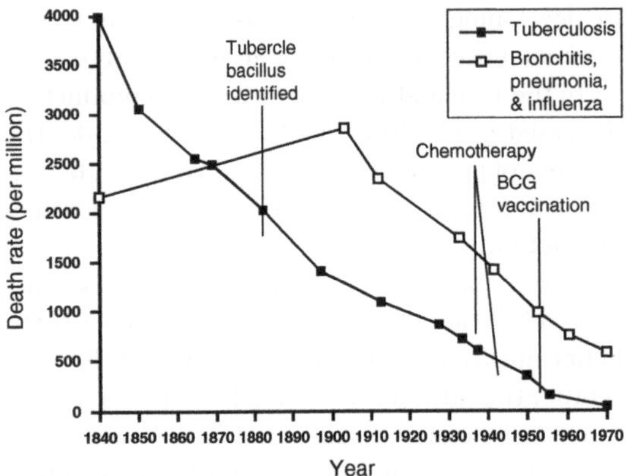

FIGURE 20.5 Pulmonary Diseases.

Source: From *Human Nature Magazine* / McKeown. *Human Nature Magazine:* Determinants of Health. © 1978 Global Rights & Permissions, a part of Cengage Learning, Inc. Reproduced by permission. www.cengage.com/permissions.

But it does not follow that these influences have the same relative importance today as in the past. In technologically advanced countries, the decline of infectious diseases was followed by a vast change in health problems, and even in developing countries advances in medical science and technology may have modified the effects of nutrition, sanitation, and contraception. In order to predict the factors likely to affect our health in the future, we need to examine the nature of the problems in health that exist today.

Because today's problems are mainly with noncommunicable diseases, physicians have shifted their approach. In the case of infections, interest centers on the organisms that cause them and on the conditions under which they spread. In noninfective conditions, the engineering approach established in the 17th century remains predominant, and attention is focused on how a disease develops rather than on why it begins. Perhaps the most important question now confronting medicine is whether the commonest health problems—heart disease, cancer, rheumatoid arthritis, cerebrovascular disease—are essentially different from health problems of the past or whether, like infections, they can be prevented by modifying the conditions that lead to them.

To answer this question, we must distinguish between genetic and chromosomal diseases determined at the moment of fertilization and all other diseases, which are attributable in greater or lesser degree to the influence of the environment. Most diseases, including the common noninfectious ones, appear to fall into the second category. Whether these diseases can be prevented is likely to be determined by the practicability of controlling the environmental influences that lead to them.

The change in the character of health problems that followed the decline of infections in developed countries has not invalidated the conclusion that most diseases, both physical and mental, are associated with influences that might be controlled. Among such influences, those which the individual determines by his own behavior (smoking, eating, exercise, and the like) are now more important for his health than those that depend mainly on society's actions (provision of essential food and protection from hazards). And both behavioral and environmental influences are more significant than medical care.

The role of individual medical care in preventing sickness and premature death is secondary to that of other influences; yet society's investment in health care is based on the premise that it is the major determinant. It is assumed that we are ill and are made well, but it is nearer the truth to say that we are well and are made ill. Few people think of themselves as having the major responsibility for their own health, and the enormous resources that advanced countries assign to the health field are used mainly to treat disease or, to a lesser extent, to prevent it by personal measures such as immunization.

The revised concept of human health cannot provide immediate solutions for the many complex problems facing society: limiting population growth and providing adequate food in developing countries, changing personal behavior and striking a new balance between technology and care in developed nations. Instead, the enlarged understanding of health and disease should be regarded as a conceptual base with implications for services, education, and research that will take years to develop.

The most immediate requirement in the health services is to give sufficient attention to behavioral influences that are now the main determinants of health. The public believes that health depends primarily on intervention by the doctor and that the essential requirement for health is the early discovery of disease. This concept should be replaced by recognition that disease often cannot be treated effectively and that health is determined predominantly by the way of life individuals choose to follow. Among the important influences on health are the use of tobacco, the misuse of alcohol and drugs, excessive or unbalanced diets, and lack of exercise. With research, the list of significant behavioral influences will undoubtedly increase, particularly in relation to the prevention of mental illness.

Although the influences of personal behavior are the main determinants of health in developed countries, public action can still accomplish a great deal in the environmental field. Internationally, malnutrition probably remains the most important cause of ill health, and even in affluent societies sections of the population are inadequately, as distinct from unwisely, fed. The malnourished vary in proportion and composition from one country to another, but in the developed world they are mainly the younger children of large families and elderly people who live alone. In light of the importance of food for good health, governments might use supplements and subsidies to put essential foods within the reach of everyone, and provide inducements for people to select beneficial in place of harmful foods. Of course these aims cannot exclude other considerations such as international agreements and the solvency of farmers who have been encouraged to produce meat and dairy products rather than grains. Nevertheless, in future evaluations of agricultural and related economic policies, health implications deserve a primary place.

Perhaps the most sensitive area for consideration is the funding of the health services. Although the contribution of medical intervention to prevention of sickness and premature death can be expected to remain small in relation to behavioral and environmental influences, surgery and drugs are widely regarded as the basis of health and the essence of medical care, and society invests the money it sets aside for health mainly in treatment for acute diseases and particularly in hospitals for the acutely ill. Does it follow from our appraisal that resources should be transferred from acute care to chronic care and to preventive measures?

Restricting the discussion to personal medical care, I believe that neglected areas, such as mental illness, mental retardation, and geriatric care, need greatly increased attention. But to suggest that this can be achieved merely by direct transfer of resources is an oversimplification. The designation "acute care" comprises a wide range of activities that differ profoundly in their effectiveness and efficiency. Some, like surgery for accidents and the treatment of acute emergencies, are among the most important services that medicine can offer and any reduction of their support would be disastrous. Others, however, like coronary care units and iron treatment of some anemias are not shown to be effective, while still others—most tonsillectomies and routine check-ups—are quite useless and should be abandoned. A critical appraisal of medical services for acute illnesses would result in more efficient use of available resources and would free some of them for preventive measures.

What health services need in general is an adjustment in the distribution of interest and resources between prevention of disease, care of the sick who require investigation and treatment, and care of the sick who do not need active intervention. Such an adjustment must pay considerable attention to the major determinants of health: to food and the environment, which will be mainly in the hands of specialists, and to personal behavior, which should be the concern of every practicing doctor.

REFERENCES

Burnet, M. 1971. *Genes, Dreams and Realities.* New York: Basic Books.

Cochrane, A. L. 1972. *Effectiveness and Efficiency.* London: Nuffield Provincial Hospitals Trust.

Dubos, R. 1971. *Mirage of Health.* New York: Harper & Row.

McKeown, T. *The Role of Medicine: "Dream, Mirage or Nemesis?* London: Nuffield Provincial Hospitals Trust.

———. 1977. *The Modern Rise of Population*. San Diego: Academic Press.

Thomas, L. 1974. *The Lives of a Cell: Notes of a Biology Watcher.* New York: Viking Press.

REYNALDO MARTORELL

21 THE NATURE OF CHILD MALNUTRITION AND ITS LONG-TERM IMPLICATIONS

Undernutrition is a major contributor to child death and is, therefore, a central issue in global health. Deaths from undernutrition are, most often, not directly caused by starvation (i.e., a lack of protein, calories, and micronutrients). Rather, undernutrition is an indirect cause of death because makes a child less likely to survive an infectious disease like measles or gastroenteritis.

Viral gastroenteral infections are very common in children living in low-income contexts. They cause diarrhea and dehydration, which increase the likelihoods of catching other diseases, experiencing delayed development, and dying. At the same time as undernutrition makes children more vulnerable to diarrheal disease, diarrhea can also make it harder for the body to absorb food, leading to undernutrition. As such, there is a vicious circle of undernutrition and diarrhea.

Diarrheal episodes and intestinal infections can cause acute dehydration and electrolyte imbalance. The short-term solution to diarrhea-related dehydration is the use of oral rehydration therapy (see Reading 5). The long-term solution, however, must be infrastructural investment for good water, sanitation, and hygiene (WASH; see Section 5) and the adoption of the World Health Organization guidelines of exclusive breast-feeding for the first six months. Breast milk contains antimicrobial agents that protect against infection, and breast-fed babies are not exposed to pathogens from bottles or from the water used to prepare formula.

Undernutrition gets attention during crises of drought and famine when images of skeletal children appear in the media. Acute malnutrition occurs as an **epidemic** *in complex humanitarian emergencies. Those skeletal babies are "wasting," and their survival demands emergency feeding with high-quality food. However, as this article demonstrates,* **endemic** *undernutrition is a more serious and widespread problem. Endemic malnutrition is widespread and has serious negative effects on individuals and populations.*

A mother's poor nutrition when pregnant is related to low-birth-weight infants. Poor nutrition in a toddler results in impaired growth and development, often marked by "stunting" (low height for age). However, as this article shows, there are a variety of other negative health effects. Malnutrition has particularly severe effects during the first 1,000 days of life. The lack of essential micronutrients in the diet—sometimes called "hidden hunger"—can result in a number of diseases from night blindness (caused by vitamin A deficiency) to anemia (iron deficiency). Interestingly, programs to decrease night blindness using Vitamin A capsules result in a significant decline in child deaths from all causes.

One of the most important take-home messages from this article is that endemic undernutrition in a society contributes to the persistence of poverty. Conversely, if a country invests in improving child nutrition, then there may be positive effects on the national economy. This has been shown by Martorell's work in Latin America, which looked at the long-term well-being of children who had been enrolled in feeding programs. Not only did those individuals benefit in health and wealth, but their children benefited too.

As you read the following article, consider these questions:

- **Why might it be in a nation's best interest to make sure that the youngest children have good diets?**
- **The author argues that the three underlying causes of undernutrition at family level are insufficient access to food; poor water, sanitation and health services; and inadequate maternal and childcare practices. Which of these do you**

Reynaldo Martorell, "The Nature of Child Malnutrition and Its Long-Term Implications." *Food and Nutrition Bulletin*, 1999, 20(3): 288–292.

think is the issue most easily addressed through a health intervention? Why?

- **This article presents evidence showing that people who were malnourished as children suffer reduced intellectual and work performance as adults. What does this tell you about genetic versus environmental influences on intelligence? What might be the large-scale societal implications of this fact?**
- **Look at the figure in the article and notice that it doesn't seem to indicate a particular box to start the cycle going. If you were working in global health, where do you think would be a good place to intervene? Why?**

CONTEXT

Reynaldo Martorell is the Robert W. Woodruff Professor of International Nutrition in the Rollins Department of Global Health at Emory University. He has been described in the *Lancet* as a "driving force in maternal and child nutrition." He has held leadership positions in the International Nutrition Foundation, the Pan American Health and Education Foundation and the Emory Global Health Institute. A prolific researcher in the Latin American context, he has also served as an advisor to UNICEF, the World Food Program, the World Health Organization, and the World Bank.

Introduction

The objective of this brief article is to review why it is important for developing countries to improve child nutrition. The reasons are simple. First, child malnutrition is a very common problem in poor countries. Second, child malnutrition has short- and long-term adverse consequences that are of great significance for the individuals affected and for the societies in which they live. Third, if the nutrition of children is improved, future generations will be healthier and more productive, and this will be an asset for national economic development.

The Nature of Malnutrition in Children

The problem of malnutrition in children is best viewed as a "syndrome of developmental impairment" caused by a complex of multifactorial factors.[1] The word "syndrome" implies that there is a group of signs and symptoms that occur together and that serve to characterize the problem of malnutrition. At the extreme of severity is severe, clinical malnutrition, illustrated by kwashiorkor and marasmus and their well-known clinical, metabolic, and anthropometric features.[2] These extreme conditions, although they are life-threatening medical problems with lifelong dysfunction for survivors, are less important, from the public health point of view, than the less severe forms of malnutrition. This is so because mild and moderate forms of malnutrition are many times more common than severe clinical malnutrition.

The hallmark of child malnutrition is growth failure, and the most commonly used indicator of growth failure is underweight, defined as a weight-for-age more than 2 standard deviations below the reference mean. In the reference curve, 2.3% of the population is below this criterion.

The Sub-Committee on Nutrition of the United Nations Administrative Committee on Coordination (ACC/SCN) estimates that 29.3% of pre-school children (i.e., < 5 years of age) in developing countries were underweight in 1995. This is lower than the 34.3% estimated for 1985. However, in absolute numbers, the number of underweight children changed little over this period, from 163.8 million in 1985 to 157.6 million in 1995. For South-East Asia, which includes Indonesia, rates of underweight are reported to have come down from 39.8% to 32.4% of pre-school children and the number of malnourished children to have decreased from 39.8 million to 32.4 million between 1985 and 1995.[3]

Many young children in developing countries also suffer from a number of nutritional deficiencies. Often, underweight and nutritional deficiencies cluster in the same villages, families, and individuals. The older literature in Latin America referred to the problem of malnutrition in young children as the *síndrome pluricarencial* or "multiple deficiency syndrome," a very apt designation. Although less than 1% of pre-school children have clinical vitamin A deficiency, many more have subclinical vitamin A deficiency. Using the cut-off point for serum retinol of less than 0.7 μmol/L to define subclinical vitamin A deficiency, many countries are found where 30% or more of children are affected; 58% of pre-school children in Indonesia, according to a 1991 survey, were affected with vitamin A deficiency.[4] Anaemia, defined as less than 11 g of haemoglobin per deciliter, is estimated to occur in more than a third of pre-school children in developing countries.[4] According to UNICEF, about a third of babies born in 1990, or some 40 million infants, were iodine deficient in utero or in early childhood, but now this figure is much less because of the widespread use of iodized salt.[5] Other nutritional problems are also common in young children and include folic acid and zinc deficiencies.[4]

Beaton et al.[1] called attention to the fact that the syndrome of child malnutrition includes, in addition to growth failure, other indications of impairment, such as delayed motor, cognitive, and behavioural development, diminished immunocompetence, and increased morbidity and mortality. The "complex of multifactorial factors" that cause child malnutrition includes three classes of underlying causes at household and family levels, which are known simply as food (i.e., insufficient access to food), health (i.e., poor water/sanitation and inadequate health services), and care (inadequate maternal and child-care practices). These in turn lead to deficient nutrient intakes and to infections and diseases, which are the immediate causes of child malnutrition[6]. Much has been learned over the last half-century about the causes of malnutrition, and this knowledge has improved our policy and programme recommendations. In the 1950s and 1960s, emphasis was placed on protein deficiency, followed by a period in the 1970s and beyond during which low energy consumption due to food insecurity was thought to be the most limiting problem in the diets of poor people. Today, poor dietary quality, which refers to inadequate concentrations of protein and micronutrients and/or to poor bioavailability, is recognized as an additional, important dietary limitation. Infections, particularly diarrhoeal diseases, are recognized as important causes of poor appetite in children and of metabolic and clinical disturbances that lead to poor nutrient utilization[6]. Finally, one of UNICEF's greatest contributions has been to underscore the role of caring behaviours in shaping the nutrition of young children.[6] Household food resources and health-care availability are necessary but not sufficient ingredients for good child health and nutrition; in addition, caretakers must use household resources wisely and meet the nutritional, health, and psychosocial needs of young children for children to be healthy and to develop normally.[7]

Windows of Greatest Developmental Vulnerability

Childhood malnutrition flourishes during periods of vulnerability. One such period is *in utero*. The prevalence of low birthweight (< 2.5 kg) is 18% in developing countries but is as high as 50% in Bangladesh.[6] These affected newborns are at high risk for serious morbidity and mortality during infancy. As adults, they tend to be smaller than others in the community by 5 cm and 5 kg, with reduced work capacity and strength.[8]

There follows a brief period of relative well-being after birth, even in settings of marked poverty, but only if babies are breastfed. At some point in early infancy, by three to six months generally, growth rates begin to falter dramatically, particularly before one year of age. By the time children are two or three years of age, many are underweight and stunted. From three years of age into the school period, children from even very poor countries will grow generally as well as children from the United States, remaining small but neither falling further behind nor catching up appreciably.[9] Some catch-up occurs in some settings during adolescence and is associated with delayed maturation[10,11]. Currently, there is no evidence that stunting can be reversed during adolescence through nutrition intervention programmes; on the other hand, adoption studies suggest that dietary interventions may accelerate maturation, shorten the adolescent growth period, and reduce final adult stature.[12]

Thus, to prevent underweight and its consequences, efforts must be made to prevent low birthweight and to promote good growth and development in the first two to three years of life.

Why are children at greater risk of malnutrition during these windows of vulnerability? *In utero* the reasons include growing up in the restricted environment provided by a stunted mother, herself the product of a malnourished childhood. Maternal reserves of fat, lean tissue, minerals, and micronutrients will be poor. In addition, dietary intakes will often be deficient in quantity and quality, and prenatal care may be poor.

Why are children less than three years of age most vulnerable to malnutrition and its effects? One reason is that growth rates in the first few years are higher than at other times after birth, and thus adverse factors have a greater potential for causing growth retardation early in life than at later years. Young children have high nutritional requirements per kilogram of body weight, in part because of their needs for growth. Another reason for the vulnerability of young children is that their immunological systems develop and mature with time; young children are more susceptible to frequent and severe infections than older children with mature immune systems. Yet another reason for the vulnerability of young children is that they are less able to make their needs known and are more vulnerable to the effects of poor parenting.[9]

Of particular relevance to the central nervous system is that the wiring of cognitive and emotional abilities, a delicate interplay of nature and nurture (i.e., stimuli), largely occurs during the early years of life. Thus, it is particularly important that young children live in an environment that provides the necessary security, experience, and stimuli for optimal growth and development of the central nervous system and associated intellectual, social, and emotional competencies.

Consequences of Childhood Malnutrition

Some years ago, Scrimshaw et al (p. 265).[13] wrote that "Synergism between malnutrition and infection is responsible for much of the excess mortality among infants and pre-school children in less developed regions." Yet, infections, rather than the underlying malnutrition, are usually regarded as the cause of mortality in young children, and for these reasons, many estimates of the relative importance of causes of pre-school mortality give little importance to malnutrition. Pelletier et al.[14] carried out an analysis demonstrating the "potentiating effect of malnutrition" on mortality rates. By their estimates, more than half of deaths among children less than five years old are due to malnutrition, mostly mild and moderate malnutrition. These estimates have received wide dissemination, and policy makers now have a better appreciation of the importance of nutrition for survival.

The improvement of vitamin A status has been demonstrated to lead to a reduction of 23% in mortality among children one to five years of age.[15] This is perhaps due to effects of vitamin A improvements on the severity of infections, particularly diarrhoeal diseases and measles. Recent research indicates that zinc supplementation in pre-school children leads to important reductions in both the number and duration of episodes of diarrhoea.[16] This probably means that improvements in zinc status have important effects on child mortality, but no studies on this question have been carried out to date.

Childhood malnutrition also leaves its imprint on the minds of those who survive it. A review of the literature reveals that poor nutrition during intrauterine life and the early years leads to profound and varied effects, which include delayed motor development, general effects on cognitive development resulting in lower IQ, and a greater degree of behavioural problems and deficient social skills at school age, as well as decreased attention, deficient learning, and lower educational achievement.[17] The bodies of survivors of child malnutrition are also affected, as demonstrated by studies conducted in rural Guatemala.[18] Improved nutrition during pregnancy and the first few years of life, achieved through the consumption of daily food supplements rich in energy, protein, and micronutrients, improved growth during early childhood and reduced stunting at three years of age. As adults, subjects who received dietary improvements were taller and had greater lean body mass, work capacity, and strength than those who did not receive dietary improvements. This is important for adults in several ways. In men engaged in hard physical labour, better work capacity and strength can lead to increased productivity. In women, more lean body mass will mean higher birthweights, and increased height and larger body frame may decrease the risk of delivery complications due to cephalopelvic disproportion. The Guatemalan study demonstrates that improving nutrition in early childhood is important, but not that improvement is necessarily achieved through food supplementation.

The benefits of improving micronutrient status are also great. Reference has been already made to some of the effects of deficiencies in vitamin A and zinc. Also important is the prevention of iron-deficiency anaemia in children and adults. Anaemia can result in impaired learning, diminished work capacity, and perhaps low birthweight and increased maternal mortality.[19] Iodine deficiency in pregnancy and early childhood, even when not severe enough to result in cretinism, can cause poor growth, delayed maturation, and diminished intellectual performance.[20]

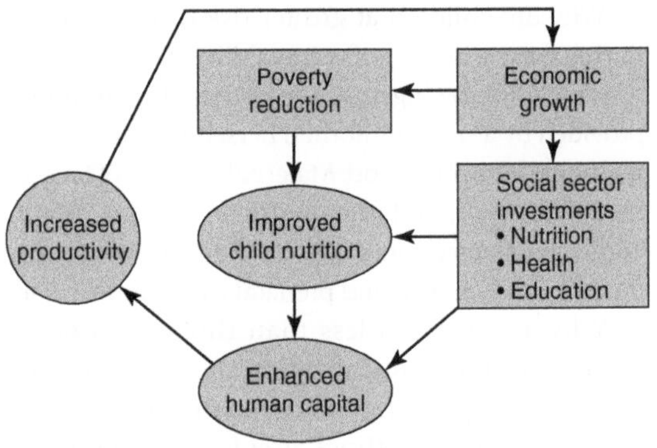

FIGURE 21.1 Human Capital Diagram.

Improved Child Nutrition and Economic Development

The relationship between improved child nutrition and economic development is shown in Figure 21.1. In this paper, the evidence justifying the arrow going from "improved child nutrition" to "enhanced human capital" has been reviewed. There is considerable evidence as well for other relationships depicted in Figure 21.1. Economic growth, particularly that which leads to poverty reduction in urban as well as in rural areas, is one of the key factors driving change in nutrition at national levels.[21] But much more can be achieved, and more quickly, if governments invest in nutrition, health, and education programmes.[21] There are examples of successful community-based programmes,[5,6,22–24] and we know much about what is needed for successful programme implementation.[25] Enhanced human capital, through improvements in nutrition and health, is thought to explain half of the economic growth of the United Kingdom, France, and other European nations in the previous two centuries.[26]

Conclusions

Three points are emphasized in this paper. First, nutritional problems are very common in poor countries. Second, these problems lead to short- and long-term functional consequences that limit human potential. Third, improving child nutrition is a national priority and an important strategy for long-term economic development. As countries face difficult choices during times of economic crisis, it becomes imperative to advocate strongly for social sector investments, including nutrition programmes for mothers and young children. Dismantling effective programmes is a counterproductive, short-term coping strategy, just as would be said in the case of households in famine-stricken areas who consume the seeds needed for future plantings and who sell their agricultural tools. In both these cases, future productive potential is compromised. Whereas options may be limited in a famine, governments in economic crises have more latitude. Public nutritionists are compelled to seek continued funding for priority programmes as well as better use of the limited resources available (i.e., increased cost-effectiveness).

REFERENCES

1. Beaton G, Kelly A, Kevany J, Martorell R, Mason J. Appropriate uses of anthropometric indices in children. ACC/SCN State-of-the-art Series Nutrition Policy Discussion Paper No. 7. Geneva: United Nations Administrative Committee on Coordination/Sub-Committee on Nutrition, 1990.
2. Jelliffe DB. The assessment of the nutritional status of the community. WHO Monograph Series No. 53. Geneva: World Health Organization, 1966.
3. Administrative Committee on Coordination/Sub-Committee on Nutrition (ACC/SCN). Update on the nutrition situation 1996. Summary of results for the third report on the world nutrition situation. SCN News, No. 14, July 1997.
4. Administrative Committee on Coordination/Sub-Committee on Nutrition (ACC/SCN). Chapter 2. Micronutrients. In: Third report on the world nutrition situation. Geneva: ACC/SCN, 1997:19–46.

5. Alnwick DJ. Combating micronutrient deficiencies: problems and perspectives. International and Public Health Nutrition Group Symposium on "Can nutrition intervention make a difference?" Proc Nutr Soc 1998;57:1–12.
6. United Nations Children's Fund (UNICEF). The state of the world's children 1998. Bringing science to bear. Oxford, UK: Oxford University Press, 1998.
7. Engle PL, Menon P, Haddad L. Care and nutrition. Concepts and measurement. Washington, DC: International Food Policy Research Institute, 1997.
8. Martorell R, Ramakrishnan U, Schroeder DG, Melgar P, Neufeld L. Intrauterine growth retardation, body size, body composition and physical performance in adolescence. Eur J Clin Nutr 1998;52(S1):S43–53.
9. Martorell R. Promoting healthy growth: rationale and benefits. In: Pinstrup-Andersen P, Pelletier D, Alderman H, eds. Child growth and nutrition in developing countries. Priorities for action. New York: Cornell University Press, 1995:15–31.
10. Martorell R, Kettel Khan L, Schroeder D. Reversibility of stunting: epidemiological findings in children from developing countries. Eur J Clin Nutr 1994;48:S45–57.
11. Simondon KB, Simondon F, Simon I, Diallo A, Bénéfice E, Traissac P, Maire B. Preschool stunting, age at menarche and adolescent height: a longitudinal study in rural Senegal. Eur J Clin Nutr 1998;52:412–8.
12. Proos LA, Hofvander Y, Tuvemo T. Menarcheal age and growth pattern of Indian girls adopted in Sweden. Acta Paediatr Scand 1991;80:852–8.
13. Scrimshaw NS, Taylor CE, Gordon JE. Interactions of nutrition and infection. WHO Monograph Series No. 57. Geneva: World Health Organization, 1968.
14. Pelletier DC, Frongillo EA, Habicht J-P. Epidemiologic evidence for a potentiating effect of malnutrition on child mortality. Am J Public Health 1993;83:1130–3.
15. Beaton GH, Martorell R, Aronson KJ, Edmonston B, McCabe G, Ross AC, Harvey B. Effectiveness of vitamin A supplementation in the control of young child morbidity and mortality in developing countries. ACC/SCN State-of-the-art Series Nutrition Policy Discussion Paper No. 13. Geneva: United Nations Administrative Committee on Coordination/Sub-Committee on Nutrition (ACC/SCN), 1993.
16. Black RE. Zinc for child health. Am J Clin Nutr 1997; 68(2S):410S–516S.
17. Martorell R. Undernutrition during pregnancy and early childhood: consequences for cognitive and behavioral development. In: Young ME, ed. Early child development: investing in our children's future. Amsterdam and New York: Elsevier Science BV, 1997:39–83.
18. Martorell R. Results and implications of the INCAP follow-up study. J Nutr 1995; 125(4S):1127S–38S.
19. Viteri FE. Prevention of iron deficiency. In: Howson CP, Kennedy ET, Horwitz A, eds. Prevention of micronutrient deficiencies. Tools for policymakers and public health workers. Washington, DC: National Academy Press, 1998:45–102.
20. Bleichrodt N, Born MP. A metaanalysis of research on iodine and its relationship to cognitive development. In: Stanbury JB, ed. The damaged brain of iodine deficiency: neuromotor, cognitive, behavioral, and educative aspects. New York: Cognizant Communication Corporation, 1994:195–200.
21. Gillespie S, Mason J, Martorell R. How nutrition improves. ACC/SCN State-of-the-art Series Nutrition Policy Discussion Paper No. 15. Geneva: United Nations Administrative Committee on Coordination/Sub-Committee on Nutrition (ACC/SCN), 1996.
22. Balachander J. Tamil Nadu's successful nutrition effort. In: Rohde J, Chatterjee M, Morley D, eds. Reaching health for all. Delhi: Oxford University Press, 1993:158–84.
23. Jonsson U, Ljungqvist B, Yambi O. Mobilization for nutrition in Tanzania. In: Rohde J, Chatterjee M, Morley D, eds. Reaching health for all. Delhi: Oxford University Press, 1993:185–211.
24. Underwood BA. Prevention of vitamin A deficiency. In: Howson CP, Kennedy ET, Horwitz A, eds. Prevention of micronutrient deficiencies. Tools for policymakers and public health workers. Washington, DC: National Academy Press, 1998:102–66.
25. Jennings J, Gillespie S, Mason J, Lotfi M, Scialfa T. Managing successful nutrition programmes. ACC/SCN State-of-the-art Series Nutrition Policy Discussion Paper No. 8. A report based on an ACC/SCN Workshop at the 14th IUNS International Congress on Nutrition, Seoul, Korea, 20–25 August 1989. Geneva: United Nations Administrative Committee on Coordination/Sub-Committee on Nutrition (ACC/SCN), 1991.
26. Fogel RW. Economic growth, population theory and physiology: the bearing of long-term processes on the making of economic policy. American Economic Review (Nashville, Tenn, USA: American Economic Association) 1994;84(3):369–95.

STEPHEN O'BRIEN

22 STATEMENT TO THE SECURITY COUNCIL ON MISSIONS TO YEMEN, SOUTH SUDAN, AND KENYA AND AN UPDATE ON THE OSLO CONFERENCE ON NIGERIA AND THE LAKE CHAD REGIONS

This is a completely different document than the others in this book. It is the transcript of a report to the Security Council of the United Nations (UN) about ongoing complex humanitarian emergencies that happened in March 2017. It is addressed to the president of the Security Council. It describes the horrendous situations of famine, **food insecurity**, *and human misery. The UN official in charge of Humanitarian Affairs and Emergency Relief reports that the worst conditions were in war-torn Yemen, South Sudan, and Somalia. However, even in peaceful Kenya, there were some 4 million citizens living with food insecurity and children experiencing chronic undernutrition. These are terrible humanitarian emergencies requiring immediate action and funding to save lives by providing food and security. Given the circumstances, Under-Secretary-General O'Brien was asking for a relatively modest amount of emergency money.*

Most Americans pay little attention to international issues until there is an emergency that gets on TV. However, given the political turmoil happening in the United States at that time, very few people were paying attention to these crises. The numbers reported in this document are staggering, and that makes it difficult to comprehend that the statistics refer to actual individual human beings with families and loved ones, with tears and fears. The document is an eyewitness account of these tragedies, and it attempts to evoke compassion by describing particular people who are in terrible circumstances. The document is a warning about a coming famine in a world that already produces enough food for everyone.

These emergencies are extremely complicated because they are politicized, and warring parties want to use (or deny) humanitarian assistance for their own strategic purposes. Obviously, violence is issue that must involve global health institutions, but the ultimate solutions require long-term political-economic actions backed by courageous political will and financial commitments. Climate change also causes droughts, famines, increasing poverty emigration (Reading 19), and that is a complicated global problem as well.

In the short run, however, essential emergency assistance seemed to be all at the UN could accomplish. This report describes the UN emergency programs that had already been undertaken. These efforts have been heroic. Aid workers have been killed; humanitarian compounds and supplies have been attacked, looted, and occupied. The UN is not the only agency involved in humanitarian relief during time of war. There are many other nongovernmental organizations, including Médecins Sans Frontières *(Doctors Without Borders; see Reading 33) as well as the International Red Cross and Red Crescent (Reading 35).*

We live in a world where some people are stuffed and others are starved. It is the responsibility of educated people in high-income countries to be aware of this paradox and understand the complexities of why it occurs in a globalized world. Finally, everyone shares a responsibility to make sure that those taking the necessary action get the support they need.

As you read the following document, consider the following questions:

- **Quite a few politicians in the United States do not support the UN, and this is a reason why the United States has not paid a significant**

Stephen O'Brien, *UN Statement to the Security Council on Missions to Yemen, South Sudan, Somalia and Kenya and an Update on the Oslo Conference on Nigeria and the Lake Chad Region*. New York: United Nations, 2017.

amount its membership dues in the past. In your opinion, why might some Americans be against the UN?

- **The document suggests three actions that need to be taken by the UN Security Council in light of the multiple humanitarian disasters. What are they? In your opinion, which is most important? Which is most difficult to accomplish?**
- **Famines are often linked to war. The editors of this book could have placed this document either in this section (Food) or Section 9 (Violence). In your opinion, are the food shortages described here primarily about food or war?**
- **What do you think are some reasons why the global market in food does not seem to work? Shouldn't the laws of supply and demand work?**
- **Why do you think most Americans do not know about the kind of humanitarian crises discussed here? Can that be fixed?**

CONTEXT

Stephen O'Brien is a British politician and diplomat who is the UN Under-Secretary-General for Humanitarian Affairs and Emergency Relief Coordinator. He assumed office in May 2015. A number of written reports, including the annual Global Humanitarian Assistance report, accompanied this verbal report to the Security Council. In 2014, UN-coordinated humanitarian appeals requested a total of US$19.5 billion, yet US$7.5 billion of the requirements went unmet.

Mr. President, Council members,

Thank you for inviting me to brief on my visits to countries facing famine or at risk of famine: Yemen, South Sudan and Somalia. I will also briefly mention the outcomes of the Oslo Conference on the Lake Chad Basin.

I need to mention that I also visited Northern Kenya where pastoralists are worst affected by the terrible drought. Over 2.7 million Kenyans are now food insecure, a number likely to reach 4 million by April. In collaboration with the Government, the UN will soon launch an appeal of $200 million to provide timely life-saving assistance and protection. For what follows however, I will focus on my other visits over the past 16 days.

Mr. President,

I turn first to Yemen. It's already the largest humanitarian crisis in the world and the Yemeni people now face the spectre of famine. Today, two-thirds of the population—18.8 million people—need assistance and more than 7 million are hungry and do not know where there next meal will come from. That is 3 million people more than in January. As fighting continues and escalates, displacement increases. With health facilities destroyed and damaged, diseases are sweeping through the country.

I spoke with people in Aden, Ibb, Sana'a and from Taizz. They told me horrific stories of displacement, escaping unspeakable violence and destruction from Mokha and Taizz city in Taizz governorate. I saw first-hand the effects of losing home and livelihood: malnourishment, hunger and squalid living conditions in destroyed schools, unfinished apartments and wet, concrete basements. In the past two months alone, more than 48,000 people fled fighting, mines and IEDs from Mokha town and the surrounding fields alone. I met countless children, malnourished and sick. My small team met a girl displaced to Ibb, still having shrapnel wounds in her legs while her brother was deeply traumatized. I was introduced to a 13-year-old girl who fled from Taizz city, left in charge of her seven siblings. I spoke with families who have become displaced to Aden as their homes were destroyed by airstrikes living in a destroyed school. All of them told me three things: they are hungry and sick—and they need peace so that they can return home.

I travelled to Aden on the first humanitarian UN flight, where I met the President, Prime Minister and Foreign Minister of the Republic of Yemen. I also met with the senior leadership of the Houthi and General People's Congress authorities in Sana'a. I discussed the humanitarian situation, the need to prevent a famine and to better respect international humanitarian law and protect civilians. I demanded full, safe and unimpeded humanitarian access. All counterparts promised to facilitate sustained access and respect international humanitarian law. Yet all parties to the conflict are arbitrarily denying sustained humanitarian access and politicize aid. Already, the humanitarian suffering that we see in Yemen today is caused by the parties and proxies and if they don't change their behaviour now, they must be held accountable for the inevitable famine, unnecessary deaths and associated amplification in suffering that will follow.

Despite the almost impossible and terrifying conditions, the UN and humanitarian partners are not deterred and are stepping up to meet the humanitarian needs across the country. In February alone, 4.9 million people received food assistance. We continue to negotiate access and make modest gains. For instance, despite assurances from all parties of safe passage to Taizz city, I was denied access and retreated to a short safe distance when I and my team came under gunfire. Yet, we managed to use this experience to clear the path for reaching people inside Taizz city with a first humanitarian truck delivery of eight tons of essential medicine on the Ibb to Taizz city road since August 2016. We will not leave a stone unturned to find alternative routes. We must prevail as so many lives depend on us, the full range of the humanitarian family.

For 2017, the humanitarian community requires US$ 2.1 billion to reach 12 million people with life-saving assistance and protection in Yemen. Only 6 per cent of that funding has been received thus far. An international ministerial-level pledging event is scheduled for 25 April, but the situation is so dire that I ask donors to give urgently now. All contributions and pledges since 1 January will be counted at the event.

I continue to reiterate the same message to all: it is only a political solution that will ultimately end human suffering and bring stability to the region. And at this stage, only a combined response with the private sector can stem a famine: commercial imports must be allowed to resume through all entry points in Yemen, including and especially Hudaydah port, which must be kept open and expanded. With access and funding, humanitarians will do more, but we are not the long-term solution to this growing crisis.

I am pleased as I said to confirm that a ministerial-level pledging event for the humanitarian response in Yemen for 2017 will take place in Geneva on 25 April. The Secretary-General will chair the event, co-hosted by the Foreign Ministers of Sweden and Switzerland, to advocate for more resources and access. For 2017, as mentioned, the Yemen humanitarian response plan asks for US $2.1 billion to assist 12 million people in need across all 22 governorates.

Mr. President,
Turning to South Sudan which I visited on 4 and 5 March. The situation is worse than it has ever been. The famine in South Sudan is man-made. Parties to the conflict are parties to the famine—as are those not intervening to make the violence stop.

More than 7.5 million people need assistance, up by 1.4 million from last year. About 3.4 million people are displaced, of which almost 200,000 have fled South Sudan since January alone. A localized famine was declared for Leer and Mayendit [counties] on 20 February, an area where violence and insecurity have compromised humanitarian access for years. More than one million children are estimated to be acutely malnourished across the country; including 270,000 children who face the imminent risk of death should they not be reached in time with assistance. Meanwhile, the cholera outbreak that began in June 2016 has spread to more locations.

I travelled to Ganyiel in Unity state where people have fled from the horrors of famine and conflict. I saw the impact humanitarians can have to alleviate suffering. I met an elderly woman with her malnourished grandson receiving treatment. I listened to women who fled fighting with their children through waist-high swamps to receive food and medicine. Some of these women have experienced the most appalling acts of sexual violence—which continues to be used as a weapon of war. Their harrowing stories are only a few among thousands who have suffered a similar fate across the country.

Humanitarians are delivering. Last year, partners reached more than 5.1 million people with assistance. However, active hostilities, access denials and bureaucratic impediments continue to curtail their efforts to reach people who desperately need help. Aid workers have been killed; humanitarian compounds and supplies have been attacked, looted, and occupied by armed actors. Recently, humanitarians had to leave one of the famine-affected counties because of fighting. Assurances by senior Government officials of unconditional access and no bureaucratic impediments now need to be turned into action on the ground.

Mr. President,
In Somalia, more than half the population—6.2 million people—need humanitarian and protection assistance, including 2.9 million who are at risk of famine and require immediate assistance to save or sustain their lives, close to 1 million children under the age of 5 will be acutely malnourished this year. In the last two months alone, nearly 160,000 people have been displaced due to severe drought conditions, adding to the already 1.1 million people who live in appalling conditions around the country.

What I saw and heard during my visit to Somalia was distressing—women and children walk for weeks in search of food and water. They have lost their livestock, water sources have dried up and they have nothing left to survive on. With everything lost, women, boys, girls and men now move to urban centres.

With the Secretary-General—his first field mission since he took office—we visited Baidoa. We met with displaced people going through ordeals none of us can imagine. We visited the regional hospital where children and adults are desperately fighting to survive diarrhoea, cholera and malnutrition. Again, as if proof was needed, it was clear that between malnutrition and death there is disease.

Large parts of southern and central Somalia remain under the control or influence of Al-Shabaab and the security situation is volatile. Last year, some 165 violent incidents—an 18 per cent increase compared to 2015—directly impacted humanitarian work and resulted in 14 deaths of aid workers. Al-Shabaab, Government Forces and other militia also continue to block major supply routes to towns in 29 of the 42 districts in southern and central Somalia. This has restricted access to markets, basic commodities and services, and is severely disrupting livelihoods. Blockades and double taxation bar farmers from transporting their grains. It is critical that AMISOM and Somali forces secure vital road access to enable both lifesaving aid and longer term recovery. A lot of hope is placed in the new Government.

The current indicators mirror the tragic picture of 2011, when Somalia last suffered a famine. It is important to add that when the famine was called at that time 260,000 had already died, this will be important in what I am about to tell you. However, humanitarian partners now have a larger footprint, mature cash programming, better data through assessments, better controls on resources and vetting of partners, as well as stronger partnership with government authorities. The Government recently declared the drought a national disaster and is taking steps to work with humanitarian partners to ensure a coordinated response. To be clear, we can avert a famine, we have a committed clear new President, a humanitarian and resilience track record, a detailed plan, we're ready despite incredible risk and danger, we have local and international leadership, we have a lot of access, now we need the international community, at the scale of you the donor agencies and nations, to invest in Somalia, its lifesaving—but we need those huge funds now.

For all three crises and North-Eastern Nigeria, an immediate injection of funds plus safe and unimpeded access are required to enable partners to avert a catastrophe; otherwise, many people will predictably die from hunger, livelihoods will be lost, and political gains that have been hard-won over the last few years will be reversed. To be precise we need $4.4 billion by July, and that's a detailed cost, not a negotiating number.

Mr. President,
Before I visited all these countries, I was in Oslo, where the governments of Norway, Germany and Nigeria, in partnership with the United Nations, organized a humanitarian conference on Nigeria and the Lake Chad region. 10.7 million people need humanitarian assistance and protection, including 7.1 million people who are severely food insecure. Humanitarian partners scaled up their response to reach the most vulnerable groups threatened by violence, food insecurity and famine, particularly in North-Eastern Nigeria.

Fourteen donors pledged a total of US$672 million, of which $458 million is for humanitarian action in 2017. This is very good news, and I commend those who made such generous pledges. More is needed however to receive the $1.5 billion required to provide the assistance needed across the Lake Chad region.

Mr. President,
We stand at a critical point in history. Already at the beginning of the year we are facing the largest humanitarian crisis since the creation of the United Nations. Now, more than 20 million people across four countries face starvation and famine. Without collective and coordinated global efforts, people will simply starve to death. Many more will suffer and die from disease. Children stunted and out of school. Livelihoods, futures and hope will be lost. Communities' resilience rapidly wilting away. Development gains reversed. Many will be displaced and will continue to move in search for survival, creating ever more instability across entire regions. The warning call and appeal for action by the Secretary-General can thus not be understated. It was right to take the risk and sound the alarm early, not wait for the pictures of emaciated dying children or the world's TV screens to mobilise a reaction and the funds.

The UN and humanitarian partners are responding. We have strategic, coordinated and prioritised plans in every country. We have the right leadership and heroic, dedicated teams on the ground. We are working hand-in-hand with development partners to marry the immediate life-saving with longer term sustainable development. We are ready to scale up. This is frankly not the time to ask for more detail or use that postponing phrase, what would you prioritize? Every life on the edge of famine and death is equally worth saving.

Now we need the international community and this Council to act:

First and foremost, act quickly to tackle the precipitating factors of famine. Preserving and restoring normal access to food and ensuring all parties' compliance with international humanitarian law are key.

Second, with sufficient and timely financial support, humanitarians can still help to prevent the worst-case scenario. To do this, humanitarians require safe, full and unimpeded access to people in need. Parties to the conflict must respect this fundamental tenet of IHL and those with influence over the parties must exert that influence now.

Third, stop the fighting. To continue on the path of war and military conquest is—I think we all know—to guarantee failure, humiliation and moral turpitude, and will bear the responsibility for the millions who face hunger and deprivation on an incalculable scale because of it.

Mr. President,
Allow me to very briefly sum up. The situation for people in each country is dire and without a major international response, the situation will get worse. All four countries have one thing in common: conflict. This means we—you—have the possibility to prevent—and end—further misery and suffering. The UN and its partners are ready to scale up. But we need the access and the funds to do more. It is all preventable. It is possible to avert this crisis, to avert these famines, to avert these looming human catastrophes.

Thank you. Thank you Mr. President.

IPPOLYTOS KALOFONOS

23 HUNGER IN THE AIDS ECONOMY OF CENTRAL MOZAMBIQUE

In a massive global effort, life-saving antiretroviral treatment for HIV/AIDS has been scaled up dramatically. In sub-Saharan Africa, the World Health Organization estimates that the percentage of HIV-positive people on treatment went from near zero to nearly 40 percent in just 10 years in the early 2000s. Around 10 million people are now on treatment in sub-Saharan Africa alone. While there is still much work to be done, this achievement—the work of many thousands of people across the world, from policymakers to local health workers—is remarkable.

But this selection by Ippolytos Kalofonos complicates that success story. While the rollout of antiretroviral medications across the world is unquestionably a good thing, this selection shows the complexities involved in providing treatment for a single disease while the factors that put people at risk for that disease—like poverty—remain unchanged. We now live in a world where millions of people are provided expensive and cutting-edge drugs free of charge, but at the same time do not have enough to eat.

The HIV epidemic has increased food insecurity in many places, notably in many areas of sub-Saharan Africa. AIDS kills people in the prime of life—people who work to earn money and get food for their families—thus many families affected by AIDS have fewer breadwinners. Also, many families have also taken on more dependents as they care for children of relatives and friends affected by AIDS. The result is fewer resources and less food per person in these families.

At the individual level, HIV makes the problems associated with being undernourished more serious. For example, HIV-infected children are more likely to experience persistent diarrhea and opportunistic infections. Because these conditions can keep the food that children eat from getting used by their bodies, they are more likely to be severely malnourished.

Taken together, these effects make HIV's impacts on food security so severe that some observers have dubbed this the "new variant famine." Discussions of HIV/AIDS treatment tend to focus on antiretroviral therapies. But for many HIV-positive people around the world, food is medicine too.

As you read this selection, ask yourself these questions:

- **Why would a person who is receiving food aid still be hungry?**
- **Why might testing positive for HIV seem "fortunate" in some cases?**
- **Kalofonos gives several examples of how food may be short and "food insecurity may drive the spread of HIV"—even for someone with food aid. Do you think there is a way around this problem?**
- **Why do you think most HIV/AIDS interventions don't provide the sort of broad social justice that Kalofonos advocates?**
- **Why do you think Kalofonos spends so much of the paper talking about historical events like colonialism and structural adjustment programs? How are those relevant to HIV/AIDS?**

CONTEXT

Ippolytos Kalofonos is an assistant professor in the Department of Psychiatry at the University of California, Los Angeles. He trained very broadly across health disciplines: he is a medical doctor, a PhD in anthropology, and he holds a master's degree in public health. His medical residency was in psychiatry. He has examined health issues through fieldwork in a variety of contexts: in Mozambique, in Brazil, and on the US–Mexico border. Currently his research focuses on ways to provide better care for people with severe mental illness.

This article is original to this volume.

The scale-up of HIV testing, care, and antiretroviral treatment (ART) in Africa is often told as a remarkable story of contemporary humanitarian intervention on a grand scale. This process is graphically depicted with charts of increasing numbers of lives saved, and visually represented with images of dramatic individual recoveries, termed the "Lazarus effect." How did the scale-up actually play out on the ground in ordinary people's lives? The massive investment in HIV treatment in one of the world's most impoverished countries resulted in the emergence of an "AIDS economy," a term that refers to the way global AIDS programs converted the HIV-positive diagnosis into a resource. The AIDS economy emerged at the intersections of the local therapeutic economy and the development economy, as an HIV diagnosis could grant access to not only medical treatment but food aid and other material benefits, and engaging in HIV care, education, and outreach could sometimes earn one a small income. In a context of great scarcity, even while this magic bullet campaign saved lives, it produced troubling social side effects. Many Mozambicans complained that while antiretroviral medications (ARVs) extended their lives, they made them hungry. Conversations such as this one were common among people on ART in Central Mozambique during the initial months of the national expansion of AIDS treatment programs:

> "Do you know what it is for your organism to be asking for food? Its wakes me in the middle of the night, and I have to eat!"
>
> "This treatment really causes hunger!"
>
> "Don't you know why? The body needs food in order to recover. The organism demands it!"
>
> "What can I do? I have nothing to eat. All I eat is ARVs!"

ART first became free and publicly available in Mozambique in early 2004. The number of people on treatment increased to over 500,000 by 2014 (UNAIDS, 2014). While those on ART were grateful for the health they regained, their chief concern was having enough to eat each day. The statement, "All I eat is ARVs" indexes two aspects of this hunger. The first is that HIV/AIDS interventions did not adequately account for hunger among the people whose lives were being saved and refers to an objective scarcity and a physiological state. The second is that ARVs seemed to create a new hunger that stands for something beyond an empty belly: the embodiment of a sense of injustice, a realization that "we are made to be hungry," that "someone is eating in my place." This critique is a reminder that, even while they save lives, AIDS treatment programs can paradoxically have dehumanizing effects if the broader social structures that contribute to suffering and impoverishment remain hidden and intact. By targeting a biological condition, political and economic concerns are sidelined, and local forms of solidarity are undermined as disease-related distinctions determine eligibility for scarce resources.

AIDS & Hunger

The coexistence of hunger and AIDS in Southern Africa is termed the "new variant famine" (De Waal and Whiteside, 2003), a vicious cycle attributed to the loss of adult labor through morbidity and mortality, an increasing burden of care on families, and deadly physiological interactions between HIV and malnutrition that increase susceptibility to infection. Hunger was a common complaint in conjunction with ART in Central Mozambique. Bodies demanded sustenance but could not afford it since they struggled to find regular work. Machambas[1] often lay fallow for several years in households afflicted by HIV/AIDS as one chronic illness in a family deprived two productive laborers: the afflicted and the caretaker. For this reason, some suppressed the possibility of illness as long as their bodies allowed, until they literally collapsed. Many initiating ARVs found themselves miraculously recovering their physical health but at rock-bottom, having sold assets to pay for treatments and sustenance, and having lost loved ones to the epidemic. Daily survival remained in question even as physical health improved.

The new variant famine does not fully account for this embodied sensation of hunger I encountered. Talk of hunger and eating in Africa is an embodied moral language that draws on popular metaphors for prosocial contributions to collective well-being and mutual aid, and illegitimate, antisocial action (Ferguson, 2006). In Northern Mozambique, West notes people "expressed ambivalence toward power in the idiom of consumption . . . they acrimoniously described the powerful in

[1] Subsistence plots urban families rely on to supplement their diets and income.

their midst . . . as 'those who eat well' or 'those who eat everything'" (2005, p. 37). Bayart's phrase "the politics of the belly" describes drives for material accumulation as well as the symbolic association of eating with political domination in West Africa (1993).

Methods

I conducted ethnographic research in Central Mozambique, based in Chimoio for 18 months over a 7-year period between 2003 and 2010, covering the initial scale-up of ART. Free testing and treatment were provided in NGO-supported AIDS speciality clinics on the grounds of public sector hospitals and clinics. I spent time in AIDS clinics, in associations of people living with HIV/AIDS (associations), and with networks of NGO-operated community home-based care (CHBC) volunteers. I explored the intersections between HIV/AIDS interventions, NGOs, local economies, and people's lives, relations, and identities. I developed a network of HIV-positive individuals and families with HIV positive members whom I visited at home and accompanied to healers, churches, clinics, and funerals. I listened to concerns beyond what people shared in clinics and NGOs. Few of these individuals had formal employment, and a minority had completed primary education. Most of my interactions in this multilingual city were in Portuguese. I had a basic competence of the most prevalent regional language, Chiteve, and I worked with a research assistant.

Legacies of Colonialism and Structural Adjustment

Capital of the central province of Manica, Chimoio, has expanded from a population of 50,000 at independence in 1975 to 238,976 in 2007 (INE, 2007). Most live in shantytown *bairros* (neighborhoods) lacking electricity and running water, called the "cane city," which ring the former colonial "cement city." Bairro households combine wage earning or income from the informal market with subsistence production on *machambas*, small plots of land outside the city.

Chimoio grew around a Portuguese textile factory built in 1944. Nationalized at independence in 1975, renamed TextÁfrica, and privatized in the late 1980s, the factory employed 2,500 to 5,000 residents before folding in 2000. This trajectory marks the major political transitions of this period. Independence initiated a period of ambitious social programs, including universal education and health care, subsidized food prices, and food rationing. This was halted by a war of destabilization initiated and supported by Rhodesia and South Africa in 1977. Communication, health, and education infrastructure were targeted as over one-third of schools and clinics were destroyed, roads were rendered impassable, and local economies collapsed. Government infrastructure was further stunted by structural adjustment reforms that initiated the transition to a free-market economy in 1986 and gained momentum with the 1992 ceasefire. Food subsidies were drastically cut and social programs were outsourced to foreign NGOs, hollowing out and fragmenting the public health sector. The number of health centers remains below prewar levels.

Mozambique is called a development success thanks to a steadily growing economy. Yet, child malnutrition and inequality have risen alongside macroeconomic indicators like gross domestic product (GDP). Chronic malnutrition levels increased from 31 percent in 1997 to 46 percent in 2006 (SETSAN, 2008). Fifty-four percent of the population lives in extreme poverty, spending less than one dollar per day, and 75% of poor family's budgets in urban Manica are spent on food (NDPB, 2004). Existing social protection programs, a food subsidy program for the elderly and the chronically ill and disabled (excluding PLWHA), reach a small percentage of those eligible and are plagued with inefficiencies (Hanlon and Smart, 2008). The International Monetary Fund recently reported: "income inequality has increased despite high rates of economic growth" and "few countries offer such a stark contrast . . . Benefits of growth have not been broadly shared and high levels of inequality hamper government policies to reduce poverty" (2016).

The poorest look to the competitive informal sector for cash earning opportunities and rely on social networks. Strain exerted on these ties has resulted in a breakdown of trust and accusations of witchcraft (Pfeiffer, 2005). Crime, sex work, and civil unrest have increased, as was evidenced by a series of public lynchings in Chimoio, Beira, and Maputo, of suspected criminals. Rising food, fuel, and utility costs in urban areas have sparked period demonstrations that erupted into violent riots in 2008 and 2010.

A small minority have become visibly wealthier, as demonstrated in Chimoio by the construction of large new houses, a strip mall, a car dealership, and a private clinic. A conspicuous culture of international development is represented by circulating SUVs emblazoned with organizational logos and bustling communities of expatriates and Mozambicans élites. Many see development projects as a source of possible material support. This expectation was projected onto HIV/AIDS interventions as they rapidly expanded.

The Disease of the Century

AIDS is called *a doença do século* ("the disease of the century"), referring to the chronological timing and the severity of the epidemic. AIDS is the leading cause of death among adults in Mozambique (UNAIDS, 2014). The availability of ART changed the stakes of the HIV diagnosis. While AIDS remained a feared disease, there was a growing awareness of the benefits associated with being HIV-positive—not only free treatment, but also food aid. Food aid from the World Food Program (WFP) was a component of the initial ART pilot programs that began in Central Mozambique in 2003. Associations, initiated to foster social support, solidarity, and activism, became known as places to seek benefits.

ART & Hunger

Associations and clinics provided presentations on nutritional education. During one such presentation in 2006, Batista observed: "my health has changed but my diet has not. There are 14 people in my house who need to eat. I appreciate the food I receive, but its not enough." Though the monthly WFP supplement was a generous amount for one person—officially 36 kg of rice, 18 kg of Corn-Soy Blend, 6 kg of beans, and 1.5 liters of oil—it rarely lasted 2 weeks when distributed among kin. Four adults and ten children, six of whom were his deceased brother's, lived in one household.

Batista had worked at TextÁfrica for 8 years. After it closed, he got by on short-term work opportunities until he fell sick. Unable to work for nearly a year, Batista sold his bicycle and his radio to pay for treatments before testing positive. He occasionally found work and the past month had been relatively profitable, as he had earned 300 meticais (US$40). This would rapidly be consumed. The estimated per person, per day basic nutritional requirements in urban Manica cost 9.6 meticais (US$0.40) (NDPB, 2004). For a family of fourteen, this would come out to just over 4 thousand meticais per month, thirteen times what Batista earned. His wife and eldest two children chipped in earnings, but the family's pooled monthly income rarely approached even even $40 a month, a quarter of the estimated amount for daily nutritional requirements.

I visited a patient named Madalena, with Cristina, a CHBC volunteer, in 2010. Cristina proudly introduced Madalena: "Here is my patient and I can tell you she is already better!" Madelena quickly added: "Yes, but my stomach hurts!" In the months since Cristina had first seen her, Madalena had tested HIV positive and begun ART. Her health and appearance had improved significantly. I assumed the stomach pain referred to hunger caused by ARVs. Madalena did comment: "this medicine bites, its not like a normal hunger. If I don't eat when I take it, I tremble and shake. It is said this medicine will kill you if you don't eat with it." She was awarded with a WFP ration card entitling her to 10 kilos of corn-soy blend and 1 kilo of legumes per month. When shared among her three children, two grandchildren, and her elderly mother, this lasted 4 days.

But Madalena's stomach pain was not simply hunger pangs. She engaged in serial short-lived sexual relationships with men who could pay and feed her. Her stomach pain was accompanied by a foul-smelling vaginal discharge that she was ashamed to reveal in the AIDS clinic lest she be rebuked for having unprotected sex. She had been diagnosed with gonorrhea in the past, and when she could afford to, she treated it with antibiotics. Cristina arranged to accompany Madalena to a clinic later that week to be assessed and receive appropriate treatment. Many PLWHA pointed to this irony—that they struggled to feed themselves and their families even while they received lifesaving pharmaceutical treatment. So even for people on treatment, food insecurity may drive the spread of HIV.

Chasing Food Aid

Nutritional supplementation was provided toward two explicit goals: improving treatment adherence and increasing weight. Attendance in the initial ART pilot programs improved dramatically when food was provided to patients. Supplements were subsequently offered to the first patients in public AIDS clinics. When the number of patients exceeded the available food, criteria were developed based on body weight, socioeconomic need, and a preference for people beginning ART. Food was provided for 6 months, a period later reduced to 3 months in order to reach more patients. Eligibility was renewed if a patient's weight did not increase.

The AIDS clinic distributed 250 food supplements among people on ART. Social workers and adherence counselors met biweekly to determine who received the monthly supplements. They periodically visited patients to see who lived in the most "vulnerable" situations: those unable to work, with multiple dependents, and little social support. They presented the cases and discussed the patients' situations to determine which were truly needy and deserved the scarce food supplements. One patient presenting herself as a single mother was declined as a counselor insisted she hid her male partner from the staff. Another was disqualified because someone had seen him working in the market. As the number on ARVs doubled, from 873 in September 2005 to 1660 in July 2006, it became impossible for the twelve adherence counselors to visit them all, but the number of food baskets available through the clinic remained the same. Set quotas were later abandoned but individuals allotments shrank—witness the difference between Batista and Madalena's shares between 2006 and 2010. Administrators were well aware of the shortfall, yet clinics lacked the space and staff to store additional food.

Patients turned down at the clinic were referred to associations and CHBC programs distributing food. CHBC volunteers tried to redistribute the supplements evenly among those they visited, but they were reprimanded and told to adhere to the programmatic priorities: people on ART received food first. In associations, distribution was awarded based on seniority and level of involvement. There was an acrimonious split in one association over the issue of benefits, as some on ART not receiving food founded a separate group: Association of People Taking Antiretrovirals.

I asked some association members how they would distribute the food if it were up to them. One declared: "Everyone wants it. I prefer either everybody received some, or nobody. It is difficult to choose. When we give it to you, who do we take it from?" This comment pointed to the conflicts caused by competition for insufficient food aid. As we left the meeting, someone lamented: "To get a card, *tem que fazer um Magaiva*" ("one must do a MacGyver[2]"): acquire it through inventiveness, resourcefulness, and initiative. Though each household was supposed to receive only one supplement from any of the multiple sources, some received more. Some employed individuals also received, while many unemployed did not.

Sacks of grain emblazoned with the donating country's flag were piled high in the distribution warehouse: Corn-Soy Blend from USAID, maize and dry beans from Canada, and rice from Algeria. The nationalized sacks seemed to confirm the impression many had of their country's relative place in the world. Recipients lined up outside, often for several hours, before entering four at a time, scooping their allotments up from piles on the floor using empty tin cans. Quantities and products varied from month to month. On one day, there was a surplus of Corn-Soy Blend, so each patient received twice the usual amount, but there was no oil. Many passed up the dry beans because cooking them consumed too much fuel. Often these products ended up being sold, an act that could disqualify the seller.

The process was a very public spectacle, from the queue to the walk home, laden with imported grains. Young men with wheelbarrows gathered outside the warehouse and carried allotments to people's homes for 10 meticais (40 cents). The coordinator commented on the state of people's grain sacks, which they poured their allotment into: "you are using such a dirty sack to carry food to your family?" When I asked her why those without clean sacks were not allowed to take an empty one from the pile that grew as grains were taken, she replied: "they would each expect a new sack every month!" All noted the bodies of those picking up food: who was fat, who was thin, who was dressed well, who was in rags, and speculated who deserved and did not deserve the food they received.

It was known food was directed toward the HIV-positive, and many were certain this motivated some to test for the disease. Activists told stories of people whom they escorted to the testing center that were brought to tears by a negative test. The limited

[2] This term comes from the American TV series "MacGyver," popular in bairro cinemas—bamboo-and-tarp structures surrounding a television. MacGuyver improvised complex devices out of improbable household items to solve apparently intractable problems.

distribution of benefits caused great disillusionment among those "fortunate" enough to test positive, however. It also generated resentment among those who were HIV-negative. A friend asked me: "why is it that the HIV-positive benefit from all these projects? Don't those of us who are healthy deserve anything?"

Food Aid, HIV/AIDS, and "Social Problems"

Representatives from government, donors, and NGOs discussed food distribution for AIDS patients. "With respect to HIV/AIDS," read the minutes of one meeting, "food should be seen as something that will assist adherence to medications and improved health, not resolve social problems." Not only were food aid programs not resolving social problems; they seemed to exacerbate them by perpetuating an economy of scarcity that provoked intense competition among PLWHA and resentment toward PLWHA from the seronegative.

Administrators and providers were constantly suspicious, looking for those who inevitably tried to *Magaiva* their way to benefits. Some NGOs abandoned food aid programs owing to both logistical problems and concerns that they fostered "corruption." One administrator felt that while her organization attempted to identify the "most vulnerable," those they served hid their assets and their spouses in order to appear as poor as possible: "I feel we are supporting the lazy and dishonest!" Another NGO stopped its program when it discovered that food aid was being sold.

Frustrations with food aid often slipped into a discourse of blame. One aid worker complained that the programs were contributing to a "learned dependence" and that people would not work in their *machambas* with food aid available: "these seropositives, they are the hardest people to work with! Always asking for things." The assertiveness of those bold enough to voice their needs was not appreciated. An accountant managing an association's micro credit project expressed his frustrations:

> Say I'm in this association. I'm given 500 meticais (20 $US) for a project. What will I do with it? I never have money. So today, I'm going to eat! Food, that is what they want. If we just distributed food, we would not have space for all the people who would show up. But when I say let's analyze our problems, no one appears. Since independence, the problem with Mozambique is that we are used to receiving, eating, and insulting the people who give.

In terms echoing colonial stereotypes, association members were seen as needy but scheming, and incapable of being trusted or thinking beyond the satisfaction of their basic needs. When asked whether associations played a role in community mobilization around HIV/AIDS, a health care provider replied: "these associations are too big to help anyone. Its just the same old people getting fat." The assessments of many working with PLWHA were tinged with moral judgment. Association members were accused of having become dependent on aid. Their stated needs were a product of laziness. In the clinic, on the other hand, those with too much agency did not receive food aid because they were not helpless enough. The search for the worthy beneficiary, the blameless sufferer, the innocent victim that could be saved by humanitarian aid, was fruitless. All involved worked in good faith—health care providers and program administrators attempted to provide what little there was to those who needed it most. Yet, the inadequate infrastructure and the overwhelming needs locked all parties into this system of triage that bred paranoia, mistrust, and competition.

Hunger as Embodied Critique

The governor of Manica spoke in Chimoio on World AIDS Day 2005. He asked how HIV prevalence in the province could be increasing despite 140 different organizations working on HIV. Serafina, the association member whom I sat next to, whispered: "they are all eating the money themselves." It was well known that HIV/AIDS issues were not just national but international priorities with considerable resources being invested in the effort. I was often asked if I knew "the secret": many were convinced that a cure for AIDS existed but was held back in order to enrich foreign organizations and their local partners as programs offering lifetime treatment expanded. PLWHA often wondered, if they were still hungry, and if AIDS treatment was a priority: "Who is eating in my place?" Serafina seemed to be answering this question when she accused the organizations of "eating the money themselves." Mozambicans pointed to the irony of how as HIV/AIDS gained prominence and importance as a national issue, the benefits somehow eluded those who suffered from the disease as the life-saving treatment inflicted hunger even while bringing health.

Joaquim remarked on the atmosphere of competition not only in the association, but within households as well:

> Here we are, positivized, but this life is taxing; what really taxes us the most, is food. We don't have any! The association will only help one person [per household], and each eats at the expense of the other. That person is eating the blood of the other. If both of us in this house had enough, for two positivized people, then we could say things were a little normal.

Joaquim referred to himself and his wife as "positivized," embracing the HIV-positive identity, but lamented that two individuals who belonged to an association, who adhered to their medications, and "lived positively" were going hungry. When I asked them if the allotment was not sufficient for two people, Rita responded: "but are we just two people? Do we not have family?" In order for one to eat, another goes hungry.

Social life in Central Mozambique revolved around food to some extent. On one visit to Rita and Joaquim, when they had no prepared food to offer, Joaquim knocked a green papaya down from a tree in his yard and offered slices with salt, which we ate together. The bread that the associations distributed at the end of their meetings similarly had a symbolic role as sharing food was a means of emphasizing solidarity. But even on this small scale, scarcity bred competition. At one meeting, when bread ran out before everyone had received some, a chaotic free-for-all broke out as the empty-handed made for the last bag. During the socialist era of the 1980s, a bulging belly served as a symbol of greed and selfishness. A protruding gut characterized the counterrevolutionary character "Xiconhoca," the antithesis of the "new man" of scientific socialism used in official government propaganda to caricature "enemies of the revolution" (Macamo, 2005). This symbol of immoral accumulation persists, as a headline for a newspaper article critical of government actions against hunger read "One Does Not Fight Hunger with a Full Belly" (Notícias, 2006). Eating is a widespread metaphor for illegitimate accumulation and corruption, as evidenced by sayings such as "a goat eats where it is tethered," referring to bureaucratic corruption. The comment who is eating in my place? was a question directed against a dysfunctional system that offered medications that extended life while exacerbating hunger. With such scarcity, fierce competition arose within the associations meant to serve as bastions of solidarity for PLWHA.

Conclusion

ARVs offer a way to commute the once certain social and biological death sentence of AIDS in Mozambique. The HIV diagnosis grants entry into a growing pool of fellow sufferers who compete for the limited material benefits available to them. The one guarantee they have, for now, if they are able overcome the considerable obstacles to make it to the AIDS clinic, is the promise of ARVs and the possibility of a few more years of life. The social networks emerging around HIV/AIDS depend upon development institutions and biomedical technologies. Those outside of the AIDS networks do not qualify for these benefits, while those within them face the grim prospects of starving while on ARVs.

There were grumblings of corruption and accusations of witchcraft among association members. When asked if she felt there was a sense of solidarity among the HIV-positive, one activist explained that on the contrary, associations saw other associations as rival political parties competing for a limited amount of resources. Associations guarded the status afforded by HIV. Three young women showed up to join the association they heard distributed food and jobs. When they could not produce proof of seropositivity, however, they were literally chased out by the jeering crowd. This may be indicative of HIV interventions that separate people into categories, who in this atmosphere of scarcity and competition, turn on each other. Scarcity can transform these potential spaces for solidarity into "Grey Zones," "morally ambiguous spaces . . . where survival imperatives overcome human solidarity as individuals jockey desperately for a shred of advantage" (Bourgois, 2005, p. 102). In the context of the local AIDS economy examined here, there were fears that only the most clever and resourceful (à la MacGuyver) could survive the sinister and shadowy forces that seemed to lie behind both the epidemic and the "fight against HIV/AIDS," leading to an atmosphere of distrust and paranoia around the treatment and food aid interventions.

While these dark visions of corruption and conspiracy may have been exaggerated, some agree that the vast funds dedicated to HIV/AIDS, dwarfing the national health budget, could be more equitably distributed (Pfeiffer, 2013). Official development assistance allocated for basic nutrition interventions decreased in the same proportion that assistance for HIV/AIDS increased between 1993 and 2003. As HIV interventions gained prominence, pro-poor interventions lost funding overall (MacKellar, 2005). Truly large-scale funding for HIV/AIDS interventions began in 2001 with funding from the World Bank, the Global Fund for Combating HIV/AIDS, Malaria, and Tuberculosis, the Clinton Foundation, and the Presidential Emergency Program For AIDS Relief (PEPFAR). While most bilateral organizations pool contributions for HIV/AIDS in a common fund jointly managed with the Ministry of Health, nearly all of the funds from the largest donor, PEPFAR, go to private and/or foreign organizations, undermining public sector services (Pfeiffer, 2013).

In Central Mozambique, inadequate attention to hunger undermines efforts to treat HIV/AIDS by inadvertently fostering conflict, competition, and suspicion. While biomedical coverage increases, overall living conditions worsen if the basic problems of hunger and economic citizenship are not addressed. The interventions can attain their stated and measured goals, while the beneficiaries of the programs continue to suffer in an environment of weakening social solidarity. This is a reminder that the technological magic bullet of ARVs alone is an insufficient intervention in the face of the increasing hunger and inequalities that continue unabated in contemporary Mozambique. AIDS treatment interventions must go beyond a vision of saving bare lives and be implemented with a broad view of social and economic citizenship.

REFERENCES

Bayart, J.-F., 1993. The State in Africa: the Politics of the Belly. Longman, London; New York.

Bourgois, P., 2005. Missing the Holocaust: My Father's Account of Auschwitz from August 1943 to June 1944. Anthropol. Theory 78, 89–123.

De Waal, A., Whiteside, A., 2003. New Variant Famine: AIDS and Food Crisis in Southern Africa. Lancet 362, 1234–1237.

Ferguson, J., 2006. Global Shadows: Africa in the Neoliberal World Order. Duke University Press, Durham [N.C.].

Hanlon, J., Smart, T., 2008. Do bicycles equal development in Mozambique? James Currey, Rochester, NY.

IMF, 2016. Republic of Mozambique—Selected Issues. IMF Ctry. Rep. 1–29.

INE, 2007. População da Província de Manica, 2007 [WWW Document]. URL http://www.ine.gov.mz/censo2007/rp/pop07prov/manica

Macamo, E., 2005. How Development Aid Changes Societies: Disciplining Mozambique Through Structural Adjustment, in: 11th CODESRIA General Assembly. Rethinking African Development: Beyond Impasse, Towards Alternatives. CODESRIA, Maputo, Mozambique.

MacKellar, L., 2005. Priorities in Global Assistance for Health, AIDS, and Population. Popul. Dev. Rev. 31, 293–312.

NDPB, 2004. Poverty and Well-Being in Mozambique: The Second National Assessment (Report). National Directorate of Planning and Budget, Ministry of Planning and Finance, International Food Policy Research Institute, Purdue University, Maputo.

Notícias, 2006. Não Combate Fome Com Barriga Cheia. Notícias.

Pfeiffer, J., 2005. Commodity Fetichismo, the Holy Spirit, and the Turn to Pentecostal and African Independent Churches in Central Mozambique. Cult. Med. Psychiatry 29, 255–283. doi:10.1007/s11013-005-9168-3

Pfeiffer, J., 2013. The struggle for a public sector: PEPFAR in Mozambique, in: Biehl, J., Petryna, A. (Eds.), When People Come First: Critical Studies in Global Health. Princeton University Press, Princeton, N.J., pp. 166–181.

SETSAN, 2008. Malnutrição Crónica Agrava-se no País [WWW Document]. URL http://www.setsan.org.mz/Index.htm

UNAIDS, 2014. MOZAMBIQUE HIV EPIDEMIC. Maputo.

West, H.G., 2005. Kupilikula: Governance and the Invisible Realm in Mozambique. University of Chicago Press, Chicago.

BENJAMIN CABALLERO

24 A NUTRITION PARADOX—UNDERWEIGHT AND OBESITY IN DEVELOPING COUNTRIES

We live in a world of underfed people and overfed people—undernourished and overnourished. At a very basic level, this is about resources—whether you can afford to have enough food. But this reading demonstrates that the situation is much more complex. The nutritional paradox in the title refers to the growing phenomenon of having undernourished children and overweight adults within a single family.

Global health has often emphasized the fight against infant and child undernutrition (see Reading 21). Undernutrition is a major factor in child mortality, so great improvements in child survival have been made by stressing the promotion of breast-feeding and the identification and supplemental feeding of children who are failing to grow properly. Infectious diseases are more dangerous for malnourished children. Growing children need proportionally more protein, vitamins, and minerals than adults, so both the quality and quantity of a diet are important.

Humans are the fattest of all land animals (in proportion to overall body size), and females generally have more fat than males do. Why? From an evolutionary point of view, carrying energy around in the form of fat is advantageous because it increases chances of survival and reproduction. Until recently, nearly all human societies experienced regular food shortages. Storing fat in times of plenty is like having "calories in the bank" for periods when there is not enough food. The average woman's body has enough stored energy to be pregnant and breast-feed even if there is a food shortage. We have a genetic predisposition to store fat.

In high- and middle-income countries, the primary health problems are being overweight or obese, which are risk factors for lethal chronic conditions like heart disease, diabetes, and stroke. This is because most people today live an "obesogenic environment," where calorie-dense foods are easily available and where demands for physical activity are low. Obesogenic environments tend to be urban ones where people work for wages and cannot grow their own food. Poor people in such a context have to spend a large percentage of their money for food—often 50% of wages. Therefore, they tend to eat cheap food that makes adults obese and leaves children undernourished. The obesogenic environment also includes technologies that reduce physical activity—like television and automobiles.

As you read this article, consider the following questions:

- **Why does the author believe that this paradox is going to get worse in the future? What do you think?**
- **Are you optimistic or pessimistic about whether global health interventions can help with this dual problem? Why?**
- **How do you interpret the graph in this article?**
- **The author states that the poor in developing countries can spend half of their budget on food. What percentage do you think your family spends on food?**
- **Many people think the current prevalence of obesity and excess weight in wealthy countries is the result of "laziness" or "gluttony." Do you agree or disagree?**
- **Some biomedical researchers have suggested that rather than trying to get people to lose weight, the goal should be to treat risk factors like hypertension and high cholesterol with medications. Do you agree or disagree? Why?**
- **Obesity is very stigmatized in the United States. Can you think of some examples of this?**

Benjamin Caballero, "A Nutrition Paradox." *New England Journal of Medicine,* 2005, 352(15): 1514–1516.

CONTEXT

Benjamin Caballero is professor of international health and pediatrics and director of the Center for Human Nutrition at the Johns Hopkins Bloomberg School of Public Health. His expertise is in international nutrition science, both in terms of public health and clinical care for children. He has been a leader in many of the professional associations in this field. The article is an opinion piece that appeared in one of the most prestigious journals in medicine, *The New England Journal of Medicine.*

A few years ago, I was visiting a primary care clinic in the slums of São Paulo. The waiting room was full of mothers with thin, stunted young children, exhibiting the typical signs of chronic undernutrition. Their appearance, sadly, would surprise few who visit poor urban areas in the developing world. What might come as a surprise is that many of the mothers holding those undernourished infants were themselves overweight.

The combination of underweight in children and overweight in adults, frequently coexisting in the same family, is a relatively new phenomenon in developing countries undergoing the nutrition transition—the changes in diet, food availability, and lifestyle that occur in countries experiencing a socioeconomic and demographic transition. In such countries, as many as 60 percent of households with an underweight family member also have an overweight one, a situation that has been dubbed the "dual burden household"[1] (see Figure 24.1). Among countries at an intermediate level of development (middle-income countries, with a per capita gross national product [GNP] of about $3,000 per year), overweight ranks fifth among the top 10 causes of disease burden—right below underweight.[2] This is the same position held by overweight as a cause of disease burden in the developed world.

Traditionally, obesity has been linked with abundance, and it was anticipated that as developing countries improved their economic status and their GNP, undernutrition would decrease and obesity would begin to appear among members of the upper socioeconomic classes. But the relationship between GNP and overweight is complex. Although being poor in the poorest countries (those with a per capita GNP of less than $800 per year) indeed "protects against" obesity, being poor in a middle-income country is actually associated with a higher risk of obesity than being richer in the same country.[3]

The reasons are not completely clear, but it is obvious that in poor countries, the dietary energy intake of the poorest people may be limited by the scarcity of food, and the high energy demands of manual labor and daily-survival activities make it difficult for people to achieve a net positive energy balance and, therefore, to gain weight. In more urbanized developing countries with a higher GNP,

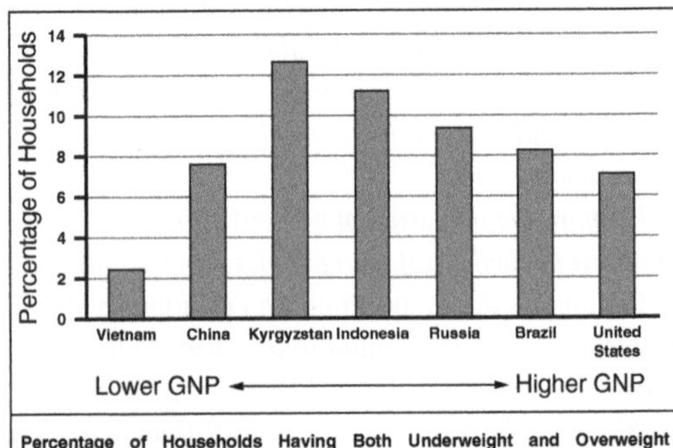

Percentage of Households Having Both Underweight and Overweight Members in Seven Countries.

The countries are arranged according to their per capita gross national product (GNP), with data adjusted for household size, from the lowest average on the left (Vietnam, $1,100) to the highest average on the right (United States, $26,250). Data are from Doak et al.[1]

FIGURE 24.1 Percentage of Households Having Both Underweight and Overweight Members in Seven Countries.

The countries are arranged according to their per capita gross national product (GNP), with data adjusted for household size, from the lowest average on the left (Vietnam, $1,100) to the highest average on the right (United States, $26,250).

Data source: C. M. Doak, Adair, L. S., Bentley, M., Monteiro, C., and Popkin, B. M. "The Dual Burden Household and the Nutrition Transition Paradox." *International Journal of Obesity and Related Metabolic Disorders,* 2005, 29: 129–136.

food scarcity may no longer be the driving factor behind energy intake. Instead, the availability of cheap, energy-dense foods (including those from street vendors and fast-food restaurants) may facilitate the consumption of more calories. Widespread access to television would favor an indoor, sedentary lifestyle, further reducing the average daily energy expenditure. In the wealthier segments of a given population, these influences may be counterbalanced by access to better education about health and nutrition, sufficient income to purchase healthier foods (which are usually more expensive), greater quantities of leisure time for physical activity, and better access to health care that would help to address problems of excess weight. The contribution of the urban environment to the underweight–overweight paradox will probably continue to increase, since it is predicted that most of the population growth in the next 30 years will occur in urban areas, and almost all these new urban areas will be located in developing countries.

These factors explain the development of obesity among people who are marginally poor. But what about the persistence of underweight? It seems evident that the improvement in per capita GNP in countries undergoing a socioeconomic transition does not benefit all citizens equally. Data from the World Bank show that the rates of poverty and underweight have actually increased among children younger than five years of age in urban areas of countries in socioeconomic transition.[4] People who move from rural to urban areas usually lose the ability to grow their own food and become dependent for their calories on a cash market. It is also more likely that women who move to the city will join the labor force and therefore become less available to prepare food at home, relying more heavily on commercially prepared foods for themselves and their families. For people with sufficient money, such a reliance may improve food choices and permit a more stable, if not better-quality, supply of dietary energy. But for those with an inadequate income, the urban environment may not offer the safety net of extended family and subsistence agriculture that is common in rural areas. These factors may explain why in Brazil women with incomes in the lowest quartile of the income distribution have a higher prevalence of underweight as well as a higher prevalence of overweight than do women with incomes in the top quartile.[5]

Because food costs consume a much larger proportion of family income in developing countries than in developed countries—more than 50 percent, in many cases—prices have a strong effect on the selection of particular foods. The globalization of food markets has resulted in the introduction of mass-produced, low-cost foods to the domestic food supply of many developing countries. This change, along with advertising campaigns, may have a powerful effect on the food choices and dietary patterns of low-income families. For example, the introduction of low-cost vegetable oils from industrialized countries greatly increased the proportion of fat calories in the average diet in countries undergoing the nutrition transition. Although many of these low-cost commercial foods are energy-dense, they may be nutrient-poor. And nutrient density is particularly important for growing children. For example, on a per-calorie basis, a five-year-old boy needs five times as much iron in his diet as a man. Cheap, energy-dense, nutrient-poor foods may adversely affect the growth of the child but may provide sufficient calories for the adult to gain excess weight.

Factors other than diet and lifestyle also link early undernutrition with overweight in adulthood. The hypothesis of "fetal origins of disease," which is supported by a number of observational epidemiologic studies, postulates that early (intrauterine or early postnatal) undernutrition causes an irreversible differentiation of metabolic systems, which may, in turn, increase the risks of certain chronic diseases in adulthood. For example, a fetus of an undernourished mother will respond to a reduced energy supply by switching on genes that optimize energy conservation. This survival strategy causes a permanent differentiation of regulatory systems that result in an excess accumulation of energy (and consequently of body fat) when the adult is exposed to an unrestricted dietary energy supply. Because intrauterine growth retardation and low birth weight are common in developing countries, this mechanism may result in the establishment of a population in which many adults are particularly susceptible to becoming obese.

The coexistence of underweight and overweight poses a challenge to public health programs, since the aims of programs to reduce undernutrition are obviously in conflict with those for obesity prevention. As pointed out by Doak et al.,[1] these programs will have to identify and consider the magnitude and demographic composition of dual-burden households at the local and regional levels and then develop more targeted interventions. It will be essential to educate health care workers about the underweight–overweight phenomenon. Fortunately, some important interventions for reducing the rate of undernutrition may also be beneficial in terms of reducing the burden of obesity: promoting breast-feeding, improving the nutritional status of women of reproductive age, and reducing the rates of fetal growth retardation and low birth weight.

Improving the "obesogenic" environment in urban areas of the developing world may be more challenging. Governments and nongovernmental organizations must play an active role in promoting and protecting an environment that supports the growth and development of infants and children, monitoring the food market, and facilitating community-based initiatives that aim to promote healthy eating and physical activity. The World Health Organization's Global Strategy on Diet, Physical Activity, and Health, endorsed by all member countries in May 2004, outlines a program and process for achieving these goals. But the other major challenge for countries in transition is to reduce socioeconomic and health disparities in urban areas. Until we close these gaps, we will continue to find malnourished children in the arms of overweight mothers.

REFERENCES

1. Doak CM, Adair LS, Bentley M, Monteiro C, Popkin BM. The dual burden household and the nutrition transition paradox. Int J Obes Relat Metab Disord 2005;29:129–36.
2. The world health report 2002: reducing risks, promoting healthy life. Geneva: World Health Organization, 2002.
3. Monteiro CA, Conde WL, Lu B, Popkin BM. Obesity and inequities in health in the developing world. Int J Obes Relat Metab Disord 2004;28:1181–6.
4. Ruel MT, Haddad L, Garrett JL. Rapid urbanization and the challenges of obtaining food and nutrition security. In: Semba RD, Bloem MW, eds. Nutrition and health in developing countries. Totowa, N.J.: Humana Press, 2001:465–82.
5. Monteiro CA, Conde WL, Popkin BM. The burden of disease from undernutrition and overnutrition in countries undergoing rapid nutrition transition: a view from Brazil. Am J Public Health 2004;94:433–4.

SECTION 6 CASES FOR TEACHING AND LEARNING

Visit the companion website, www.oup.com/us/brown-closser, for direct links to the featured online resources.

Lisa Armstrong, *Voluntary or Regulated? The Trans Fat Campaign in New York City*
Students consider different approaches to regulating trans fats in restaurants. This case requires students to consider political aspects of public health regulation.

Treeby Brown, *Tackling Childhood Obesity: A Case Study in Maternal and Child Health Leadership*
In this case study, students consider the political dynamics surrounding an effort to address childhood obesity in the American South. The case is designed to help students think about leadership around food-access issues in the United States. It would be best for older students who have some experience with workplace dynamics and politics.

Cornell University's Food Policy Case Studies
This excellent series of case studies gives students background information on a food security issue, presents policy options to address the issue, and then asks students to make recommendations on policy. Many of these cases cover issues also addressed in the readings in this section. Here is a sampling of cases dealing with issues covered in this book, but there are many more:

HIV/AIDS, Gender, and Food Security in Sub-Saharan Africa
Food Security, Nutrition, and Health in Costa Rica's Indigenous Populations
Developing a National Food Fortification Program in the Dominican Republic
Biofortification in a Food Chain Approach in West Africa
The Impact of Food for Education Programs in Bangladesh
The Nutrition Transition and Obesity in China
Food Advertising Policy in the United States
Surviving Shocks in Ethiopia: The Role of Social Protection for Food Security
Niger's Famine and the Role of Food Aid

Philips and Rhatigan, *Treating Malnutrition in Haiti with Ready-to-Use Therapeutic Foods*
This case describes a disagreement between Médecins Sans Frontières (Doctors Without Borders) and the Haitian government over the best use of Plumpy'Nut, a nutritionally supplemented peanut paste, in Haiti. Students must consider strategies for dealing with malnutrition, as well as ways to fund those strategies.

SNAP Challenge
Students (and instructors!) can engage in the SNAP challenge, where participants feed themselves on a SNAP budget for a week. Hunger Free Vermont has clear instructions for the challenge.

As they engage in the challenge, students may also want to consider online critiques and debates over the SNAP Challenge approach. This activity may not be appropriate for all students.

Wachter et al., *Reducing Child Malnutrition in Maharashtra, India*
In this case, students learn about and analyze a successful intervention to address child malnutrition in Maharashtra, which was a part of India's Integrated Child Development Services program. They consider what would be required to scale the program up.

SECTION 6 VIDEOS AND WEB RESOURCES

Visit the companion website, www.oup.com/us/brown-closser, for direct links to the featured online resources.

Food Insecurity in the United States – Feeding America
An interactive map of food insecurity in the United States. Students can explore rates of food insecurity in their home counties and compare them with other areas of the country.

Obesity Prevalence Maps – CDC
These maps of obesity prevalence in the United States are especially interesting paired with the information on food insecurity. Students can examine and discuss the significant differences in rates of obesity in different states.

The State of Food Insecurity in the World 2015 – Food and Agriculture Organization
Interactive maps show rates of food insecurity globally. Students can compare these with rates of poverty and water insecurity in the maps in the Conceptual Tools for Sections 3 and 4.

***A Silent Epidemic* – PBS**
Photojournalists describe a project in collaboration with Médecins Sans Frontières (Doctors Without Borders) documenting global malnutrition. The film covers many key issues, including the invisibility of much malnutrition and the nature of food aid. (13 min)

***Undernutrition: Understanding the Context* – United Nations REACH**
This participatory film made in Bangladesh underlines the social determinants of hunger. The introduction and a short excerpt from the film (e.g., from about 15:00–20:00) can be shown in class to illustrate key issues. (24 min)

***Food, Inc.* – Robert Kenner**
This 2009 feature-length documentary explores Big Food in the United States.

***Cooked* – Michael Pollan**
This 4-hour Netflix documentary explores many aspects of food and cooking. Episode 2, "Water," dovetails well with many issues of global Big Food explored in this textbook.

***Super Size Me* – Morgan Spurlock**
In this 2004 feature-length documentary, Morgan Spurlock eats only McDonald's food for 30 days. While less academic than other films on this list, it is accessible and entertaining.

PART

3

Social Determinants of Health

SECTION

7

Inequalities and the Social Gradient

Which one will tell you more about an individual's health and life chances: ZIP Code or genetic code? Molecular biology is a cutting-edge science, but it may not reveal the most important determinants of health. While DNA sequences may predict some particular predispositions to health-related conditions, the place where you live is a much stronger predictor of how you will live—and how you will die.

Social stratification means that there are groups within a society that have unequal access to strategic resources like money and loans, higher education, social connections, property, ways to make a living, access to quality health care, and access to good health information. In agrarian societies, the most important strategic resource is land, but many farmers throughout the world do not own their own land and must pay rent to landlords.

So far in this book, we have talked about the *material* determinants of health, like air, water, and food; the articles in this section are about the *social* determinants of health. The social determinants of health are things like social class, **gender**, ethnicity, education, and so forth. The material and social determinants of health are connected: poor people are more likely to have trouble accessing good food and water.

In American culture, many people do not like to think or talk about our severely stratified social system. Some people actually deny the existence of social class and inequality; most Americans think they belong to the middle class, even if, in reality, they are in the upper-or lower-wealth quintiles.

The United States does not collect epidemiological statistics with social class as a variable. Instead, American epidemiologists use indirect measures like ZIP Code, race or ethnicity, and education. From an epidemiological point of view, the geographical place where we live—our ZIP Code—is a good indicator of where we are on the "socio-economic ladder" of inequality. Britain, on the other hand, has collected social class data for a long time; that is a reason why many of the articles in this section were written by scholars from England.

Epidemiological data clearly show that, on an individual level, there is a strong relationship between a person's position on the social ladder and his or her health status. Poor people have shorter and harder lives than those who are rich. Poor people, and groups that experience discrimination, suffer from more diseases and die earlier. The social system itself is an inherent—and often invisible—cause of health problems.

» CONCEPTUAL TOOLS «

The Socioeconomic Gradient

- **Absolute poverty—for example, not having enough money to buy sufficient healthy food to eat—deeply affects health.** Over a billion people on Earth are living in what the World Bank calls "extreme poverty," subsisting on less than $1.25 a day. More than 10% of the world's population is malnourished. Poor nutrition and poverty have severe impacts on well-being and health (as is discussed in Section 6, which is about food).

  Comparing the average life expectancy in countries with different levels of income (GDP per capita) clearly shows the effects of absolute poverty on health. Figure CT7.1 shows the situation in 2000; you can also explore historical and more recent data at http://www.gapminder.org.

  The take-home message here is that up to about $4,000 per person per year in GDP country wealth affects average life expectancy in dramatic ways: increases in GDP lead to increases in life expectancy. However, above about $4,000 in GDP more money doesn't seem to have a great effect on average life expectancy across the whole country.

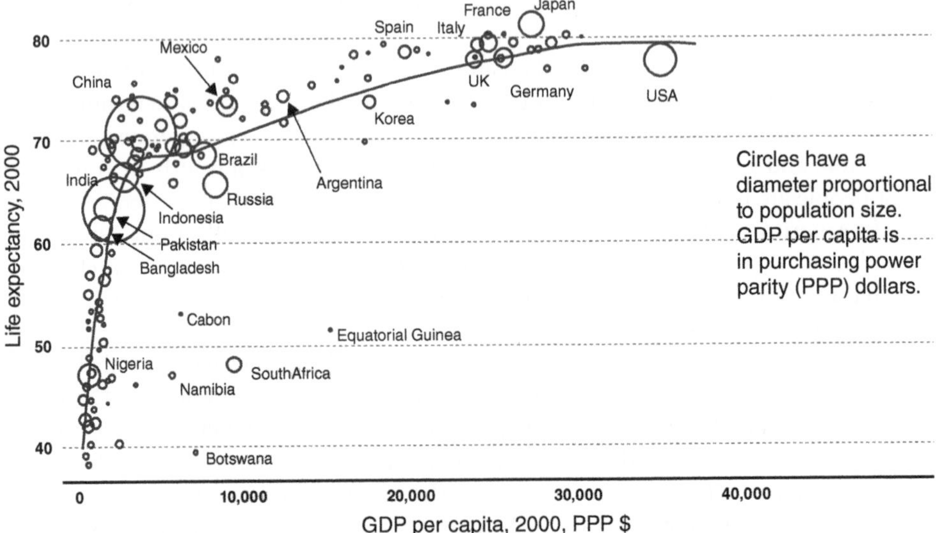

FIGURE CT7.1 The Preston Curve in 2000.

Image source: World Health Organization Commission on Social Determinants of Health. *Closing the Gap in a Generation*, http://apps.who.int/iris/bitstream/10665/43943/1/9789241563703_eng.pdf.

- **Relative poverty also affects life expectancy, even when basic needs for survival are fulfilled.** Nearly everywhere in the world, there is a **socioeconomic gradient** in health: as income increases, life expectancy increases. Wealthy people in a given country live longer and healthier lives (on average) than middle-income people in that same country, who, in turn, live longer and healthier lives than poor people.

  These trends hold across the world. Figure CT7.2 shows an example of infant mortality rates varying by income within different countries.
- **Because of the socioeconomic gradient, it cannot be assumed that someone in a rich country will be better off health-wise than someone in a poor country.** Poor people in wealthy countries may have worse health outcomes than wealthy people in poor countries. Figure CT7.3 is from a classic study comparing life expectancy in Matlab, Bangladesh, and Harlem, New York, published in 1990. As you can see, child mortality was higher in Bangladesh, but men in Bangladesh were more likely than men in Harlem to be alive after the age of 40. The death rates in Harlem were so high in large part because of cardiovascular disease.
- **The socioeconomic gradient in health outcomes is real in countries across the world, but the causes of health disparities are complex.** Some researchers have suggested that stress is a major cause of high rates of death like those seen in Harlem. In studies done in humans, as well as other primates and mammals, researchers have found that being lower in social status can lead to higher stress that contributes to chronic disease.

  One explanation for this is that a lack of respect and autonomy is very stressful. This type of stress may be very different than the stress that high-status

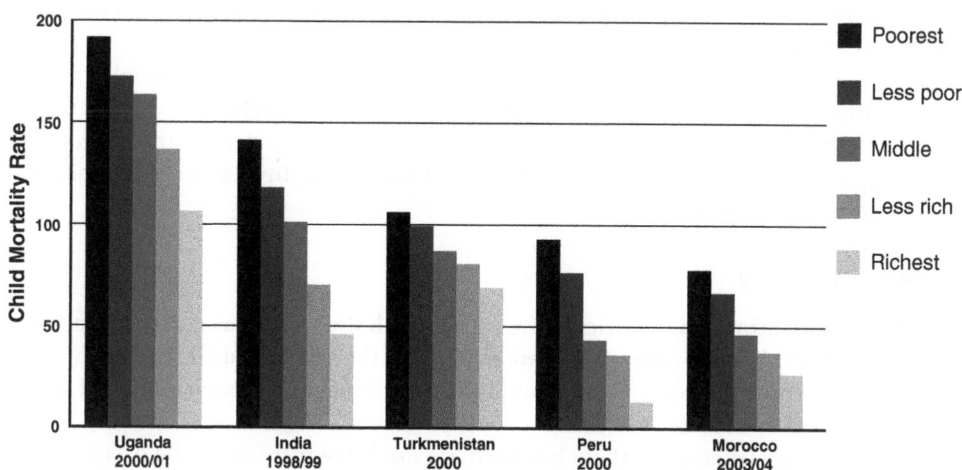

FIGURE CT7.2 Under-Five Mortality Rate per 1,000 Live Births by Level of Household Wealth.

Data source: D. R. Gwatkin, Rutstein, S., Johnson, K., et al. (2007). *Socio-Economic Differences in Health, Nutrition and Population within Developing Countries.* Washington, DC: World Bank, using DHS data.

Image source: World Health Organization Commission on Social Determinants of Health. *Closing the Gap in a Generation,* http://apps.who.int/iris/bitstream/10665/43943/1/9789241563703_eng.pdf.

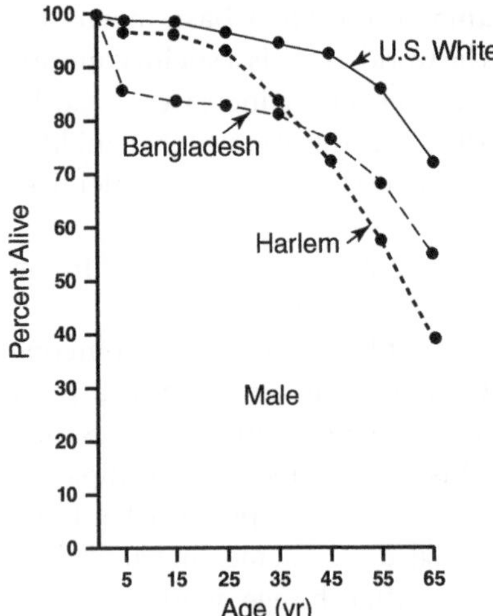

FIGURE CT7.3 Age-Adjusted Death Rates in Harlem (1960–1980) and the United States (1930–1980).

Image source: C. McCord, and Freeman, R. "Excess Mortality in Harlem." *New England Journal of Medicine*, 1990, 322: 173–177.

individuals experience: for example, you may experience some stress in getting all your work done in college, but you still probably have relative control over that situation. The stress experienced by low-status individuals with little control appears to have greater impacts on health. Chronic lack of respect can take its toll on the body—a thousand small stresses can accumulate in significant harm.

Stress is likely a part of the explanation for why people of lower social status live shorter lives, but there are likely many other factors that contribute to this as well. As Part 2 of this book shows, for example, the quality of human environments and food shape human health in profound ways. Figure CT7.4 shows some of the many ways that socioeconomic inequality can affect health.

One striking example of social inequality affecting health is going on right now in the United States. Mortality rates across groups have been falling in the United States and in other wealthy countries for decades. However, around 2000, these trends reversed for just one group: **white middle-aged men and women in the United States saw their mortality rates rise.** This trend, which includes striking increases in suicide and drug- and alcohol-related deaths, continues today. Alongside these rising mortality rates are rising rates of morbidity in this group, including rising rates of chronic pain.

This rise in mortality is strongly linked to income—rich white people are not affected this way. These "deaths of despair," as the researchers who study them call them, affect mostly white people without a college degree and reflect the increasing lack of available good jobs and social mobility for people in this demographic category.

Global Inequality

- **Globalization is a historical process by which the world has gotten "smaller."** The term **"globalization"** became popular in the 1990s, but the origins of this process are much older—the world has been connected through trade and colonization for hundreds of years.

  In the 21st century, there has been a remarkable increase in the exchange of knowledge, goods, and economic capital throughout the world. This process has been accelerated by new technologies, like the Internet, and the spread of economic policies, like free-market economics. Some believe that globalization is inevitable and is basically a good thing, because free markets have spread new scientific and cultural achievements worldwide and have lifted many people out of poverty.

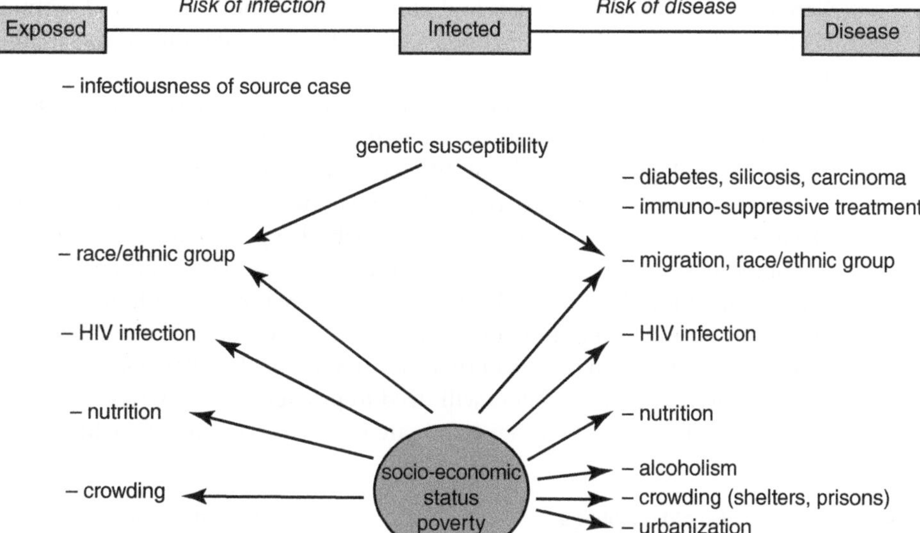

FIGURE CT7.4 Impact of Environmental Factors on the Risk of HIV Infection and Development of HIV/AIDS Disease after Infection.

Source: Epidemiologic Reviews Copyright © 2001 by the Johns Hopkins University Bloomberg School of Public Health All rights reserved Vol. 23, No. 2 Printed in U.S.A. From Exposure to Disease: The Role of Environmental Factors in Susceptibility to and Development of Tuberculosis Christian Lienhardt.

Other people think globalization is a bad thing because it has perpetuated inequality in the world rather than reducing it: the rich are becoming richer. However, both sides agree that globalization has made everyone more interdependent.

- **"Third World" is an outdated term.** During the era of the Cold War (1947–1991), political scientists referred to capitalist United States and Europe as the "first world" and the USSR and other communist countries as the "second world." The "first world" and the "second world" were in competition for worldwide influence over impoverished, unaligned, ex-colonial countries. "Third world" became a term for these poor and "underdeveloped" nations. This term is problematic because of the value judgement in the numbering system and because it implies that somehow these "worlds" are not connected. Today, international agencies categorize nations in terms of average income (i.e., low-, middle-, and high-income countries). This categorization is preferable to the terms "developed" and "underdeveloped," which hide historical and current patterns of trade and exploitation between rich and poor countries.

Gender

- **Other social factors in addition to income also affect health outcomes. One of these is gender. Gender** and sex are different things. In general, *sex* refers to biological differences between men and women, and *gender* refers to the pervasive social, cultural, economic, and political differences between men and women.

Gender is a cultural construct, and cultural ideas about men's and women's health, and men's and women's bodies, differ from social group to social group and across historical periods.

There are significant health consequences of the cultural constructions of gender differences. Prevalence of disease is often different for women and men, often not because of biology but because of differential exposures or access to resources. There are also problems of underreporting and underrecognition of some diseases, like heart disease in women. There is little doubt that gender affects health.

Sometimes, different values placed on male and female children can affect health outcomes. Figure CT7.5, from the same area of Bangladesh and in the same time period as the study in Figure CT7.3, shows the risk of dying for boys and girls depending on the sex of their siblings. In much of Bangladesh, girls are very expensive, because parents will need to provide large dowries for them to get married. Boys, on the other hand, are often an economic benefit, because

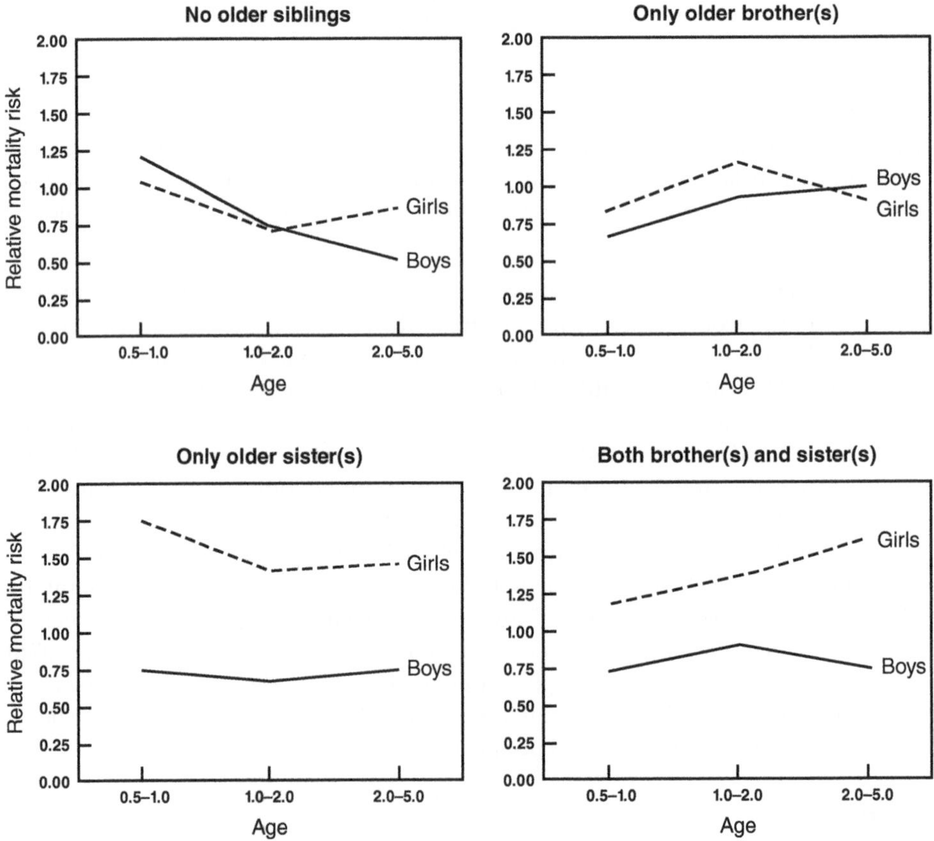

FIGURE CT7.5 Relative Mortality Risk by Age, Sex, and Family Composition.

Standard = mortality of all children in relevant age interval.

Source: P. K. Muhuri, and Preston, S. H. "Effects of Family Composition on Mortality Differentials by Sex Among Children in Matlab, Bangladesh." *Population and Development Review,* 1991, 17(3), 415–434.

usually they will live with their parents in the joint family system and support them as they age. Does this help explain the patterns?

Little girls with older sisters were probably less likely to get special items like extra food or medical care. The results were high death rates for girls with older sisters.

- **An important critique of the literature on women's health is that women have been "essentialized" as reproducers: health interventions have often been focused on their ability to reproduce.** Women's health is often equated with reproductive health, and other aspects of health are underemphasized.
- **Men have gender too, and this affects their health.** Sometimes the word "gender" in global health has referred only to issues of women's health. But gender issues do not only pertain to women; male gender roles and expectations are also culturally constructed. This may be part of the reason why men have lower life expectancies than women in every country reporting vital statistics to the World Health Organization. Men have higher rates of alcohol abuse, suicide, road traffic fatalities, and death from violence. But, male gender and the health impacts of masculinity have not been studied thoroughly.

Race

- **Race is not a useful biological category.** Most people believe the word "race" is a scientific term with a specific biological meaning. But the concept of race is biologically meaningless in humans. Human biologists have found that the categories people in the United States use to categorize race, like eye shape and skin color, cannot be used to predict a person's underlying genetic make-up (aside from the genes determining eye shape and skin color, of course). All groups of people (or "races") contain great amounts of genetic diversity, while there are only relatively tiny genetic differences *between* these groups.

  The term "race" is a historical artifact from archaic biological beliefs. The idea that there are a few "races"—white, black, red, yellow—or their scientific-sounding equivalents—Caucasoid, Negroid, Mongoloid—simply doesn't make scientific sense or serve a useful purpose in biological explanations.
- **The North American rule of racial hypodescent is one indication of the social construction of race.** Racial hypodescent means that if a child has parents of two different races, they will be classified as the lower-status race. For example, in the United States, a child who has one African-American parent and one white parent is socially classified as an African-American. This does not make biological sense, because the child inherits one-half of her genes from each parent. The same rule functions for children of mixed-caste marriages in India. There are historical reasons for racial hypodescent in the United States: slave children became material property of the slave owner, even if he was the biological father. Different societies with their own histories and economics have different social rules of racial classification.
- **Race affects health outcomes because of its importance as a social category.** While race is meaningless biologically, race as a social category is of incredible importance. Race has been used to rationalize exploitation (like slavery) or socioeconomic injustice (racism).

And while race is not a valid biological category, it does have real biological consequences. Race affects the environment and socioeconomic realities of people, which then influence health outcomes—for example, higher disease rates and lower life expectancies for members of some minority groups. These differences in life expectancy can be striking, even controlling for income. The experience of racism is an important stressor with negative impacts on health (Reading 26).

- **Ethnicity is a useful and important social construct.** Often, when people in the United States use the term "race," they are actually referring to social categories of identity and subcultural differences that should be called **ethnicity**. Ethnic categories are based on cultural distinctions of history, religion, language, and so forth. People identify with their own ethnic group, and they are identified by others as members of that group. At the same time, however, the boundaries between ethnic groups are permeable, flexible, and socially constructed.

  As is so evident in today's world, ethnic groups are often the focus of ethnocentrism, bigotry, and political violence. Ethnicity affects health.
- **Ethnicity interacts with social class.** People may use the term "race" when they are actually referring to differences in social class—that is, differences in access to material resources like money, property, and education. The United States is a highly stratified society in terms of wealth. And this economic stratification often runs along ethnic lines. Members of ethnic minorities are more likely to be poorer and less powerful. Racist beliefs on the part of the dominant white ethnic groups exacerbate the problems of socioeconomic inequity.

Addressing Inequality

- **Because inequalities have such profound impacts on health, we can think of them as disease-causing agents.** Social inequalities can be thought of as **macroparasites**—they cause disease in a way just as real as the disease caused by microparasites (like, say, malaria).
- **Inequalities are a product of human social structures, and we humans can change our social structures.** Changes in taxation policy are one example of a way that people can increase or decrease inequality. Such changes in social structure are also likely to change health outcomes.
- **Some health programs include "empowerment" of poor people or women as part of their agenda because if those people have more power to make choices in their lives, they are likely to have better health outcomes.** Many women's empowerment programs in health, however, are "empowerment lite": they aim to give women more power within the family, but give no attention to the larger structures of economic inequality that keep them, their families, and their children poor.
- **Access to medical care is a part of what causes socioeconomic inequalities in health, but only a small part.** As Part 2 of this book shows, the determinants of health—access to water, food, and a healthy environment—are more critical in determining health outcomes. But, access to medical care is an important issue too.

RICHARD WILKINSON AND MICHAEL MARMOT, EDITORS

25 SOCIAL DETERMINANTS OF HEALTH: THE SOLID FACTS

So far, this book has emphasized the biological factors affecting our physical health, primarily focusing on people's interactions with their environments. However, the World Health Organization (WHO) definition of health also includes our social and mental well-being (see Reading 1). And, as this selection explains, social factors affect our physical health. As such, it is important to have a bio-psycho-social perspective for understanding health and medicine.

The social determinants of health form an area of global health that is incredibly important and well researched. This reading comes from a WHO report summarizing eight social variables that clearly show that an individual's socioeconomic position affects their physical and mental health. The underlying concept is called the "social gradient." This means that people who find themselves lower on the social hierarchy suffer from more disease and illness and consequently do not live as long. This reading also uses the current evidence to make public policy recommendations.

The social gradient was first recognized in Great Britain. This was for two reasons. First, it is a comparatively wealthy country with universal access to quality medical care and a good system for social welfare. Second, the British have always been more open about the existence of social class, so they collect epidemiological data with the variable of social class—a factor that is not completely captured by simply looking at income. The first important research on this topic—the Whitehall studies, beginning in 1967—focused on male civil employees whose jobs were categorized in six grades. Directors at the top of the civil service had the best health, and the lower the job grade, the worse the men's health. This is a clear example of the social gradient. What was surprising was how clearly this worked in a stair-step fashion; the differences between the different social grades were extremely clear and sharp. Yet none of these employees were extremely rich nor extremely poor. And because of the British National Health Service, all of them had access to medical care.

After that first study, the social gradient was found all over the world. However, the gradient was much steeper in nations with more social inequality, like the United States.

More recent research has focused on income inequality as a social determinant of health. The experience of poverty is not only absolute poverty but relative deprivation and social status. There are differences in health and life expectancy even between people with high income and those with even higher income. In some nations, income inequality has skyrocketed over the past quarter century.

Explaining how social inequalities are transformed into health disparities is a topic of ongoing research. In other words, how does inequality "get under the skin?" One mechanism is stress. Stress is not necessarily a bad thing in itself. It is part of a fight-or-flight response that evolved for a reason in humans. But when stress is chronic and ongoing, it causes damage to physical and mental health. Adverse childhood experiences, like being subjected to violent abuse, affect health in the long run. So do experiences like unemployment and food insecurity. Having a job that is unpleasant because it has low control is also unhealthy.

Social support can help decrease stress, and having no social support is very bad for health. People who are excluded from society, like the homeless, have much shorter life expectancies. Finally, people who are experiencing stress or unhappiness are much more likely to become addicted to alcohol or drugs, and these habits are harmful to one's health.

Excepts from *Social Determinants of Health: The Solid Facts*, edited by R. Wilkinson and M. Marmot. 2d ed. Copenhagen: World Health Organization Europe, 2003.

As you read the following article, consider the following questions:

- **Were you surprised by where the United States ranked in the figure about proportion of children living in poor households? As a critical reader of epidemiological research, what weakness might you see in how this chart was made?**
- **There was a crisis in heroin overdose death in the United States in 2016 and 2017. How might you describe the social epidemiological distribution of this health problem? How might this epidemic be related to the information about the social determinants of health?**
- **Why might national levels of income inequality be correlated with national measures of population health? What do you think might be a practical solution to this problem? What would be the obstacles in making that solution happen?**
- **There are other social determinants of health, like differential access to transportation, quality food, or higher education. Draw a diagram showing how these determinants are connected to health on biomedical pathways and social-psychological ones.**
- **Why is social support important to your own health? Think of this both in terms of prevention as well as when you are sick.**
- **Why did the authors entitle this piece "solid facts"?**

CONTEXT

This WHO report was actually written by a consortium of thirteen social epidemiologists from Great Britain. The original report (available on the Internet) cites many different studies that support the facts reported here. The two editors of this pamphlet are the most famous scholars in the world in regards to the social determinants of health: Richard Wilkinson and Sir Michael Marmot. Rickard Wilkinson is both a scholar and advocate who had been a Professor of Social Epidemiology at the University of Nottingham. His book with Kate Pickett, *The Spirit Level* (New York: Bloomsbury, 2009), argues that societies with more equal distribution of incomes have better health, fewer social problems, and are more cohesive than ones in which the gap between the rich and poor is greater. Sir Michael Marmot is a professor at University College London and the Director of the UCL Institute of Health Equity. He has led research groups on health inequalities for over 35 years and was chair of the WHO Commission on Social Determinants of Health. In addition to his numerous scholarly publications and official reports, he has also written a book for the public entitled, *The Status Syndrome: How Your Social Standing Directly Affects Your Health and Life Expectancy* (London: Bloomsbury, 2004).

1. The Social Gradient

Life expectancy is shorter and most diseases are more common further down the social ladder in each society. Health policy must tackle the social and economic determinants of health.

What Is Known

Poor social and economic circumstances affect health throughout life. People further down the social ladder usually run at least twice the risk of serious illness and premature death as those near the top. Nor are the effects confined to the poor: the social gradient in health runs right across society, so that even among middle-class office workers, lower ranking staff suffer much more disease and earlier death than higher ranking staff (Figure 25.1).

Both material and psychosocial causes contribute to these differences and their effects extend to most diseases and causes of death.

Disadvantage has many forms and may be absolute or relative. It can include having few family assets, having a poorer education during adolescence, having insecure employment, becoming stuck in a hazardous or dead-end job, living in poor housing, trying to bring up a family in difficult circumstances and living on an inadequate retirement pension.

These disadvantages tend to concentrate among the same people, and their effects on health accumulate during life. The longer people live in stressful economic and social circumstances, the greater the physiological wear and tear they suffer, and the less likely they are to enjoy a healthy old age.

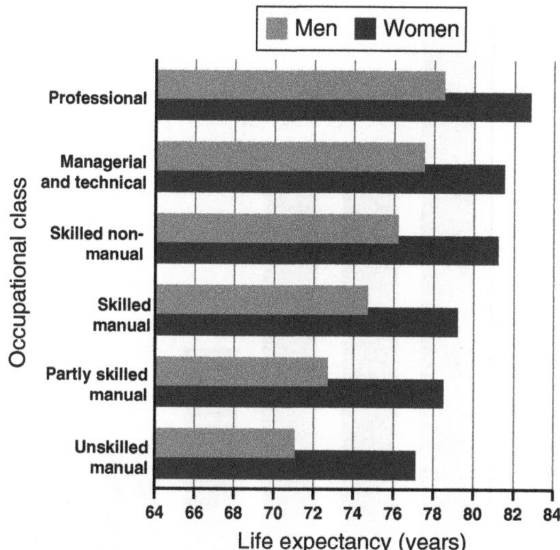

FIGURE 25.1 Occupational Class Differences in Life Expectancy, England and Wales, 1997–1999

Policy Implications

If policy fails to address these facts, it not only ignores the most powerful determinants of health standards in modern societies, it also ignores one of the most important social justice issues facing modern societies.

- Life contains a series of critical transitions: emotional and material changes in early childhood, the move from primary to secondary education, starting work, leaving home and starting a family, changing jobs and facing possible redundancy, and eventually retirement. Each of these changes can affect health by pushing people onto a more or less advantaged path. Because people who have been disadvantaged in the past are at the greatest risk in each subsequent transition, welfare policies need to provide not only safety nets but also springboards to offset earlier disadvantage.
- Good health involves reducing levels of educational failure, reducing insecurity and unemployment and improving housing standards. Societies that enable all citizens to play a full and useful role in the social, economic and cultural life of their society will be healthier than those where people face insecurity, exclusion and deprivation.

2. Stress

Stressful circumstances, making people feel worried, anxious and unable to cope, are damaging to health and may lead to premature death.

What Is Known

Social and psychological circumstances can cause long-term stress. Continuing anxiety, insecurity, low self-esteem, social isolation and lack of control over work and home life, have powerful effects on health. Such psychosocial risks accumulate during life and increase the chances of poor mental health and premature death. Long periods of anxiety and insecurity and the lack of supportive friendships are damaging in whatever area of life they arise. The lower people are in the social hierarchy of industrialized countries, the more common these problems become.

Why do these psychosocial factors affect physical health? In emergencies, our hormones and nervous system prepare us to deal with an immediate physical threat by triggering the fight or flight response: raising the heart rate, mobilizing stored energy, diverting blood to muscles and increasing alertness. Although the stresses of modern urban life rarely demand strenuous or even moderate physical activity, turning on the stress response diverts energy and resources away from many physiological processes important to long-term health maintenance. Both the cardiovascular and immune systems are affected. For brief periods, this does not matter; but if people feel tense too often or the tension goes on for too long, they become more vulnerable to a wide range of conditions including infections, diabetes, high blood pressure, heart attack, stroke, depression and aggression.

Policy Implications

Although a medical response to the biological changes that come with stress may be to try to control them with drugs, attention should be focused upstream, on reducing the major causes of chronic stress.

- In schools, workplaces and other institutions, the quality of the social environment and material security are often as important to health as the physical environment. Institutions that can give people a sense of belonging, participating and being valued are likely to be healthier places than those where people feel excluded, disregarded and used.

- Governments should recognize that welfare programmes need to address both psychosocial and material needs: both are sources of anxiety and insecurity. In particular, governments should support families with young children, encourage community activity, combat social isolation, reduce material and financial insecurity, and promote coping skills in education and rehabilitation.

3. Early Life

A good start in life means supporting mothers and young children: the health impact of early development and education lasts a lifetime.

What Is Known

Observational research and intervention studies show that the foundations of adult health are laid in early childhood and before birth. Slow growth and poor emotional support raise the lifetime risk of poor physical health and reduce physical, cognitive and emotional functioning in adulthood. Poor early experience and slow growth become embedded in biology during the processes of development, and form the basis of the individual's biological and human capital, which affects health throughout life.

Poor circumstances during pregnancy can lead to less than optimal fetal development via a chain that may include deficiencies in nutrition during pregnancy, maternal stress, a greater likelihood of maternal smoking and misuse of drugs and alcohol, insufficient exercise and inadequate prenatal care. Poor fetal development is a risk for health in later life (Figure 25.2).

Infant experience is important to later health because of the continued malleability of biological systems. As cognitive, emotional and sensory inputs programme the brain's responses, insecure emotional attachment and poor stimulation can lead to reduced readiness for school, low educational attainment, and problem behaviour, and the risk of social marginalization in adulthood. Good health-related habits, such as eating sensibly, exercising and not smoking, are associated with parental and peer group examples, and with good education. Slow or retarded physical growth in infancy is associated with reduced cardiovascular, respiratory, pancreatic

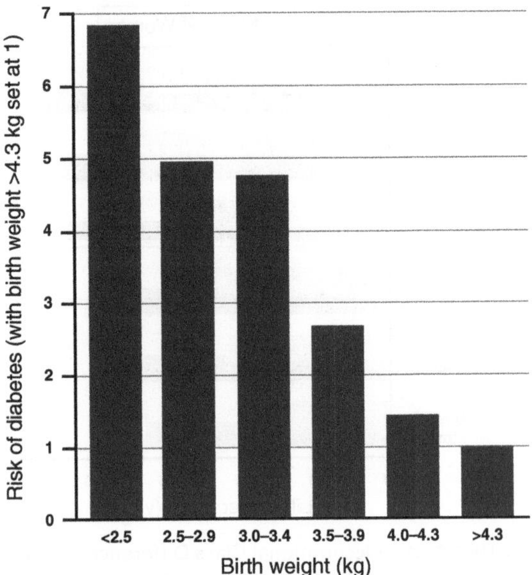

FIGURE 25.2 Risk of Diabetes in Men Aged 64 Years by Birth Weight
Adjusted for body mass index.

and kidney development and function, which increase the risk of illness in adulthood.

Policy Implications

These risks to the developing child are significantly greater among those in poor socioeconomic circumstances, and they can best be reduced through improved preventive health care before the first pregnancy and for mothers and babies in pre- and postnatal, infant welfare and school clinics, and through improvements in the educational levels of parents and children. Such health and education programmes have direct benefits. They increase parents' awareness of their children's needs and their receptivity to information about health and development, and they increase parental confidence in their own effectiveness.

Policies for improving health in early life should aim to:

- increase the general level of education and provide equal opportunity of access to education, to improve the health of mothers and babies in the long run;
- provide good nutrition, health education, and health and preventive care facilities, and adequate social and economic resources, before

first pregnancies, during pregnancy, and in infancy, to improve growth and development before birth and throughout infancy, and reduce the risk of disease and malnutrition in infancy; and
- ensure that parent–child relations are supported from birth, ideally through home visiting and the encouragement of good parental relations with schools, to increase parental knowledge of children's emotional and cognitive needs, to stimulate cognitive development and pro-social behaviour in the child, and to prevent child abuse.

4. Social Exclusion

Life is short where its quality is poor. By causing hardship and resentment, poverty, social exclusion and discrimination cost lives.

What Is Known

Poverty, relative deprivation and social exclusion have a major impact on health and premature death, and the chances of living in poverty are loaded heavily against some social groups.

Absolute poverty—a lack of the basic material necessities of life—continues to exist, even in the richest countries of Europe. The unemployed, many ethnic minority groups, guest workers, disabled people, refugees and homeless people are at particular risk. Those living on the streets suffer the highest rates of premature death.

Relative poverty means being much poorer than most people in society and is often defined as living on less than 60% of the national median income. It denies people access to decent housing, education, transport and other factors vital to full participation in life. Being excluded from the life of society and treated as less than equal leads to worse health and greater risks of premature death. The stresses of living in poverty are particularly harmful during pregnancy, to babies, children and old people. In some countries, as much as one quarter of the total population—and a higher proportion of children—live in relative poverty (Figure 25.3).

Social exclusion also results from racism, discrimination, stigmatization, hostility and unemployment. These processes prevent people from participating in education or training, and gaining access to services and citizenship activities. They are socially and psychologically damaging, materially costly, and harmful to health. People who live in, or have left, institutions, such as prisons, children's homes and psychiatric hospitals, are particularly vulnerable.

The greater the length of time that people live in disadvantaged circumstances, the more likely they are to suffer from a range of health problems, particularly cardiovascular disease. People move in and out of poverty during their lives, so the number of people who experience poverty and social exclusion during their lifetime is far higher than the current number of socially excluded people.

Poverty and social exclusion increase the risks of divorce and separation, disability, illness, addiction and social isolation and vice versa, forming vicious circles that deepen the predicament people face.

As well as the direct effects of being poor, health can also be compromised indirectly by living in neighbourhoods blighted by concentrations of deprivation, high unemployment, poor quality housing, limited access to services and a poor quality environment.

Policy Implications

Through policies on taxes, benefits, employment, education, economic management, and many other areas of activity, no government can avoid having a major

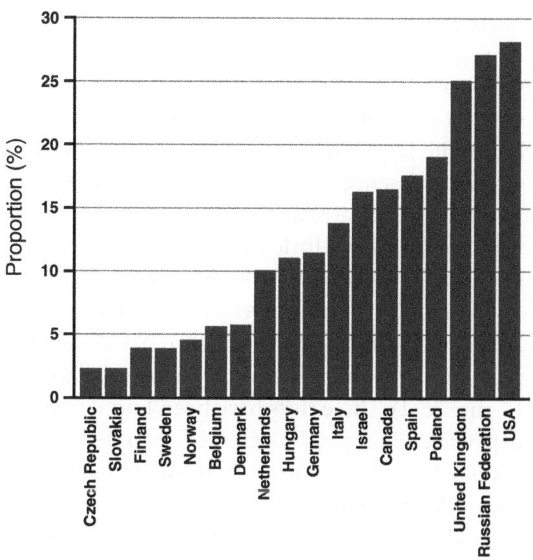

FIGURE 25.3 Proportion of Children Living in Poor Households (Below 50% of the National Average Income).

impact on the distribution of income. The indisputable evidence of the effects of such policies on rates of death and disease imposes a public duty to eliminate absolute poverty and reduce material inequalities.

- All citizens should be protected by minimum income guarantees, minimum wages legislation and access to services.
- Interventions to reduce poverty and social exclusion are needed at both the individual and the neighbourhood levels.
- Legislation can help protect minority and vulnerable groups from discrimination and social exclusion.
- Public health policies should remove barriers to health care, social services and affordable housing.
- Labour market, education and family welfare policies should aim to reduce social stratification.

5. WORK

Stress in the workplace increases the risk of disease. People who have more control over their work have better health.

What Is Known

In general, having a job is better for health than having no job. But the social organization of work, management styles and social relationships in the workplace all matter for health. Evidence shows that stress at work plays an important role in contributing to the large social status differences in health, sickness absence and premature death. Several European workplace studies show that health suffers when people have little opportunity to use their skills and low decision-making authority.

Having little control over one's work is particularly strongly related to an increased risk of low back pain, sickness absence and cardiovascular disease (Figure 25.4). These risks have been found to be independent of the psychological characteristics of the people studied. In short, they seem to be related to the work environment.

Studies have also examined the role of work demands. Some show an interaction between demands and control. Jobs with both high demand and low control carry special risk. Some evidence indicates that social support in the workplace may be protective.

Further, receiving inadequate rewards for the effort put into work has been found to be associated with increased cardiovascular risk. Rewards can take the form of money, status and self-esteem. Current changes in the labour market may change the opportunity structure, and make it harder for people to get appropriate rewards.

These results show that the psychosocial environment at work is an important determinant of health and contributor to the social gradient in ill health.

Policy Implications

- There is no trade-off between health and productivity at work. A virtuous circle can be established: improved conditions of work will lead to a healthier work force, which will lead to improved productivity, and hence to the opportunity to create a still healthier, more productive workplace.
- Appropriate involvement in decision-making is likely to benefit employees at all levels of an organization. Mechanisms should therefore be developed to allow people to influence the

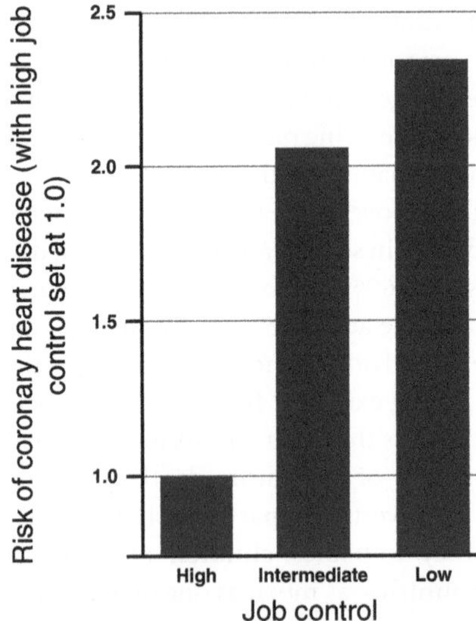

FIGURE 25.4 Self-Reported Level of Job Control and Incidence of Coronary Heart Disease in Men and Women. Adjusted for age, sex, length of follow-up, effort/reward imbalance, employment grade, coronary risk factors and negative psychological disposition.

design and improvement of their work environment, thus enabling employees to have more control, greater variety and more opportunities for development at work.

- Good management involves ensuring appropriate rewards—in terms of money, status and self-esteem—for all employees.
- To reduce the burden of musculoskeletal disorders, workplaces must be ergonomically appropriate.
- As well as requiring an effective infrastructure with legal controls and powers of inspection, workplace health protection should also include workplace health services with people trained in the early detection of mental health problems and appropriate interventions.

6. UNEMPLOYMENT

Job security increases health, well-being and job satisfaction. Higher rates of unemployment cause more illness and premature death.

What Is Known

Unemployment puts health at risk, and the risk is higher in regions where unemployment is widespread. Evidence from a number of countries shows that, even after allowing for other factors, unemployed people and their families suffer a substantially increased risk of premature death. The health effects of unemployment are linked to both its psychological consequences and the financial problems it brings—especially debt.

The health effects start when people first feel their jobs are threatened, even before they actually become unemployed. This shows that anxiety about insecurity is also detrimental to health. Job insecurity has been shown to increase effects on mental health (particularly anxiety and depression), self-reported ill health, heart disease and risk factors for heart disease. Because very unsatisfactory or insecure jobs can be as harmful as unemployment, merely having a job will not always protect physical and mental health: job quality is also important (Figure 25.5).

During the 1990s, changes in the economies and labour markets of many industrialized countries increased feelings of job insecurity. As job insecurity continues, it acts as a chronic stressor whose effects grow with the length of exposure; it increases sickness absence and health service use.

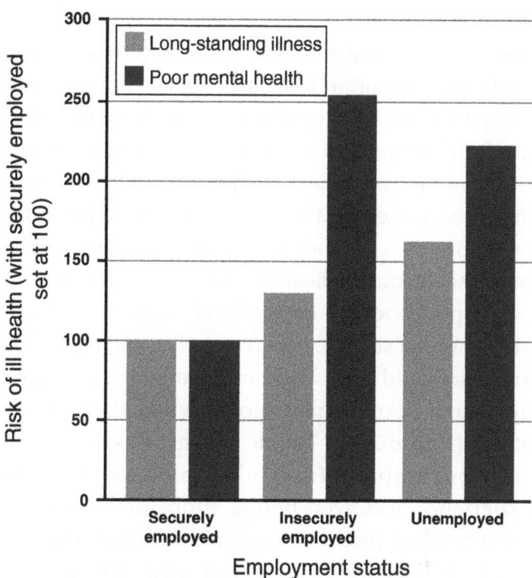

FIGURE 25.5 Effect of Job Insecurity and Unemployment on Health.

Policy Implications

Policy should have three goals: to prevent unemployment and job insecurity; to reduce the hardship suffered by the unemployed; and to restore people to secure jobs.

- Government management of the economy to reduce the highs and lows of the business cycle can make an important contribution to job security and the reduction of unemployment.
- Limitations on working hours may also be beneficial when pursued alongside job security and satisfaction.
- To equip people for the work available, high standards of education and good retraining schemes are important.
- For those out of work, unemployment benefits set at a higher proportion of wages are likely to have a protective effect.

7. SOCIAL SUPPORT

Friendship, good social relations and strong supportive networks improve health at home, at work and in the community.

What Is Known

Social support and good social relations make an important contribution to health. Social support helps give people the emotional and practical resources they need. Belonging to a social network of communication and mutual obligation makes people feel cared for, loved, esteemed and valued. This has a powerful protective effect on health. Supportive relationships may also encourage healthier behaviour patterns.

Support operates on the levels both of the individual and of society. Social isolation and exclusion are associated with increased rates of premature death and poorer chances of survival after a heart attack (Figure 25.6). People who get less social and emotional support from others are more likely to experience less well-being, more depression, a greater risk of pregnancy complications and higher levels of disability from chronic diseases. In addition, bad close relationships can lead to poor mental and physical health.

The amount of emotional and practical social support people get varies by social and economic status. Poverty can contribute to social exclusion and isolation.

Social cohesion—defined as the quality of social relationships and the existence of trust, mutual obligations and respect in communities or in the wider society—helps to protect people and their health. Inequality is corrosive of good social relations. Societies with high levels of income inequality tend to have less social cohesion and more violent crime. High levels of mutual support will protect health while the breakdown of social relations, sometimes following greater inequality, reduces trust and increases levels of violence. A study of a community with initially high levels of social cohesion showed low rates of coronary heart disease. When social cohesion declined, heart disease rates rose.

Policy Implications

Experiments suggest that good social relations can reduce the physiological response to stress. Intervention studies have shown that providing social support can improve patient recovery rates from several different conditions. It can also improve pregnancy outcome in vulnerable groups of women.

- Reducing social and economic inequalities and reducing social exclusion can lead to greater social cohesiveness and better standards of health.
- Improving the social environment in schools, in the workplace and in the community more widely, will help people feel valued and supported in more areas of their lives and will contribute to their health, especially their mental health.
- Designing facilities to encourage meeting and social interaction in communities could improve mental health.
- In all areas of both personal and institutional life, practices that cast some as socially inferior or less valuable should be avoided because they are socially divisive.

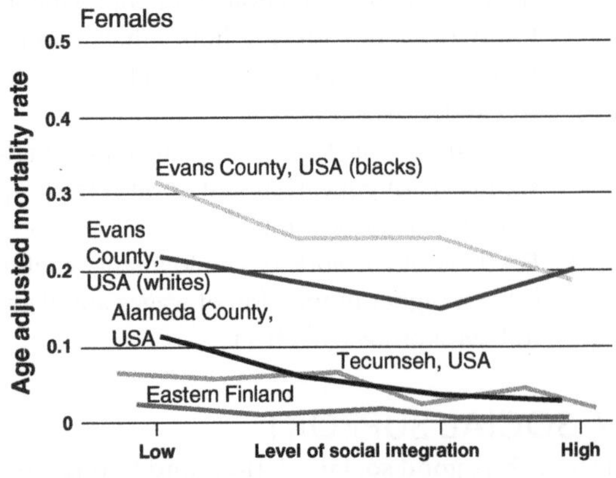

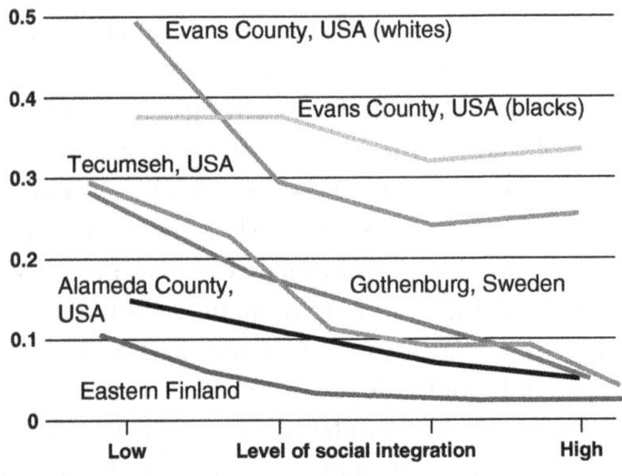

FIGURE 25.6 Level of Social Integration and Mortality in Five Prospective Studies.

ALAN GOODMAN

26 DISEASE AND DYING WHILE BLACK: HOW RACISM, NOT RACE, GETS UNDER THE SKIN

In the United States, "race" is an extremely important social concept that permeates national politics and culture. It is also a fundamental aspect of socioeconomic inequality and, therefore, a social determinant of health. Race is important in the United States because of the tragic history of slavery that has been followed by more than 150 years of brutal oppression and discrimination. The reading argues that race is a worthless category for understanding human biological variation. Race is a cultural creation, not a reality of biology. On the other hand, racism *is an undeniable fact that has huge consequences for health and well-being. "Racism" refers to prejudice, discrimination, or antagonism directed against someone of a different "race" based on the belief that one's own group is superior. Ultimately, racism is based on a dangerously incorrect belief of biological inferiority.*

Skin color is a salient aspect of human biological variation worldwide. Variations in skin color—determined by the size of melanin globules in the epidermis—are hard not to notice. Obviously, there is a spectrum of skin colors among human beings, and this spectrum is, in large measure, caused by genetic variations resulting from natural selection. Human genetic variations occur in a wide range of attributes, from height, to bone density, to blood characteristics such as sickle-cell trait. These variations, too, are a result of evolution through natural selection. This means that certain genetic traits are advantageous *for particular environments.*

Genetic variation across a range of phenotypic traits do exist in humans, but these traits are not linked to race in the way many Americans imagine. The vast majority of genetic variation in humans exists in all races. Knowing someone's skin color does not allow us to predict their genetic make-up.

This reading argues that it is inappropriate to ascribe racial disparities in health to genes. This is a hard thing for some people to swallow because the cultural ideas of race, biology, skin color, and genes seem so obvious, particularly for European Americans. Racism is classic example of structural violence (see Reading 32).

Unfortunately, epidemiologists have often fallen into the trap of treating race as if it referred to biology. In the past, race was erroneously used as a scientific explanation for differences in disease prevalence between social groups. For example, it was once believed that higher rates of tuberculosis in African Americans were due to some unidentified inherited biological weakness—instead of conditions of poverty that increased transmission and of chronic undernutrition that exacerbated the expression of disease. Similarly, psychiatrists once described a so-called mental illness in slaves called "drapetomania," a condition that caused slaves to want to run away from plantations!

This assumption has resulted in health data in the United States being collected with race or ethnicity as a standard variable. This subsequently reinforced the notion that race has a biological basis. On the other hand, the United States has never collected very good health data on socioeconomic class, and race can sometimes be used as a rough proxy. However, racial categories often lump groups of people with very different experiences of class together.

The social inequalities of "race" and ethnicity continue to cause great differences in health outcomes not only in the United States but also in many countries throughout the world. The way that racial categories are constructed, however, depends on the country. Most often, lighter skin colors are considered superior. This colorism exists even within so-called racial groups. In Latin America, India, and many other parts of the world, skin color may contribute to determining one's position in the social hierarchy. Like with

Alan Goodman, "Disease and Dying While Black." In *New Directions in Biocultural Anthropology*, edited by Molly K. Zuckerman and Debra L. Martin, 67–87. Hoboken, NJ: Wiley, 2016.

American race, being low on that hierarchy causes stress and its associated severe health consequences.

Some epidemiologists say that one can predict more about an individual's health status by knowing their ZIP Code than their genetic code. It is important to recognize that health disparities based on racism can be addressed by changing cultural attitudes, behaviors, and social structures. Racism is both a sociopolitical and moral problem in the United States; it has been this way since the beginning of the country. Social change requires both cultural and political willingness to change. African Americans have experienced some improvements in health and well-being since the civil rights movement of the 1960s, but the health gaps remain unacceptable.

As you read this selection, consider these questions:

- **Why is race not a useful way to think about human biological variation?**
- **If the author is right about genes, why are there inequalities in health measures between different racial and ethnic groups? What about economic classes?**
- **Why isn't their more focus on social inequality rather than genetics as the source of health disparities?**
- **Does the Black Lives Matter movement concern health? If so, how?**
- **Some people say that the negative health effects of racism is like "death from a thousand paper cuts." What might that mean? How might it be related to "micro-aggressions"?**
- **What might be the effects of racism on risk of disease or access to health care?**

CONTEXT

Alan Goodman, a biological anthropologist, teaches at Hampshire College. Dr. Goodman's research has used the methodologies of skeletal biology and paleopathology to examine nutritional stress in prehistoric populations. He has compared the nutritional stresses in the past with those of contemporary people in low-income countries. He is an expert in nutritional anthropology. He also works to educate the general public on the current science regarding the race concept, for example, through coauthoring the book *Race: Are We So Different?* (Malden, MA: Wiley Blackwell, 2012).

In the middle of the 20th century and going back at least to the early 1600s, race was unquestionably real: it was deep, matter of fact, and biological. In academic circles, race was the same as the same as human biological variation. As human biological variation, race explained deep differences in many key aspects of life, from educational attainment and intelligence to violence and crime, to wealth and health. This dominant worldview in the West was comforting in the sense that those differences were inherited, unchangeable, and natural facts of life. Differences in wealth and health were not seen as due to differences in power, racism, prejudice, or unequal treatment.

But were we missing something? The 1960s and civil rights movement made clear that something else might also be at work: whites and individuals of color inhabited different and unequal worlds. From segregation laws, to subordinate schools and hospitals, individuals of color occupied an inferior position. Although slavery had been abolished for a century, a racial worldview and institutional racism persisted.

Growing up in the 1960s, I knew that racism was everywhere. Books and daily conversations in the United States were saturated with the worldview about the relative inferiority of nonwhite races. These discussions sounded a lot like Nazi racial propaganda against the Jews from the 1930s. Moreover, I knew that the conditions of life were so varied by race that they must contribute to and widen differences in life outcomes. They were also unjust.

In a sense, the argument as to the cause of racial differences in health, the topic of this article, is a version of the nature-versus-nurture argument. The nature side viewed racial differences as due to genetic variation, whereas the nurture side viewed these differences as primarily due to the environmental conditions: poor schools, disadvantaged neighborhoods, and the like.

My personal epiphany came in 1973. It was in a class that destroyed the nature side of the argument. The professor, George Armelagos, explained that the idea of race as an explanation and synonym for human biological variation was once universally accepted in anthropology and that it had spread to other sciences and practices such as medicine and public health. But it proved to be a false theory. It wasn't so much that nurture topped nature but that we had misunderstood the nature of human biological variation.

Professor Armelagos explained that human biological variation is continuous, complex, and ever changing. As a static and typological concept, race is inherently unable to explain the complex and changing structure of human biological variation, and, by extension, race (as a genetic construct) could not explain health variation. To begin to comprehend human biological variation required an evolutionary theory and mechanisms of evolutionary change. Professor Armelagos went on to say that race is still real. But that race, rather than being genetically based, is a cultural ideal—with biological consequences. The ideology of race is necessary for racism. Students' responses ranged from disbelief to transformation. Many in the room could not accept Armelagos's claim that races-as-genetics was an outmoded idea. Others misunderstood his message, thinking he was denying the reality of biological variation itself.

I was one of the transformed students. I grew up in a working class family in a town that comprised mostly second-generation immigrants from Italy and Ireland. I was aware that I was perceived as Jewish and different from my Irish and Italian friends in some fundamental way. Yet when I attended a more diverse university, something striking happened: I became "white." I was no longer perceived as very distinct from other students of European descent. It was then that I learned about the fluidity of race. The color line demarcating races changes to fit the circumstances.

I was aware of the power of race as a worldview in 1973. But what I understood less was the idea's ability to persist after it had been proven unscientific. If asked in the 1970s if race would survive as a way to think about human biological variation in 2015, I would have answered a definitive "No!" I was naive to the durability of an economically useful idea.

In this article I explore two causal pathways used to explain health inequalities by race: (1) genetic differences in disease susceptibility among races and (2) variation in lived experiences of discrimination, including subtle and more overt forms of racism, among socially ascribed races. I argue that a genetic explanation is both epistemologically and epidemiologically flawed: human genetic variation maps poorly onto racial groups, and genetic differences rarely work in isolation. Conversely, the preponderance of evidence suggests that racial differences in health are rooted in conditions that expose persons and communities of color to a life of increased stress, pollution, and poor health care. These everyday discriminations and institutionalized racisms have profound health consequences.

"Race" and Health Inequalities: Two Causal Pathways

There is a striking consistent, persistent, and deep disparity in nearly every indicator of health by race in the United States (Kochanek, Arias, and Anderson 2013; Olshansky et al. 2012; Smedley, Stith, and Netson 2003). In particular, whites do best and African Americans do worst on nearly every indicator of health from prevalence and incidence of infant to chronic diseases to infant mortality and life expectancy (Kochanek, Arias, and Anderson 2013; Sacher et al. 2005). That is inequality. That is differential suffering and loss of life.

Why is it that such differences in health and disease persist among races? For well over a century, occasional debates—or more accurately, parallel arguments—have continued in scientific literatures and among various publics. Two arguments predominate: In one argument, racial differences in health are traced back to the god- given or evolutionary development of racial differences in genetics. This "raciogenetics" perspective accepts that race is a viable substitute or shorthand for genetic variation between populations, and such genetic differences are assumed to be causes of disease as well as other racial differences.

In the more recent counterargument, race-based health inequalities are causally traced to variation in the "lived experience" of those assigned to different racial categories. Here, *lived experience* refers to the totality of everyday conditions that are embedded into the fabric of social, personal, and institutional relationships. Some of these experiences are rather subtle personal interactions that communicate values based on phenotypic appearances, and others still are more deeply and profoundly personal experiences of racism (Krieger et al. 2011).

In the following sections I outline the raciogenetic argument and then the lived experience/racism argument. I conclude with a critique of the compromise position that both racial biology and lived experiences are important and with a call for greater clarity as to what we mean by *race* when it is used in public health research and practice.

The Raciogenetic Perspective

The worldview that racial differences in health are due to natural or inborn factors is an old one that extends back to at least the early 19th century. Frederick Hoffman (1896), for example, published a wealth of data on race differences in health in the United States. His influential treatise suggested that the increased morbidity and mortality of African Americans in northern U.S. cities resulted from their collective, inborn inabilities to survive the rigors of the contemporary world. Hoffman predicted their eventual demise.

At the time Hoffman was writing, many physicians felt that races were differentially susceptible to disease, and therefore particular races were more likely to suffer from particular diseases. So, for example, once sickle cell disease was identified in African Americans, it was assumed to be a race-specific disease (Tapper, 1999 and Wailoo 1997). When Europeans began to present with symptoms of sickle cell anemia in the 1920s and 1930s physicians thought that they must be part "negro." The possibility that sickle cell had nothing to do with race, but much to do with evolution and genetics, was not considered until the middle of the 20th century (Livingstone 1958).

In the 21st century, the idea that germs obey the color line, or that diseases are specific to one race or the other, had been dismissed. But the remnants persist that races are quasiscientific units with separate disease susceptibilities. Indeed, raciogenetics persists as a dominant explanation for variation not just in conditions such as sickle cell anemia that are caused by a single allele variants but also for variation in complex metabolic conditions such as diabetes and heart disease (Goodman 2000 and Sankar 2004). In 2005 the U.S. Food and Drug Administration approved the medication BiDil for use in African-Americans, presumably because it was effective in combating congestive heart failure in this group for reasons that were thought to be intrinsic to that group (Temple and Stockbridge 2007).

Finally, it is clear that we live in an age of genetics, a time in which genetics has taken hold as the dominant explanation for most behaviors and conditions. Certainly, genetic medicine is big business. And so it follows that genetics might explain variation in health among races (Goodman et al. 2003).

The Lived Experience of Racialization and Racism

In part because of the emergence of social epidemiology in the later part of the 20th century (Krieger 2001), the effects of dietary habits, stress, pollutants, work conditions, and other aspects of daily life on health are clearer. Part of the work in this field has pointed toward how life-long differences in living conditions might explain the bulk of the variation in health among races (see, for example, Geronimus 1992; Williams, Jackson, and Anderson 1997). Social class and racism are closely intertwined, and both interact to affect life courses, determining exposure to, among other things, healthy foods, pollutants, and experiences of discrimination and rendering people differentially vulnerable to risk factors (Krieger 2003).

In some sense, the lived experience hypothesis is so strong and obvious and fits the data so well that even those who strongly back genetic explanations acknowledge the importance of lived experience (Satel 2002). Yet, for reasons noted shortly, the tendency is not to drop a genetic explanation entirely but to acknowledge a role for both lived experience and raciogenetics (Satel 2002). The problem with this compromise position is that it says little about underlying etiology. Ultimately, if one wishes to address health inequities, the relative importance of these distinct etiologic pathways must be determined.

The debate continues. It is both scientific and political in the sense that each hypothesis points toward a series of actions that have political and ethical implications. In the following section, I present reasons why race should not be used as shorthand for human genetic variation. If race maps poorly onto genetic variation, as it does, then the raciogenetic explanation is fatally flawed.

Why "Race" ≠ Human Genetic Variation

Race is a powerful idea and a worldview that was invented and reified to explain variation in human biology, culture, and behavior (Smedley 1999). The underpinnings of this idea can be traced to classic Greek philosophical notions of ideal types and Christian ideas about a great chain of being. However, in the view of most historians of race and slavery, the idea of biologically based human races was itself a more recent invention (Smedley 1999). With the development of transoceanic travel and international migration, human differences were magnified. Politics and ideology went hand in hand. Colonialism and the desire to exploit lands and people clearly contributed to the tendency toward value-laden, racialized thinking. Starting in the 18th century, natural historians such as Linnaeus began to classify humans into subspecies or races. These classifications persist today. However, we now know that the raciogenetics

- is antithetical to the idea of evolution;
- does not fit the measurable reality of the structure of human variation;
- does not translate into a concept that is epidemiologically repeatable; and
- leads to a series of conflations that inhibit understanding of the cause, treatment, and prevention of disease.

The Idea of Race versus Evolution

Race, as noted, is largely a socially constructed idea about how human genetic variation is structured. It is, in fact, an idea that should have been cast aside with the development of evolutionary thinking (Goodman 1997). What is perhaps most problematic about the idea of race is that it is not a process; rather, it is cast as a thing or an end result of a process. To say that race differences exist because of race is a tautology. There are in these explanations no explicitly theorized arguments relating to the processes by which race differences came into being. Yet we know now that genetic variation arose and is a result of human evolution and history. The idea of race, of stable and unchanging types, inhibits rather than advances studies of the evolution of human differences.

The Structure of Human Variation

If the idea of race—dividing humans into some three or more racial groups—approximated in a useful way the geographic structure of human variation, then one might support the notion that race is an imperfect but acceptable stand-in for human genetic variation. So framed, the association of place and genetic variation does not explain everything, but it is a sort of "quick and dirty" approximation (Satel 2002). This position may have been defensible before the application of modern genetics to human evolutionary studies. However, it is not defensible now for the following rules of human variation.

Human variation is continuous

Allelic and phenotypic frequencies tend to vary gradually across human populations. Definitions of race as a discontinuous category, reflecting clear "breaks," are thus conceptually flawed: It is impossible to identify where one race begins and another ends. Skin color, for example, varies widely by latitude and degree of exposure to ultraviolet. Since Africa covers such a wide span of latitude, it is reasonable that African groups exhibit a wide range of skin colors that overlap tremendously with individuals from other continents (Jablonski 2012).

Human traits vary independently from one another

Traits tend to vary independently of other traits. Race categories will therefore vary by the traits used to classify. A classification based on sickle cell trait might include equatorial Africans, Greeks, and Turks, while another classification based on lactase enzyme deficiency might include eastern and southern Africans with southern Europeans, Japanese, and Native Americans. There is no possibility for consistency. Because skin color is correlated only with a few other phenotypic traits such as hair and eye color, it is true to say that "race is only skin deep" (Diamond 1994).

Within-race-group genetic variation is much greater than variation among "races"

Starting with Lewontin (1972), studies have statistically apportioned variation in different genetic systems to different levels: among "races" and within "races" and smaller populations such as the Hopi, the Ainu, and the Irish. Lewontin collected data on blood group polymorphisms in different groups and races. He found that blood group variation between races statistically explains only about 6% of the total variation. These results show that if one is to adopt a racial paradigm, one must acknowledge that race will statistically explain only a small proportion of genetic variation. Moreover, this small variation is better explained by geographic distance (Templeton, 1998).

Yu, Chen, and Ota (2002) more recently compared a large sequence of DNA, 25,000 letters, or base pairs, long, of 10 individuals from each of the three main "races" typically used in medical studies: Asian, European, and African. They counted out the number of differences between any two individuals and found that the average number of differences between any two individuals from Africa was greater than the average number of differences between an African and a European or Asian. These results support the understanding that there is greater genetic variation in Africa because of the increased evolutionary time humans have spent in Africa. Most startling perhaps is that Europeans and Asians, rather than being genetically separable, appear more accurately to be subsets of Africans. We truly are, it seems, all Africans.

Race: An Unrepeatable Explanatory Variable

Race is impossible to define in a stable and universal way because "race as biology" varies with place and time, and the socially determined color line is even more dynamic. Other continuous variables such as head and foot size are classified into hat sizes and shoe sizes, and these systems work. A problem with race in practice is that there is no agreed-on "race scale" as there are hat and shoe size scales. Ideas about race are fluid and based on different phenotypic cues. The salient cues change over time, place, and circumstance and are subject always to social and cultural processes.

Race: Conflating Lived Experience and Genetics

Other key methods of classification such as social class may also differ widely. Although always imperfect, measures of social class begin to provide a glimpse at the underlying processes through which social and economic positions affect lived experience and health. Where race critically differs is in the breadth of potential interpretations of the underlying processes. As previously noted, some individuals view racial differences in disease as due to genes, while others view race differences as the consequence of the lived experience of race and racism. Obviously, this confusion has serious implications for theory and practice. One cannot do predictive science based on a changing and indefinable cause.

Conflating Human Genetic Variation and Race

Human genetic variation does exist: It is real and measurable. But it is also more dynamic than one might assume. For example, the genetics of Amherst, Massachusetts, in 1615 was very different from those of 1815 and 2015. And the road from genetic factors to complex diseases and behaviors is exceedingly interactive and less than fully determined. Where we end up—whether a behavior or disease becomes manifest—is undoubtedly related, though partly and incompletely, to genetics. But none of this has anything to do with race.

A reasonable compromise position would be to accept the fact that racial inequalities in health are likely a result of both causal pathways: genetic and lived experience. In fact, this is precisely the position advocated by Francis Collins (2004), the powerfully placed head of the U.S. National Institutes of Health. But Sankar and colleagues (2004) argue that such a position has the real consequence of overstating the importance of genetics, as well as continuing to conflate race with human genetic variation. In their analysis, such a position is likely to divert research funds from studies of socioeconomic causes of health disparities.

Conclusion

No single reason noted here may be sufficient to throw race as genetics, or raciogenetics, onto the scrap heap of surpassed scientific ideas. But considered in combination, the critical discussion clearly suggests that it is time to move beyond raciogenetic thinking in the health sciences. Such a move not only finally jettisons an outdated paradigm, it also provides the space to explore more fully the complex and critical connections between the experience of racism and health and, ultimately, the full range of causes of health inequities.

REFERENCES

Collins, F. S. 2004. What We Do and Don't Know about 'Race,' 'Ethnicity,' Genetics, and Health at the Dawn of the Genome Era, *Nature Genetics* 36 (supplement 111): S13–S15.

Diamond, J. 1994. Race without Color. *Discover* (November): 83–89.

Geronimus, A. T. 1992. The Weathering Hypothesis and the Health of African-American Women and Infants: Evidence and Speculations. *Ethnicity & Disease* 2(3): 207–21.

Goodman, A. H. 1997. Bred in the Bone? *Sciences*: 20–25; March/April.

Hoffman, F. 1896. Race Traits and Tendencies of the American negro. *Publications of the American Economic Association* 11: 1–329.

Jablonski, N. G. 2012. *Living Color: The Biological and Social Meaning of Skin Color.* Berkeley and Los Angeles: University of California Press.

Kochanek, K. D., Arias, E., and Anderson, R. N. 2013. How Did Cause of Death Contribute to Racial Differences in Life Expectancy in the United States in 2010? NCHS Data Brief, No. 125 (July): 1–7.

Krieger, N. 2001. Theories for Social Epidemiology in the 21st Century: An Ecosocial Perspective. *International Journal of Epidemiology* 30: 668–77.

——. 2003. Does Racism Harm Health? Did Child Abuse Exist before 1962? On Explicit Questions, Critical Science, and Current Controversies: An Ecosocial Perspective. *American Journal of Public Health* 93: 194–99.

Krieger, N., et al. 2011. Exposing Racial Discrimination: Implicit and Explicit Measures: The My Body, My Story Study of 1,005 U.S.-Born Black and White Community Health Center Members. *PLoS One* 6(11).

Lewontin, R. 1972. The Apportionment of Human Diversity. *Evolutionary Biology* 6: 381–98.

Livingstone, F. B. 1958. Anthropological Implications of Sickle Cell Gene Distribution in West Africa. *American Anthropologist* 60(3) (June): 533–62.

Olshansky, S. J., et al. 2012. Differences in Life Expectancy Due to Race and Educational Differences Are Widening, and Many May Not Catch Up. *Health Affairs* 31(8): 1803–13.

Sacher, D., et al. 2005. What If We Were Equal? A Comparison of the Black-White Mortality Gap in 1960 and 2000. *Health Affairs* 24(2): 459–64.

Sankar, P., Cho, M. K., Condit, C. M., et al. 2004. Genetic Research and Health Disparities. *Journal of the American Medical Association* 291(24): 2985–89.

Satel, S. L. 2002. I Am a Racially Profiling Doctor. *The New York Times*, May 5.

Smedley, A. 1999. *Race in North America: Evolution of a Worldview.* Boulder, CO: Westview Press.

Smedley, B. Stith, A. Y. and Netson, A. C. 2003. *Unequal Treatment: Confronting Racial and Ethnic Disparities in Health Care.* Washington, D.C.: National Academies Press.

Tapper, M. 1999. *In the Blood: Sickle Cell Anemia and the Politics of Race.* Philadelphia: University of Pennsylvania Press.

Temple, R., and Stockbridge, N. 2007. BiDil for Heart Failure in Black Patients: The U.S. Food and Drug Administration Perspective. *Annals of Internal Medicine* 146(1): 57–62.

Templeton, A. 1998. Human Races: A Genetic and Evolutionary Perspective. *American Anthropologist* 100: 632–50.

Wailoo, K. 1997. *Drawing Blood.* Baltimore: Johns Hopkins Press.

Williams, D. R., Yu, Y., Jackson, J., and Anderson, N. 1997. Racial Differences in Physical and Mental Health: Socioeconomic Status, Stress, and Discrimination. *Journal of Health Psychology* 2: 335–51.

Yu, N., Chen, F.-C., Ota, S., et al. 2002. Greater Genetic Differences within Africans Than between Africans and Eurasians, *Genetics* 161: 269–74.

SECTION 7 CASES FOR TEACHING AND LEARNING

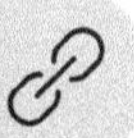

Visit the companion website, **www.oup.com/us/brown-closser**, for direct links to the featured online resources.

California Newsreel, *Debating Policy Proposals to Improve Population Health: A Case Study and Simulation of the Marshall Islands*

In this case study, designed to be used with the movie *Unnatural Causes*, students evaluate proposals for a World Health Organization grant to improve population health in the Marshall Islands, examining the determinants of health, as well as health issues like tuberculosis. The early activities in the case are a bit simple for college students, but the simulation where students evaluate intervention proposals from the perspective of different stakeholders that is appropriate for the college classroom.

California Newsreel, *Place Matters: Researching Our Neighborhoods*
Students gather online data about their own neighborhoods to examine the impact of neighborhood on health outcomes. Instructors may also choose to include an interview component, where students interview neighborhood residents about their experiences. This case is designed to be used with the movie *Unnatural Causes* but could also function independently of the movie.

Leigh Gantner, *PROGRESA: An Integrated Approach to Poverty Alleviation in Mexico*
Students learn about Mexico's Conditional Cash Transfer program, which gave cash incentives to rural poor families if their children attended school and health education sessions. Students consider the successes and challenges of this program and consider how it might be adapted to other contexts.

Lane et al., *Racial and Ethnic Disparity in Birth Weight in Syracuse, NY*
In this case, students examine the demographics of infant mortality in Syracuse, New York. They calculate infant mortality rates and relative risk for African-American and white infants. They also calculate attributable risk and population attributable risk for tobacco use. Another version of the case, set in North Carolina, is also available online.

Talbot and Rhatigan, *Multidrug-Resistant Tuberculosis Treatment in Peru*
This case study describes Partners in Health's groundbreaking project to treat multidrug-resistant tuberculosis in Peru; the project included steps designed to mitigate economic barriers to treatment. This case is useful for helping students think about how the determinants of health might be addressed in an intervention. It could also be paired with Chapter 12, which discusses Partners in Health's work in Haiti.

SECTION 7 VIDEOS AND WEB RESOURCES

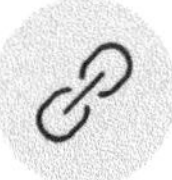

Visit the companion website, www.oup.com/us/brown-closser, for direct links to the featured online resources.

***Unnatural Causes* – California Newsreel**
This seven-part documentary works wonderfully in the classroom. It clearly lays out the social determinants of health, with engaging case studies and interviews with prominent public health experts in the field. Episodes cover aspects of socioeconomic and racial health disparities in depth. While showing the entire documentary would take too much class time for most instructors, each episode can stand alone, and each one can be shown within a class period.

Harlem Public Health Commute

This website, created by an MD/MPH student to help medical students understand public health concepts relevant to working in Harlem Hospital, has sections with engaging videos and links on the social determinants of health; race and health; health systems; injuries and violence; substance use; alternative health systems; environmental health; and sexual health. Each section collects engaging short videos and other resources from around the Web.

***How Economic Inequality Harms Societies* – Richard Wilkinson**

This TED talk by the groundbreaking researcher Richard Wilkinson outlines issues of economic inequality and health. It very clearly explains the concept of the social gradient. (17 min)

The Rich Live Longer Everywhere. For the Poor, Geography Matters – *New York Times*

These interesting interactive maps and graphs analyze the interaction between poverty, neighborhood, and health—specifically looking at areas where poor people live longer. The *New York Times* is paywalled, but a few article views per month are free, and most universities have access to it.

Same City, but Very Different Life Spans – *New York Times*

These maps of life expectancy by neighborhood in New York City, Chicago, Atlanta, and Richmond, Virginia, show how powerfully ZIP Code can affect life expectancy. They are especially interesting for students with familiarity with these cities.

A particularly detailed map of northern Virginia (which includes information on income, race, and education, as well as life expectancy), and less detailed maps of additional cities are also available via links on the companion website.

Health Equity Monitor – WHO Global Health Observatory

This health inequality visualization tool allows students to explore changes over time in inequality in reproductive, maternal, newborn, and child health in the world or within a particular country.

Inequality Is Real

An engaging interactive website exploring income inequality in the United States. It does not directly address issues of health but would be a good activity for a class looking closely at US health disparities.

***The Biology of Skin Color* – Howard Hughes Medical Institute**

This accessible short video explains how the range of skin color seen in modern humans evolved. (19 min) There are also assignments on the website appropriate for students with some basic background in genetics.

SECTION

8

Sex and Reproduction

This section is about the fundamental facts of life—sex and reproduction. The health consequences of sex, maternity, and childbirth are central concerns of contemporary global health.

In the history of global health and economic development (see Reading 35), overpopulation and population control were very important themes. While there is a demand for family planning services and their overall health benefits, the delivery and acceptability of birth control can be very complicated. Sometimes people have compelling economic reasons to want large families.

Students in rich countries often take it for granted that sex and reproduction are very different things and that unwanted pregnancies can be avoided. Those same students are usually aware that sex can be a route of transmission for infectious diseases, yet, sexually transmitted infections (STI) like chlamydia can be common on college campuses.

The most important STI of the late 20th century is HIV/AIDS, and the expansion of global health has been, in part, a reaction to that crisis. Because of scientific research and public health prevention efforts, rates of HIV/AIDS mortality have declined remarkably, and the disease has morphed from a death sentence to a manageable chronic disease. Nevertheless, HIV rates in sub-Saharan Africa have been unacceptably high. This section has two readings that deal with the question of HIV/AIDS in Africa. We recommend that you read them back to back and come to your own conclusions.

This section also has an article about the controversial topic of female genital modification (FGM) surgeries. There are many people who want to end this practice; the reading by Hoodfar (Reading 29) demonstrates that the issue is quite complicated.

The last reading in this section is about a successful program for reducing deaths during and after childbirth in Sri Lanka. This is a wonderful and positive case study that is a success story of tackling a serious global health problem.

» CONCEPTUAL TOOLS «

- **Sex can be good for your health**. Sex can give pleasure and cement intimate social relationships. It can provide a biological underpinning of a positive emotion called love and is responsible for the basic human grouping—the family.

As such, sex can contribute to social support, mental health, and general well-being. Sex and reproduction are necessary for the continuation of life on earth.

- **Sex can be bad for your health.** Sex is one mode of transmission of infectious disease, including HIV/AIDS and a variety of other sexually transmitted infections (STI). Unwanted sex is interpersonal violence that can result in physical or mental damage. Sex without contraception can result in pregnancy, and childbirth (while it is often a much-desired outcome) carries risks of death, injury, and reduced life expectancy—much higher risks in places without access to quality medical services before and during birth.
- **Women are more vulnerable to the negative health effects of sex for biological reasons.** In vaginal intercourse, females have greater exposure than men to fluids (such as semen) that may carry viruses or bacteria. Because of the mechanics of vaginal sex, they may experience micro-abrasions during sex so that disease transmission is more likely.
- **Women are also more vulnerable to the negative health effects of sex for sociocultural reasons.** Unwanted sex reflects differences in social power and physical strength. Socioeconomic and cultural factors may mean that women do not always have the freedom or power to refuse sex or to demand the use of condoms. Simply being married can also be a risk factor for HIV infection or experience of violence. Many societies also place a great deal of pressure on women to refrain from having sex outside of marriage or to submit to it without complaint within a marriage. In some cases, this can create significant mental health problems.
- **Infertility and fertility are important concerns of local people, as well as global health theorists, but for different reasons.** In many low- and middle-income countries, infertility is feared and stigmatized. Failing to conceive a child (especially a male) can be a terrible thing. Having many children can be a valuable asset in agricultural societies, and in places without stable social security programs, many people must rely on their children for support in old age. However, before the 1990s, international health was (overly) concerned with family planning and population growth and focused on preventing pregnancy.

  This mismatch between local interests and global or governmental agendas has sometimes led to distrust of health agencies. For example, coercive tactics used in India to sterilize people in the 1970s led to violent protests and a long-term legacy of distrust.
- **FGM refers to surgeries done for aesthetic and cultural reasons. It is very controversial.** The practice is also called cutting, circumcision, and mutilation. There are a wide range of practices in different parts of the world; some much more extensive than others. Although many people in the United States have a hard time believing it, parents have their daughters undergo FGM surgeries because they love them and want them to be normal, beautiful, and marriageable. This is a reason why FGM persists despite being illegal and opposed by many international organizations.
- **Research on the harmful medical effects of FGM is inconclusive because of variations in hygienic contexts of operations and the types of surgeries.** International opposition to FGM focuses on both health questions and human rights issues. The operations can have negative health effects, although this is often the result of unhygienic surgical conditions.

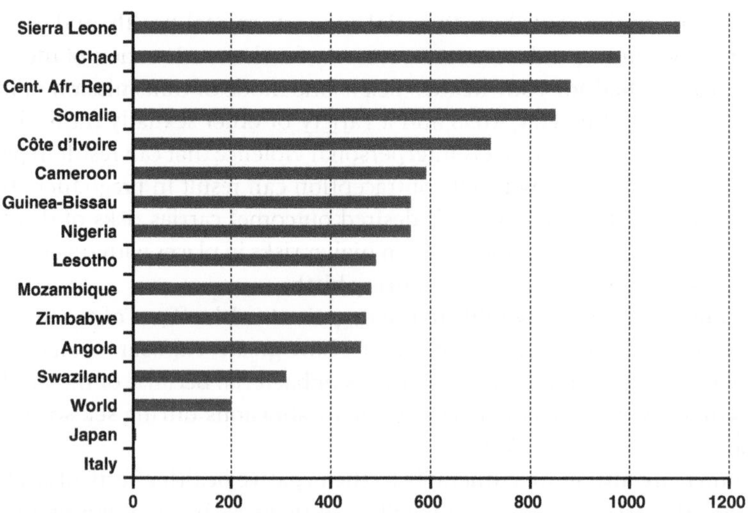

FIGURE CT8.1 Maternal Mortality for Thirteen African Countries, the World, Italy, and Japan: 2013 (Maternal Deaths per 100,000 Births).

Source: J. Chamie. "All in Africa: The World's 13 Highest Mortality Countries." PassBlue, January 16, 2016, http://www.passblue.com/2016/01/06/the-worlds-13-highest-mortality-countries-all-in-africa/.

Maternal Mortality

- **Maternal mortality rates are unacceptably high in the Global South.** The risk of dying during or soon after childbirth is 20 times higher in poor countries than rich ones, although there is much variation within countries. As seen in Figure CT8.1, sub-Saharan African countries have the highest risk of maternal death. The chances of death are highest among the rural poor.
- **Maternal mortality is represented using the maternal mortality ratio (MMR).** This allows direct comparisons between different places. The MMR is the ratio of the number of pregnancy-related deaths per 100,000 live births. MMR reflects access to quality obstetric services and a nation's health services in general (Figure CT8.2; Table CT8.1).
- Although they are particularly severe in the developing world, maternal mortality and morbidity remain a challenge in the United States. Between 1990 and 2013, the MMR increased in the United States, putting the country on the opposite track from other high-income countries and most of the world.

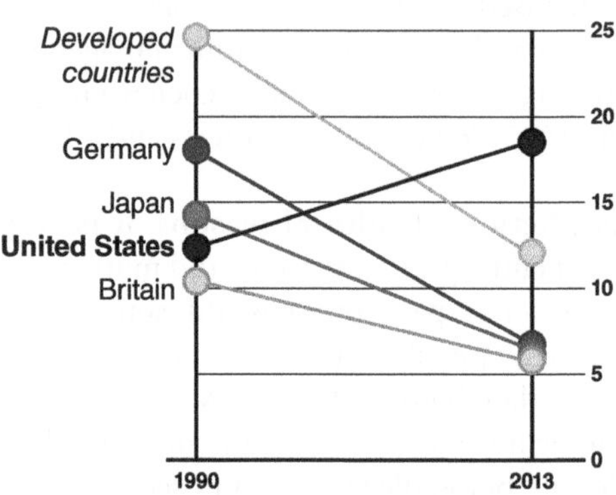

FIGURE CT8.2 Maternal Mortality Rate, per 100,000 Live Births.

Source: N. J. Kassebaum, Barber, R. M, Bhutta, Z. A., et al. "Global, regional, and national levels of maternal mortality, 1990–2015." *Lancet*, 2016, 388(10053): 1775–1812.

TABLE CT8.1 MMR by Country for 2015.

Country	MMR
Central African Republic	882
Nigeria	814
Afghanistan	396
Haiti	359
Ethiopia	353
India	174
Indonesia	126
Iraq	50
Brazil	44
Malaysia	40
Mexico	38
China	27
Iran	25
Russian Federation	25
Chile	22
Thailand	20
Turkey	16
United States of America	14
Bosnia and Herzegovina	11
Libya	9
United Kingdom	9
Japan	5
Austria	4
Kuwait	4
Finland	3

Data source: World Bank and UNICEF. *Trends in Maternal Mortality: 1990 to 2015*, http://apps.who.int/iris/bitstream/10665/194254/1/9789241565141_eng.pdf.

- **Contraception and family planning are good for the health of both mothers and children.** Babies are healthier when they are wanted, well fed, and born with sufficient space between siblings. Family planning and birth spacing are generally good for a woman's mental and physical health, although there are circumstances in which there may be compelling social and economic reasons for a woman to want many children.
- **Reduction in maternal mortality requires more than skilled attendants and clean, safe childbirth facilities.** As seen in Figure CT8.3, safe motherhood needs to be based on gender equity, primary health care, and knowledge. The health-care system must offer a range of obstetrical services. Figure CT8.3 includes abortion care; this is because unsafe abortions are a major cause of maternal mortality.
- **Delay can occur in three different parts of the birth process, increasing the risk of injury or death in childbirth**: deciding to get care, transportation to medical facilities, and delayed treatment within a facility. Safe motherhood requires knowledge, infrastructure, and preparation for emergencies. Figure CT8.4 shows the factors that can cause such delays.

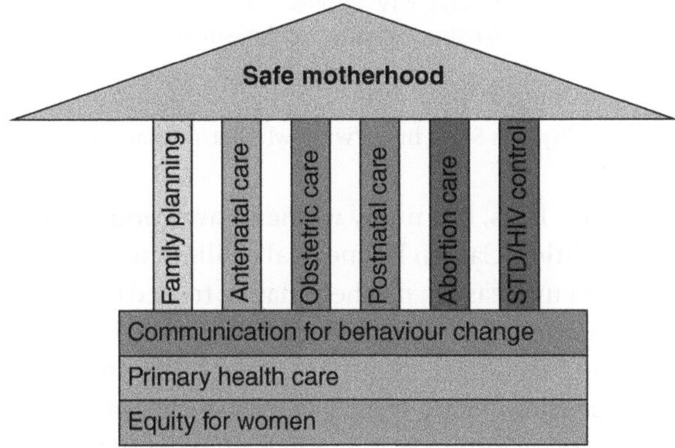

FIGURE CT8.3 Pillars of Safe Motherhood.

Source: Essentials of Safe Motherhood, Dimensions of Public Health (blog), https://publichealthinnepal.blogspot.it/2016/05/essentials-of-safe-motherhood.html.

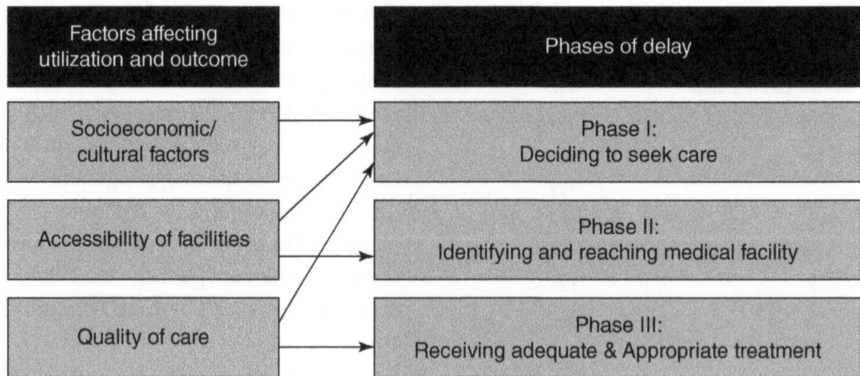

FIGURE CT8.4 Phases of Delay Related to Maternal Mortality: A Conceptual Model.
Source: MEASURE Evaluation, University of North Carolina at Chapel Hill, www.measure-evaluation.org.

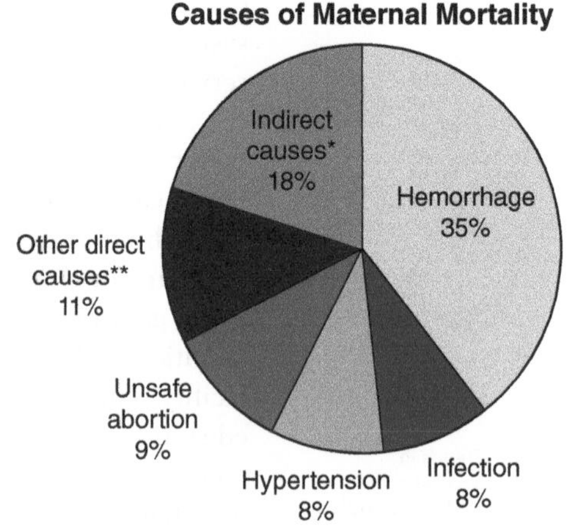

FIGURE CT8.5 Causes of Death in Childbirth.
Source: WHO Maternal Mortality Fact Sheet http://www.who.int/mediacentre/factsheets/fs348/en/

- **Facility births save lives, but many women have good reasons to choose not to give birth in facilities.** Care in biomedical facilities may be very expensive, facilities may be dirty or unpleasant, mothers may be treated badly, or their local hospital may prevent them from having family members with them at the time of birth.

  Births outside of facilities can be made safer by having trained attendants. **Traditional birth attendants** are often enthusiastic about learning more skills and gaining access to more resources that will lead to better birth outcomes.
- **The primary cause of death in childbirth is excessive bleeding.** This is seen in Figure CT8.5. Direct causes of death include obstructed labor and embolisms; indirect causes include infections with malaria, HIV, and accidents.

HIV and Other STIs

- **AIDS is caused by the HIV virus and is transmitted through sex or blood.** HIV/AIDS was first recognized among gay men in the United States in the 1980s, and, at the time, it was almost universally lethal. It was, therefore, associated with much stigma and fear. Globally, HIV is primarily transmitted through heterosexual sex, although it can be transmitted by other exchanges of fluids.
- **Roughly 35 million people have died from AIDS,** and 40 million people are living with the HIV virus in 2017. Most of those people live in Africa.
- **The context of HIV/AIDS changed drastically with the invention of anti-retroviral therapy (ART).** HIV/AIDS can now be a manageable chronic disease. The challenge of the pandemic is both of prevention and of disease management with anti-retroviral therapies.
- **The underlying reasons for higher HIV prevalence in Africa are debatable.** Some researchers believe that it is primarily about patterns of sexual behavior, while others emphasize the context of poverty, different viral strains, and endemic diseases that may lower immune function. You can read about these different perspectives in Chapters 27 and 28.
- **There are certain social groups that have higher risk of HIV infection,** including men who have sex with men and commercial sex workers. The control of HIV requires understanding of both sexual behavior and the socioeconomic constraints that shape sexual decision-making.
- **In addition to HIV, there are many other sexually transmitted infections (STIs).** The health effects of many STIs are preventable but can be serious. For example, human papillomavirus (HPV) is a sexually transmitted virus that can cause cancer if not prevented through vaccination or detected early through Pap smears, and chlamydia is a sexually transmitted infection that can cause infertility if not promptly treated.

  HPV can be prevented with a new vaccine. Because it is expensive (in stark cost/benefit calculations), it is likely that the vaccine will not reach poorer populations for a long time. However, some countries like Rwanda are implementing widespread vaccination for HPV.
- **Some cultural traditions may reduce risk of sexually related health problems, although they did not originate for medical reasons.** Male circumcision has been shown to reduce risk of HIV/AIDS transmission (and other STIs). Cultural rules that enforce modesty or virginity, as well as discourage extramarital relationships, may also have similar functions. At the same time, these same traditions can increase stigma for those with HIV or other STIs.

DANIEL HALPERIN AND HELEN EPSTEIN

27 WHY IS HIV PREVALENCE SO SEVERE IN SOUTHERN AFRICA?

Note: This article should be read in conjunction with Reading 28.

HIV/AIDS was the most important pandemic of the later 20th century. In the 30-plus years since the disease (AIDS) and its cause (HIV virus) were first identified in the 1980s, this single disease has attracted more scientific attention and funding for both basic research and intervention studies than any other disease in history. The epidemic has been a true tragedy that continues today (Peter Brown, one of the authors of this textbook, lost two brothers to the disease). Roughly 35 million people have died from AIDS, and 40 million are currently living with HIV; about 70% of the infected live in Africa. Most HIV transmission today is related to sexual intercourse, primarily heterosexual sex, although it can also be transmitted by other methods of fluid exchange, such as sharing needles.

While the disease is probably much older, it was first identified in the early 1980s among men who have sex with men in the United States and Europe as well as intravenous drug users. Because these were socially stigmatized groups, and because the disease was almost universally fatal, HIV/AIDS was highly stigmatized. The health crisis also triggered political activism for gay rights and accelerated research to find a treatment.

In the mid-1990s, antiviral drug therapies began to be available at very high prices that only the wealthy could afford. Clearly this was a morally unacceptable situation, and the international community eventually created funding mechanisms (including UNAIDS, the Global Fund, and PEPFAR) to make antiviral drug therapies available where they are most needed. Once treatment (and survival) was a possibility, HIV testing became more widespread, and AIDS incidence decreased. The epidemiological character of the disease varies from country to country, but it is surprising to many people in upper-income countries that simply being a married woman in Africa can be a significant risk factor.

This article examines the question about why the rates of HIV/AIDS are so much higher in Southern Africa than any other part of the world. It is based on the recommendations of a conference of experts in 2006 that identified concurrent sexual relationships and lack of male circumcision as proximate behaviors as key factors explaining the geographically unequal distribution of HIV. Concurrency refers to a pattern where people have multiple sex partners over a period of time. It is different from serial monogamy, in which people have multiple sex partners but only one at a time. The concurrency hypothesis was popularized in a 2008 book called The Invisible Cure: Why We Are Losing the Fight against AIDS in Africa *by Helen Epstein (New York: Picador, 2008). While concurrency clearly plays some role in HIV/AIDS transmission in some areas, using it as an explanation for why HIV/AIDS rates are so high in sub-Saharan Africa remains very controversial—as explained in the next article.*

Successful global health interventions require efforts for both prevention and treatment. This article addresses prevention. In the past, prevention messages emphasized the ABCs: A*bstinence,* B*e faithful, and use* C*ondoms. The idea is that these strategies are in order of effectiveness: if you cannot do the first one, then follow the second, and finally revert to the third. The evidence in this article is substantial, but is the story it tells about HIV/AIDS in Africa correct?*

D. Halperin and H. Epstein, "Why Is HIV Prevalence So Severe in Southern Africa?" *Southern Africa Journal of HIV Medicine*, 2007 (March), 19–25.

As you read the following article, consider the following questions:

- **In your opinion, what does it mean to be "promiscuous"? Is there a gendered component to this cultural conception?**
- **What do you think might be logical or practical reasons why a married woman would have continuing affairs with other men?**
- **Are you surprised to learn that African men and women do not have more lifetime sexual partners than people in other places? Why might some people be surprised?**
- **Do you think it is naïve to think that longstanding sexual behaviors can be changed through health education? Do you think adult men will line up to get circumcised? (Check out the evidence on that one.)**
- **In your opinion, do you think the ABC strategy can work? In what contexts?**

CONTEXT

Daniel Halperin is an adjunct full professor at the Gillings School of Global Public Health, University of North Carolina, Chapel Hill, as well as a visiting senior researcher at Florida International University. Previously, he worked at the Harvard School of Public Health. Trained in medical anthropology and epidemiology, he did extensive research in Latin America before turning his attention to HIV/AIDS prevention. He is co-author with Craig Timberg of an award-winning book *Tinderbox: How the West Sparked the AIDS Epidemic and How the World Can Finally Overcome It* (New York: Penguin, 2012), as well as over sixty scientific articles. Helen Epstein is an American writer, molecular biologist, and consultant specializing in public health in developing countries. Author of *The Invisible Cure: Why We Are Losing the Fight Against AIDS in Africa* (New York: Picador, 2008), she has done research on reproductive health and AIDS in Africa for such organizations as the Rockefeller Foundation, the Population Council, and Human Rights Watch. Her research interests include the right to health care in developing countries and the relationship between poverty and health in industrialized countries. This article appeared in the *Southern African Journal of HIV Medicine* in 2007.

A 'Think Tank' meeting on AIDS prevention in the high HIV prevalence countries in southern Africa, convened in Lesotho in May 2006 by SADC and UNAIDS, concluded that 'high levels of multiple and concurrent sexual partnerships by men and women with insufficient consistent, correct condom use, combined with low levels of male circumcision are the key drivers of the epidemic in the subregion.'[1] The top two 'key priority interventions' recommended by the HIV-AIDS, reproductive health, epidemiological and other experts participating in the Think Tank meeting were: (*i*) 'Significantly reduce multiple and concurrent partnerships for both men and women', and (*ii*) 'Prepare for the potential national roll out of male circumcision ... depending on the outcome of the [now successfully completed] Kenya and Uganda randomized trials'. Various other factors in the region's HIV epidemic, including a range of gender issues, especially the need for greater male involvement in HIV prevention, high prevalence of sexual violence, low HIV risk perception, and pervasiveness of transactional sex among young people, especially young women, were also discussed, and continued promotion of primary abstinence, greater access to HIV counselling and testing and access to condoms, especially in high-risk situations, were also recommended. This paper, however, focuses on the evidence underlying the Prevention Think Tank Meeting's two main conclusions.

The highly generalised HIV epidemic in southern and parts of east Africa is uniquely severe. Elsewhere, HIV transmission continues to be strongly associated with especially high-risk activities, namely use of injectable drugs, male-to-male anal sex, and sex work, and the most effective means of prevention are now generally recognised.[2] Although HIV has been present for nearly two decades in much of Asia, Latin America and eastern Europe, extensive heterosexual spread has seldom occurred in those regions.[3–6] While there is concern over the possibility that it could still occur, for the foreseeable future southern Africa will certainly remain by far the most severely affected region of the global pandemic.[6–9]

Although there has been some decline in HIV in parts of eastern Africa, rates remain extremely high in much of southern Africa.[2,7–9] The overwhelming burden of HIV is still concentrated in this region, home to less than 2% of the global population but at least one-third of all HIV-infected people. Infection rates among adults in South Africa, Swaziland, Botswana and western Kenya range from 20% to at least 30%, roughly an order of magnitude higher than anywhere else in the world, outside of Africa.[2]

What might account for this pervasive discrepancy? The now conclusive body of epidemiological and biological evidence confirming the strong association between lack of male circumcision and HIV[10–15] is increasingly understood to explain much of the roughly fivefold difference in HIV rates between southern and western Africa[7,16] (Figure 27.1). In 2005, a randomised clinical trial of male circumcision for HIV prevention in Orange Farm, South Africa, found that the procedure reduced a man's risk of infection by at least 60%, and two similar clinical studies in Kenya and Uganda were recently halted prematurely, also due to such robust findings.[17–19] However, this key driver does not explain why HIV has spread so much more extensively in southern Africa than in India or in Europe, where circumcision is similarly uncommon. Although sexual cultures do vary from region to region,[20] these differences have not been studied in sufficient depth and their significance is not so obvious. For example, Demographic and Health Surveys and other studies suggest that, on average, African men typically do not have more sexual partners than men elsewhere.[21] A comparative study of sexual behaviour, conducted by the World Health Organization (WHO) in the 1990s, found that men in Thailand and Rio de Janeiro were more likely to report five or more casual sexual partners in the previous year than were men in Tanzania, Kenya, Lesotho, or Zambia. And very few women in any of these countries reported five or more partners a year.[22,23] Men and women in Africa report roughly similar, if not fewer, numbers of lifetime partners than do heterosexuals in many Western countries.[21,24–26]

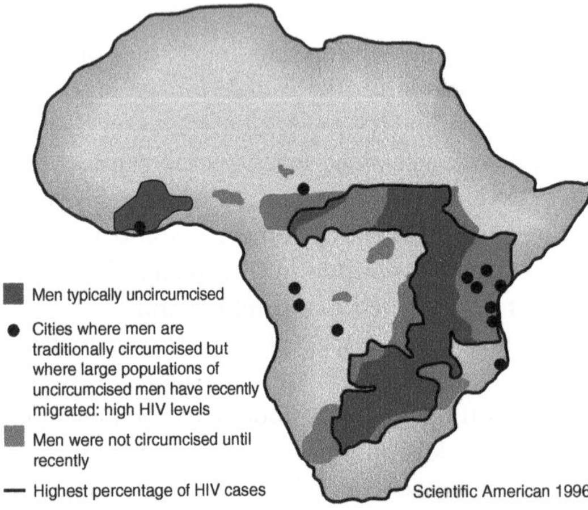

FIGURE 27.1 Male Circumcision and HIV in Africa. Regions in Africa where most men are uncircumcised. *Source:* J. C. Caldwell, and P. Caldwell. "The African AIDS Epidemic." *Scientific American*, 1996, 274 (3): 62, 66–68.

Of increasing interest to epidemiologists is the observation that in Africa men and women often have more than one – typically two or perhaps three – concurrent partnerships that can overlap for months or years. For example, according to the WHO study, 18%, 22% and 55% of men in Tanzania, Lusaka (Zambia) and Lesotho, respectively, reported having two or more *regular*, ongoing (lasting at least a year) sexual partnerships in the previous year, compared with only 3% and 2% of men in Thailand and Sri Lanka. Among women, 9%, 11% and 39% in Tanzania, Lusaka and Lesotho reported two or more regular partnerships in the previous year, compared with just 0.2% and 1% of women in Thailand and Sri Lanka[22,23] (Fig. 27.2). This pattern of concurrent partnerships differs markedly from that of the pattern of serial monogamy more common in the West – i.e. the tendency to have one relatively long-term (a few months or longer) partner after another

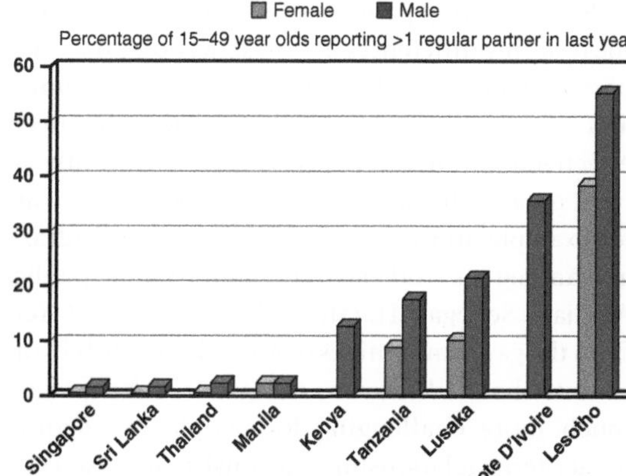

FIGURE 27.2 Concurrent Partnerships Globally. Percentage of fifteen to forty-nine-year-olds reporting greater than one *regular* partner in last year.

Source: M. Carael 1995: Halperin and Epstein 2004.

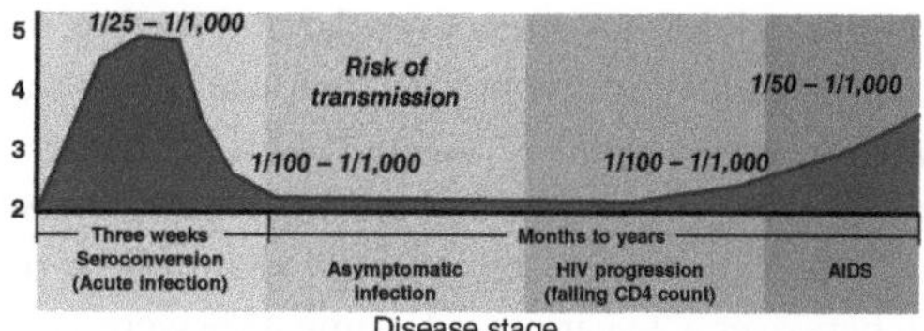

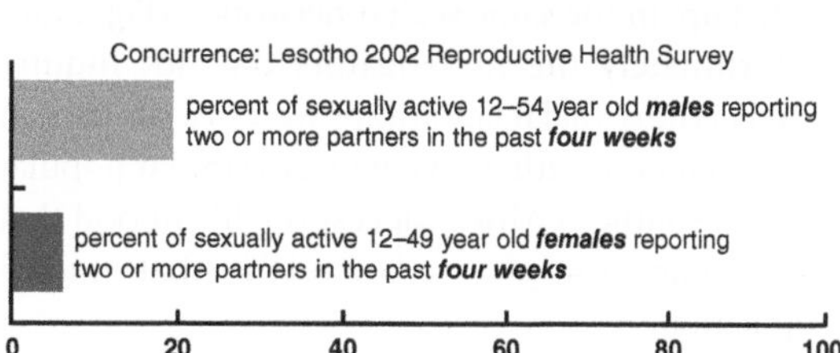

FIGURE 27.3 "Acute Infection" and Concurrence.

Source: Lesotho 2002 Reproductive Health Survey.

– or the more 'one-off' casual and commercial sexual encounters that occur everywhere.[23,27,28]

Morris and Kretzschmar used mathematical modelling to compare the spread of HIV in two populations, one in which serial monogamy was the norm and one in which long-term concurrency was common.[28] Although the total number of sexual relationships was similar in both populations, HIV transmission was much more rapid with long-term concurrency – and the resulting epidemic was some 10 times greater. The effect that Morris and Kretzschmar measured was due to the impact of sexual networking alone; they assumed that the infectiousness of HIV did not vary over time. However, it is now established that viral load, and thus infectivity,[15] is much higher during the 'acute infection' window period (typically about 3 weeks long) initially following HIV infection.[27,29,30] The combined effects of sexual networking and the acute infection spike in viral load means that as soon as one person in a network of concurrent relationships contracts HIV, everyone else in the network is placed at risk. In Lesotho, for example, according to a national Reproductive Health Survey conducted in 2002, 20% of men and nearly 10% of women reported having two or more partners during the past 4 weeks[31] (Fig. 27.3). And in the 2005 national, population-based 'Nelson Mandela' serosurvey in South Africa, among youth aged 15 - 24 about 40% of males and almost 25% of females reported having more than one current sexual partner. In contrast to this pattern of concurrent partnerships, serial monogamy traps the virus within a single relationship for months or years, so when a new partner is engaged the acute infection period of unusually high HIV infectivity has usually passed.

Morris subsequently studied sexual networks in Uganda, Thailand, and the USA.[28] She found that Ugandan men reported fewer lifetime sexual partners than Thai men, but while the Thais mainly had one-off encounters with sex workers, the Ugandan men's relationships tended to be of much longer duration. Given that the per-act probability of heterosexual HIV transmission is, on average, very low,[15] the much higher number of cumulative sexual acts – and hence the likelihood of transmission – within any given relationship was much greater in Uganda than in Thailand or the USA. In addition, except for sex workers, very few Asian women have concurrent partners, whereas a larger proportion of African women do. Even though the Ugandan women in Morris's study reported fewer concurrent relationships than Ugandan men, the multiple partnerships that some of them did have helped importantly to maintain the extensive interlocking sexual networks which facilitate the generalised spread of HIV.[23,28]

Although most African women in concurrent partnerships are not sex workers, such relationships often include a powerful element of sexual-economic exchange, related to issues of gender and income inequality, sexual culture, poverty, and the globalisation of consumerism.[32,33] A recent study from Malawi found that among some 1 000 adult villagers, whose sexual relationships were carefully mapped by researchers over a 2-year period, some 65% were 'connected up' in the same sexual network[34] (Fig. 27.4). Unfortunately the investigators did not inquire whether the sexual relationships were of a concurrent or serial nature, although data from similar populations in southern Africa suggest the likelihood that concurrency also plays a key role in that Malawi population.[1,2]

Although polygamy, and therefore a type of concurrency, is common in much of north and west Africa, as well as in other Muslim regions of the world, HIV infection rates tend to be considerably lower there. The most likely explanation is twofold: first, in most of west Africa and in all Muslim countries, nearly all men are circumcised.[5,6,9,13] Secondly, large-scale heterosexual concurrency networks can only emerge if a significant proportion of women are also engaging in multiple, longer-term relationships. But in Muslim societies generally, women's sexual behaviour tends to be under strict surveillance, which limits the extent of sexual networks.

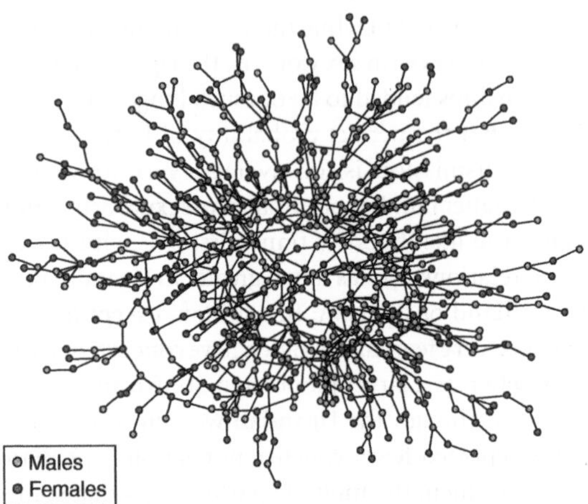

FIGURE 27.4 Sexual Networking in Likoma, Malawi.

Source: S. Helleringer, and Kohler, H. P. *The Structure of Sexual Networks and the Spread of HIV in Sub-Saharan Africa: Evidence from Likoma island (Malawi).* University of Pennsylvania Population Aging Research Center, Working Paper Series 06–02.

Such differing patterns of sexual behaviour and the resulting differences in sexual networks have important implications for HIV prevention programmes and outcomes. Consistent use of condoms has been effectively promoted in Asia's organised brothels, most notably in Thailand and Cambodia, as well as, for example, in the Sonagachi project in Calcutta,[35] and among sex workers in the Dominican Republic, Abidjan, Senegal, Harare and elsewhere.[36–38] Yet, from the gay communities of Australia and San Francisco to the market towns of Uganda, it has proved much more challenging for people in ongoing longer-term relationships to consistently use condoms[37–43] (Fig. 27.5). In southern Africa – unlike in most of Asia or Latin America – such longer-term relationships are typically the ones in which HIV transmission takes place. For years, condom promotion has been a mainstay of donor-funded HIV prevention in Africa, yet a comprehensive review commissioned by UNAIDS concluded that, although condoms are highly effective when used correctly and consistently, 'no clear examples have emerged yet of

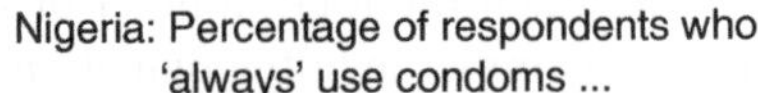

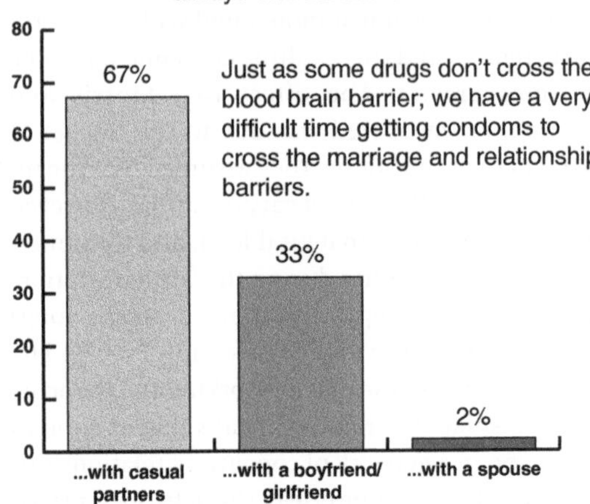

FIGURE 27.5 Condom Use in Longer versus Shorter-Term Relationships.

Just as some drugs don't cross the blood brain barrier, we have a very difficult time getting condoms to cross the marriage and relationship barriers.

Source: D Stanton 2006; Van Rossem et al. *AIDS Educ and Prev. 2001.* 13(3):252–267.

a country that has turned back a generalized epidemic primarily by means of condom promotion.'[37]

Furthermore, a large experts' meeting convened by WHO in July 2006 concluded that, although treatment of sexually transmitted (bacterial) diseases continues to be an important public health measure, the impact on preventing HIV transmission, especially in high HIV prevalence, more generalised epidemics, is likely to be fairly minimal[31] (WHO Report forthcoming). And perhaps even more sobering, several meta-analyses and other rigorous reviews of the data on the impact of HIV testing and counselling on preventing HIV infection, particularly in Africa, so far tend to similarly suggest the likelihood of limited impact (especially for individuals who test HIV negative), although access to testing is clearly very important for various other reasons, including as an entry point for care and treatment.[44–46]

Thus while condoms (and STI treatment and HIV testing) remain important interventions, there is considerable evidence that people worldwide are more likely to use condoms during commercial and casual sexual encounters than in longer-term relationships, in which there is a sense of commitment and trust.[1,37–40,42,43] Also, because HIV can spread so efficiently through populations in which concurrent partnerships are common, everyone's risk is thereby increased, including persons who are commencing a sexual relationship, those who are monogamous with a partner who is not, or people who practise 'serial monogamy'. It is hoped that wider understanding of the dangers of longer-term concurrency could lead to a shift in social norms emerging from a deeper appreciation of the importance of avoiding and addressing concurrency, not only for those whose behaviour is 'risky' according to conventional standards, but also for those whose behaviour is not considered risky, such as monogamous women.

Although clearly no simple solution exists to this complex problem, it appears imperative that in addition to condom availability and other prevention approaches in Africa, there needs to be franker discussion and concerted public-health efforts addressing the dangers of having more than one longer-term sexual partner at a time, or of having a partner who has more than one longer-term partner. Because most Africans do not have high numbers of partners, they may not realise the special dangers of having long-term concurrent partners, especially in regions of high HIV prevalence. In much of southern Africa, even people with only two lifetime partners – hardly high-risk behaviour by Western standards – need to appreciate just how risky that one extra partner can be, for themselves and others, if the relationships are long-term and concurrent.

At a SADC/UNAIDS-organised regional consultation on social change communication for HIV prevention, held in Swaziland in October 2006, it was concluded that the focus of communications programmes across the region over the next 5 years should be on partner limitation.[47] Because in many African countries cultural practices and traditional policies allow and sometimes even encourage multiple partnerships for men, communications programmers will need to work closely with local leaders in order to get the messages right.

In addition, it was agreed that expanded and improved male circumcision services will need to be placed within a broader framework of male reproductive and sexual health.[1,47] Future communications programming will also need to emphasise that while male circumcision is protective, it certainly is not fully protective. Therefore messages which combine information about male circumcision along with promotion of partner limitation and consistent condom use will be essential.

It may seem simplistic to expect people to change their sexual behaviour, once they learn how dangerous it is to have multiple concurrent partnerships in areas of high HIV prevalence. There are, after all, numerous social, cultural and economic reasons why multiple concurrent partnerships exist. In many societies, having multiple partners is a powerful signifier of masculinity, and a relatively wealthy man may even be expected to have more than one wife or girlfriend as long as he can afford to do so.[48] It is also the case that many women in Africa – especially poor women – may be compelled to rely on multiple partners for support, and often have little power to negotiate with their partners about the timing of sex, use of condoms, etc. A detailed exploration of sexual culture in southern Africa is beyond the scope of this paper, but any HIV prevention strategy to address partner reduction and faithfulness should also take place within a wider campaign to address gender issues and to raise the status of women generally.[49]

Despite such important limitations, there is evidence that focused, clearly articulated partner reduction campaigns can make a difference, even in countries where traditional norms would seem to militate against behaviour change. The 'Zero Grazing' (partner reduction and faithfulness) campaign in Uganda,[31,33,37,39,50–53] coupled with evidence from other places such as Kenya and Addis Ababa,[54,55] suggests that fundamental society-wide changes in sexual norms and resulting declines in HIV rates can occur in Africa, just as they did in highly affected communities in north America and Europe in the 1980s.[56,57] Large surveys conducted in Uganda by WHO/the Global Programme on AIDS indicate that between 1989 and 1995 there was a 60% decline in the percentage of people reporting two or more sexual partners in the past 12 months.[41,50] The proportion of men reporting three or more partners fell even more dramatically[41,51] (Figure 27.6).

These behavioural changes are believed to explain much of the decline in HIV *prevalence* that occurred during the 1990s, which modelling studies suggest was preceded by a steep decline in *incidence* – or the rate of new infections – during the late 1980s, when the Zero Grazing campaigns were at their height.[8,50–53] A sampling of newspaper articles on HIV-AIDS in Kampala's main English language paper, *The New Vision*, between 1987 and 1992 found that of 20 articles in the period 1987–1989, 12 mainly addressed behaviour change (partner reduction-related issues in particular), whereas of 25 articles from 1990 to 1992, only 2 did so (although several in the latter period addressed issues such as increasing the condom supply). For example, a long piece on 'zero grazing' and other 'B' types of behaviour change, titled 'Slim [AIDS] is forcing people to change social habits', from 23 October 1987, contained this anecdote: 'In Bugolobi, a young housewife with three children declared, with a gleam in her eye, "My husband stays at home much more. And I encourage him to do so by enthusiastically keeping him informed of the latest gossip about Slim victims."'[51] An 11 November 1989 editorial in *The New Vision* concluded, 'AIDS has no cure. Protect yourself by zero-grazing.'

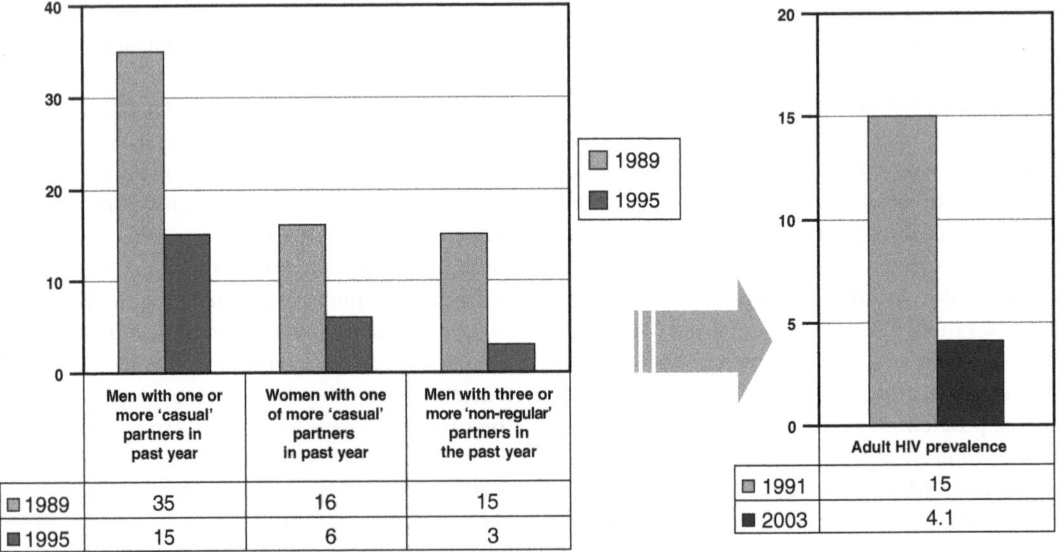

FIGURE 27.6 Behavioral and HIV Trends in Uganda.
Source: World Health Organization/Global Programme on AIDS surveys.

Recently, attention has been drawn to the reversal of the prevention success in Uganda, where there are some indications that HIV prevalence has increased.[2] This has been variously attributed to temporary shortages of condoms, or the expansion of abstinence-until-marriage programmes conducted by evangelical churches that may promote unrealistic standards of sexual behaviour.[58,59] However, the stagnant and worsening trends in Uganda date from about 2000, significantly before either the condom shortages or the proliferation of such abstinence-only programmes. Another possibility is that these negative HIV trends are due, at least in part, to the phasing out of the 'Zero Grazing' and other partner reduction/fidelity-focused campaigns of the late 1980s.[60–62] Indeed, Demographic and Health Surveys conducted between 1995 and 2005 suggest that there has been a considerable increase in the number of sexually active adults reporting multiple partners. The recognition that partner reduction has been neglected in Uganda's more recent prevention programmes, and that it must be a central theme of future campaigns, was emphasised in the final recommendations of a 3-day research symposium, organised by Makerere and Harvard universities, which was held in Kampala in December 2006.[63]

The Ugandan case is not unique. In Kenya, where HIV prevalence has also declined considerably, albeit more recently,[2] the percentage of men reporting two or more sexual partners in the last year fell very sharply, according to Demographic and Health Surveys conducted between 1993 and 2003.[31,38] A study in rural Zimbabwe found an approximately 50% decrease in the percentage of men reporting a new sexual partner in the last month over a roughly 3-year period, coinciding with a significant decline in HIV prevalence and incidence[64] (Fig. 27.7). In Swaziland, where the government recently began aggressively promoting messages such as 'I Choose to Have Only One Sexual Partner' and 'Your Secret Lover Can Kill You', preliminary data from large surveys conducted in 2005 and 2006 found that after only 1 year, the percentage of adults reporting two or more partners in the last 4 weeks had fallen by approximately half.[65–67] This 4-week indicator roughly covers the 'acute infection' period, also approximately 3–4 weeks, and so may provide some measure of the degree of sexual networking in the population and the potential for highly efficient transmission of HIV.

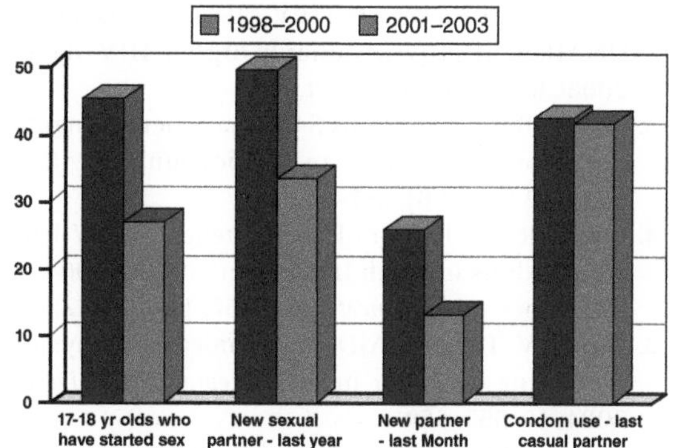

FIGURE 27.7 Behavior Change among Males in Manicaland, Zimbabwe.

Source: S. Gregson, Garnett, G. P., Nyamukapa, C. A., et al. "HIV Decline Associated with Behavior Change in Eastern Zimbabwe." *Science*, 2006, 311: 664–666.

In conclusion, although partner reduction/faithfulness approaches have received relatively little attention in most of Africa,[68,69] they appear to be feasible and epidemiologically crucial. The experiences of Uganda and some other places, where campaigns emphasising 'B' appear to have been associated with population-wide declines in HIV,[31,33,38,39,41,50–53] suggest there is empirical validity to the common-sense notion of emphasising partner limitation – in addition to other crucial approaches, such as the promotion of consistent condom use and increased access to safe and affordable voluntary male circumcision – for HIV prevention.[70,71]

REFERENCES

1. *Experts Think Tank Meeting on HIV Prevention in High-Prevalence Countries in Southern Africa*. Southern African Development Community (SADC). Meeting Report, May 2006. Gaborone: SADC HIV and AIDS Unit. http://www. sadc.int/attachments/news/SADCPrevBrochure.pdf.

2. UNAIDS. *Global Report on HIV-AIDS, 2006*. Geneva: UNAIDS. http://www.unaids.org/en/HIV_data/2006GlobalReport/default.asp.
3. Chin J, Bennett A, Mills S. Primary determinants of HIV prevalence in Asian-Pacific countries. *AIDS* 1998; 12 (suppl B): S87–91.
4. Kumar R, Jha P, Arora P, *et al.* Trends in HIV-1 in young adults in south India from 2000 to 2004: a prevalence study. *Lancet* 2006; 367: 1164–1172.
5. Short RV. The HIV/AIDS pandemic: new ways of preventing infection in men. *Reprod Fertil Devel* 2004; 16: 555–559.
6. Cohen J. Asia and Africa: on different trajectories? *Science* 2004; 304: 1932–1938.
7. Asamoah-Odei E, Garcia Calleja JM, Boerma JT. HIV prevalence and trends in sub-Saharan Africa: no decline and large subregional differences. *Lancet* 2004; 364: 35–40.
8. Shelton JD, Halperin DT, Wilson D. Has global HIV incidence peaked? *Lancet* 2006; 367: 1120–1122.
9. Halperin DT, Post GL. Global HIV prevalence: the good news might be even better. *Lancet* 2004; 364: 1035–1036.
10. Halperin DT. Male circumcision: A potentially important new addition to HIV prevention. Contact (*'HIV Prevention: Current Issues and New Technologies'*) 2006; 82: 32–36, World Council of Churches, Toronto. http://www.wcc-coe.org/wcc/news/con-182.pdf
11. Bailey RC, Plummer FA, Moses S. Male circumcision and HIV prevention: current knowledge and future research directions. *Lancet Infect Dis* 2001; 1: 223–231. http://www.ingentaconnect.com/content/els/14733099/2001/00000001/00000 004/art00117
12. Weiss HA, Quigley MA, Hayes RJ. Male circumcision and risk of HIV infection in sub-Saharan Africa: a systematic review and meta-analysis. *AIDS* 2000; 14: 2361–2370.
13. Halperin DT, Bailey RC. Male circumcision and HIV infection: ten years and counting. *Lancet* 1999; 354: 1813–1815. http://www.circumcision-info.com/halperin_bailey.html
14. Donoval BA, Landay AL, Moses S, *et al.* HIV-1 target cells in foreskins of African men with varying histories of sexually transmitted infections. *Am J Clin Pathol* 2006; 125: 386–391.
15. Quinn TC, Wawer MJ, Sewankambo N, *et al.* Viral load and heterosexual transmission of human immunodeficiency virus type 1. *N Engl J Med* 2000; 342: 921–929.
16. Potts M. Male circumcision and HIV infection. *Lancet* 2000; 355: 926.
17. Auvert B, Taljaard D, Lagarde E, Sobngwi-Tambekou J, Sitta R, Puren A. Randomized, controlled intervention trial of male circumcision for reduction of HIV infection risk: the ANRS 1265 Trial. *PLoS Med* 2005; 2: 1–11. http://medicine.plosjournals.org/perlserv/?request=get-document&doi=10.1371/journal.pmed.0020298.
18. McNeil D. Circumcision's anti-AIDS effect found greater than first thought. *New York Times* 2007; February 23. http://www.nytimes.com/2007/02/23/science/23hiv.html.
19. Williams BG, Lloyd-Smith J O, Gouws E, *et al.* The potential impact of male circumcision on HIV in sub-Saharan Africa. *PLoS Med* 2006; 3: e262. http://medicine.plosjournals.org/perlserv/?request=get-document&doi=10.1371/journal.pmed.0030262.
20. Caldwell JC, Caldwell P, Quiggin P. The social context of AIDS in sub-Saharan Africa. *Popul Dev Rev* 1989; 15: 185–234.
21. Wellings K, Collumbien M, Slaymaker E, Singh S, Hodges Z, Patel D, Bajos N. Sexual behaviour in context: a global perspective. *Lancet* 2006; 368: 1706–1728.
22. Carael M. Sexual behaviour. In: Cleland JG, Ferry B, eds. *Sexual Behaviour and AIDS in the Developing World*. London: Taylor & Francis, 1995.
23. Halperin D, Epstein H. Concurrent sexual partnerships help to explain Africa's high HIV prevalence: implications for prevention. *Lancet* 2004; 363: 4–6.
24. Santelli JS, Brener ND, Lowry R, *et al.* Multiple sexual partners among U.S. adolescents and young adults. *Fam Plann Perspect* 1998; 30: 271–275.
25. Morris M. A comparative study of concurrent sexual partnerships in the United States, Thailand and Uganda. Published abstract, American Sociology Association Annual Meeting, Anaheim, California, 18 - 21 August 2002: session 409.
26. Pettifor AE, Rees HV, Steffenson A, *et al.* HIV and sexual behavior among young South Africans: a national survey of 15 - 24-year olds. Reproductive Health Research Unit, University of the Witwatersrand, Johannesburg, 2004. http://www.rhru.co.za/site/publications.asp.
27. Hudson CP. AIDS in rural Africa: a paradigm for HIV-1 prevention. *Int J STD AIDS* 1996; 7: 236–243.
28. Morris M, Kretzschmar M. Concurrent partnerships and the spread of HIV. *AIDS* 1997; 11: 681–683.
29. Pilcher CD, Tien HC, Eron JJ, *et al.* Brief but efficient: acute HIV infection and the sexual transmission of HIV. *J Infect Dis* 2004; 189: 1785–1792.

30. Wawer MJ, Gray RH, Sewankambo NK, *et al.* Rates of HIV-1 transmission per coital act, by stage of HIV-1 infection, in Rakai, Uganda. *J Infect Dis* 2005; 191: 1403–1409.
31. Halperin DT. Evidence-based behavior change HIV prevention approaches for Sub-Saharan Africa. Presentation at Harvard Medical School, 17 January 2007. http://www.globalhealth.harvard.edu/HUPASeminar_Halperin.html.
32. Leclerc-Madlala S. Transactional sex and the pursuit of modernity. *Social Dynamics* 2003; 29: 1–21.
33. Epstein H. The fidelity fix. *New York Times Magazine* 2004; 13 June: 54–59.
34. Helleringer S, Kohler HP. The structure of sexual networks and the spread of HIV in Sub-Saharan Africa: evidence from Likoma island (Malawi). University of Pennsylvania Population Aging Research Center, *Working Paper Series* 06–02.
35. Jana S, Bandyopadhyay N, Mukherjee S, Dutta N, Basu I, Saha A. STD/HIV intervention with sex workers in West Bengal, India. *AIDS* 1998; 12 (suppl B): S101–108.
36. Ghys PD, Diallo MO, Ettiegne-Traore V, *et al.* Increase in condom use and decline in HIV and sexually transmitted diseases among female sex workers in Abidjan, Cote d'Ivoire, 1991–1998. *AIDS* 2002; 16: 251–258.
37. Hearst N, Chen S. Condom promotion for AIDS prevention in the developing world: is it working? *Stud Fam Plann* 2004; 35: 39–47.
38. Shelton J. Confessions of a condom lover. *Lancet* 2006; 368: 1947–1949.
39. Green EC. *Rethinking AIDS Prevention*. Westport, Conn: Praeger, 2003.
40. Ahmed S, Lutalo T, Wawer M, *et al.* HIV incidence and sexually transmitted disease prevalence associated with condom use: a population study in Rakai, Uganda. *AIDS* 2001; 15: 2171–2179.
41. Bessinger R, Akwara P, Halperin DT. Sexual behavior, HIV and fertility trends: a comparative analysis of six countries; phase I of the ABC study. Chapel Hill, North Carolina: Measure Evaluation, 2003. http://www.cpc.unc.edu/measure/publications/pdf/sr-03-21b.pdf.
42. Meekers D, Klein M, Foyet L. Patterns of HIV risk behavior and condom use among youth in Yaounde and Douala, Cameroon. *AIDS Behav* 2003; 7: 413–420.
43. Flood M. Lust, trust and latex: why young heterosexual men do not use condoms. *Culture Health Sexuality* 2003; 5: 353–369.
44. Glick P. Scaling up HIV voluntary counseling and testing in Africa: what can evaluation studies tell us about potential prevention impacts? *Evaluation Review* 2005; 29: 331–357.
45. Matovu JK, Gray RH, Makumbi F, *et al.* Voluntary HIV counseling and testing acceptance, sexual risk behavior and HIV incidence in Rakai, Uganda. *AIDS* 2005; 19: 503–511.
46. Corbett EL, Makamure B, Cheung YB, *et al.* HIV incidence during a cluster-randomized trial of two strategies providing voluntary counselling and testing at the workplace, Zimbabwe. *AIDS* 2007; 21: 483–489.
47. *SADC Regional Consulation on Social Change Communication for HIV Prevention*. 3 - 4 October 2006, Ezulwini, Swaziland. Meeting report. Gaborone: SADC HIV and AIDS Unit.
48. Hunter M. Cultural politics and masculinities: multiple-partners in historical perspective in KwaZulu-Natal. *Culture, Health and Sexuality* 2005; 7: 389–403.
49. Epstein H, Kim J. Fighting back against gender violence in South Africa. *New York Review of Books*. January 2007. http://www.nybooks.com.
50. Stoneburner R, Low-Beer D. Population-level HIV declines and behavioral risk avoidance in Uganda. *Science* 2004; 304: 14–18. http://www.sciencemag.org/cgi/data/304/5671/714/DC1/1.
51. Shelton J, Halperin DT, Nantulya V, Potts M, Gayle HD, Holmes KK. Partner reduction is crucial for balanced 'ABC' approach to HIV prevention. *BMJ* 2004; 328: 891–894. http://bmj.bmjjournals.com/cgi/content/full/bmj;328/7444/891.
52. Green EC, Halperin DT, Nantulya V, Hogle, JA. Uganda's HIV prevention success: The role of sexual behavior change and the national response. *AIDS and Behavior* 2006; 10: 335–346. http://www.springerlink.com/content/h00r4n 6521805w27/fulltext.html.
53. Slutkin G, Okware S, Naamara W, *et al.* How Uganda reversed its HIV epidemic. *AIDS and Behavior* 2006; 10: 351–360. http://www.springerlink.com/content/7024v857p67q0220/fulltext.pdf.
54. Cheluget B, Baltazar G, Orege P, Ibrahim M, Marum LH, Stover J. Evidence for population level declines in adult HIV prevalence in Kenya. *Sex Transm Infect* 2006; 82: Suppl 1, i21–26.
55. Mekonnen Y, Sanders E, Aklilu M, *et al.* Evidence of changes in sexual behaviours among male factory workers in Ethiopia. *AIDS* 2003; 17: 223–231.
56. Becker MH, Joseph JG. AIDS and behavioral change to reduce risk: a review. *Am J Public Health* 1988; 78: 394–410.

57. Winkelstein W Jr, Wiley JA, Padian NS, *et al.* The San Francisco Men's Health Study: Continued decline in HIV seroconversion rates among homosexual/bisexual men. *Am J Public Health* 1988; 78: 1472–1474.
58. Bass E. Fighting to close the condom gap in Uganda. *Lancet* 2005; 365: 1127–1128.
59. Good in parts: the latest UNAIDS report suggests a little hope is justified. *The Economist* 2006; 21 November. http://www.economist.com/node/8313767?zid=&ah=ac379c09c1c3fb67e0e8fd1964d5247f.
60. Epstein H. God and the fight against AIDS. *New York Review of Books* 2005; 52: 28 April. http://www.nybooks.com/articles/17963.
61. Epstein H. *The Invisible Cure: Africa, the West and the Fight Against AIDS.* New York: Farrar Straus & Giroux. In press, May 2007.
62. Symposium Resolutions and Recommendations. African Successes: Can Behavior-Based Solutions Make a Crucial Contribution to HIV Prevention in Sub-Saharan Africa? Meeting held 17–20 December, Kampala, Uganda. http://ugandasymposium.jot.com/WikiHome.
63. Timberg T. Uganda's early gains against HIV eroding; message of fear, fidelity diluted by array of other remedies. *Washington Post* 2007; 29 March, p. A1. www.washingtonpost.com/wp-dyn/content/article/2007/03/28/AR 2007032802510. html?referrer=email.
64. Gregson S, Garnett GP, Nyamukapa CA, *et al.* HIV decline associated with behavior change in eastern Zimbabwe. *Science* 2006; 311: 664–666.
65. Halperin D, Andersson N, Mavuso M, Bicego G. Assessing a national HIV behavior change campaign focusing on multiple concurrent partnerships in Swaziland. International AIDS Conference Oral Presentation Abstract, Toronto, August 2006. http://www.iasociety.org/abstract/show.asp?abstract_id=2199617; http://today.reuters.co.uk/news/articlenews.aspx?type=healthNews&storyID=2006-08-15T132307Z_01_COL548149_RTRIDST_0_HEALTH-MULTIPLE-PARTNERSHIPS-DC.XML&archived=False.
66. IRIN News Service. Swaziland: AIDS campaign induces behaviour change. *IRIN*, 27 October 2006. http://www.alertnet.org/thenews/newsdesk/IRIN/bee9c252234f045d1275451934ae1c5.htm.
67. Timberg C. In Swaziland, 'secret lovers' confronted in fight against AIDS. *Washington Post* 2006; 29 October, p. A15. http://www.washingtonpost.com/wp-dyn/content/article/2006/10/28/AR2006102800445.html.
68. Timberg C. Speeding HIV's deadly spread: multiple, concurrent partners drive disease in southern Africa. *Washington Post* 2007; 2 March, p. A1. http://www. washingtonpost.com/wp-dyn/content/article/2007/03/01/AR2007030101607. html.
69. Epstein H. Africa's lethal web net of AIDS: the quiet acceptance of informal polygamy is spreading the risk. *Los Angeles Times* 2007; 15 April. http://www.latimes.com/news/opinion/commentary/la-op-epstein15apr15,0, 4906338.story?coll=la-news-comment-opinions.
70. Halperin DT, Steiner M, Cassell M, Green EC, Hearst N, Kirby D, Gayle H, Cates W [149 signers in total]. The time has come for common ground on preventing sexual transmission of HIV. *Lancet* 2004; 364: 1913–1915. http://www. iasociety.org/images/upload/Lancet%20HIV%20prevention.pdf.
71. McNeil D. W.H.O. urges circumcision to reduce spread of AIDS. *New York Times* 2007; March 29. http://www.nytimes.com/2007/03/29/health/29hiv.html?ei=5070&en=4f962a3432644116&ex=1176091200&adxnnl=1&adxnnlx=1175993826-3EZSrZjKPHqukXlhQfU/+Q (also: http://www.sfgate.com/cgi-bin/article. cgi?f=/c/a/2007/03/29/MNG5LOTIV21.DTL&hw=circumcision&sn= 002&sc= 772).

EILEEN STILLWAGGON AND LARRY SAWERS

28 UNDERSTANDING HIV/AIDS IN THE AFRICAN CONTEXT

Note: This article should be read in conjunction with Reading 27.

Understanding HIV/AIDS in the African context is a complicated endeavor. This article provides a serious contrast to the previous reading, which emphasized the issue of concurrency in sexual relationships in southern Africa. In contrast, this article considers many broader interacting factors that provided conditions to make the HIV/AIDS epidemic spread in sub-Saharan Africa.

Epidemics do not occur simply because a pathogen crosses some geographical or biological barrier. Rather, the overall context must be conducive to an epidemic. This is one reason why epidemics are often associated with wars (see Reading 32).

Like other sexually transmitted infections (STIs), HIV/AIDS is only partially about sex. A variety of contextual factors including nutrition, hygienic conditions, and poverty that can constrain the behavior of individuals also affect disease transmission. Answering the question of why there is such a high rate of HIV/AIDS in sub-Saharan Africa requires an understanding and serious consideration of the contexts—both epidemiological and socio-economic. It is not sufficient to focus only on individual behavior. If we look only at individual behavior, we are likely to exaggerate the ability of people to make choices within particular social and economic contexts and also likely to underestimate the power of structural violence (see Reading 34).

This article first considers the disease burden and the ecology of poverty in populations with high rates of HIV. These factors make an individual more likely to become infected, because undernutrition and infectious diseases, such as other STIs, malaria, and schistosomiasis, lead to burdens on a person's immune system.

The health systems in many sub-Saharan African countries are so inadequate that the initial arrival of HIV/AIDS was barely recognized—quite unlike the United States. African health-care systems and epidemiological surveillance systems are overburdened and underfunded. Clinics often lack simple equipment like clean hypodermic needles. There are so many variables interwoven in the causation of the HIV/AIDS epidemic that it is probably impossible to measure them all in randomized controlled studies. It is certainly the case that the most basic epidemiological methods (like the 2×2 table) are inadequate for explaining the complex interaction of causes.

Science, including research on the causes of disease, is often polluted by the scientists' preexisting cultural assumptions and prejudices. This may be the case with assumptions about the sexual behavior of the other societies—in this case, the historical stereotype of Africans as hypersexualized may have led to an overemphasis on sexual explanations for the spread of HIV/AIDS.

This tendency to discover things that we already believe to be true is called confirmation bias. The only way to circumvent such bias is through repeated study and reanalysis. This article interrogates the concurrency hypothesis by critically examining the methods used by other researchers. Such arguments about methods sometimes seem unnecessarily trivial to students. In reality, however, looking at the methods that studies use is critical to understanding whether their findings are actually correct.

Remember that this article should be read in conjunction with the previous reading (Reading 27).

As you read this piece, consider the following questions:

- **The previous article concluded with two concrete recommendations for future HIV/AIDS prevention programs, but this article does not. In your opinion, what do you think that the authors would propose as solution(s) to the complexity of the epidemic?**

This article is original to this volume.

- **In your opinion, why has HIV/AIDS received more attention than "old" health challenges like undernutrition, malaria, schistosomiasis, or the neglected tropical diseases?**
- **Consider the difference that the authors propose between causes of cases and causes of incidence. Might this difference reflect the way that clinical doctors think, as opposed to people who practice public health?**
- **In your opinion, are there really "methodological handcuffs" that can hamper progress in health improvements? If so, what is the solution?**
- **Do you think that an incomplete consideration of a complex web of causation, as described here, can be considered "false facts?"**
- **The authors of this article are economists. Do you think that this makes a difference in their approaches to global health?**

CONTEXT

Eileen Stillwaggon is a professor of economics and Benjamin Franklin Professor of Arts and Sciences at Gettysburg College. Her primary interest has been on the relationship between health and economic development, described in her book, *Stunted Lives, Stagnant Economies: Poverty, Disease, and Underdevelopment* (New Brunswick, NJ: Rutgers University Press, 1998). Recognizing the problems with an individualized behavior approach to health interventions for HIV/AIDS, she wrote *AIDS and the Ecology of Poverty* (Oxford: Oxford University Press, 2006)—about the same time as the popular book discussed in Reading 27. She has also done research on economic development in Native American communities and in Latin America. Larry Sawers is a professor of economics at American University, Washington, DC. His major research interests are in the causes of economic underdevelopment, one of which is poor health, and economic development policy. He has been a Senior Fulbright Scholar in Tanzania, Ecuador, and Lithuania. His books include *The Other Argentina: The Interior and National Development* (Boulder, CO: Westview, 1996) and *Emerging Financial Markets in the Global Economy* (co-editor with Daniel Schydlowsky and David Nickerson; River Edge, NJ: World Scientific, 2000).

Large events are almost never like a meteor hitting the earth. They arise over time, from multiple, often interacting causes. Wars result from the combined effects of economic, political, and sometimes natural events. Famines reflect the inability to buy food due to income loss as well as supply factors, such as crop failures and logistical obstacles. Traditional epidemiology has always recognized that outbreaks of disease occur in a specific context of environmental, social, and economic conditions. For an individual, as for a population, "the epidemiology of an infectious disease reflects complex interactions between the infectious agent, the host, and the environment".[1]

We know a great deal about why epidemics spread. Random introductions of pathogens into human populations occur continually, but they rarely lead to epidemics or pandemics. Favorable conditions are necessary for a microbe to make a person sick or for the disease to spread throughout a population. Plague was introduced numerous times into Europe before 1348 without pandemic spread. But 30 years of falling per capita food consumption had weakened the population and provided the conditions needed for the Black Death.[2,3] For 100 years before 1991 there was no cholera outbreak in the Americas, although cholera *vibrio* was introduced into coastal waters throughout the region on countless occasions. The return of cholera to the hemisphere followed substantial deterioration in sanitary conditions throughout Latin America during the "lost decade" of the 1980s, a period of economic crisis, decreased government social expenditures, falling incomes, and increasing inequality. From one squalid slum to another, cholera spread north and south from Peru across Latin America.[4]

Epidemiological, clinical, and laboratory evidence show that HIV infection is influenced by the same factors that promote transmission of other infectious diseases. People with nutritional deficiencies, with parasitic diseases, whose general health is poor, who have little access to health-care services, or who are otherwise economically disadvantaged have greater susceptibility to infectious diseases, whether they are transmitted sexually or by food, water, air, or other means. This essay examines the spread of HIV/AIDS in sub-Saharan Africa using this perspective, and shows how much writing about AIDS in Africa has neglected to take these factors into account.

The Health Environment of African AIDS

At the time the HIV epidemic was spreading in Africa, the real annual income of the average person in the United States was more than 60 times that of the average Tanzanian or Malawian.[5] Calorie intake per person in sub-Saharan Africa had not increased from 1970 to 2000 and was still only 70 percent of the consumption level of industrialized countries. Public and private spending on health services in Canada was 200 times what it was in Ethiopia.[5] Malnutrition and parasite infection contribute to greater susceptibility to any infectious disease, including those transmitted sexually. There are also certain diseases prevalent in Africa, but rare in the rest of the world, that sharply increase the probability of transmission of HIV.

When HIV emerged in the early 1980s, it was barely noticed in some African countries because of the routine enormity of suffering. Even today, HIV is far from the only threat to poor people in the region. When the HIV epidemic was already advanced in Malawi, a study of a plantation there reported three deaths per month from AIDS, certainly a terrible toll. But there were six non-AIDS deaths of adult workers per month, and 15 deaths per month of workers' dependents.[6] HIV flourishes where people are dying of other diseases. That is not mere coincidence.

Nutrition

From 1988 to 1998, when emerging or localized HIV epidemics developed into generalized epidemics in sub-Saharan Africa, 30 percent of the population of the region was malnourished.[7] Malnutrition increases vulnerability to infectious and parasitic diseases generally, increases HIV viral load and viral shedding, and undermines the integrity of the skin and mucosa, thereby increasing sexual and vertical transmission of HIV.[8–15] (For numerous additional sources on nutrition, see.)[16] Malnutrition alone cannot explain differences in HIV epidemics across the globe, but, given the well-understood connection between immune status and malnutrition, it surely played a role in accelerating the spread of HIV in sub-Saharan Africa.

Malaria

When generalized epidemics of HIV were developing in the region, there were nearly 200 million cases of malaria in Africa every year and nearly 1 million deaths.[17,18] At the time, Uganda, Tanzania, and Mozambique had the highest incidence of malaria in the world, and Malawi, Zambia, and Zimbabwe were not far behind.[19] Then as now, more than 90 percent of acute infections and deaths from malaria were in sub-Saharan Africa.[17] Malaria increases HIV viral load up to ten times for as much as seven weeks after an episode of fever, and that can more than double heterosexual transmission.[20–22] An HIV-infected person could have elevated viral load for more than half of every year since people are repeatedly reinfected in highly endemic areas. Malaria also leads to anemia and impairs immune response, both of which make those with HIV more contagious.[23] Malaria is especially dangerous in areas of southern Africa where it occurs in seasonal epidemics (Botswana, Zimbabwe, Swaziland, South Africa, and Namibia), which are also the countries with the highest rates of HIV.[24]

Helminths

Infection with helminths, or parasitic worms, impairs immune response and increases HIV viral load, increasing transmission of HIV and accelerating progression to AIDS.[25–28] Because helminth infection is so prevalent in sub-Saharan Africa, even a small additional risk of HIV transmission due to helminth infection could mean many additional HIV infections overall. A double-blind, controlled trial found that treating worm infections in HIV-infected persons results in a statistically significant improvement in immune system functioning.[29,30] That suggests that a simple, inexpensive (2 US cents) and effective deworming medication could allow HIV-infected people to be healthier while reducing the risk of infecting a partner, especially when antiretroviral treatment for HIV may be unavailable.

Schistosomiasis

Nearly 90 percent of cases of the parasitic disease, urogenital schistosomiasis, occur in sub-Saharan Africa, where it afflicts 120 million people.[31,32] Schistosomiasis is highly prevalent in almost every country in sub-Saharan Africa. Schistosome worms and their eggs colonize the reproductive tract in men and women, causing inflammation, viral shedding, and genital ulcers, all of which increase the transmission efficiency of HIV.[33–36] In endemic areas, from 33 to 75 percent of women have genital lesions and inflammation resulting from schistosome eggs.[37] The presence of eggs causes inflammation in the urogenital system and breaches in the integrity of the epithelial layer and the protective mucosal surface.[32,37,38] Women with genital ulcers of schistosomiasis have three to four times the risk of being infected with HIV as women in the same village without genital ulcers of schistosomiasis.[37–40]

Treatment with praziquantel is effective in killing the worms and stopping egg production and is safe even in pregnancy and during lactation. Lack of access to treatment can produce irreversible damage to the reproductive tract. Praziquantel costs US $0.30 per treatment, and even a single treatment in childhood can reduce adult disease by half. Fewer than 8 percent of people in need are treated although mass drug administration is feasible and inexpensive.[32,41]

Other Sexually Transmitted Infections

Sub-Saharan Africa has the highest burden of sexually transmitted infections (STIs) of all of the world's regions.[19,42] In 2004, the mean burden of STIs in sub-Saharan Africa [measured in disability-adjusted life years (DALYs) per 100 000] was nearly six times the mean burden outside the region, and all 47 sub-Saharan African countries for which there were data were among the world's 52 countries with the highest STI burden.[19] Poor access to health care services, antibiotics, and antivirals contributes to the persistence and spread of STIs in the region,[43] in spite of unexceptional or even conservative sexual behavior documented in empirical studies (see below).

Some STIs produce ulceration of the genitals that are open pathways for transmission of HIV. All sexually transmitted infections produce inflammation, increased HIV shedding, and increased viral load, all of which have been shown to increase the risk of HIV transmission. Numerous observational studies since the late 1980s demonstrate that STI coinfections make persons with HIV more contagious and make STI-infected persons more vulnerable to HIV acquisition.[27,43–48] STI diagnosis and treatment have been standard parts of the HIV prevention toolkit since the 1980s.

Non-Sexual Transmission

In addition to diseases that can increase HIV transmission rates during heterosexual and mother-to-child exposure, non-sexual modes of transmission could play an especially important role in sub-Saharan Africa and among other poor populations. There are numerous, common medical blood exposures (for example, injections with unsterilized syringes, blood transfusions, catheter and intravenous placements, and internal obstetrical examinations) and non-medical blood exposures (for example, barbering and hairdressing, tattooing, scarification, injections given by non-medical personnel, and intravenous recreational drug use) that can potentially transmit HIV.[49–51] Even if each one of those possible non-sexual routes of transmission produces only a small share of new infections, together they would play an important role in the epidemics of sub-Saharan Africa, where sterilization equipment in clinics could be lacking.

AIDS Policy in Africa

Since the argument above is well supported in mainstream epidemiology and in scientific research over the past four decades, why is it not reflected in AIDS policy for sub-Saharan Africa? Why does funding for HIV prevention not cover prevention of co-factor infections, including malaria, urogenital schistosomiasis, and STIs?

There are several reasons for the departure of AIDS research from traditional epidemiology. Over the course of the twentieth century, the emphasis of medical research shifted from environmental and population-level factors to individual-level theories of disease causation,[16,52–54] and that change became evident in the evolution of AIDS discourse towards a focus on individual factors, in particular sexual behavior. We return to those methodological issues later in the essay. Here we examine the overwhelming emphasis on sexual behavior in HIV-prevention policy.

In the 1980s and 1990s, the enormity and speed of the AIDS pandemic were menacing. An incurable disease was spreading both in the West and in Africa, and ignorance of Africa served to allay Western fear by constructing AIDS as a disease of the social Other. Western stereotypes had long portrayed Africans as exotic and hypersexualized. Notions of racial difference pervaded the social science literature on AIDS in Africa and were especially explicit during the first 15 years of the epidemic. No one used the word race, but the notion entered into the discourse as "culture." Racial "science" in an earlier epoch and popular racial stereotypes that persist to the present day stress sexual differences between the races and portray sub-Saharan Africans as exotic, strange, and even disturbing.[55–57]

By the late 1980s, the presumption, promoted in scholarly and popular literature, that the extraordinary nature of heterosexual behavior in sub-Saharan Africa explained the high prevalence of HIV in the region became widely accepted among researchers and policy makers. Influential and frequently cited works were characterized by sweeping statements about pan-African sexuality, either without evidence or with only anecdotal evidence dating from the 1920s to the 1970s. Through suggestive language and innuendo, they conveyed the impression of Africans bent on self-destruction because of cultural factors that differentiated them from everyone else. (See among others.[58,59] For extensive discussion of racial innuendo in AIDS discourse, see).[16,60]

Racial stereotypes continue to pervade Western culture, casting their shadow over scholarship and public policy, even among persons who, on a conscious level, vigorously and sincerely oppose racial discrimination. The influence of notions of "race" in both the popular mind and in the imagery of science is insidious and difficult to counter because so much of racial stereotyping is in the "unstated assumptions and unthinking responses",[61] rather than in explicit postulates. That is aggravated by the tendency for both academic and journalistic writing about sub-Saharan Africa to consist of a "repertoire of amazing facts".[62] Writing about sub-Saharan Africans, popular and scholarly, almost always emphasizes how they are different from others, not their commonality with people everywhere.

Western researchers, editors of academic journals, bilateral donor agencies, and international organizations framed the spread of AIDS in sub-Saharan Africa in behavioral terms, neglecting the health environment in which the epidemic unfolded in the region. The power to define the causes of HIV in exclusively behavioral terms narrowed the research questions and policy responses. In spite of the lack of evidence, the theme in much AIDS scholarship and policy literature remains that "Africans are not like everyone else."

Inconsistencies in the Behavioral Paradigm

Serious researchers naturally sought data on sexual behavior to test the proposition that differences in sexual behavior could explain 50-fold differences in HIV prevalence between some African countries and the rest of the world. The UN Global Programme on AIDS, the Demographic and Health Surveys (DHS) funded by USAID, and numerous other researchers have produced a substantial body of survey research on sexual behavior in Africa and elsewhere. The surveys demonstrate that within every country there is considerable variation in sexual behavior—some people have many partners, for example, but most people have one, very few, or none—and prevalence of HIV across the globe and within sub-Saharan Africa does not correlate with patterns of risky behaviors. Evidence from those surveys showed that in sub-Saharan Africa sexual behavior was more conservative than in Europe, the United States, Canada, and Latin America, whether measured by average age of sexual debut, prevalence of pre- or extra-marital sex, average number of partners, visits to commercial sex workers, or average number of partners in one year or over a lifetime.[63,64] (For extensive documentation, see).[16,65]

In the 1990s, a second important finding further undermined the validity of the behavioral paradigm. Researchers found that HIV is not a particularly virulent pathogen and that per-act transmission rates are quite low between otherwise healthy adults in heterosexual contacts, though somewhat higher during the first few weeks after initial infection.[66–70] Thus, empirical evidence on both the behavior and the biology needed for a behavioral explanation was lacking. Nevertheless, AIDS had become associated in the popular imagination, including that of researchers, as an exceptional, African behavioral phenomenon. Because asking how Africans are different from everyone else seemed so reasonable to most people, a new variant, the concurrency hypothesis, became the conventional wisdom without credible empirical support.

Concurrency to the Rescue

In the early 1990s, a few researchers proposed that long-term overlapping partnerships—also called multiple concurrent partnerships, or concurrency—might explain the difference in HIV prevalence between Africa and the rest of the world.[71,72] A decade later, it was clear that other forms of heterosexual behavior could not account for the extraordinarily high HIV prevalence in the region, and concurrency emerged as the dominant explanation.[73–75] It was argued that concurrency—in contrast to one-time or short-term sexual encounters—could permit sufficiently frequent sexual exposures during the first few weeks of HIV infection, when transmission efficiency is highest, to provide the missing engine capable of driving the African HIV epidemics.

The promoters of this updated version of the behavioral paradigm asserted that long-term concurrent partnerships are unusually common in sub-Saharan Africa.[73–79] Furthermore, they asserted that concurrent partnerships spread HIV much more effectively than sequential multiple partnering.[75] If either assertion is incorrect, then the concurrency hypothesis fails. We argue that neither is correct.

Is Concurrency More Common in Sub-Saharan Africa?

In 2010, we reviewed more than three dozen studies that proponents of the concurrency hypothesis had presented as evidence of extraordinarily high concurrency prevalence in sub-Saharan Africa.[65] We found more than 100 errors in their reporting of the results of those surveys. Moreover, most of the surveys recruited (rather than randomly sampled) a small number of respondents, often in a single neighborhood or village, so the results could not be generalized to the larger population.[65] The few surveys that randomly sampled a large population used a measure of concurrency that has been judged unreliable by the UNAIDS Reference Group on Estimates, Modelling and Projections.[80] None of the studies provided credible evidence that concurrency was unusually high in sub-Saharan Africa.[65] In 2010, the DHS (Demographic and Health Surveys) began to measure concurrency using the questionnaire proposed by the UNAIDS Reference Group. There are now surveys from 31 countries in sub-Saharan Africa that interviewed a representative national sample of adults, all using the same definition of concurrency.[81,82] The average prevalence of concurrency (having overlapping sexual partnerships six months prior to the interview) was 8.3 percent for men and 1.0 percent for women, or 4.7 percent for all adults age 15 to 49. Concurrency prevalence in the United States and several European countries is in the same range as the numbers from sub-Saharan Africa, though perhaps higher for women and lower for men.[83–85]

Is Concurrency Especially Effective in Spreading HIV?

One cannot conduct trials with humans to test if concurrency is an especially effective mechanism for spreading HIV, so to explore the issue one must use mathematical modeling of sexual networks, specifically using a technique called individual-based stochastic simulation modeling. The modeling takes a number of factors into account, including the average length of each partnership, the likelihood of forming a concurrent partnership, and the daily risk or probability of acquiring HIV (which in turn implicitly assumes the frequency of sexual contact in each partnership). For the modeling to generate useful results, these parameters must be based on reasonable estimates from survey research or clinical studies. Early modeling appeared to show that HIV spreads far more rapidly with concurrent partnering than with serial monogamy.[75] Those results were cited by the modelers themselves and many others to make the claim that concurrency explained exceptionally high rates of HIV in sub-Saharan Africa. That proposition soon became widely accepted.

The original model, however, depended on parameters that were simply implausible. The modelers assumed that every person, male or female, had sex with every partner every day, with up to four partners. Moreover, they assumed that each day, in each sexual partnership, there was a 5 percent chance of HIV transmission. That 5 percent transmission risk is nearly 100 times larger than the consensus risk estimate of experts on the subject. Eaton and colleagues[86] adapted the original model's code and assumed an evidence-based per-day transmission risk. They found that HIV either does not spread through sexual networks at all or spreads far more slowly than the original model found.

We built on Eaton's work by assigning realistic values for other model parameters. Based on survey research in sub-Saharan Africa, we assumed that partnerships there, like everywhere else, last for many years. We also assumed that secondary partnerships have shorter durations on average and lower frequency of sexual contact than primary (marital or cohabiting) partnerships. With all of those errors corrected, the restructured model cannot generate *any* HIV epidemic that does not move to extinction, that is, the epidemic collapses on itself. That remains so whatever level of concurrency one assumes, even levels far above those considered in the original model and far above levels reported in the DHS surveys in sub-Saharan Africa.[81,82,87]

In sum, when properly measured, levels of concurrency in sub-Saharan Africa are not unusually high and, when properly modeled, concurrency at even implausibly high levels cannot produce sustainable simulated HIV epidemics. Thus, the concurrency hypothesis, the last bulwark of the behavioral paradigm, is without empirical or theoretical validity. And yet, HIV-prevention policy is still rooted in a behavioral, rather than a biomedical model.

What Should Inform AIDS Policy?

We have discussed how Western stereotypes of a hypersexualized pan-African culture, rooted in a belief that Africans are not like other people, allowed behavioral explanations to dominate the search for causes of high rates of HIV in sub-Saharan Africa. There are, however, methodological obstacles that also have prevented epidemiologists and public health practitioners from using the biomedical evidence described earlier in this essay. The increasingly individual-level focus of medicine and public health was aggravated by the excessive reliance on experimental and statistical methods that intentionally omit from consideration the context in which individual illness or population-wide outbreaks occur.

AIDS discourse about Africa and HIV-prevention policy are derailed by confusion over what Rose calls "causes of cases and causes of incidence".[52] Individual risk factors that are associated only with one proximate cause (such as sex) do not fully explain why one individual becomes infected and another does not, nor do they explain why one population has higher incidence than another.

Poor nutrition, malaria, helminths and STIs make each sex act and each birth more risky in sub-Saharan Africa and accelerate epidemics of HIV in the region. By targeting only one proximate cause, sex, policy makers ignore the fundamentally different distribution of risk factors between sub-Saharan Africa and affluent, temperate-zone regions. The 'background noise' of an environment teeming with bacterial, viral, and parasitic cofactors is the appropriate object of study to understand causes of elevated HIV risk for individuals and higher incidence in sub-Saharan Africa.

Methodological Handcuffs

Any causal explanation must involve some simplification, but randomized controlled trials (RCTs) are designed to evaluate the effects of just one singular cause. RCTs are essential in the evaluation of new drugs for which the effectiveness and harmful effects are unknown, but they are blunt instruments for understanding infections or other pathologies that arise from multiple interacting causes, or evaluating public health interventions.[88,89] Epidemics are complex systems; trials that attempt to change one part of that system may show unreliable results because of multiple causes and delayed effects.[90,91]

Trials of vitamin A supplementation for HIV-infected pregnant women reveal the difficulty of attempting to isolate one factor in a complex terrain. Observational studies indicated that women who were deficient in vitamin A were more likely to transmit HIV to their infants,[92] but most trials of vitamin A supplementation failed to demonstrate a statistically significant difference in newborn infection,[93] although one trial supported the hypothesis.[94] Erroneously, some concluded that it is pointless to provide supplements to pregnant, vitamin-A deficient, HIV-infected women, in spite of known benefits of supplementation for women's health. Trial design permits only the conclusion that an intervention is or is not a unique solution. The trial cannot evaluate partial solutions or contributing causes. It does not matter how precise the answers are in such trials; their results are inaccurate because they do not include all causes. They are what physicists have called "not even wrong," because they do not ask the right questions and thus omit relevant data.

The STI–HIV Treatment Trials: Where Context Is Everything

Another example of the attempt to understand HIV without understanding its context is the case of the STI-HIV treatment trials. In the 1990s, a randomized controlled trial showed that even modest efforts to improve the quality of diagnosis and care for STIs in Mwanza, Tanzania led to a nearly 40 percent lower HIV incidence in communities with those interventions than in communities without the interventions.[95] Nevertheless, nine subsequent trials in diverse locations in sub-Saharan Africa using a variety of interventions did not find a statistically significant difference in HIV incidence between two or more randomly selected groups. There were, however, methodological flaws in each of those trials that make it invalid to draw policy conclusions from them. (For citations to all trials, see.)[48]

RCTs require clinical equipoise, which means that the researchers really do not know if the intervention is beneficial, considering both its efficacy and its side effects. STIs are serious, sometimes devastating diseases. Medications to treat almost all STIs were shown in earlier trials to be effective and have few side effects. Observational data and the Mwanza trial indicated, moreover, that STI treatment could decrease HIV incidence. Consequently, ethical conduct in all the trials after Mwanza required that participants in both intervention and control groups in the study received STI treatments. There was thus little difference in exposure (the interventions being tested) between the intervention and control groups and so one could expect little difference in HIV incidence between the two groups. In statistical terms, the post-Mwanza trials were underpowered to detect a statistically significant difference in HIV incidence. Since it is impossible to construct ethical and meaningful RCTs to measure the impact of STI treatment on HIV transmission, it was inappropriate to throw out evidence from scores of observational studies that demonstrated the efficacy of STI treatments and the likelihood of reducing HIV incidence. STI treatment is a neglected intervention in HIV prevention and public health generally. (For examination of numerous other methodological problems with the 9 post-Mwanza trials, see.)[48]

Many policymakers also dismiss treatment of schistosomiasis as an HIV-prevention strategy, citing those same STI trials. There is no doubt that treating schistosomiasis would alleviate substantial urogenital morbidity and other health problems at low cost. What is contested is whether praziquantel should be a standard part of HIV prevention. The observed three- to four-fold increase in HIV acquisition in several studies[39,96] suggests substantial attributable risk and should be sufficient to warrant wide implementation of praziquantel treatment. Given the high prevalence of schistosomiasis, over 120 million infected in sub-Saharan Africa, even a small increase in risk of HIV transmission would generate very large numbers of new HIV infections.

When an intervention is beneficial in itself, is safe, inexpensive, and logistically simple to administer in resource-poor settings, it does not make sense to impose the same burden of proof as one would for an intervention that is untested, or risky, or expensive, or complicated, such as for new drugs in the research phase.[97–99]

Emerging Understanding of Emerging Infectious Diseases

The mucosa of the genital tract is not a mere mechanical barrier. It is more accurate to refer to the microbial community of the genital tract as the ecosystem in which sex takes place. Poor genital health constitutes a disruption of vaginal microbial communities.[91] STIs can cause lesions that later become infected with staphylococci and streptococci. Antibiotics for bacterial STIs are ineffective in treating those secondary infections. Treating schistosomiasis, or STIs, is clearly beneficial, as it begins the restoration of genital health. But each treatment taken in isolation might not register as statistically significant due to the presence of inflammation or lesions from other causes. Recovery of the environmental balance may well exceed the time frame of an RCT. The response to an inadequate statistical methodology should not be to reject a beneficial intervention.

The multiplicity of environmental risks could seem like an insurmountable barrier to HIV prevention. On the contrary, it presents a range of opportunities. Even small improvements in the health of 'sick populations' could have large population-wide effects on HIV spread.[52] In complex systems, small differences in initial conditions can result in large differences in outcomes. Moreover, multiple interactions provide multiple entry points to improve health and improve resistance to new threats.[90]

In order to implement integrated disease prevention and treatment, changes are also needed in the methods of health economic analysis. Just as health research has been limited by a silo approach, economic studies attempt to measure the costs and benefits of interventions in isolation. Treatment for schistosomiasis or STIs, for example, has spillover effects on vulnerability to other diseases, the benefits of which are not generally considered in an economic analysis of a single intervention. This is true for spending outside the health sector as well. One intervention—in sanitation, education, health, job creation—can have multiple beneficial effects that are mutually reinforcing.[100,101] Recognition of spillover benefits and financing interventions across multiple budgets would enable policymakers to have a greater impact in choosing interventions with high impact at lower cost. Solutions to global health problems are easier to identify and cheaper to implement with recognition of the interaction among pathogens, hosts, and the environment, which shapes the context of health and disease.

REFERENCES

1. Hahn BH, Shaw GM, De Cock KM, Sharp PM. AIDS as a zoonosis: scientific and public health implications. Science (New York, NY). 2000;287 (5453):607–14.
2. Pounds NJG. An Economic History of Medieval Europe. London: Longman; 1994.
3. Fischer D. The Great Wave: Price Revolutions and the Rhythm of History. Oxford: Oxford University Press; 1996.
4. Stillwaggon E. Stunted Lives, Stagnant Economies: Poverty, disease, and underdevelopment. New Brunswick, N.J.: Rutgers University Press; 1998. xv, p.342.
5. UNDP (United Nations Development Programme). Human Development Report. New York: United Nations; 2004.
6. Morris C. Workplace HIV Programs in Malawi: A Case Study and Review of Evidence Based Interventions in HIV Care, Support, and Prevention. In: Kosanovich W, editor. Bureau of International Labor Affairs Research Symposium Papers, Vol 2, HIV/ AIDS and the Workplace in Developing Countries. Washington: U.S. Department of Labor; 2003. p. 165–88.
7. World Bank. Nutritional Status and Poverty in Sub-Saharan Africa. Findings Washington, DC: Knowledge Networks, Information and Technology Center; 1998 [Available from: http://www.worldbank.org/afr/findings/english/find108.htm.
8. Beisel W. Nutrition and Immune Function: Overview. Journal of Nutrition. 1996;126:2611S–115S.

9. Chandra RK. Nutrition and the immune system: an introduction. American Journal of Clinical Nutrition. 1997;66(2):460S-3S.
10. Fawzi WW, Hunter DJ. Vitamins in HIV disease progression and vertical transmission. Epidemiology. 1998;9(4):457–66.
11. Friis H, Michaelsen KF. Micronutrients and HIV Infections: A Review. European Journal of Clinical Nutrition. 1998;52:157–63.
12. John GC, Nduati RW, Mbori-Ngacha D, Overbaugh J, Welch M, Richardson BA, et al. Genital shedding of human immunodeficiency virus type 1 DNA during pregnancy: association with immunosuppression, abnormal cervical or vaginal discharge, and severe vitamin A deficiency. Journal of Infectious Diseases. 1997;175(1):57–62.
13. Landers D. Nutrition and Immune Function II: Maternal Factors Influencing Transmission. Journal of Nutrition. 1996;126:2637S–40S.
14. Nimmagadda A, O'Brien W, Goetz M. The Significance of Vitamin A and Carotenoid Status in Persons Infected by the Human Immunodeficiency Virus. Clinical Infectious Diseases. 1998;26:711–8.
15. Semba R, Miotti P, Chiphangwi JD, Saah AJ, Canner JK, Dallabetta GA, et al. Maternal Vitamin A deficiency and mother-to-child transmission of HIV-1. Lancet. 1994;343:1593–7.
16. Stillwaggon E. AIDS and the Ecology of Poverty. New York: Oxford University Press; 2006.
17. WHO (World Health Organization). Number of malaria deaths, global health observatory (GHO) data: WHO (World Health Organization); 2017 [cited 2017 March 3, 2017]. Available from: http://www.who.int/gho/malaria/epidemic/deaths/en/.
18. WHO. World Malaria Report Geneva: World Health Organization; 2008 [Available from: www.who.int/malaria/wmr2008/malaria2008.pd.
19. WHO (World Health Organization), Department of Measurement and Health Information. Global Burden of Disease Estimates, Death and DALY estimates for 2002 by cause for WHO Member States, Table 4. Estimated DALYs per 100,000 population by cause and member state 2002 Geneva: WHO (World Health Organization); 2004 [Available from: http://www.who.int/healthinfo/bodestimates/en/index.html.
20. Abu-Raddad L, Patnaik P, Kublin JG. Dual Infection with HIV and Malaria Fuels the Spread of Both Diseases in Sub-Saharan Africa. Science (New York, NY). 2006;314:1603–6.
21. Hoffman IF, Jere CS, Taylor TE, Munthali P, Dyer JR, Wirima JJ, et al. The Effect of *Plasmodium falciparum* Malaria on HIV-1 RNA Blood Plasma Concentration. AIDS. 1999;13(4):487–94.
22. Whitworth J, Morgan D, Quigley M, Smith A, Mayanja B, Eotu H, et al. Effect of HIV-1 and increasing immunosuppression on malaria parasitaemia and clinical episodes in adults in rural Uganda: a cohort study. Lancet. 2000;356(9235):1051–6.
23. Gonzalez R, Ataide R, Naniche D, Menendez C, Mayor A. HIV and malaria interactions: where do we stand? Expert review of anti-infective therapy. 2012;10(2):153–65.
24. Korenromp EL, Williams BG, de Vlas SJ, Gouws E, Gilks CF, Ghys PD, et al. Malaria Attributable to the HIV-1 Epidemic, Sub-Saharan Africa. Emerging Infectious Diseases. 2005;11(9):1410–9.
25. Borkow G, Bentwich Z. HIV and Helminth Coinfection: Is Deworming Necessary? Parasite Immunology. 2006;28:605–12.
26. Walson JL, John-Stewart G. Treatment of Helminth Co-Infection in Individuals with HIV-1: A Systematic Review of the Literature. PLoS neglected tropical diseases. 2007;1(3):e102.
27. Modjarrad K, Vermund SH. Effect of Treating Co-infections on HIV-1 Viral Load: A Systematic Review. Lancet Infectious Diseases. 2010;10:455–63.
28. Mkhize-Kwitshana ZI, Taylor M, Jooste P, Mabaso ML, Walzl G. The influence of different helminth infection phenotypes on immune responses against HIV in co-infected adults in South Africa. BMC Infectious Diseases. 2011;11(273).
29. Walson JL, Otieno PA, Mbuchi M, Richardson BA, Lohman-Payne B, Macharia SW, et al. Albendazole treatment of HIV-1 and helminth co-infection: a randomized, double-blind, placebo-controlled trial. AIDS. 2008;22(13):1601–9.
30. Walson JL, John-Stewart G. Treatment of helminth co-infection in HIV-1 infected individuals in resource-limited settings. Cochrane Database of Systematic Reviews. 2008(1):CD006419.
31. WHO (World Health Organization). Current Estimated Total Number of Individuals with Morbidity and Mortality Due to *Schistosomiasis Haematobium* and *S. Mansoni* Infection in Sub-Saharan Africa Geneva2008 [Available from: http://www.who.int/schistosomiasis/epidemiology/table/en/index.html.
32. WHO (World Health Organization). Statement—WHO Working Group on Urogenital Schistosomiasis and HIV Transmission, 1–2 October 2009

Geneva: WHO; 2009 [Available from: http://www.who.int/neglected_diseases/integrated_media_urogenital_schistosomiasis/en/index.html.

33. Attili VR, Hira S, Dube MK. Schistosomal Genital Granulomas: A Report of 10 Cases. British Journal of Venereal Disease. 1983;59:269–72.

34. Feldmeier H, Poggensee G, Krantz I, Helling-Giese G. Female Genital Schistosomiasis. New Challenges from a Gender Perspective. Tropical and Geographical Medicine. 1995;47(2 Suppl):S2–15.

35. Leutscher P, Ravaoalimalala VE, Raharisolo C, Ramarokoto CE, Rasendramino M, Raobelison A, et al. Clinical Findings in Female Genital Schistosomiasis in Madagascar. Tropical Medicine and International Health. 1998;3(4):327–32.

36. Marble M, Key K. Clinical Facets of a Disease Neglected Too Long. AIDS Weekly Plus. 1995(August 7):16–9.

37. Kjetland EF, Leutscher PD, Ndhlovu PD. A review of female genital schistosomiasis. Trends in Parasitology. 2012;28(2):58–65.

38. Mbabazi PS, Andan O, Fitzgerald DW, Chitsulo L, Engels D, Downs JA. Examining the Relationship between Urogenital Schistomiasis and HIV Infection. PLoS NTDs. 2011;5(12).

39. Kjetland EF, Ndhlovu PD, D. P, Gomo E, Mduluza T, Midzi N, et al. Association between genital schistosomiasis and HIV in rural Zimbabwean women. AIDS. 2006;20(4):593–600.

40. Downs JA, Mguta C, Kaatano GM, Mitchell KB, Bang H, Simplice H, et al. Urogenital schistosomiasis in women of reproductive age in Tanzania's Lake Victoria region. American Journal of Tropical Medicine and Hygiene. 2011;64(3):364–9.

41. WHO (World Health Organization). Number of people treated for schistosomiasis and reported coverage of treatment (%), by WHO region, 2006–2008. Working to overcome the global impact of neglected tropical diseases. Geneva: World Health Organization, 2010.

42. WHO) World Health Organization. Sexually Transmitted Infections: WHO) World Health Organization; 2017 [Available from: http://apps.who.int/iris/bitstream/10665/75838/1/WHO_RHR_12.31_eng.pdf.

43. Fleming D, Wasserheit J. From Epidemiological Synergy to Public Health Policy and Practice: The Contribution of Other Sexually Transmitted Diseases to Sexual Transmission of HIV Infection. Sexually Transmitted Infections. 1999;75:3–17.

44. Rotchford K, Strum AW, Wilkinson D. Effect of Coinfection with STDs and of STD Treatment on HIV Shedding in Genital-tract Secretions: Systematic Review and Data Synthesis. Sexually Transmitted Diseases. 2000;27(5):243–8.

45. Røttingen J-A, Cameron W, Garnett G. A systematic review of the epidemiologic interactions between classic sexually transmitted diseases and HIV: How much really is known?". Sexually Transmitted Diseases. 2001;28(10):579–97.

46. Glynn JR, Biraro S, Weiss HA. Herpes simplex virus type 2: a key role in HIV incidence. AIDS. 2009;23(12):1595–8.

47. Hayes R, Watson-Jones D, Celum C, Wijgertd Jvd, Wasserheit J. Treatment of sexually transmitted infections for HIV prevention: end of the road or new beginning? AIDS. 2010;24(Supplement 4): S15–S26.

48. Stillwaggon E, Sawers L. Rush to judgment: the STI-treatment trials and HIV in sub-Saharan Africa. J Int AIDS Soc. 2015;18:19844.

49. Brewer DD, Brody S, Drucker E, Gisselquist D, Minkin SF, Potterat JJ, et al. Mounting anomalies in the epidemiology of HIV in Africa: Cry the beloved paradigm. International Journal of STDs and AIDS. 2003;14:144–7.

50. Deuchert E, Brody S. The role of health care in the spread of HIV/AIDS in Africa: evidence from Kenya. International Journal of STDs and AIDS. 2006;17(11):749–52.

51. Gisselquist D. Points to Consider: Responses to HIV/AIDS in Africa, Asia, and the Carribean. London: Adonis and Abbey; 2008.

52. Rose G. Sick Individuals and Sick Populations. International journal of epidemiology. 1985;14(1):32–8.

53. Susser M. Epidemiology in the United States after World War II: The Evolution of Technique. Epidemiological Review. 1985;7:147–77.

54. Schwartz S, Carpenter K. The Right Answer for the Wrong Question: Consequences of Type III Error for Public Health Research. American journal of public health. 1999;89:1175–9.

55. Gilman S. Difference and pathology: Stereotypes of sexuality, race, and madness. Ithaca, NY: Cornell University Press; 1985.

56. Gilman S. 'I'm Down on Whores': Race and gender in Victorian London. In: Goldberg D, editor. Anatomy of racism. Minneapolis: University of Minneapolis; 1990.

57. Gilman S. Black bodies, white bodies: Toward an iconography of female sexuality in the late nineteenth-century arts. In: Donald J, Rattansi A, editors. "Race," culture and difference. London: Sage; 1992. p. 171–97.
58. Caldwell J, Caldwell P. The cultural context of high fertility in sub-Saharan Africa. Population and Development Review. 1987;13(3):409–37.
59. Caldwell J, Caldwell P, Quiggin P. The social context of AIDS in sub-Saharan Africa. Population and Development Review. 1989;15(2):185–234.
60. Stillwaggon E. Racial Metaphors: Interpreting Sex and AIDS in Africa. Development and Change. 2003;34(5):809–32.
61. Dubow S. Scientific racism in modern South Africa. Cambridge: Cambridge University Press; 1995.
62. Coetzee JM. White Writing: On the culture of letters in South Africa. New Haven: Yale University Press; 1988.
63. Cleland J, Ferry B, editors. Sexual Behaviour and AIDS in the Developing World. London: Taylor and Francis for the World Health Organization; 1995.
64. Wellings K, Collumbien M, Slaymaker E, Singh S, Hodges Z, Patel D, et al. Sexual Behaviour in Context: a Global Perspective. Lancet. 2006; 368(9548):1706–28.
65. Sawers L, Stillwaggon E. Concurrent sexual partnerships do not explain the HIV epidemics in Africa: a systematic review of the evidence. Journal of the International AIDS Society. 2010;13(34).
66. Chan DJ. Factors Affecting Sexual Transmission of HIV-1: Current Evidence and Implications for Prevention. Current HIV Research. 2005;3:223–41.
67. Boily M-C, Baggaley RF, Wang L, Masse B, White RG, Hayes RJ, et al. Heterosexual risk of HIV-1 infection per sexual act: systematic review and meta-analysis of observational studies. Lancet Infectious Diseases. 2009;9(2):118–29.
68. Gray RH, Wawer MJ, Brookmeyer R, Sewankambo NK, Serwadda D, Wabwire-Mangen F, et al. Probability of HIV-1 transmission per coital act in monogamous, heterosexual, HIV-1-discordant couples in Rakai, Uganda. Lancet. 2001;357(9263):1149–53.
69. Wawer MJ, Gray RH, Sewankambo NK, Serwadda D, Li X, Laeyendecker O, et al. Rates of HIV-1 transmission per coital act, by stage of HIV-1 infection, in Rakai, Uganda. Journal of Infectious Diseases. 2005;191(9):1403–9.
70. Hollingsworth TD, Anderson R, Fraser C. HIV-1 Transmission, by Stage of Infection. Journal of Infectious Diseases. 2008;198:687–93.
71. Hudson CP. Concurrent partnerships could cause AIDS epidemics. International Journal of STD and AIDS. 1993;4(5):249–53.
72. Watts CH, May RM. The influence of concurrent partnerships on the dynamics of HIV/AIDS. Mathematical Biosciences. 1992;108(1):89–104.
73. Halperin DT, Epstein H. Concurrent Sexual Partnerships Help to Explain Africa's High HIV Prevalence: Implications for Prevention. Lancet. 2004;364(9428):4–6.
74. Halperin DT, Epstein H. Why is HIV Prevalence so Severe in Southern Africa? Southern African Journal of HIV Medicine. 2007(March):19–25.
75. Morris M, Kretzschmar M. Concurrent Partnerships and the Spread of HIV. AIDS. 1997;11(5):641–8.
76. Morris M, Epstein H, Wawer M. Timing Is Everything: International Variations in Historical Sexual Partnership Concurrency and HIV Prevalence. PLoS One. 2010;5(11):1–8.
77. Epstein H, Halperin D. Global sexual behaviour. Lancet. 2007;369(9561):557; author reply
78. Mah TL, Halperin DT. Concurrent Sexual Partnerships and the HIV Epidemics in Africa: Evidence to Move Forward. AIDS and Behavior. 2008.
79. Epstein H. AIDS and the irrational. Bmj. 2008;337:a2638.
80. UNAIDS Reference Group on Estimates MaP. Consultation on Concurrent Sexual Partnerships. Nairobi, Kenya: UNAIDS, 2009 30 November 2009. Report No.
81. Sawers L, Isaac A. Partnership duration, concurrency, and HIV in sub-Saharan Africa. African Journal of AIDS Research. 2017; 16(2):155-64.
82. Sawers L. Measuring and modelling concurrency. J Int AIDS Soc. 2013;16:17431.
83. Adimora AA, Schoenbach VJ, Bonas DM, Martinson FE, Donaldson KH, Stancil TR. Concurrent sexual partnerships among women in the United States. Epidemiology. 2002;13(3):320–7.
84. Adimora AA, Schoenbach VJ, Doherty IA. Concurrent sexual partnerships among men in the United States. American journal of public health. 2007;97(12):2230–7.
85. Leridon H, van Zessen G, Hubert M. The Europeans and their Sexual Partners. In: Hubert M, Bajos N, Sandfort T, editors. Sexual Behaviour and HIV/AIDS in Europe: Comparisons of National Surveys. London: UCL Press; 1998. p. 165–96.
86. Eaton J, Hallett T, Garnett G. Concurrent Sexual Partnerships and Primary HIV Infection: A Critical Interaction. AIDS and Behavior. 2010;15(4):687–92.

87. Sawers L, Isaac AG, Stillwaggon E. HIV and concurrent sexual partnerships: Modelling the role of coital dilution. Journal of the International AIDS Society. 2011;14(44).
88. Pearce N. Traditional Epidemiology, Modern Epidemiology, and Public Health. American journal of public health. 1996;86(5):678–83.
89. Habicht JP, Victora CG, Vaughan JP. Evaluation designs for adequacy, plausibility and probability of public health programme performance and impact. International journal of epidemiology. 1999;28(1):10–8.
90. Stillwaggon E. Complexity, cofactors, and the failure of AIDS policy in Africa. Journal of the International AIDS Society. 2009;12(12):1–9.
91. Stillwaggon E. Living with uncertainty. Trends in Parasitology. 2012;28(7):261–6.
92. Dreyfuss ML, Fawzi WW. Micronutrients and vertical transmission of HIV-1. Am J Clin Nutr. 2002;75(6):959–70.
93. Wiysonge CS, Shey MS, Sterne JA, Brocklehurst P. Vitamin A supplementation for reducing the risk of mother-to-child transmission of HIV infection. Cochrane Database of Systematic Reviews. 2005(4):CD003648.
94. Coutsoudis A, Pillay K, Spooner E, Kuhn L, Coovadia HM. Randomized trial testing the effect of vitamin A supplementation on pregnancy outcomes and early mother-to-child HIV-1 transmission in Durban, South Africa. South African Vitamin A Study Group. AIDS. 1999;13(12):1517–24.
95. Grosskurth H, Todd J, Senkoro K, Newell J, Klokke A, Changalucha J, et al. Impact of Improved Treatment of Sexually Transmitted Diseases on HIV Infection in rural Tanzania: Randomised Controlled Trial. Lancet. 1995;346(8974):530–6.
96. Downs JA, van Dam GJ, Changalucha JM, Corstjens PLAM, Peck RN, de Dood CJ, et al. Association of schistosomiasis and HIV infection in Tanzania. American Journal of Tropical Medicine and Hygiene. 2012;87(5):868–73.
97. Victora CG, Habicht JP, Bryce J. Evidence-based public health: moving beyond randomized trials. American journal of public health. 2004;94(3):400–5.
98. Black N. Why we need observational studies to evaluate the effectiveness of health care. Bmj. 1996;312(7040):1215–8.
99. Hill AB. The Environment and Disease: Association or Causation? Proceedings of the Royal Society of Medicine. 1965;58:295–300.
100. Stillwaggon E. Better economic tools for evaluating health and development investments. AIDS. 2014;28(3):435–7.
101. Remme M, Vassall A, Lutz B, Luna J, Watts C. Financing structural interventions: going beyond HIV-only value for money assessments. AIDS. 2014;28(3):425–34.

HOMA HOODFAR

29 WHY CIRCUMCISION?

In the discipline of global health, which looks at health issues in societies around the world, it is common for people to encounter cultural ideas and practices that are very alien to their own ideas of normal. This can be personally challenging because others' practices might offend our own notions of morality, propriety, and social justice. How can one distinguish between cultural difference and structural violence? In working in global health, it is important to ask the question: do we seek to change others' behaviors because they are actually unhealthy or is it because of our own cultural perspective?

The topic of this reading is a controversial one, which makes some students uncomfortable or angry. Surgeries involving female genital cutting have many names—including female circumcision (FGC), female genital mutilation (FGM), and female genital modification (FGM). These different names reflect different attitudes of the people using the terms. Within the world of global health, there are activist groups who have a goal of eradicating this cultural practice. There are several reasons given for such strong opposition: it is surgery done on girls too young to consent; it results in a lack of sexual enjoyment; it is oppressive of women; or it is medically dangerous. Opponents conclude that the practice is a violation of human rights.

One important issue is the degree to which the practice is medically dangerous. Is the pain and risk of infection because of the surgery itself or because of the lack of anesthetics and a sterile context? From an epidemiological standpoint, the answer to that question is highly contested, and good data are scarce.

Anthropologists do know a good deal about the cultural practice—why people do it, what the variations of the practice are, and where it is most common. There are several common misconceptions about FGC in Europe and North America. First, the practice is not required by Islam in some general sense. Many Muslim cultures around the world don't engage in this practice at all, and some Christian cultures do. Second, the practice is motivated by notions of beauty, marriageability, and what is normal and expected. Third, there are active discussions about the practice, even in societies with high rates of the surgery, and there are indications that the custom is changing—not necessarily because of international campaigns but because of modernization in general.

One question is "Whose business is this?" In global health, this might be a question of how much medical or psychological harm is being done. From a local point of view, this may be an issue of cultural tradition.

This selection describes what some women in Cairo had to say about the practice when the anthropologist Homa Hoodfar worked there in the 1980s. Hoodfar made friendships with and hung out with lower-middle-class women in Cairo to learn about the dynamics of their marriages. One of the things that came up as a topic of conversation was circumcision. These conversations reveal perspectives that can be surprising to many Americans.

As you read this selection, ask yourself the following questions:

- **Women in societies that practice FGM/FGC are motivated, in part, by questions of beauty and aesthetics. Given that fact, can you think of practices of body modification done in North America for the same reason?**
- **For women who have gone through this procedure, what might it mean that people from other societies call them "mutilated"?**
- **Can you think of ways in which health risks might be reduced?**

Excerpted from *Between Marriage and the Market*, by Homa Hoodfar. Berkeley: University of California Press, 1997, 256–262.

- **What are the linkages between FGM/FGC and patriarchy? Is the custom supported by women, men, or both? Is this a violation of human rights?**
- **Why might this custom persist?**

CONTEXT

Homa Hoodfar is an emerita professor of anthropology at Concordia University in Montreal. In addition to the book that this excerpt is drawn from, *Between Marriage and the Market* (1997), Hoodfar has written extensively about women's experiences in both Egypt and Iran. In 2016, Hoodfar was visiting Iran and was arrested for charges tied to being a feminist. She was held for 3 months before being released after negotiations with the Canadian government. (Hoodfar is a dual citizen of Canada and Iran.) She has said she survived her imprisonment by using her research skills—after her release, she told the Guardian newspaper, "I decided, I'm an anthropologist and I'm here, so I can use this as a method of doing anthropological fieldwork. It wasn't fieldwork that I had chosen, it was not a project I wanted to write, but there I was."

Although femininity and masculinity are viewed as natural phenomena in men and women, nonetheless, it is assumed that children's sexuality can be enhanced through appropriate social and cultural practices. Thus an important responsibility of parents is to ensure that their children are socialized into proper gender roles and appropriate sexual desires. In this context, circumcision is viewed as a crucial channel through which the sexuality of boys and girls is enhanced, which in turn is a step toward ensuring a successful marriage and family life for them. Circumcision, or *tahur* (literally, an act of purification), is just such a vehicle. In fact, some parents were convinced that circumcision was the single most important factor in producing sexually healthy children, particularly daughters. It was considered the most important event in the lives of boys and girls between birth and marriage.

All boys in the neighborhood were circumcised by the time they reached the age of seven or eight. Men and women were aware that male tahur was not a universal practice despite its wide use in the Middle East. However, all Muslims were conscious that Islam requires boys to be circumcised to confirm their membership in the male Muslim community. Several fathers pointed out that overlooking this important *wagib* (duty) is considered a great sin. A few mentioned that even Americans have realized the health benefits of circumcision and many have their sons circumcised. In contrast to the discussions of female circumcision, however, there were no direct references to a connection between circumcision and fertility or masculinity; rather the stress was put on health issues and Islamic requirement.

Many people described the elaborate ceremonies and feasts traditionally held for boys' circumcisions, particularly eldest sons', which took place when boys were about eight or nine. Today, however, the situation is very different, and few people in Cairo throw such parties. In fact, among the families I lived with, boys whose birth was attended by a doctor (at the hospital or at home) were circumcised at birth; others underwent the operation within the first few years of life with a minimum of ceremony.[1] Several families with sons around the same age arranged to take the boys to a hospital, or sometimes to a *hakim* (a traditionally trained health practitioner). The boys were kept in bed, or at least indoors for a few days, and they would be given sweets and sometimes a new toy. A favorite meat dish, usually chicken, was prepared for them. Neighbors would visit and congratulate the family; one or two close friends might bring candy or pastries. People refrained from mentioning the boys' pain and discomfort. Fathers were actively involved in decisions regarding their sons' circumcision, particularly for boys older than two.

[1] During the two and a half years I spent in the field, there were none of the elaborate parties I had been told about. Some of the women explained that if they had more money, they would have given the boys a party; they believed that the rich still held lavish circumcision parties and feasts.

On the whole, relative to girls' circumcision, the boys' circumcisions were nonevents.

All girl children in the neighborhoods were circumcised, usually between the ages of eight and twelve, to ensure femininity and fertility and as part of their preparation for marriage and motherhood. Although female circumcision has been prohibited and the Egyptian government launched a campaign against it in the sixties, all the women I met in the neighborhoods, regardless of regional, educational, and family backgrounds, were circumcised (or at least claimed to be), and none objected to or suggested not doing the same with their daughters.[2] Most women were aware of the law, but they either did not take the ban seriously or considered that such matters were none of the government's business. Nonetheless, it was commonly known that in many cultures, especially in Western societies, women are not circumcised. To justify female circumcision, women initially explained it to me as an Islamic practice. When I reminded them that people in Iran or Saudi Arabia and many other Muslim countries do not practice it, they then suggested it was part of Egyptian culture. Occasionally, in support of this view, the women added that Christian Copts also share this Egyptian tradition. It was common knowledge that there are different degrees of circumcision (infibulation) and that a more severe type, which they did not approve of and referred to as Pharaonic, was practiced among the Sudanese. As in the case of males, circumcision was considered purification, and the process involved removing all or part of the clitoris to make women feminine and sexually more receptive to men as well as to improve fertility.[3]

In discussing why women need to be circumcised, I was struck by the way it was described to me: "It makes a woman clean, soft, and feminine. It makes a woman desire a man and be receptive to his seed, and it increases her chances of getting pregnant." Women frequently stated that the clitoris, were it not removed, would continue to grow and become like a penis, making women cold to men. Apparently, it was for this reason that circumcision of women was often delayed until the girls were older, for the clitoris might grow again and women would have to undergo a second operation. In support of their belief, my female informants explained that upper-class women (who are not circumcised due to the influence of the West) often marry very late and frequently have unhappy marriages, sometimes resulting in divorce. They suggested that this was because uncircumcised women are too cold sexually and are not receptive to their husbands' sexual demands. Some women used my own case to prove their point. They remarked that at the age of twenty-seven my spinsterhood was attributable to the fact that my parents had chosen not to have me circumcised, and I had thus grown cold to men.[4]

As the only uncircumcised woman, I was often the subject of jokes and teasing. Frequently friends jokingly suggested that they organize a circumcision for me before my return to England so as to ensure my eventual marriage and pregnancy. In fact, I was taken by surprise when close to my departure from Cairo in 1986, one of the older neighborhood women who had become fond of me and treated me like her daughter took me aside. She suggested, seriously, that maybe I should consider having a circumcision if I was interested in family life, which she thought I must be since my research and studies dealt primarily with women, family life, and children. She said that, of course, if my own mother had been there she would have discussed it with her since no woman should organize her own circumcision. I politely refused, saying that no women in my family, or in our Iranian tradition, were circumcised and that all modern medical sciences (in which they had a great

[2] More educated women said that in the old days, when hygiene was poor, many women had complications but added that nowadays few women face these problems because of improved cleanliness during the procedure. They pointed out that if young girls do experience infection after the operation, they are easily treated with injections of penicillin or other antibiotics.

[3] Although I received an invitation to accompany two girls who were to be circumcised to the home of the hakima, I refused on the grounds that it was un-Islamic and that I could not bear to see the little girls suffer so much pain. The neighborhood women thought that I was too sensitive.

[4] In fact, at the time I was not twenty-seven but thirty-three. I had discovered early in my fieldwork that at my age, the neighborhood women would find my choice to remain unmarried not just anomalous but suspicious. Therefore, in 1983 when in a guessing game they could not believe that I was more than twenty-four, I did not correct them. My apparent lack of interest in men was viewed as a lack of femininity, which only confirmed their views about uncircumcised women.

deal of trust) indicated that circumcision was bad for a woman's health and had a negative impact on reproductive health. She looked at me in disbelief and said that the doctors must have looked at the Sudanese type of circumcision, not at the Egyptian. She then asked me why Egypt has the largest population if circumcision is bad, and why it is that throughout the Arab world men want to marry Egyptian women.[5] My explanation that the cost of marriage was lower in Egypt than in Iraq, Kuwait, and Saudi Arabia was dismissed, as she pointed out that the cost of marriage in those places had gone up only recently, but the preference for Egyptian women goes back centuries. After a few seconds of silence, she told me that even the Egyptian men who go to Europe and marry Europeans with white skin and yellow hair divorce these wives after a while and marry Egyptian women because they make men happy (meaning sexually) and are very good mothers. Unfortunately, the news of my marriage, to a man who my friends in the neighborhoods decided was much older than I by looking at his photograph, later combined with the fact that I had no children after four years of marriage, only served to confirm their views (see also Sholkamy 1994; Inhorn 1996: 29–37).

Apparently, female circumcision in the past occasioned a celebration for women neighbors and relatives, and the circumcised girls were given small gifts. The celebrations are now much more modest and, like boys' circumcision parties, generally consist of visits from close friends and relatives of the mother who may or may not offer a little present to the circumcised girl. If the family's budget allows, the girl might receive a new dress or other item of clothing, or maybe a small piece of jewelry such as earrings. She rests for a week or so and is given nourishing food; chicken or pigeon is prepared if the family can afford it. Traditionally, girls bathed in the Nile River after circumcision; now, I was told, the girls throw the piece of flesh into the Nile (see also Early 1993: 102–106).

Fathers remained aloof during their daughters' circumcision, their role being limited primarily to paying the bills. As a young Muslim woman, it was not appropriate for me to discuss these issues with men. However, most women I spoke with said that their husbands had no opinion on the subject. On a couple of occasions men brought up the subject themselves, having heard that I was opposed to the practice as "un-Islamic." One man who had migrated to several Gulf countries and knew that the circumcision of women has nothing to do with Islam but is an African tradition told me that when he tried to convince his wife that perhaps the operation was unnecessary for their daughter, his wife accused him of being cheap and not wanting to pay the expenses. So he gave in and his daughter was circumcised.

Some of the men who were among the more educated persons of my sample explained to me that they were not sure of the wisdom of the practice but had been persuaded by their womenfolk that it would be a shame for daughters to grow up uninterested in men and have unhappy marriages. At least in two cases women also told the fathers who were reluctant to perform the circumcision that they would have to accept the responsibility if their daughters could not find suitors because everyone would know if their daughters were not circumcised. Fathers were reminded that there are few men who would want to marry an uncircumcised woman. This, of course, was an effective threat since no father wanted to jeopardize his daughter's chances of finding a good husband. As one woman who had just circumcised her daughter and knew of my reservations told me, "The fact is that men who have reservations about circumcision would marry circumcised women, but those who see circumcision as necessary for women would not marry uncircumcised women." Fertility and marriage are so important that few parents will risk allowing their daughters to go uncircumcised, lest it endanger her marriageability and chances of motherhood.

Moreover, circumcision, for boys and especially for girls, was an important event in other social and individual respects.[6] Contrary to my expectation

[5] There is a strong assumption among Egyptian women, but also men, that Arab men are particularly fond of Egyptian women and prefer to marry them. With the advent of migration and more contact with the Arab world, many non-Egyptian Arab men have chosen to marry Egyptian women, often because the cost of marriage in their own countries is very high. Additionally, Egyptian movies, television soap operas, and music have given a certain cachet to Egyptian/Cairene women, who are assumed to be more assertive and outspoken.

[6] See Lightfoot-Klein 1989 and Toubia 1993, 1995 for a thorough study of circumcision in Africa.

based on my reading of the feminist literature,[7] I found women often shared their circumcision experiences and talked light-heartedly of the shock and pain they went through. In a way, this common experience of women was a rite of passage to the feminine world. None felt bitter about it, although all knew that many Muslim and non-Muslim women were not circumcised. A few women pointed out that both girls and boys have to experience pain and discomfort to appreciate sexual pleasure in adulthood.

My observations and the many discussions I had with women on the subject of female circumcision contradicted almost everything I had heard or read about the topic in England. I realized, despite the impression fostered in the literature and through feminist lectures I had attended, that men actually had a minimal direct role in female circumcision. Moreover, women's unreserved and open discussion about sexual pleasure clearly contradicted the common assumption about the loss of sexual interest and feeling among circumcised women, which included my entire sample.[8] What is significant is that women's perceptions of their situation contradict the widely held belief that circumcision is meant to control women's sexuality.[9] Those who practiced circumcision in these low-income communities of Cairo believed that circumcision makes women more sexually receptive to men and is an important catalyst for creating a healthy sexual relationship between a husband and wife.[10] Given the extremely wide gap between the women's perception of circumcision and the perceptions of those who advocate its abolition, it is not surprising that the campaign for the eradication of female circumcision has not been successful. Views of women who practice female circumcision and see it as an integral part of their lives have not been taken into consideration in devising strategies that would convince them to stop the practice for their own good. Unfortunately, neither the government nor its critics have used the legitimacy of Islam to discourage women from practicing female circumcision.

REFERENCES

Abdalla, Raqiya. 1982. *Sisters in Affliction: Circumcision and Infibulation of Women in Africa.* London: Zed Press.

Early, Evelyn A. 1993. *Baladi Women of Cairo: Playing with an Egg and a Stone.* Boulder, Colo.: Lynne Rienner.

Hayes, Rose Oldfield. 1975. "Female Genital Mutilation, Fertility Control, Women's Roles and Patrilineage in Modern Sudan: A Functional Analysis." *American Ethnologist* 2: 617–633.

Inhorn, Marcia. 1996. *Quest for Conception: Gender, Infertility, and Egyptian Medical Traditions.* Philadelphia: University of Pennsylvania Press.

Lightfoot-Klein, Hanny. 1989. "A History of Clitorial Excision and Infibulation Process in the Western World." In Lightfoot-Klein, *Prisoners of Ritual: An Odyssey into Female Genital Circumcision in Africa.* New York: Haworth Press.

Sa'dawi, Nawal el-. 1980. *The Hidden Face of Eve: Women in the Arab World.* London: Zed Press.

Sholkamy, Hania. 1994. "The Quest for Fertility." Paper presented at the Annual Meeting of the American Anthropological Association, Atlanta.

Toubia, Nahid. 1993. *Female Genital Mutilation: A Call for Global Action.* New York: Women Ink.

Toubia, Nahid. 1995. *Female Genital Mutilation.* New York: Rainbo.

[7] See, for instance, Hayes 1975; el-Sa'dawi 1980; Abdalla 1982.

[8] Obviously, this study has not been a medical one. Neither has it been a comparative one with a control sample of uncircumcised women. I am relying only on what I have observed. However, I have come across at least one case study in Sudan that has confirmed that circumcised women do experience orgasm (Lightfoot-Klein 1989).

[9] This view of circumcision is perhaps more true for Western culture than for the Middle East. In the nineteenth and early twentieth centuries clitoridectomy was practiced in North America to curb women's sexual desire (Lightfoot-Klein 1989).

[10] This belief is so strong that young men who seem to be uninterested in women and sexually less inclined are said to be better off marrying uncircumcised women, who are assumed to be less interested in men.

30 SAVING MOTHERS' LIVES IN SRI LANKA

The United Nations' Millennium Development Goal 5 was to "improve maternal health." One specific target was to reduce maternal mortality by 75% between 1990 and 2015. While the progress made toward that goal was very impressive, the goal was not reached; the decline in maternal mortality was around 45% on a global level. Nearly all countries made maternal deaths decline, although the United States is one glaring exception.

On a worldwide basis there remain huge differences between countries in maternal mortality ratios (MMR: deaths per 100,000 live births). The five worst MMRs in African countries are all over 800 (meaning that nearly one in one hundred births results in the mother dying). Given this level of risk, it is no wonder that women can be very afraid of childbirth. Women in high-income countries are often concerned about optimizing their "birth experience;" in other countries, the concern is avoiding death.

In contrast, the risk of death during childbirth in high-income countries is generally extremely low; for example, the MMR in Greece is three. The exception is the United States, where the MMR has risen from twelve in 1990 to twenty-eight in 2013; this means that the United States ranks forty-eighth globally in this important measure of the accessibility of prenatal care and childbirth. As this article describes, this ratio is quite close to the MMR in Sri Lanka. The US MMR has risen even though childbirth in the United States costs an average of $3,000 to $4,500 for uncomplicated vaginal births and between $7,500 and $10,500 for cesarean births. (The cost variation between states is remarkable: New Jersey rates are about $10,000 higher than the national average—and higher-cost areas do not necessarily have lower rates of maternal death.)

Maternal mortality is a global health issue that has attracted much attention from donors. It is possible to decrease these deaths to very low rates since the vast majority of such deaths or childbirth injuries are preventable. There are several common reasons for death during childbirth. The primary cause is excessive bleeding in the postpartum period. Many countries with high MMRs either have very dispersed populations or an inadequate number of health facilities. A woman at risk of death during childbirth needs to receive adequate obstetric care, and this is only possible when the right equipment and staff are available. In a sense, MMR can be considered a proxy measure for the availability and quality of obstetric services and health services in general.

In the past, global health efforts emphasized the training of traditional birth attendants in biomedically proper sterile procedures. Now, the emphasis is on having births in medical facilities. In addition to this, communities need to be prepared for the danger of excessive bleeding and the necessity of emergency transportation; this means that men need to be educated too.

One model country for improving maternal health is Sri Lanka, and its success is described in this article. Sri Lanka's MMR was 405 in 1955 and was reduced to 32 by 2013. In contrast, India's MMR in 2013 was 189 and Nepal's was 291. Sri Lanka is a lower middle-income country with a notable family health program in which a midwife/primary health-care worker is assigned to every 3,000 citizens. As described here, nearly all births in Sri Lanka occur in medical facilities. In addition, nearly all new mothers are visited at home by a midwife within one week of birth.

As you read this article, consider the following questions:

- **What impacts did the determinants of health have on changes in maternal mortality in Sri Lanka? What impacts did the provision of medical care have?**
- **What role might gender equity and women's education play in maternal mortality rates? What might be the exact mechanisms by which they affect maternal mortality?**

Ruth Levine and the What Works Working Group, "Saving Mother's Lives in Sri Lanka." In *Millions Saved: Proven Successes in Global Health*. Washington, DC: Center for Global Development, 2007.

- **Ask a mother if she was ever worried about the possibility of her own death when her child was born. What were her major worries? Why do you think she felt that way?**
- **This article identifies reasons for the success in Sri Lanka as being related to access to facilities, professionalization of midwifery, public education and institutional organization, and a commitment to quality improvement. In your opinion, which of these is the most important? Why?**

CONTEXT

This article is a case study from the book *Millions Saved: Global Successes in Global Health* (2007), edited by Ruth Levine and published by the Center for Global Development. This book, currently in its second edition, includes twenty case studies from around the world. All of the cases were judged to be effective, cost-efficient, based on real partnerships, and having measurable results. Most of the cases tend to involve single disease oriented "vertical" programs instead of ones involving primary health care. The Center for Global Development (www.cgdev.org) is an excellent source of information in global health and economic development. Ruth Levine, a health economist, is currently the program director of Global Development and Population at the William and Flora Hewlett Foundation.

The reduction in deaths during pregnancy and delivery has long been held out as a major international public health goal, but many countries have had difficulties making progress toward it. Most observers now agree that there are no quick fixes, and that the solution will come with the strengthening of now-failing health systems in many poor countries, building up the training of professional and paraprofessional health workers, improving access to both basic and higher-level services, and ensuring the availability of basic medical supplies and medications to deal with obstetric problems. The case of Sri Lanka demonstrates how rapidly progress can occur when those fundamental building blocks are in place.

Mothers Shouldn't Die in Childbirth

Pregnancy and childbirth are natural events and typically require little or no medical intervention for either mother or baby. But in about 15 percent of all pregnancies, a severe complication affects the woman—for example, maternal diabetes or dangerously high blood pressure sets in, excessive bleeding occurs during childbirth, or the mother suffers from a serious postpartum infection. In about 1 to 2 percent of the cases, women often require major surgery and may die without effective treatment of these complications.

Over and above the baseline risk of pregnancy, women are in danger of dying during pregnancy and childbirth if their general health is poor. Malnutrition, malaria, immune system deficiency, tuberculosis, and heart disease all contribute to maternal mortality. In addition, use of unsafe abortion services is a major risk factor for maternal death.

Maternal mortality,[1] the death of a woman while pregnant or within about two months after the end of the pregnancy, echoes through families for many generations. Women who die are in the prime of their lives and are likely to be leaving behind one or more children—a loss that places at risk those children's social development, health, education, and future life chances. The death of a woman in childbirth is highly correlated with the survival of the child she is bearing; the risk of a child dying before age 5 is doubled if the mother dies in childbirth. At least one fifth of the burden of disease for children

[1] The official definition of the maternal mortality ratio is the number of maternal deaths for every 100,000 live births. "Maternal" death refers to a death during pregnancy or within 42 days after the end of the pregnancy from a cause related to the pregnancy or its management. Thus, the death of a pregnant woman from an accident or an infectious disease not specifically related to the pregnancy would not count in the numerator.

under 5 is associated with poor maternal health.[1] Because poor women are far more likely to die than better-off women, maternal mortality is one of the factors contributing to the transmission of poverty from one generation to the next.

Interventions to detect pregnancy-related health problems before they become life threatening, and to manage major complications when they do occur, are well known and require relatively little in the way of advanced technology. What is required, however, is a health system that is organized and accessible—physically, financially, and culturally—so that women deliver in hygienic circumstances, those who are at particularly high risk for complications are identified early, and help is available to respond to emergencies when they occur. Although some maternal deaths are unavoidable even under the most favorable circumstances, the vast majority can be prevented through systematic and sustained efforts.

Because of overall high health risks and weak health systems, almost all maternal deaths take place in developing countries. Ninety-nine percent of the 585,000 maternal deaths each year occur in poor nations.

The extremes tell the story: Women in the poorest sub-Saharan countries have a 1 in 8 chance of dying during their lifetime because of pregnancy; Western European women have a risk of 1 in 4,800. And in the developing world, maternal death is very much the tip of the iceberg: For each maternal death, somewhere between 30 and 50 other women experience serious injury or infection because of pregnancy and childbirth. In developing countries, more than 40 percent of pregnancies lead to complications, illness, or permanent disability in the mother or child.[2]

During the past several decades, as child health indicators have generally improved in the developing world and even as fertility rates have fallen, the WHO estimates that maternal mortality has remained relatively unchanged at a high level. Some countries, however, have been able to make significant and sustained progress toward making pregnancy safer for women, even beyond what would be expected with general improvements in living conditions and female health. The lessons from those settings are now informing the approaches international agencies promote.

Sri Lanka's Public Health Traditions

Sri Lanka, an ethnically diverse country of almost 20 million people living on a densely populated island in South Asia, has a storied history of public-sector commitment to human development. Although it is (and always has been) a poor country, with a current average annual per capita income of $740, the development of social services even before independence in 1948 has far exceeded the gains made in countries at similar economic levels. Access to public education was rapidly expanded during the first half of the 1900s, and schooling of girls has long been much more common in Sri Lanka than in neighboring countries in the region. As a result, 89 percent of Sri Lankan adult women are literate, compared with a South Asian average of 43 percent.[3]

Health services, too, have benefited from strong public-sector leadership. Going back to the 1930s, the government focused on expanding free health services in rural areas, with attention given to preventive services and especially control of major communicable diseases. Financing for this effort was derived largely from income taxes. Currently, life expectancy in Sri Lanka is 71 years for men and 76 for women, compared with 57 for men and 58 for women on average in low-income countries.[3]

One unusual asset to which Sri Lanka lays claim is a good civil registration system, which has been in place since 1867. This system, which first started recording maternal deaths around 1900, has provided valuable information for planning and monitoring progress. So, unlike in most poor countries where maternal mortality estimates are based on very imperfect sources and methods, Sri Lanka benefits from relatively good data and a tradition within the public administration of using it.

Elements of Success

Sri Lanka's success in reducing maternal deaths is attributed to widespread access to maternal health care, which is built upon a strong health system that provides free services to the entire population, the professionalization and broad use of midwives, the systematic use of health information to identify problems and guide decision making, and targeted quality improvements. These elements have been introduced in steps, with emphasis first on improving overall (and particularly rural) access to both lower- and higher-level facilities, then on reaching particularly vulnerable populations, and later on quality improvements.[2]

Access

The first challenge in this country that is largely rural was access. The creation of a basic health service infrastructure, starting in the 1930s, extended access across rural areas to a range of preventive and curative services, enabling initial improvements in maternal health. At the lowest level, the infrastructure consisted of health units staffed by a medical officer, who was responsible for serving the population within a given area. Within each of these health areas, public health midwives provided care for all pregnant women.

A viable referral system for both pregnancy-related and other health problems was established from the early days. The health units were—and continue to be—supported by cottage hospitals designed to offer very basic services; rural hospitals and maternity homes at a primary level; district hospitals and peripheral units at the secondary level; and tertiary provincial hospitals with specialist services, teaching hospitals, and specialist maternity hospitals.

At both the lower and higher levels, the number of facilities was expanded rapidly, increasing from 112 government hospitals in 1930 (about 182 beds per 100,000 people) to 247 hospitals in 1948 (close to 250 beds per 100,000). The secondary and tertiary institutions also underwent expansion in the 1950s.

No referral system works without accessible transportation—a need that was identified relatively early in Sri Lanka's health system development. Between 1948 and 1950, the national ambulance fleet was increased from 12 to 67 ambulances. All provincial hospitals had between three and five ambulances each, as did major district hospitals and those in more remote areas.[4]

Professionalization of Midwifery

While the basic health infrastructure was being developed, specific attention was paid to the problem of who would deliver what type of services and, in particular, how maternal health services would be delivered. The path chosen was to depend on a large number of clinically qualified midwives. This strategy has proved successful both in Sri Lanka and elsewhere (see Box 30–1).

From early days, public health midwives have underpinned the health unit network. Each midwife serves a population of 3,000 to 5,000 and lives within the local area. Midwives' duties include visiting pregnant women at home, registering them for care, encouraging them to attend antenatal clinics, and working with the doctor who runs those clinics. The midwives are considered to be one of the most important elements in the excellent health performance of the country. Supervision and a referral network back up midwives, who undergo an 18-month training program. They report to supervisors, typically nurse-midwives, who have nursing training in addition to the basic midwife preparation; the supervisors then report to the medical officer. Established procedures for service delivery and supervision, along with frequent in-service training, help midwives stay current and deliver high-quality services.

Importantly, public health midwives are part of both the health system and their local communities and thus provide a valuable link between the women and the health units. Even when a midwife does not attend a birth, the family knows how to find her in the event of a problem. It is widely maintained that the public health midwives are key to sustaining the population's confidence in and satisfaction with the public maternal health care services.

The growth in the number of midwives was rapid, while at the same time fertility was falling. As a result, while in 1935 there were 219 live births per government midwife on average, by 1960 the ratio had fallen to 143 live births per midwife and by 1995 to 51 live births per midwife (see Table 30–1).

[2] Our understanding of the pace and causes for decline in maternal mortality is due to a study by Pathmanathan and colleagues (2003), which sheds light on the main factors of success. Unless otherwise noted, information in this case study is drawn from that source.

BOX 30.1 The Midwife Approach

The relationship between low maternal mortality and extensive use of professional midwives to deliver antenatal, birthing, and postpartum services, which is seen in the developing world today, has been observed historically in the industrialized world. In countries where doctors predominantly assisted births in the period around 1920, such as the United States, New Zealand, and Scotland, the maternal mortality ratio was 600 or more per 100,000 live births. During the same period, in countries where doctors and midwives equally attended births, including France, Ireland, Australia, and England, maternal mortality was lower, averaging around 500 per 100,000 live births. And strikingly, during the same period, in countries where midwives attended most births—Norway, Sweden, the Netherlands, and Denmark—the maternal mortality ratio was very low, between 200 and 300 per 100,000 live births.

Professional midwives have special training to acquire clinical competence, are licensed or registered by public authorities and are given support, in the form of regular supplies as well as supervision. They also are linked to a functional referral system, so they know precisely where higher-level care can be obtained when women face obstetric emergencies.

Midwives are trusted frontline workers who have the distinct advantage of being close to where births are taking place—within the community—and thus even if they are not called in for each normal birth, they are available when the unexpected occurs.

Moreover, because midwives can be trained and supported at relatively low cost, and have salaries that are far lower than medical doctors, the effective use of this cadre of health workers is one of the keys to saving mothers' lives within a modest budget.

TABLE 30.1 Development of Government-Employed Birth Attendants, Sri Lanka, 1930–1995.

Year	Live Births per Government Midwife	Population per 1,000 Government Doctors	Government Nurses per Government Doctor	Specialist Obstetricians in Government Hospitals per 100,000 Live Births
1930	405	15.4	n.a.	n.a.
1935	219	n.a.	n.a.	n.a.
1940	n.a.	14.8	n.a.	n.a.
1945	186	n.a.	n.a.	n.a.
1950	163	11.4	1.7	n.a.
1955	157	9.2	2.3	n.a.
1960	143	8.4	2.8	n.a.
1965	n.a.	7.5	2.4	n.a.
1970	n.a.	6.5	2.9	n.a.
1975	n.a.	6.4	2.7	n.a.
1980	125	7.2	3.3	14.0
1985	85	7.4	3.8	15.0
1990	68	7.0	2.7	20.0
1995	51	4.0	2.9	23.0

Note: n.a. = not available

Source: I. Pathmanathan, Lijestrand, J., Martins, J. M., et al. (2003). *Investing in Maternal Health: Learning from Malaysia and Sri Lanka.* Washington, DC: World Bank.

Largely because of the focus on midwifery—combined with access to higher-level services—more than in many other countries, women in Sri Lanka rapidly became accustomed to the notion of attended births and, increasingly, births in hospitals. Up until 1940, skilled attendants assisted only about

30 percent of the births. By 1950, after the implementation of policies to introduce and expand the cadre of public health midwives, this percentage had doubled. Concurrently, the proportion of babies delivered in government health care facilities increased from 6 percent in 1940 to 33 percent 10 years later. Currently, skilled practitioners attend to 97 percent of the births, and the majority are in hospitals.

Information and Organization

Effective management, including the use of information for monitoring and planning, reinforced the two early building blocks of Sri Lanka's success in reducing maternal deaths—access to basic health services and professional midwifery. In the 1950s, the health education division was formed within the Ministry of Health, and medical officers of maternal and child health were designated to coordinate maternal and child health services in each district.

Quality Improvements, Including Targeting of Vulnerable Groups

In part because of the information and close monitoring provided, in the 1960s and 1970s the government identified several ways to improve the system. The Ministry of Health systematically used maternal death inquiries to identify problems in the delivery of care—for example, the reason a problematic delivery was not detected in time to save a life. The Ministry of Health would then circulate information about how to prevent similar problems.

The government's program to reach women on the tea estates—farming operations that contracted South Asian labor in large numbers—provides another example of a targeted effort to ensure good quality services for all. Women on the large, privately owned tea estates were particularly isolated, socially and physically. Once the estates were nationalized in the 1970s, the government assumed responsibility for health services, and medical officers (with transport) and public health nurses established a network of polyclinics to provide integrated maternal and child health services, including family planning services, to the tea estates. Estate management gave the women paid leave to attend the monthly polyclinics.

Bringing these women into the public health system paid off. Between 1986 and 1997, the number of women from the estates delivering in hospitals increased dramatically, from 20 percent to 63 percent.

Steady, Impressive Declines

While the maternal mortality ratio (the number of deaths during pregnancy or immediately afterward divided by the number of births) has persisted at high levels in many poor countries, Sri Lanka has been able to halve the maternal deaths (relative to the number of live births) every six to 12 years since 1935.

In the 1930s, the maternal mortality ratio in Sri Lanka was estimated to be over 2,000 per 100,000 live births. By the 1950s, the rate had declined to less than 500 per 100,000. Although data limitations prevent a full explanation of the source of these improvements, it is widely believed that successful efforts to combat malaria and the introduction of modern medical practices deserve much of the credit during this phase.

The steep decline in the maternal mortality ratio that was observed from the 1930s to the early 1950s has been attributed largely to the all-out war on malaria.[5] DDT spraying commenced in 1945 and led to a rapid decline in malaria incidence within a few years. In addition to the highly successful malaria control program, control of hookworm infection and general improvements in sanitation might also have contributed to improvements in maternal health before 1950.[6] Moreover, the rapid decline in maternal mortality during the early 1950s could be attributed to the introduction of modern medical treatment, such as antibiotics, through a health service network established in the pre-1950s era and having considerable reach in rural areas.

The maternal mortality ratio was halved again during the following 13 years, up until 1963, when the government made special efforts to extend health services, including critical elements of maternal health care, through a widespread rural health network. In the decades that followed, the public sector systematically applied stepwise strategies to improve organizational and clinical management, reducing the maternal mortality ratio by 50 percent every 6 to 12 years. And among women working on tea estates, the maternal mortality ratio declined from 120 in 1985 to 90 in 1997 as the polyclinic system was developed.

In total, this has meant a decline in the maternal mortality ratio from between 500 and 600 maternal deaths per 100,000 live births in 1950 to 60 per 100,000 today.[7]

Did Targeted Efforts Make the Difference?

The declines in maternal mortality are clear, as is information about efforts the government made to build the overall health system and to address the problem of maternal deaths in particular. A reasonable question to ask, then, is whether the system changes caused the health improvements, or just happened at the same time. Tackling this question—using data that span some 60 years—requires piecing together several types of epidemiologic evidence. And doing so yields a convincing answer.

One way to answer the question of whether system changes caused declines in maternal deaths is to compare the overall decline in female deaths with deaths due to maternal causes. Such a comparison is enlightening because overall female mortality can be assumed to be related, in large measure, to improvements in living conditions and in the general health system. In 1950, maternal deaths accounted for 19 percent of deaths among women aged 15 to 49 years. By 1996, while both maternal and all female deaths declined, maternal causes accounted for only 1.2 percent of all female deaths in the reproductive age range.

Another way to understand the cause-effect relationship is to look at the changes in maternal deaths due to individual causes known to be associated with specific health care delivery strategies. So, for example, deaths due to hypertensive disease and sepsis—two causes that are associated throughout the world with lack of access to skilled attendance—declined dramatically during the 1940s, when emphasis was being placed on increasing the availability of midwives and skilled attendants at birth. In contrast, hemorrhage did not decline significantly during the early years studied (1930–1950), when the major approaches the government took were the overall development of an accessible health care system, the control of malaria, and decreasing the proportion of home births. But between 1950 and 1970, as the government emphasized blood transfusion services and other strategies to address the problem, maternal deaths due to hemorrhage decreased from 113 to 45 per 100,000.

The main conclusion from this type of analysis is that the actions of the health system, rather than improvements in general living conditions, led to a large share of the improvements in maternal health that occurred over 60 years in Sri Lanka. The finding is reinforced by a parallel analysis of a similar trajectory of maternal mortality decline in Malaysia, which was similarly successful in achieving a sustained, long-term reduction in maternal deaths over several decades (although starting from a lower initial level). In the case of Malaysia,[8] public health researchers have drawn the link between overall and cause-specific changes in maternal mortality and implementation of a similar set of strategies: professionalizing midwifery, expanding access, mobilizing women and communities, and improving management and the ability to reach the poorest.

In Sri Lanka, the story of improvement in maternal health goes far beyond the health system itself. Mothers' health significantly benefited from effective public investment in basic health services, in improving basic living standards, and in high levels of female education. But the Sri Lankan case, like a very different experience in Honduras (see Box 30–2), reveals ways in which specific strategies to address the problem of maternal deaths greatly augmented the health benefits that would have resulted solely from broad improvements in welfare.

Relatively Low Cost

Sri Lanka has achieved much better health status and steeper declines in maternal mortality than countries at comparable income and economic growth levels—and it has done so while spending relatively little on health services, compared with those same countries. In India, for example, the maternal mortality ratio is more than 400 per 100,000 live births, and spending on health constitutes over 5 percent of GNP. In Sri Lanka, the maternal mortality ratio is less than one quarter of that, and the country spends only 3 percent of GNP on health.

BOX 30.2 The Honduran Experience

In Honduras, one of the poorest countries in the Western Hemisphere, the maternal mortality ratio declined by 38 percent between 1990 and 1997, from 182 to 108 maternal deaths per 100,000 live births. This remarkable achievement, which surprised many observers, was the result of a concerted effort by government officials and development agencies to address maternal mortality.

Although expanding access to essential health services had been a government priority since the 1980s, a study of maternal health in the early 1990s that revealed a serious problem of maternal mortality served as a "rude awakening" to the Ministry of Health, according to Dr. Isabella Danel, US Centers for Disease Control and Prevention expert on maternal health, now posted at the World Bank. This study stimulated a new focus on safe motherhood programs and the inclusion of specific maternal health priorities in the national health policy. Importantly, the government used information about differentials among geographic areas to target its efforts.

By the mid-1990s, a three-part strategy was well into implementation. The first part of the strategy was a reorganization of health services, intended to increase access to skilled care for pregnant women. This included the inauguration of community health clinics, with traditional birth attendants supervised by auxiliary nurses; the construction of maternity waiting homes attached to public hospitals; the establishment of birthing centers supervised by nurse midwives in rural areas; and the expansion of the basic health center and hospital infrastructure.

As a result of these efforts, between 1990 and 1997, Honduras' health infrastructure was expanded by 7 new area hospitals, 13 birthing centers, 36 health centers, 266 rural health centers, and 5 maternity waiting homes.

The second dimension of the strategy was the training of health workers in specific areas: Traditional birth attendants and public health system staff were trained to recognize high-risk pregnancies and deal with both routine births and obstetric emergencies. Traditional birth attendants were encouraged to accompany women with emergencies to the hospital. The final part of the strategy was community participation, in which local communities were provided with the opportunity to describe and identify solutions to their own health problems and, through newly implemented decentralization policies, were given more decision-making authority. Although this was very much a government strategy, resources from a variety of donors were channeled into its support.

Between 1990 and 1997, maternal mortality across Honduras declined, with the biggest reductions in some of the poorest and most remote areas. So while overall skilled birth attendance changed little during the period, the number of maternal deaths declined from 381 in 1990 to 258 in 1997 due to better referral of women with complications before, during, and after delivery.

The experience of Honduras, like that of Sri Lanka, challenges the notion that little can be done to act on the problem of poor maternal health in poor countries. Success depends neither on major technological innovation nor on high levels of spending, but rather on a combination of three factors: government commitment, which is often spurred by quantifying the problem; targeted actions to improve referrals and emergency services in hospitals; and expanded access to well-trained birth attendants within the community, supported by higher levels of care.[9]

Major expenditures, aside from the health infrastructure that served a variety of purposes other than maternal care, are on skilled labor. In Sri Lanka, as in other poor countries, labor is relatively cheap, and in fact, salaries for civil servants have been declining in relative terms. The country could afford widespread access to maternal health care by using a mix of health personnel: Most of the maternal health workers are well-trained but low-cost midwives and who are described as extremely dedicated. They are closely supervised by nurse-midwives, who in turn are supported by a small number of medical doctors.

Most remarkably, Sri Lanka's success has been achieved on a decreasing budget. Between 1950 and 1999, the proportion of the national budget spent on maternal health services has steadily fallen, from 0.28 percent of GDP in the 1950s to 0.16 percent in the 1990s. Originally, this was due to efficiency gains made in the 1950s and 1960s.

More recently, because salaries of government health staff have been falling, overall expenditures have declined. In addition, expenditures on private services have become relatively more important in the health sector as a whole: In 1953, an estimated 38 percent of total expenditures were private; by 1996, about half of the total spending was from private sources.[10]

Major Lessons

Sri Lanka's achievements in reducing the toll of pregnancy have been impressive and correspond to a setting where the public sector has for many decades placed priority on the population's health and education. But others can take inspiration from the country's record: In the late 1950s, when the first efforts were made to address the problem of maternal deaths, the GNP of Sri Lanka was equivalent, in constant dollars, to the national income of Bangladesh, Uganda, and Mali today and far lower than that of Pakistan, Egypt, or the Philippines. In relative terms, Sri Lanka has spent less on health—and achieved far more—than any of these countries.

The gains that Sri Lanka made were reinforced in many ways by good education, an emphasis on gender equity, and broad health system development—but the specific actions that were taken to solve the problem of maternal deaths had a separate and identifiable positive impact. In Sri Lanka, the basic health system served as an essential platform from which to work but did not itself generate the impressive results. Those were due to a step-by-step strategy to provide broad access to specific clinical services, to encourage utilization of those services, and to systematically improve quality.

REFERENCES

1. World Bank. *Safe Motherhood and the World Bank: Lessons from 10 Years of Experience.* Washington, DC: World Bank; 1999.
2. World Health Organization. *Maternal Mortality in 1995: Estimates Developed by WHO, UNICEF, and UNFPA.* Geneva, Switzerland: World Health Organization; 2001.
3. World Bank. *World Development Indicators.* Washington, DC: World Bank; 2003.
4. Wickramasinghe WG. *Administration Report of the Director of Medical and Sanitary Services for 1951.* Colombo, Sri Lanka: Ceylon Government Press; 1952.
5. Abeyesundere ANA. *Recent Trends in Malaria Morbidity and Mortality in Sri Lanka: Population Problems of Sri Lanka.* Sri Lanka: Demographic Training and Research Unit, University of Colombo; 1976.
6. Wickramasuriya GAW. Maternal mortality and morbidity in Ceylon. *J Ceylon Branch British Med Assoc.* 1939;36(2):79–106.
7. United Nations. *Human Development Report.* New York, NY: United Nations; 2003.
8. Pathmanathan I, Liljestrand J, Martins JM, et al. *Investing in Maternal Health: Learnings from Malaysia and Sri Lanka.* Washington, DC: World Bank; 2003.
9. Danel I. *Maternal Mortality Reduction, Honduras, 1990–1997: A Case Study.* Washington, DC: World Bank, Latin America and Caribbean Region; 1999.
10. Hsiao W. *A Preliminary Assessment of Sri Lanka's Health Sector and Steps Forward.* Cambridge, Mass: Harvard University and Institute of Policy Studies; 2000.

SECTION 8 CASES FOR TEACHING AND LEARNING

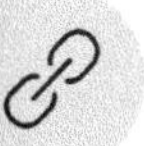

Visit the companion website, www.oup.com/us/brown-closser, for direct links to the featured online resources.

Charumilind et al., *HIV in Thailand: The 100% Condom Program*

Students examine an HIV-prevention program in Thailand and consider methods for condom promotion, particularly among sex workers. There is also a follow-up case online.

Chera et al., *Understanding and Developing Conceptual Frameworks and Causal Models in Maternal and Child Health Programming*
Students learn about the Canadian bilateral aid organization's approach to maternal and child health, specifically the use of conceptual frameworks and causal models. They explore how these conceptual frameworks and causal models might shape a maternal and child health intervention in Mali.

Cole et al., *HIV Prevention in Maharashtra, India*
Students learn about a program of peer education for HIV prevention in India. They are asked to consider the complexities of the process of transitioning the program from a nongovernmental organization to a government run model. There is also a follow-up case online, entitled *The Avahan India AIDS Initiative: Managing Targeted HIV Prevention at Scale.*

Linda Foster, *Tackling Infant Mortality at the Local Level: A Case Study in Maternal and Child Health Leadership*
This case, which takes place in a fictitious town in Virginia, is designed to help students think about leadership around infant mortality in the United States. It would be best for older students who have some experience with workplace dynamics and politics.

Beth Knowlton, *Guatemala, Reproductive Health and the UNFPA*
Students consider the complexity of building political alliances to support reproductive health legislation in Guatemala in the early 2000s.

Novick et al., *Sexually Transmitted Disease (STD) in Adolescents*
This case, set in New York State, begins with a clinical discussion of gonorrhea and chlamydia, and moves to discussions of mandatory reporting, behavioral counseling, and partner notification.

Sullivan et al., *Botswana's Program in Preventing Mother-to-Child HIV Transmission*
This case incudes a wealth of information on Preventing Mother-to-Child HIV Transmission (PMTCT). Students engage questions of maternal health care, record-keeping, and child survival.

SECTION 8 VIDEOS AND WEB RESOURCES

Visit the companion website, www.oup.com/us/brown-closser, for direct links to the featured online resources.

Maternal Mortality and Childbirth

Maternal Mortality Ratio – The World Bank
This site includes graphs of the maternal mortality ratio over time in a variety of countries, as well as graphs of attended births and prenatal care. Other health indicators are also covered. Students can easily compare trends over time in a variety of countries.

***What's Behind America's Rising Maternal Mortality Rate* – NPR/ProPublica**

This ten-minute radio piece explores why American women die at much higher rates than in other wealthy countries, and why that rate is rising. The touching and well-researched program follows the death of a neonatal nurse as a way to illustrate larger trends.

Sister

Following women and health workers in in Ethiopia, Cambodia, and Haiti, this feature-length documentary explores maternal mortality through personal stories. It includes a focus on the structural issues underlying maternal deaths.

A Walk to Beautiful

This full-length documentary is about obstetric fistula in Ethiopia. The film follows rural women with fistula who travel to Addis Ababa to get treatment.

Population

***Don't Panic: The Facts about Population* – BBC/Hans Rosling**

In this engaging documentary, Hans Rosling uses data to describe population growth over the last thousand years and argues that the view many people hold of population growth in the world is outdated. He explores patterns of resource use and population change globally. Other, shorter videos are also available on the Gapminder website. (1 hour)

HIV/AIDS

***The Lazarus Effect* – HBO and (Red)**

This moving short film explores the impact of the rollout of anti-retroviral therapy in sub-Saharan Africa. (30 min)

A Closer Walk

This powerful full-length documentary about the global AIDS epidemic follows people living with HIV/AIDS in a variety of contexts across the world. Although some of the facts in this documentary are a bit dated (it was made in 2003, before antiretroviral therapy was available to many people in sub-Saharan Africa), showing segments of the film in class can be a compelling way to illustrate some of the key issues associated with the global HIV/AIDS epidemic.

The Bloody Truth

This interactive website (and associated film, *Rise of the Killer Virus*) takes a historical perspective to tie the rise of HIV to structural issues including colonialism, as well as factors such as blood transfusions and unsterile needles. Students can compare the explanatory framework in this documentary with those in Chapters 27 and 28.

Also see the video resources on HIV/AIDS in Sections 1 and 12 of this book.

SECTION

9

Violence

This section of the book considers violence, an important and challenging problem in global health. Experiencing violence can be harmful to your health, just as suffering from a disease can be. Three levels of violence cause a massive amount of mortality, morbidity, and suffering today throughout the world: **interpersonal violence**, **social violence**, and **structural violence**. The distinctions between these levels were identified by John Galton, a leader in the field of peace studies.

The three articles in this section explore these three different types of violence. Reading 31 is about a type of interpersonal violence—**intimate partner violence (IPV)**. IPV is common everywhere in the world; in fact, physical violence against one's spouse is legal in some places.

The second type of violence is between different social groups—from local gangs to national armies. Reading 32 is about war and public health. Levy and Sidel argue that people working in global health have an ethical obligation to do everything possible to prevent or mitigate social violence. As we will see in the next section of this book (Section 10), many global health institutions arose because of war and violence. Reading 33 explores the example of Doctors Without Borders (Médecins Sans Frontières), and describes the challenges and frustration of disaster relief in war zones and refugee camps.

Finally, Reading 34 discusses structural violence. This type of violence is often invisible because it is taken for granted as a sociocultural norm. The institution of slavery is an extreme example. Social structures create and reinforce inequalities, and as Section 7 of this book explored in detail, social inequalities lead to poor health outcomes for those with less power.

» CONCEPTUAL TOOLS «

Interpersonal Violence and Intimate Partner Violence

- **Interpersonal violence** between individuals includes homicides, beatings, psychological attacks, and intimate partner violence. The most common victims of interpersonal violence are women, and perpetrators tend to be men. The prevalence of interpersonal violence is higher within disadvantaged groups.

- **Gun control is a public health issue.** The availability of firearms directly affects the likelihood of interpersonal violence leading to death.
- **Intimate Partner Violence (IPV) and sexual violence are serious, preventable public health problems that affect millions of people throughout the world.** IPV describes physical, sexual, or psychological harm by a current or former partner or spouse. IPV is a human rights violation.
- **IPV is more common than many people think.** While the prevalence of IPV is difficult to measure because of cultural differences and stigma, the WHO estimates that about one-third of women worldwide over age fifteen have experienced either physical and/or sexual intimate partner violence in their lifetime. Physical security of women is not found in any country of the world. Men are also victims of IPV, but it is less common. Figure CT9.1 shows the prevalence of IPV in the United States.
- **Risk factors** associated with IPV include being young, having low income, being food or housing insecure, abusing alcohol, having had exposure to violence as a child, and holding attitudes accepting of violence and gender inequality. Factors that protect against IPV include women's social and economic empowerment.

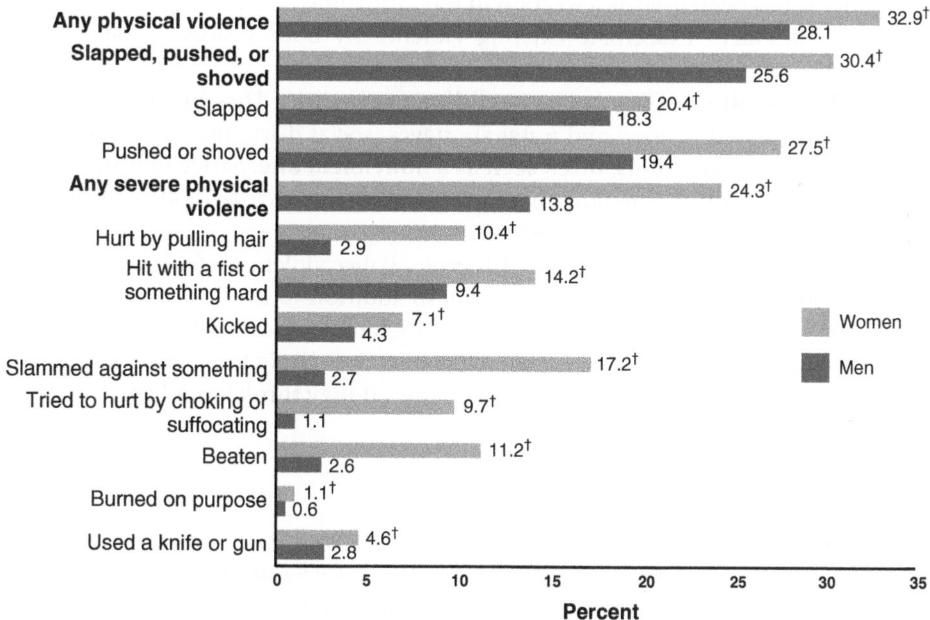

FIGURE CT9.1 Lifetime Prevalence of Physical Violence by an Intimate Partner—U.S. Women and Men.

Source: Centers for Disease Control. *National Intimate Partner and Sexual Violence Survey:* 2010, https://www.cdc.gov/violenceprevention/pdf/nisvs_report2010-a.pdf.

SOCIAL VIOLENCE

- **Social violence** occurs between social groups and includes war, terrorism, and genocide. Nation-states organize and maintain armies and police to enforce order within their territories, as well as to wage war on enemy groups. Governments often sanction social violence, and nonstate actors also use violence for political goals. While soldiers are often killed or disabled in war, the primary victims of social violence are noncombatants.
- **War kills and disables more people than many major diseases.** War is often not conceptualized as a health problem, but its health effects go far beyond the battlefield and into the future. Civilians are the major casualties in contemporary wars.
- **War is the antithesis of global health** as seen in Table CT9.1.
- **The modern technologies of violence have become more available and more lethal.** High-income countries sell sophisticated weapons throughout the world and have flooded the earth with guns. Both high- and low-income countries spend large amounts of their budgets to buy deadly inventions of the "military industrial complex"—assault rifles, bombs, aircraft, drones, or nuclear missiles—and tend to spend less on programs for health and social welfare. This is particularly the case with the United States (Figure CT9.2).
- **Rape has been used as a weapon of war.** Situations of conflict, postconflict, and displacement exacerbate existing violence by both strangers and intimate partners.
- **The casualties of war go beyond direct casualties.** They include illness and death caused by food and water shortages, social disruption, and human displacement. **Sanctions, often seen as a nonviolent alternative to war, can also cause casualties.** Sanctions that limit populations' access to food, medicine, and economic growth have health impacts.
- **Police violence is a public health issue.** Police violence is frequently directed at socially marginalized groups and, in addition to its direct negative health effects, can exacerbate other health problems. For example, police violence against injecting drug users can make them less likely to practice harm reduction practices like obtaining clean needles if they think it might attract police attention.

TABLE CT9.1. Effects of War vs Global Health Programs.

War and Violence	Global Health and Development
Kills people, both combatants and civilians	Saves lives and improves health
Maims people both physically and mentally	Reduces physical and mental suffering
Destroys infrastructure	Builds infrastructure
Exacerbates poverty	Invests in health for economic development
Increases hate and intolerance	Enhances education and understanding
Forces migration and displacement	Builds communities and cooperation
Destroys the future for individuals	Allows individuals to build a better future

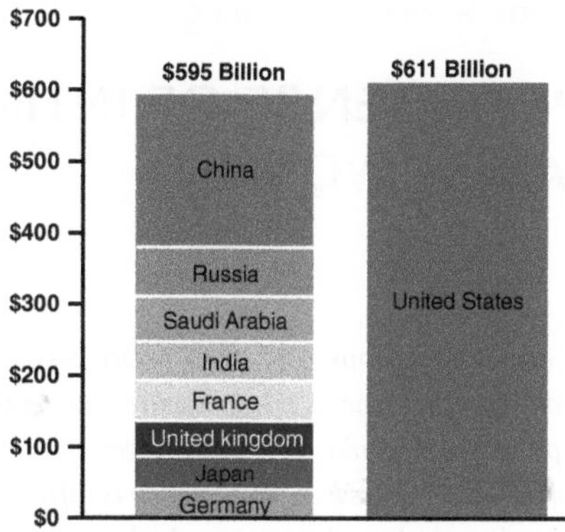

FIGURE CT9.2 The United States Spends More on Defense than the Next Seven Countries Combined.

Source: Stockholm International Peace Research Institute, SIPRI Military Expenditure Database, April 2017. Data are for 2016. Compiled by PGPF. © 2017 Peter G. Peterson Foundation.

STRUCTURAL VIOLENCE

- **Structural violence** is a more hidden type that includes systemic, taken-for-granted institutional arrangements of exploitation aimed against certain groups. Both laws and customs promote racism, sexism, classism, and ethnic discrimination that, in turn, cause physical and mental health problems. Slavery represents an extreme form of structural violence. Health inequalities are also a reflection of structural violence: the high rate of heart disease in poor communities in the United States is one example of how the effects of social structure can hurt or kill people in relatively powerless groups.
- **Cultural explanations for health disparities can cover up structural violence.** Often, widely accepted explanations for why poor people might be sicker blame the victims. For example, in the United States, people who are obese are often thought of as lazy and undisciplined and thus to blame for the health problems associated with obesity. In India, where open defecation is common, some decision makers say that there is a "culture" of open defecation among the poor, when, in most cases, the inability to afford clean safe toilets is more likely to be the cause. These broadly accepted (yet often untrue) ideas make it harder to see the ways that poverty and inequality powerfully shape risks for disease.

K. M. DEVRIES, J. Y. T. MAK, C. GARCÍA-MORENO, M. PETZOLD, J. C. CHILD, G. FALDER, S. LIM, L. J. BACCHUS, R. E. ENGELL, L. ROSENFELD, C. PALLITTO, T. VOS, N. ABRAHAMS, AND C. H. WATTS

31 THE GLOBAL PREVALENCE OF INTIMATE PARTNER VIOLENCE AGAINST WOMEN

This reading is a systematic review of a very serious global health problem. The authors combined information from a number of separate research projects to provide a cross-national study of the prevalence of intimate partner violence (IPV). The review included 141 studies conducted in eighty-one countries. In the past, IPV was often called "wife beating" or domestic violence, but the current definition of IPV includes physical, sexual, or emotional abuse occurring in any relationship. IPV is a problem on US college campuses, as well as everywhere else in the world.

There have been many international agreements condemning IPV, including the Declaration on the Elimination of Violence against Women in 1993. In the United States, IPV was legal in some states as recently as 1920, and federal legislation was only passed in 1994. The United Nations estimates that over 600 million women live where IPV is not considered a crime. Despite national laws and international agreements, IPV is one of the world's most important health issues.

It is difficult to compare the prevalence of IPV across cultures, primarily because the way women answer surveys is strongly influenced by local cultural attitudes about the acceptability of admitting to having been a victim. Where society accepts violent behavior as a "normal" part of marriage, women themselves may feel that they deserved to be beaten or raped by their husband. Alternately, if there is a stigma associated with being the victim of IPV, that may also discourage admitting that it happens. As such, global health experts assume that there is underreporting.

The fact that the meaning of emotional abuse is vague also causes methodological difficulties. Therefore, most studies focus on the physical and sexual forms of violence. Some types of IPV are very clear—in terms of homicide, for example, women are more likely to be murdered by their intimate partner than by anyone else.

This short reading summarizes a huge amount of data. Worldwide, the authors conclude that around 30% of women experience IPV at some time in their life. Lifetime experience is different than the incidence rate in a single year, which would be lower.

The chart in this article is very interesting because it shows worldwide variation in IPV rates, although it does not explain the reasons for this variation. Global health research demonstrates that IPV rates can be correlated with a number of variables, including alcohol use, childhood exposure to violence, a lack of education for women, and poverty. These factors could explain some of these differences. The differences could also be a result of cultural norms leading to different rates of women being willing to report they have experienced IPV.

This article concludes on a hopeful note by describing some successful programs focused on changing social norms that have had a significant effect of reducing rates of IPV.

As you read this article, consider the following questions:

- **When researchers focus solely on emotional/psychological violence, there is little difference between what is experienced by women and men. However, men are much less likely to be injured as a result of IPV, and men are much more likely to escalate a verbal battle into violence using a lethal weapon. Why do you think that is the case?**
- **Why might being a victim of IPV be stigmatized?**
- **How is IPV an example of a health problem that is not primarily medical? If a physician or police officer sees evidence of IPV, what do you think they should do?**

K. M. Devries, J. Y. T. Mak, C. García-Moreno, et al. "The Global Prevalence of Intimate Partner Violence against Women." *Science*, 2013, 340(28): 1527–1528.

- **Many women cannot or do not leave abusive relationships, even when their lives are in danger. Why might that be the case?**
- **There seems to be no universal relationship between IPV and women's employment. It depends on the particular sociocultural context. How do you think employment may either increase or decrease risk of IPV?**

CONTEXT

This reading appeared in *Science*, the premier journal of the American Academy for the Advancement of Science. There are fourteen co-authors, all of whom are experts in the field; many of them work at the London School of Tropical Medicine and Hygiene. A systematic review of a complex topic like IPV requires the synthesis of research studies that often use different methodologies.

Violence against women is a phenomenon that persists in all countries.[1] Since the 1993 World Conference on Human Rights and the Declaration on the Elimination of Violence against Women, the international community has acknowledged that violence against women is an important public health, social policy, and human rights concern. However, documenting the magnitude of violence against women and producing reliable comparative data to guide policy and monitor progress has been difficult.

The most common form of violence that women experience is from an intimate partner (IPV). This violence may be physical, sexual, or emotional. Most research to date has focused on assessing the prevalence and impacts of physical and/or sexual violence by partners. The short- and long-term health impacts of women's exposures to physical and/or sexual IPV are multiple.[2] For example, it is a leading cause of homicide death in women globally[3] and is associated with increased levels of depression and suicidal behaviors.[4] Prospective research from South Africa and Uganda shows that women exposed to physical and/or sexual IPV are more likely to acquire HIV infection.[5,6] The health and social impacts result in substantial economic costs, with one study estimating the cost of IPV at more than £15 billion in England and Wales in 2009 alone.[7]

There are high-level global commitments to addressing violence against women and gender inequality, including IPV. The 2013 United Nations Commission on the Status of Women focused on prevention and elimination of all forms of violence against women and girls; the UN Secretary General's UNiTE Campaign focuses on ending violence against women; and Millennium Development Goal 3 aims specifically "to promote gender equality and empower women." Similarly, many national governments have laws that explicitly criminalize intimate partner violence.

There is growing consensus in the research community on how to document the prevalence of women's exposures to physical and/or sexual partner violence in an ethically responsible way.[8] "Gold standard" research methods include the conduct of one-on-one interviews in private, where women are asked direct, specific questions about their experience of a range of violent acts, including slaps, punches, kicks, the use of weapons, and forced or coerced sex.[9]

As a result of this consensus and a greater global commitment to addressing violence against women, over the past decade, there has been a rapid expansion in the number of population studies examining IPV prevalence. However, existing surveys vary considerably in the specific measure of exposures to violence used, the populations sampled, and other characteristics. This has resulted in a large body of available prevalence data, but underlying challenges in interpretation, because of the lack of comparability across studies. We here present a synthesis of current evidence that provides new estimates of global and regional prevalence of IPV against women.

Synthesizing Evidence to Estimate Prevalence

Our research involved two main steps. First, we did a systematic review of all available global prevalence data from studies representative at national or subnational levels. We searched 26 medical and social science databases, performed additional analysis of the WHO Multi-Country Study on Women's Health and Domestic Violence (10 countries), and requested additional analysis of the International Violence Against Women Surveys (8 countries); Gender, Culture and

Alcohol: An International Study (16 countries); and the Demographic and Health Surveys to 2009 (20 countries) to obtain further prevalence estimates.

Second, we used classical meta-regression methods to estimate women's lifetime prevalence of IPV. We modeled estimates for 21 global regions, adjusted for differences in study quality and characteristics, and provide age-standardized estimates, which reflect country age- and sex-specific population structures in 2010.

Data from 141 studies in 81 countries informed our estimates. Studies provided data on physical or sexual partner violence, or both, of different severity levels, occurring over different time periods and for age groups. The earliest study collected data in 1983; however, 96% of estimates that informed our model came from studies with data collected in 1999 or later. In all, 80% of estimates used a gold standard definition of IPV measurement.

The results show that globally, in 2010, 30.0% [95% confidence interval (CI) 27.8 to 32.2%] of women aged 15 and over have experienced, during their lifetime, physical and/or sexual intimate partner violence. There is considerable regional variation in the prevalence of physical and/or sexual partner violence (see Figure 31.1).

Implications for Policy

Given the high prevalence of IPV in all regions of the world, a greater focus on primary prevention is urgently needed alongside the provision of health, social, legal, and other support services.[10] The prevention field is still in its nascence, but emerging evidence suggests several promising areas of intervention.

The strong association between exposure to violence in childhood and later experiences or perpetration of violence highlights the potential importance of interventions to prevent child maltreatment and witnessing of violence by their parents.[10] For example, parenting interventions and social norm change to reduce the use of violence against children[10] and the provision of support to children living in violent families are possibilities.

Secondary education for women is consistently associated with lower levels of IPV, but women's employment has been shown to have the potential to either reduce or increase risk, depending upon geocultural context. In rural South Africa, an intervention that combined economic and social change program components showed a 55% reduction in past year levels of IPV over 2 years.[11]

At the societal level, there is a need to challenge social norms that may condone some forms of IPV

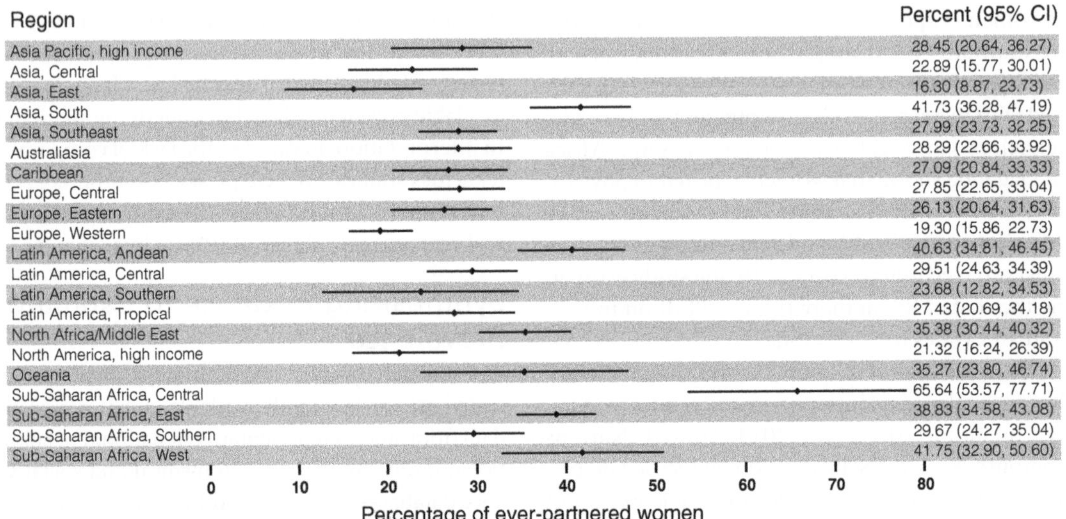

FIGURE 31.1 Regional Prevalence of IPV, Percentage of Ever-Partnered Women.

Source: K. M. Devries, Mak, J. Y., García-Moreno, C., et al. "Global Health. The Global Prevalence of Intimate Partner Violence against Women." *Science*, 340: 1527–1528.

and male control over women, as well as norms that result in IPV being seen as a private issue, rather than a public concern. There are many promising social change interventions, including initiatives to support increased local activism against violence, to engage men and boys in violence prevention, and to use the media to promote nonviolent and gender equitable relationships and encourage neighbors to take action when violence occurs.[10] Interventions to challenge social norms that promote problematic alcohol use among men, which is commonly associated with an increased severity and frequency of perpetration of IPV against female partners, are also needed.[12]

The UN estimates that more than 600 million women live in countries where domestic violence is not considered a crime.[13] Laws are important both to symbolize the unacceptability of IPV, as well as to provide a potential mechanism of legal recourse for women. At the national level, there is a need also to promote equal economic rights and entitlements for women—including equal access to formal wage employment, equal participation in schooling, and access to secondary education—and to address potentially discriminatory family law that may limit women's ability to divorce or maintain custody of their children.[14]

Given the impacts and high prevalence of IPV it is likely that many women using health services are experiencing or have histories of abuse. The WHO, along with other professional health bodies, have produced guidance on how best to provide health care and support to women who have experienced violence.[15] This work highlights the potential for health services to help identify, support, and refer women who are experiencing IPV and the need to support children growing up in households where there is IPV. It also identifies potential health sector entry points for an effective response.

IPV is a complex issue, and there are no quick-fix solutions. However, the global variation in the levels of violence highlight that IPV is not inevitable. There are multiple, important intervention entry points, and a concerted, multisectoral response is needed. Alongside the provision of services, an increased investment in violence prevention should form a central part of an expanded response. Research has a central role in this initiative, to support learning about the impact of different promising interventions being implemented globally, their costs, and how to take interventions to scale. Without such investments, the high levels of IPV documented here may continue unabated. The international community must honor commitments it has made over the past decade and devote resources to reducing violence against women, including IPV.

REFERENCES

1. C. Watts, C. Zimmerman, *Lancet* **359**, 1232 (2002).
2. J. C. Campbell, *Lancet* **359**, 1331 (2002).
3. H. Stöckl *et al.*, *Lancet* (2013). 10.1016/S0140-6736(13)61030-2
4. K. M. Devries *et al.*, *PLoS Med.* **10**, e1001439 (2013).
5. R. K. Jewkes *et al.*, *Lancet* **376**, 41 (2010).
6. F. G. Kouyoumdjian *et al.*, *AIDS* **27**, 1331 (2013).
7. S. Walby, *The Cost of Domestic Violence: Up-date 2009* (Lancaster Univ., Lancaster, UK, 2010); www.lancs.ac.uk/fass/doc_library/sociology/Cost_of_domestic_violence_update.doc.
8. Department of Gender, Women, and Health, WHO, *Putting Women First: Ethical and Safety Recommendations for Research on Domestic Violence Against Women* (WHO, Geneva, 2001).
9. C. García-Moreno *et al.*, *Science* **310**, 1282 (2005).
10. L. Heise, *What Works to Prevent Partner Violence? An Evidence Overview* (STRIVE, London School of Hygiene and Tropical Medicine, London, 2011).
11. J. C. Kim *et al.*, *Am. J. Public Health* **97**, 1794 (2007).
12. K. Graham *et al.*, *J. Interpers. Violence* **26**, 1503 (2011).
13. L. Turquet *et al.*, *Progress of the World's Women 2011–2012: In Pursuit of Justice* (UN Women, New York, 2013).
14. L. Heise, *Determinants of Partner Violence in Low and Middle-Income Countries: Exploring Variation in Individual and Population Level Risk* (London School of Hygiene and Tropical Medicine, London, 2012).
15. WHO, "Responding to intimate partner and sexual violence against women: WHO clinical and policy guidelines" (WHO, Geneva, 2013).

Acknowledgments: We thank S. Kishor, K. Graham, H. Johnson, L. Heise, L. Petre, J. Astbury, J. Campbell, L. Davidson, M. Ellsberg, R. Jewkes, R. Naved, J. Mercy, H. Resnick, L. Sadowski, L. B. Schraiber, A. Taket, M. Yoshihama, the Economic and Social Research Council, Sigrid Rausing Trust, and the UN Development Programme, UN Population Fund, WHO, World Bank Special Programme of Research, Development, and Research Training in Human Reproduction.

BARRY S. LEVY AND VICTOR W. SIDEL

32 WAR AND PUBLIC HEALTH: AN OVERVIEW

The first paragraph of this reading is stunning. War is terrible, period. Given nuclear weapons, war threatens the survival of our species and the planet. As noted in the Conceptual Tools for this section of the book, war can be seen as the antithesis of global health in both its aims and effects.

How many of your fellow students know that there are ten official wars and eight active military conflicts happening in the world today? And those are just the "official" ones recognized by the US government. Other unofficial violent conflicts are ongoing in sixty-four countries and involve 576 militias or separatist groups. In fact, four ongoing conflicts (Syria, South Sudan, Iraq, and the drug war in Mexico) are each resulting in over 10,000 casualties per year (as of 2014). Throughout the world, new technologies mean that armed conflict is killing more and more civilians, while the risks to soldiers has decreased. Although social scientists like Steven Pinker have argued the prevalence of violence in the world has declined throughout history, the human costs of war remain intolerable.

There have been continuous wars involving the United States and allies during the last 15 years, with little domestic social opposition. The Vietnam War was the last time the United States experienced widespread social unrest from an antiwar movement. One difference between then and now is the fact that there is an all-volunteer army, and only a small percentage of Americans know someone serving in the military. University students do not face the draft, so wars can seem distant to them.

This article provides an overview of the direct and indirect effects of war on population health and welfare. The list is depressingly incomplete because the long-term effects may continue long after active fighting has ceased. For example, inexpensive land mines regularly maim or kill children playing in fields that can no longer be used for agriculture; safely removing those landmines is extremely expensive.

The article is written for public health practitioners and, therefore, emphasizes the practical things that people in the profession can do. Given human nature and the contemporary sociopolitical context, it is overly idealistic to believe that wars can simply be stopped. But there is much the global health community can do to reduce unnecessary suffering and encourage the prevention of violence and the peaceful resolutions of disputes. When examining group violence, it is obvious that global health must be political.

As you read this selection, consider the following questions:

- **Of all the negative effects of war that are listed in this article, what do you think is the worst? Which is an effect that you may never have thought about?**
- **If men are usually the combatants in armed conflicts, why do the authors say that women are particularly vulnerable to the negative effects?**
- **From a global health perspective, can you think of a scenario where war may have positive effects on a population's health?**
- **Epidemiologists in federal institutions like the Centers for Disease Control and Prevention and the National Institutes of Health are not permitted to be actively involved in political advocacy (or they may lose their jobs). What do you think of this policy?**

CONTEXT

This is the first chapter of book *War and Public Health* (2007), which was edited by two famous public health physicians, political activists, and past presidents of the American Association of Public Health. Together, they have edited other books about public health, social injustice, and climate change. Barry Levy worked at the Centers for Disease Control and Prevention early in his career and currently teaches at Tufts School of Public Health. He is also a well-known researcher in maternal health. Victor Sidel is the Distinguished University Professor of Social Medicine at Montefiore Medical Center and the Albert Einstein College of Medicine in the Bronx, New York. He has been a key leader in the advocacy organization Physicians for Social Responsibility and as co-founder of the organization International Physicians for the Prevention of Nuclear War—an organization that received the Nobel Peace Prize in 1985.

War accounts for more death and disability than many major diseases combined. It destroys families, communities, and sometimes whole cultures. It directs scarce resources away from protection and promotion of health, medical care, and other human services. It destroys the infrastructure that supports health. It limits human rights and contributes to social injustice. It leads many people to think that violence is the only way to resolve conflicts—a mindset that contributes to domestic violence, street crime, and other kinds of violence. And it contributes to the destruction of the environment and overuse of nonrenewable resources. In sum, war threatens much of the fabric of our civilization.

War has been conventionally defined as armed conflict conducted by nation-states. The term is also used to describe an armed conflict within a nation (a "civil war" or a "war of liberation") and armed action by a clandestine group against a government or an occupying force (a "guerrilla war" or "intifada"). *Public health* has been defined as "what we, as a society, do collectively to assure the conditions in which people can be healthy."[1] War is generally anathema to public health.

Some of the impacts of war on public health are obvious, but others are not. The direct impact of war on mortality and morbidity is apparent. An increasing percentage of those killed or injured during war have been civilians. An estimated 191 million people died directly or indirectly as a result of conflict during the 20th century, more than half of whom were civilians.[2] The exact figures are unknowable because of poor recordkeeping in many countries and its disruption in times of conflict.[3]

Civilians are increasingly affected by war. There is evidence that in some wars 90 percent or more of the people killed were noncombatants.[4] Many of them were innocent bystanders, caught in the crossfire of opposing armies; others were civilians who were specifically targeted during wars. During each year of the past decade, there have been approximately 20 wars, mainly civil wars that are infrequently reported by the news media in the United States. For example, almost 4 million people died during the civil war in the Democratic Republic of Congo, and 1 million people, about half of whom were civilians, died in the 30-year civil war in Ethiopia.[5]

Since 1999, the number of major armed conflicts has steadily decreased. There were 17 major armed conflicts in 16 locations worldwide during 2005—the lowest number since the end of the Cold War in 1990. Most conflicts in recent years have been civil wars within nations. For example, in the 1990–2005 period, only 4 of 57 active conflicts were armed conflicts between nations: between Eritrea and Ethiopia in 1998–2000; between India and Pakistan in 1990–1992 and again in 1996–2003; between Iraq and Kuwait (and a large coalition of nations) in 1991; and the Iraq War starting in 2003. (The last of these wars has evolved into sectarian conflict.) Of the remaining 53 conflicts within nations during this period, 30 were fought for control over government and 23 were fought for control over territory.[6] Some enduring conflicts have taken place in recent years in the same locations as they did in the 1960s, such as the conflicts between Israel and the Palestinians, between India and Pakistan for control over the territory of Kashmir, in the Democratic Republic of Congo, and in Colombia.[7]

There have been some encouraging developments in recent years. Despite continuing violence in Iraq and Darfur, during the 2002–2005 period the number of wars being fought worldwide decreased from 66 to 56, with the greatest reduction in sub-Saharan Africa. Battle-related deaths during the same period are estimated to have declined by almost 40 percent. More wars are ending in negotiated settlements instead of being fought to the bitter end—a trend that reflects increased commitment of the international community to peacemaking.[8]

There have also been some discouraging developments, however. In four regions of the world, the number of armed conflicts increased between 2002 and 2005. International "terrorist" incidents tripled between 2000 and 2005, with an even greater relative increase in the number of deaths. And the number of organized violence campaigns against civilians annually rose by 56 percent between 1989 and 2005.[8]

Given the brutality of war, many people survive wars only to be physically or mentally scarred for life. Millions of survivors are chronically disabled from injuries sustained during war or the immediate aftermath of war. Approximately one-third of the soldiers who survived the civil war in Ethiopia, for example, were injured or disabled, and at least 40,000 individuals lost one or more limbs during the war.[5] Antipersonnel landmines represent a serious threat to many people.[9] For example, in Cambodia, 1 in 236 people is an amputee as a result of a landmine explosion.[10]

Millions more people are psychologically impaired from wars, during which they have been physically or sexually assaulted or have physically or sexually assaulted others; have been tortured or have participated in the torture of others; have been forced to serve as soldiers against their will; have witnessed the death of family members; or have experienced the destruction of their communities or entire nations. Psychological trauma may be demonstrated in disturbed and antisocial behaviors, such as aggression toward family members and others. Many soldiers, on returning from military action, suffer from posttraumatic stress disorder (PTSD), which also affects many civilian survivors of war.

Women are especially vulnerable during war. Rape has been used as a weapon in many wars—in Korea, Bangladesh, Algeria, India, Indonesia, Liberia, Rwanda, Uganda, the former Yugoslavia, and elsewhere. As acts of humiliation and revenge, soldiers have raped the female family members of their enemies. For example, at least 10,000 women were raped by military personnel during the war in Bosnia and Herzegovina.[11] The social chaos brought about by war also creates situations and conditions conducive to sexual violence.

Children also are especially vulnerable during and after wars. Many die as a result of malnutrition, disease, or military attack. Many are physically or psychologically injured. Many are forced to become soldiers or sexual slaves to military officers. The health of children suffers in numerous other ways, as reflected by increased mortality rates among infants and young children and decreased rates of immunization coverage.[12,13]

The infrastructure that supports social well-being and health—including medical care facilities, electricity-generating plants, food supply systems, water treatment and sanitation facilities, and transportation and communication systems—has been destroyed during many wars, so that many people have inadequate access to food, clean water, medical care, or other conditions necessary for public health. Economic sanctions can have a similar effect. For example, the United Nations Children's Fund (UNICEF) has estimated that between 350,000 and 500,000 excess child deaths occurred in Iraq between 1991 and 1998, many due to inadequate nutrition, contaminated water, and shortages of essential medicines, all of which were worsened by international economic sanctions imposed on Iraq.

Many people during wartime flee to other countries as refugees or become internally displaced persons within their own countries, where it may be difficult for them to maintain their health and safety. Refugees and internally displaced persons are vulnerable to malnutrition, infectious diseases, injuries, and criminal and military attacks. A substantial number of the approximately 12 million refugees and 20 to 25 million internally displaced persons in the world today were forced to leave their homes because of war or the threat of war.[14,15]

In addition to the direct effects of war, there are three categories of indirect and less obvious impacts on health of war and preparation for war: diversion of resources, domestic and community violence, and damage to the environment.

Many countries spend large amounts of money per capita for military purposes. The countries with the highest military expenditures are shown in Table 32–1. War and the preparation for war divert huge amounts of resources from health and human services and other productive societal endeavors.[16–18] This diversion of resources occurs in many countries. In some less developed countries, national governments spend $10 to $20 per capita on military expenditures but only $1 per capita on all health-related expenditures. The same type of distorted priorities also exist in more developed countries. For example, the United States ranks first among nations in military expenditures and arms exports, but 38th among nations in infant mortality rate and 45th in life expectancy at birth. Since 2003, during a period when federal, state, and local governments in the United States have been experiencing budgetary shortfalls and finding it difficult to maintain adequate health and human services, the U.S. government has spent almost $500 billion for the Iraq War, and is spending (in 2007) more than $2 billion a week on the war.

Weapons represent a large portion of expenditures for military purposes. Availability of weapons, especially small arms and light weapons, often increases the likelihood of armed conflict. Between

TABLE 32.1 The 15 Countries with the Highest Military Expenditures in 2005.

Country	Spending (in Billions of Dollars)	Spending per Capita (in Dollars)	World Share of Spending (Percent)
United States	478	1,604	48
United Kingdom	48	809	5
France	46	763	5
Japan	42	329	4
China	41	31	4
Germany	33	401	3
Italy	27	468	3
Saudi Arabia	25	1,025	3
Russia	21	147	2
India	20	19	2
South Korea	16	344	2
Canada	11	327	1
Australia	11	522	1
Spain	10	230	1
Israel	10	1,430	1
Total of top 15	840*	—	84*
All countries	1,001	155	100

*Because of rounding, this total is not the sum of above numbers.

Source: Omitoogun W, Sköns E. Military expenditure data: a 40-year overview. In Stockholm International Peace Research Institute. SIPRI Yearbook 2006: Armaments, Disarmament and International Security. Oxford: Oxford University Press, 2006, p. 302.

2003 and 2004, there was a substantial increase in international arms sales worldwide, from $233 to $268 billion (not including China). The United States accounted for approximately 63 percent of these international arms sales, the United Kingdom about 19 percent, and France about 12 percent.[19]

War often creates a cycle of violence, increasing domestic and community violence in the countries engaged in war. War teaches people that violence is an acceptable method for settling conflicts. Children growing up in environments in which violence is an established way of settling conflicts may choose violence to settle conflicts in their own lives. Teenage gangs may mirror the activity of military forces. Men, sometimes former military servicemen who have been trained to use violence, commit acts of violence against women; there have been instances of men murdering their wives on return from the battlefield.

Finally, war and the preparation for war have profound impacts on the physical environment. The disastrous consequences of war for the environment are often clear. Examples include bomb craters in Vietnam that have filled with water and provide breeding sites for mosquitoes that spread malaria and other diseases; destruction of urban environments by aerial carpet bombing of major cities in Europe and Japan during World War II; and the more than 600 oil-well fires in Kuwait that were ignited by retreating Iraqi troops in 1991, which had a devastating effect on the ecology of the affected areas and caused acute respiratory symptoms among those exposed. Less obvious are the environmental impacts of the preparation for war, such as the huge amounts of nonrenewable fossil fuels used by the military.

Roles of Public Health Professionals in Preventing War and Its Health Consequences

Like most public health problems, war and its health consequences are preventable. There are several roles that public health professionals can play in preventing war and its consequences. These roles include

- Participating in surveillance and documentation of the health effects of war and of the factors that may cause war
- Developing and implementing education and awareness-raising programs on the health effects of war
- Advocating policies and promoting actions to prevent war and its health consequences
- Working directly in actions to prevent war and its consequences.

The basic principles of prevention are applicable to the prevention of war and the minimization of its consequences. In this context, we define

- *Primary prevention* as preventing war or causing a halt to a war that is taking place
- *Secondary prevention* as preventing and minimizing the health and environmental consequences of war once it has begun
- *Tertiary prevention* as treating or ameliorating the health consequences of war.

Many of the roles for public health professionals in secondary and tertiary prevention take place in war zones, where there is a narrow line between protecting and serving people on the one hand and supporting the war effort on the other.

In terms of tertiary prevention, there are roles that public health professionals can play in caring for victims of war, including assisting and providing health and medical care services for all dis-placed persons and prisoners of war. Health professionals can also help to document the dangers that refugees would face if they were forced to return to their home countries.

Conclusion

War is the one of the most serious threats to public health. Public health professionals can do much to prevent war and its health consequences. Preventing war and its consequences should be part of the curricula of schools of public health, the agendas of public health organizations, and the practice of public health professionals. Activities by public health professionals to prevent war and its health consequences are an essential part of our professional obligations.

The greatest threat to the health of people worldwide lies not in specific forms of acute or chronic diseases—and not even in poverty, hunger, or homelessness. Rather, it lies in the consequences of war.

As stated in a resolution adopted by the World Health Assembly, the governing body of the World Health Organization: "The role of physicians and other health workers in the preservation and promotion of peace is the most significant factor for the attainment of health for all."[20]

War is not inevitable. For perhaps 99 percent of human history, people lived in egalitarian groups in which generosity was highly valued and war was rare. War first occurred relatively recently in human history along with changes in social organization, especially the development of nation-states. Even at present, when war seems ever-present, most people live peaceful, nonviolent lives. If we can learn from history, we may be able to move beyond war and create a culture of peace.[21]

REFERENCES

1. Institute of Medicine, Committee for the Study of Public Health. The Future of Public Health. Washington, DC: National Academy of Sciences, 1988.
2. Rummel RJ. Death by Government: Genocide and Mass Murder Since 1900. New Brunswick, NJ, and London: Transaction Publications, 1994.
3. Zwi A, Ugalde A, Richards P. The effects of war and political violence on health services. In Kurtz L (ed.). Encyclopedia of Violence, Peace and Conflict. San Diego, CA: Academic Press, 1999, pp. 679–690.
4. Garfield RM, Neugut AI. The human consequences of war. In Levy BS, Sidel VW (eds.). War and Public Health. New York: Oxford University Press, 1997.
5. Kloos H. Health impacts of war in Ethiopia. Disasters 1992;16:347–354.
6. Harbom L, Wallensteen P. Patterns of major armed conflicts, 1990–2005. In Stockholm International Peace Research Institute. SIPRI Yearbook 2006: Armaments, Disarmament and International Security. Oxford, UK: Oxford University Press, 2006, p. 108.
7. Holmqvist C. Major armed conflicts. In Stockholm International Peace Research Institute. SIPRI Yearbook 2006: Armaments, Disarmament and International Security. Oxford, UK: Oxford University Press, 2006, pp. 77–107.
8. The Human Security Brief 2006. Vancouver, Canada: University of British Columbia, 2006. Available at: http://www.humansecuritygateway.info/ (accessed June 4, 2007).
9. Stover E, Cobey JC, Fine J. The public health effects of land mines. In Levy BS, Sidel VW (eds.). War and Public Health. New York: Oxford University Press, 1997, pp. 137–148.
10. Stover E, Keller AS, Cobey J, Sopheap S. The medical and social consequences of land mines in Cambodia. JAMA 1994;272:331–336.
11. Ashford MW, Huet-Vaughn Y. The impact of war on women. In Levy BS, Sidel VW (eds.). War and Public Health. New York: Oxford University Press, 1997, pp. 186–196.
12. Mann J, Drucker E, Tarantola D, et al. Bosnia: The war against public health. Medicine and Global Survival 1994;1:140–146.
13. Horton R. On the brink of humanitarian disease. Lancet 1994;343:1053.
14. Reed J, Haaga J, Keely C (eds.). The Demography of Forced Migration: Summary of a Workshop. Washington, DC: National Academy Press, 1998.
15. Hampton J (ed.). Internally Displaced People: A Global Survey. London: Earthscan, Norwegian Refugee Council and Global IDP Survey, 1998.
16. Macrae J, Zwi A. Famine, complex emergencies and international policy in Africa: An overview. In Macrae J, Zwi A (eds.). War and Hunger: Rethinking International Responses to Complex Emergencies. London: Zed Books, 1994, pp. 6–36.
17. Brauer J, Gissy WG (eds.). Economics of Conflict and Peace. Aldershot: Avebury, 1997.
18. Cranna M (ed.). The True Cost of Conflict. London: Earthscan and Saferworld, 1994.
19. Dunne JP, Surry E. Arms production. In Stockholm International Peace Research Institute. SIPRI Yearbook 2006: Armaments, Disarmament and International Security. Oxford, UK: Oxford University Press, 2006, pp 387–430.
20. World Health Assembly. Resolution 34.38. Geneva: World Health Organization, 1981.
21. Fry DP. Beyond War: The Human Potential for Peace. New York: Oxford University Press, 2007.

PETER REDFIELD

33 BEYOND HAPPY ENDINGS

There are many nongovernmental organizations (NGOs) that send humanitarian aid after natural disasters like hurricanes and earthquakes. However, there are far fewer NGOs that work in dangerous war-torn areas with refugees and internally displaced people. This article is about one of the most famous NGOs in global health, Médecins Sans Frontières *(MSF, or Doctors Without Borders), which provides medical services in "complex humanitarian emergencies."*

MSF provides massive amounts of free medical care to people whose lives are in crisis. Since it was founded in 1971 as a reaction to the terrible war in Biafra, Nigeria, MSF has provided services to more than 100 million patients. In 2015 alone, MSF provided 8.6 million medical consultations.

This NGO was given the Nobel Peace Prize in 1999. However, it strongly resists being associated with labels like heroism, charity, development, or relief. The organization is fiercely independent, international, and willing to criticize. It is nomadic—ready for the next crisis and unwilling to form permanent local partnerships. While MSF members save many lives and witness terrible human suffering, they do not have solutions or a plan to save the world. MSF follows violence and tries to patch up individuals whose bodies and lives have been torn up by war.

This article considers the questions of optimism, pessimism, and pragmatism in the moral mandate of global health. The author of this selection is an anthropologist who wanted to understand the cultural ethos and daily lives of people working with MSF. The reading has a philosophical orientation, beginning on some observations about optimism and naïveté as portrayed in Voltaire's Candide.

As you read this article, consider the following questions:

- **The last sentence of this article is, "Surely there is more to life than saving it." In the context of war and violence, do you think the narrow goals of MSF—"just" saving lives in a crisis—make working for the NGO frustrating?**
- **Must humanitarian assistance be apolitical? Why do some people think it should be?**
- **In your opinion, what are some characteristics of MSF than seem to make it unique?**
- **From a global health perspective, is it right to say that there are "no happy endings" in war?**

CONTEXT

Peter Redfield is a professor of anthropology at the University of North Carolina, Chapel Hill, where he also leads an interdisciplinary working group Moral Economies of Biomedicine. His expertise includes the anthropology of humanitarianism and human rights; ethics; studies of medicine, science, and technology; and NGOs. This article is original to this volume but is based upon research described in his book *Life in Crisis: The Ethical Journey of Doctors Without Borders* (2013). He is currently working on a project dealing with the design of technologies of global health interventions for clean water and sanitation.

Modified version of Chapter 9 of *Life in Crisis: The Ethical Journey of Doctors Without Borders,* by Peter Redfield. Berkeley: University of California Press, 2013.

"There aren't any happy endings. You need to learn that first thing in college and get on with it."

—MSF PROJECT COORDINATOR, New York, 2006

When I began studying the organization Médecins Sans Frontières (Doctors Without Borders or, in aid world acronym, MSF), it struck me how persistently people who had spent a long time with the group would downplay any suggestion that their work was in any way heroic. "We're not saving the world" went the gist of their refrain, often expressed with wry humor, and sometimes more than a trace of anger. Such a claim stood in contrast to the rosy glow suffusing most public portrayals of humanitarian action, including some of MSF's own fundraising appeals, replete with urgent exhortations to save lives. It also diverged sharply from the earnest language of problem solving so prominent in international development and global health.

It has grown difficult to discuss any issue without offering a solution. Our era prizes the idiom of problem solvers, no matter how often or how spectacularly they might fail. Particularly in the contemporary United States, good will and earnest effort remain deeply held articles of faith, and the suggestion that they might not ultimately prevail nears heresy. When faced with unpleasant questions or facts related to values they hold dear, people often react with predictable dismay. Sometimes they will dismiss them. At other times they resort to a more sweeping form of defense: how dare one reject optimism, the faith in success against all odds? Without hope of success, after all, what is the use of even trying? In historical terms this reaction exhibits a strikingly narrow sense of ethical possibility, devoid of noble defeats or unrewarded virtue. Nonetheless it remains insistent, heartfelt, and not simply a norm of legendary American naiveté. Surely action demands hope and hope demands optimism, if not a fully articulated utopia. A solution *must* lie in the future, and so be implied even when raising a question.

The trajectory of MSF, however, suggests anything but a straight line or obvious conclusion. However seductively simple the group's message may be, it has yielded no clear solutions. Indeed, the record offers few examples of "success" in any grand sense. Its classic mode of emergency action responds to immediate needs, after all, and makes few claims about anything beyond survival. Even when venturing beyond emergency settings, the group encounters the broader wasteland of human need. There its machinery—often impressive at an individual level—appears suddenly frail and miniature. Even its best projects rarely yield lasting results; when handed over to states or less well-funded organizations they frequently dissipate. Sustainability, so easy to desire, remains hard to achieve. Moreover, the group's commitment to mobility dictates against permanent partnerships. Having defined itself "without borders" it remains fundamentally nomadic, and hence a creature of transitory relations. Sympathies aside, it does not claim to promote social justice beyond medical issues, let alone to save the world.

Nonetheless, MSF undeniably does save lives. A survey of details evokes more than such a stock phrase. The organization's balance sheet of activities for 2005, for example, included a full 10 million outpatient consultations and close to 400,000 clinical admissions worldwide. These figures encompass a range of medical activities, both exceptional and routine. The group conducted 75,000 major surgeries, 8,000 for trauma suffered in conflict. It delivered 91,000 babies. It oversaw 161,000 people with HIV-AIDS, and supplied 60,000 of these with antiretroviral drugs. It also cared for 22,000 cases of tuberculosis, and well over two million of malaria. It provided 806,000 vaccinations for measles and 361,000 for yellow fever. Some 130,000 children received therapeutic feeding and 12,000 women treatment for sexual violence. Nearly 150,000 patients benefited from mental health services of some kind.[1] Such statistics aggregate specific stories, some happier than others. Even the few individual narratives selected for the organization's reports suggest different outcomes that stretch beyond the moment—dramatic recovery, mundane survival, continuing despair. But the raw force of the combined result remains: among the many facing likely

[1] MSF Activity Report 2005–6, p. 84.

death, a few more lived. What might appear modest for a horizon of world history, can measure the very limits of a personal one.

Thus while MSF may offer no grand solution, it certainly addresses an impressive array of smaller problems. Indeed, the group defines itself explicitly in terms of action, and the language of engagement. It runs projects and prides itself on being operational. Its version of humanitarianism demands activity for its claim to moral worth. Still it views abstract advocacy with suspicion, feeling that authority derives from presence in "the field." Resolutely secular, its rhetorical practice nonetheless positions field missions as something like sacred sites. Truth itself derives from action, not contemplation.[2] At the same time the group's tradition favors argument, dispute and a measure of self-reflection. Its self-presentation includes not only the arrogance of moral claims, but also restlessness and discontent. One finds few traces of optimism here.

The work of MSF, then, provides an example of acting in the absence of expected solutions, and indeed while questioning the action itself.[3] However much specific conduct may vary, the very ethos remains interesting. What might happen to the status of a category like "hope" in such circumstances? To approach this question, I first detour through one small moment in the history of optimism, both to decouple that term from hope, and to recall that people have long grappled with how to respond to suffering and injustice.

After Optimism

> "'What's optimism?' said Cacambo. 'Alas,' said Candide, 'it is a mania for saying things are well when one is in hell.'"
>
> —VOLTAIRE, *Candide*, 1759

During the period Europeans consider their Enlightenment, the contrarian French writer Voltaire penned his most celebrated work, a scathing indictment of rosy outlooks. Entitled *Candide*, and subtitled *Optimism*, it featured a sublimely naïve protagonist, stumbling through a cascade of mishaps large and small. Voltaire gave this hapless youth an even more resilient mentor: Dr. Pangloss, the notoriously monotone philosopher who persistently interpreted every event in light of his favored maxim—that we indeed inhabit "the best of all possible worlds." The book's satire indicted the views of Gottfried Leibniz and Alexander Pope, and more broadly any form of theological optimism that would soothingly suggest that all events reflect a masterful divine plan, no matter how unfortunate they may appear. Partly inspired by the Lisbon earthquake of 1755, *Candide* grapples with what would later become the loadstone of humanitarian ethics. How to respond to tragedy? How to live with a shortage of happy endings?

Voltaire's famously ambiguous answer undercuts philosophical reflection with a note of pragmatism. The survivors of his epic tour of suffering finally reunite in Turkey, where, fortunes won and lost, they work a small farm together. There, each learns to exercise a particular talent, and all prove useful. Pangloss offers one final, grand summation, demonstrating how they have reached this happy state only by enduring their many misadventures. Candide affably acknowledges his teacher's conclusion as "very well put," but then reiterates his new, prosaic maxim: "we must cultivate our garden."[4] How precisely to read this statement, however, remains unclear. Would it imply a final acceptance of things as they are? Or conversely, would it signal continued skepticism, and a rejection of any philosophical justification of the status quo? Satire resists simple summation.

Alluding to this now distant juncture of European thought serves as a reminder that current predicaments are rarely entirely new. It also helps distinguish between varieties of optimism and hope. Voltaire's Panglossian caricature offers one optimistic extreme, insisting everything will turn out for the best. Humanitarians of MSF's variety tend to peer through a darker lens, perceiving what Fiona Terry calls—contra Pangloss—a "second best

[2] See Arendt 1998 on action and contemplation.

[3] See Fassin 2012: 246 on the condition of simultaneously acting and expressing "ambivalence or disappointment."

[4] The work's closing passages as cited in this paragraph are from Voltaire 1991: 75.

world."[5] Humanitarian rhetoric, after all, specializes in issuing calls to arms rather than reassurance. Only a quick response promises to "save lives" amid needless suffering. What lies beyond this moment of rescue grows less clear. The life saved is simply a continuing future, one that may prove as dark as the past that precedes it. There are no sure grounds for optimism in life itself. Moreover, few members of the group profess much faith in either capitalism or human nature. Confronting repeated panoramas of human agony, they reject the economic theodicy that the market remained an absolute good, no matter what casualties it might produce. They also recognize that civilian suffering inspires political manipulation as well as human sympathy. Morality is never pure or certain; sometimes it flows in contradictory, and even damaging ways. By the time of my research, a chorus of observers had warned of the "dilemmas" and "hard choices" of international aid for many years, some of the most withering analyses coming from former adherents.[6]

Nonetheless, humanitarianism remains a favored screen for projections of something like a happy ending, particularly in settings otherwise devoid of them. MSF's oppositional legacy hardly serves to immunize it from this affliction. Indeed, if anything it would appear to add a patina of rebellious flair in heroic affirmation of life. Profiles of the group regularly play on this redemptive theme, well summarized by the evocative title of a lucid Canadian study of MSF: "Hope in Hell."[7] Along with countless humanitarian fundraising brochures, this title implies the possibility of redemption through sufficient generosity coupled with energetic action. But what sort of hope could exist in hell? Or more accurately, what might follow optimism in a second best world?

In the centuries after Voltaire mocked theological complacency, secular versions of a happy ending generally took political form. For classic liberalism faith resided in individual liberty and the wonders of market innovation. Leftist alternatives endorsed a harder line of revolutionary upheaval, seeking to reshape the social order. Utopian visions could endow suffering with worldly meaning; one died for the greater good. Even where revolutionary fires burned low, the modernist political idiom remained that of progressive change and the redemption of remaking. It had little patience for traditions of charity, or any activity that implied an acceptance of given conditions and existing inequalities.

The generation that brought MSF into being inherited this wider political sensibility. Key figures had activist biographies, and the organization itself emerged at a time of social and political turmoil. Being "without borders" was a claim to conceptual as well as geographic liberation; its members would refuse complacency and remain rebellious. I was initially surprised by the degree to which the group avoided terms like "charity" and "relief" (memorably, the then director of the Amsterdam office excised such offending language from my proposal with a red pen). I subsequently realized that the aid world had its own shifting sense of vocabulary, within which MSF saw itself as an oppositional conscience. However much they might act like a charity in delivering aid, they had no desire to be one.

Nonetheless, veterans of the organization rarely sounded sanguine about either the state of the world, or the greater benefits of their work. When I asked the head of communications of the Paris office about his views on hope in 2005, he responded in the following way:

> Hope? Hope for whom? The beneficiaries? Those in contact with MSF for sure, it helps them with living conditions, health, etc. Hope for global society or something like that? Well, that's putting a lot of hope in something that doesn't really have this pretense. We deliver the means of life survival, tents, water, medicine. That's our objective, being rescue workers.

Warming to the topic, he then enlarged the reflection to more general analysis of the limits of any nongovernmental organization:

> The have been surveys that show people putting MSF on a pedestal, "a factor for peace" and things

[5] Terry 2002: 216.

[6] The list of warning titles runs remarkably long. For two relevant examples see e.g. Brauman 1996; Rieff 2002; Terry 2002. Hugo Slim provides an incisive discussion of "dilemmas" (Slim 1997).

[7] Bortolotti 2004.

like that. But it's absurd to pretend that NGOs can be a factor of peace. NGOs can be a safety net of sorts, but to replace states? No, not in any systematic way. Privatization and all that, it's just not very realistic. If you look at the beneficiaries of specific programs, suffering from a specific problem, like AIDS, malaria and so on then we can talk about hope. But that's specific to this NGO, not anything grand like solidarity or a global village. Fighting poverty, or something like that, that's way beyond our reach. We're like rescue workers on a highway after a car crash. Should they stop just because tomorrow there will be another crash? MSF tried to narrow what we mean by humanitarianism. Not health for everyone, that's political, that has to be dealt with at a political level. Humanitarianism should be the third party in the battlefield. It can extend beyond war to other crises, pandemics like AIDS, etc. But change the world? That's something else.

As befit this individual's professional role as a spokesman, the comments struck common themes. Although the group might be a frequent recipient of laudatory approval, its members generally resisted any heroic mantle. Instead, when commenting at this level they emphasized their limitations and the inherent modesty of the enterprise. Aware of the charge that humanitarianism served as either a handmaiden for the status quo or a mask for imperial designs, they deliberately deflated its role, repeatedly insisting on realism.

In addition to avoiding abstract language and utopian claims, MSF's variant of realism stressed action, less in the sense of any grand gesture than in that of daily practice. A former member of the group later answered my query by email with a particularly memorable deflating comparison:

> I don't really know how to respond to "hope" in a humanitarian context. My instinctive reaction is allergic, I confess . . , in the big scheme of things, humanitarians are "a sparrow fart in the winds of history," as a friend says. I prefer the view that humanitarians are really no different than any other kind of social work, or even menial labor, like janitorial work. It's just cleaning up other people's messes. Maybe there's some remotely ethical dimension to that kind of work, and if so it's no different than the remotely ethical dimension of humanitarianism.

Such a comment may go to extreme lengths in its rhetorical refusal of heroic rescue, and in its portrayal of humanitarianism as routine maintenance work. The sort of mess confronting humanitarianism would appear far more morally charged than that usually facing a janitor. Yet its author had considerable experience with several other humanitarian organizations and was obviously quite committed to this activity at the level of practice. Moreover, he was well read in philosophy. One wall of his Amsterdam office even featured a quotation from Theodor Adorno's *Minima Moralia*: "The only philosophy which can be responsibly practiced in the face of despair is the attempt to contemplate all things as they would represent themselves from the point of redemption."[8]

What then to make of such statements? Do they express contradictions, false modesty or sincere turmoil? Even taken at a literal level they signal an abiding ambivalence about the expectations placed on humanitarian work, expectations that the urgent language of fundraising only helped promote. Whatever else, humanitarianism constitutes a sensibility, like environmentalism, one that similarly lends itself to moral feeling and public campaigns. People readily contribute to save lives, whereas they rarely do so to perform routine maintenance. And yet emergency response only addresses problems that remain narrowly defined. By itself it offers little in the way of an agenda, and hardly substitutes for political platforms or social policies. Reflective individuals who have spent considerable time doing such aid work fully recognize this limitation.

Simply put, MSF has no plan. That is not to suggest that it lacks specific goals, strategies, projections and expectations, nor that it avoids "planning" at the level of ordinary bureaucratic procedures. The complex, plural federation of national sections produces an endless supply of documents both short and long to track the present, evaluate the past and anticipate the future. But unlike most governmental agencies—and even philanthropic donors like the

[8] Adorno (1974 [1951]).

Gates Foundation—it does not attempt to steer a certain predetermined course. Rather, the group responds to specific situations, while maintaining a looser version of Red Cross principles. Its action thus remains reactionary in the technical sense, defined against given pre-existing conditions rather than imagining hypothetical alternatives.

The group's emergence, furthermore, coincided with a period of political disillusionment, and an erosion of intellectual faith in the prospect of Marxist revolution, the romance of decolonization—even politics itself. The original French branch took form against the human wreckage of conflicts in Nigeria and Bangladesh, followed by the excesses of revolution in settings like Cambodia, Ethiopia. Amid the debris of political regimes its members found refuge in medical work, and asserting the value of human life. In concert with an expanding consortium of quarreling cousins, they gradually defined an uneasy ethical stance around this minimalist moral principle, eventually designated as "an ethic of refusal." The group would focus on political failure, and reject justifications for human suffering. In making pronouncements, however, it would resist straying far from actually existing problems or health affairs.

Nonetheless, MSF's adherents are radically egalitarian in at least one respect: they wish for a world where all humans would receive equal care, no matter their location or the nature of their suffering. No one should die a needless death. Many also believe in an active welfare state, at least in the sense of expressing dismay in its absence, and a resulting failure to provide populations with adequate medical services. In this sense they may participate in the "neoliberal" moment—even embodying certain aspects of its forms—but they do so with reluctance and suspicion. Moreover, the group's inherited ethos remains that of rebellion. Like the range of its actions, the field of political desire running through MSF quite exceeds its self-representation. Its members alternately embrace moral minimalism and rebel against it.[9] Thus an organization established to defy borders finds itself perpetually proclaiming and debating limits.

[9] See Brauman 1996: 65.

Residual Hope and Discontent

> "Hope is definitely not the same thing as optimism. It is not the conviction that something will turn out well, but the certainty that something makes sense, regardless of how it turns out."
>
> —VACLAV HAVEL, 1986

The administrator in MSF's New York office who complained to me about the desire for happy endings was discussing the organization's struggle to retain good people, despite having an oversupply of eager volunteers. "Younger people do one mission and then are off," she observed. "How to disabuse them of the notion that this might be glamorous and attractive, but at the same time instill real spirit?" Her comments echoed those of other experienced members, contemplating inheritance and the future of the organization. At first glance, MSF hardly suffered from a recruitment problem. They regularly received far more inquiries than they could ever accept, turning away the vast majority of applicants. Most of these eager souls, however, were people without experience. They would require training and orientation, not only with technical skills but also with organizational culture. In addition they began as unknown elements, whose personal qualities remained to be tested, and might unbalance a team. Some regularly proved to have unrealistic expectations, of both the world and themselves. The divide between "first mission" volunteers and veterans could thus at times loom almost as large as that between expatriate and national staff. Within the structure and logic of the organization, only experienced members—with tested international perspective—possessed the requisite knowledge and judgment to fill leadership roles.

MSF's problem was that not enough of those who survived their initiation continued on into other missions. Those who did struggled not only with career concerns but questions of burnout as well. The life proved demanding and the work all-consuming. One could always do more, and yet results remained elusive. At the same time, the thought that this would become just a job haunted the organization and unsettled many within it. MSF feared complacency, to the extent that it institutionalized turnover. Just as it fretted about naive children of privilege, it also worried about national staff from poor countries, and anyone else suspected of joining for a paycheck. Neither group was certain to display the proper spirit or tireless commitment.

For their part experienced members of the organization vacillate between expressions of abiding loyalty and deep frustration. The pages of its internal newsletters include exhortations and denunciations, tributes and dark humor. After hours discussions, particularly at mission sites, regularly involve banter and often self-interrogations or confessions of doubt. I was warned early on not to take these moments too seriously, since the same individuals would rise the next day and return to work. Nonetheless the pattern remains. So does a record of fiercer dispute, sometimes leading to angry rupture. An impressive number of MSF's pioneers stormed away from the organization, some more than once. Although life might now be calmer than in the era of the "dinosaurs" (as aging veterans are known), the well of emotional tensions remains. Most of the organization's missions raise as many questions as they resolve. Indeed, recognizing that might at times appear something like a rite of passage.

Sample scene: an MSF compound in Northern Uganda, with a Canadian doctor, on her first mission, a visiting Canadian journalist, a Ugandan driver and this anthropologist. We have recently returned from a visit to a clinic in a distant refugee camp, and the others turn contemplative after asking about my research.

> Doctor: Should we all just leave? The project is great when there, but it's clear it will collapse when we leave. (She looks at the driver, who merely smiles and shakes his head).
>
> Journalist: The problem is a nonfunctioning government. That's the issue.
>
> Doctor: But people at home are thinking it's all such great work. That we're making a real difference.
>
> Anthropologist (trying out a new question): Do you need to feel optimistic to act?
>
> Doctor: I think it's easier as a doctor, being on the medical side of MSF. People going to die no matter what, you know that, but you can still work for health.
>
> Journalist: I won't agree that development is a failure. The problem is the government.
>
> Doctor: Then maybe we should just stay on and on.
>
> Journalist: The new missionaries?
>
> Doctor: It took me five years to find someone to fill in for six months!

The moment passes, as such moments do, and we return to other topics and our respective roles. Nothing has been resolved. Nonetheless, the exchange touches the undercurrent of uncertainty running through MSF's larger enterprise.

I should add that this particular project seemed more promising than many; the population had clear needs, and no one else stood ready to supply them. Unlike the mission's other project site, a camp nearer to the regional town and swarming with jockeying organizations, it was not yet "aid-fucked," in the pungent description of the group's field coordinator. The doctor liked to work there, feeling useful. It was precisely because the project seemed promising that it raised anxieties about its future. We all knew that MSF would pull back when the crisis eased. It was not a development organization. It did not wish to substitute for a state. Its project remained a small one, with limited goals. None of this, however, felt particularly satisfying. Of the individuals present, only the driver had a direct stake in the Uganda's government. While judiciously silent during this discussion, his earlier remarks suggested he personally had little faith in the political future. Indeed, as several other Ugandans reminded me at various junctures, "change" could always mean things getting worse as well as getting better.

"Africans must solve African problems," an Argentinean doctor proclaimed a few years later, sitting at a bar in the same town. "That's why I want to return to Argentina. The medical staff I worked with today were good—as good as I am or better." He seemed to be speaking to himself as much as the others around the table, affirming a strongly held belief shared by many within MSF. A newcomer who had just started in a larger clinic, Ernesto was acutely aware that his medical degree gave him little real advantage among less credentialed but more experienced Ugandan colleagues. Brought up with leftist political sympathies, and also facing a tight job market for young doctors in his home country, he had decided to volunteer for international work. MSF was a famous and professional organization, even paying for the plane ticket that allowed him to interview. So far he was glad he had joined; he wanted to practice real medicine among people who needed it. However, solidarity should only be taken so far. Ultimately he was not a Ugandan, and it was not his place to dictate a lasting solution. Local professionals should take the lead.

"We have to accept that we're not fixing anything, just working on something and moving all the time," a more weathered coordinator told me emphatically at their Brussels office in 2003. "To think that we're fixing anything is wrong." His point nicely summarized the organization's moral minimalism. One should act for the best, but without undue expectations. Together with Ernesto's anti-colonial sensibility, it outlined a limit of what MSF should attempt as a mobile entity driven by emergency. What about hope, however? Might it hold any residual place within a recipe of acting with minimal expectations? Beyond pointing to small triumphs of individual lives saved, MSF members sometimes indicated another potential benefit of action: one never quite knew where it would lead. Refugee camps were hardly sterile spaces, after all, as another old hand reminded me in Brussels. Amid all the problems they generated they also could, from time to time, "accelerate history." Once people had enjoyed better health care, they might expect more, and so demand more of their political leaders. A space of "normality" amid crisis might help restore a sense of dignity, and with it the possibility of greater self-determination.

I stress that such claims emerge made in a qualified way—as a possibility, not a given certainty. Often the speaker would point to a specific case known to collective experience, but whether as exception or a rule was not always clear. Rather than any sure chain of causality, they indicated a more fundamental dynamic of uncertainty in practice. Members of MSF recognize the gap between intention and deed, and through it, a glimmer of hope. The fact that the group is there has effects, never fully predictable beforehand. This unpredictability leaves room for small countercurrents, exceptions amid a larger pattern of setbacks. Should its engagements fail to affect public health at a population level, they might still achieve disruptive significance through their clinical outcomes, defending human life and dignity "one patient at a time." Thus something like hope becomes embodied and realized in specific individuals and actual lives. The results may not establish good public policy, but they potentially disrupt the bad, while benefiting a tangible few in the process.

What I am describing as moral minimalism and residual hope resides at the intersection of a concern for values and effects. As Craig Calhoun notes, humanitarianism labors beneath Max Weber's distinction between value rationality and instrumental rationality, phrased as a question of whether to favor good deeds for themselves, or to concentrate on their outcomes.[10] Within the contemporary aid world, the categorical concern for life and suffering that motivates humanitarian organizations encounters expectations of accounting and demonstrating results. From a humanitarian perspective to let people suffer would be wrong. But what if trying to help only makes things worse? In embracing action and an ethic of refusal, MSF seeks to limit abstraction and emphasize practice. To accept justifications for suffering, even in the name of other goods, would risk leaving true humanitarianism behind.

Such austere minimalism, however, is not easy to maintain. Members of MSF frequently chafe at the restrictions of their own organization. Field teams are often loath to leave mission settings after the official crisis is over, and look for other reasons to stay. Moreover, individuals regularly denounce aspects of the group's positions they found wanting. MSF's tradition of internal discussion and debate absorbs much of this turmoil, sometimes redirecting it into new projects that can extend well beyond emergency care. But other concerns raise more

[10] Calhoun 2008: esp. 89–94. Also see Bornstein 2009.

fundamental questions for those with a progressive conscience. Why does MSF keep insisting it is not a pacifist organization when it constantly finds itself in warzones? Why is it so tentative about issues related to poverty and so allergic to development? Why not claim human rights or social justice? Why not embrace movements to counter existing forms of globalization? Even experienced members wonder aloud from time to time within their continuing commitment. Humanitarianism, it seems, always leaves one wanting more.

MSF's chosen path leads to a resolutely bleak horizon. Once there many eventually leave for other endeavors, a few taking the more haunting exit of suicide. Some soldier on, however, even in the face of repeated failure. "The hopelessness of human beings is not a reason to abandon them," a Spanish doctor proclaimed at a public forum in Amsterdam. "Should we only get involved in beautiful, sexy emergencies or also in hopeless places? Our work is to keep trying amid pessimism." His words echo famous formulations of others who saw the world darkly while actively engaging it: Antonio Gramsci's motto "pessimism of the intellect, optimism of the will" or Michel Foucault's self-description as a "hyperactive pessimist."[11] Similarly, MSF keeps acting amid dissatisfaction. It thus reluctantly participates in the greater humanitarian illusion that "something is being done." One saving grace might rest in the slight uncertainty of between action and outcome. Another could reside in dissatisfaction itself, and a continuing attitude of restless refusal.

Two moments may help outline this ethos of continuing discontent. On one of my initial visits to MSF, in this case an office in Amsterdam, I interviewed a veteran staff member, then readying to work for another organization. After a lengthy discussion of the politics of intervention, he paused, lit another cigarette and noted with a wry smile: "The beauty of MSF is the anarchy as well. We're not always consistent." The comment stayed with me throughout subsequent research. Beyond reflecting the essential style of the group, it also summed up and celebrated its de facto embrace of contradiction. Keeping things unsettled was a moral ethos as well as a way of life.

Several years later I found myself at a party in Kampala. Near its end, amid empty bottles of wine and eddies of conversation, the local heads of MSF-France and MSF-Switzerland discussed the state of affairs of their larger organization. They agreed that people were now being pushed too quickly into leadership roles. To really take up the charge one needed self-confidence, and a full grasp of the habits of a complex, far-flung entity, something hard to develop without four or five years of experience. Most crucially of all, one needed a visceral understanding of MSF's calling. Both were native French speakers, and they used a term I hadn't heard before: *hargne*, or irascibility. For them the MSF spirit went beyond passionate commitment. It required an ever-cantankerous edge, not for its own sake but as an aversion to accepting things as they were. The fact that these two individuals were known for their calm and cheerful personalities only underscored that the latter point. Here again the official, circumscribed ethical stance did not translate simply into practice. Nor did it satisfy the larger hunger to appear rebellious and questioning, to convert crisis back into critique. One might not know what to say or do, but one should stay irascible.

Who can argue with water, hygiene and basic health care? A clean tap, a latrine, a simple clinic. These are all essentially good things in their way, especially when surrounded by glaring absence. Of course meager, temporary presence only highlights the continuing inequality of circumstances. Charity offers only minor ameliorations, not justice. Too, the delivery of any good has multiple effects, and mingles care with control. All generate new possibilities for regulation: a tap can be turned on and off, a latrine requires maintenance and a clinic preaches the gospel of healthy behavior. Such control extends to the basic functions and conditions of life—life in its most elemental and animal form. It is precisely this aspect of life that MSF often confronts, both literally and rhetorically. At our present moment it produces a compelling vision, matters of life and death, the raw stuff of personal concern filtered through mass media. But it remains important to recall that humans have prized other values,

[11] Gramsci 1994: 299–300 for a formulation and potential debt to the French writer Romain Rolland; Foucault 1984: 343.

sometimes deeming them a worthy trade for existence. Love, honor, belief, utopian futures—the list runs through the moral range of causes for which people have both killed and died, sacrificing being for something else. Humanitarians have good reason to remain discontent, not only with others but also themselves. Surely there is more to life than saving it.

REFERENCES

Adorno, Theodor. 1974 [1951]. *Minima Moralia: Reflections from Damaged Life.* London: NLB.

Arendt, Hannah. 1998 [1958]. *The Human Condition.* Second ed. Chicago: University of Chicago Press.

Bornstein, Erica. 2009. "The Impulse of Philanthropy." *Cultural Anthropology* 24 (4).

Bortolotti, Dan. 2004. *Hope in Hell: Inside the World of Doctors Without Borders.* Buffalo, NY: Firefly Books

Brauman, Rony. 1996. *Humanitaire, le dilemme.* Paris: Editions Textuel.

Calhoun, Craig. 2008. "The Imperative to Reduce Suffering: Charity, Progress and Emergencies in the Field of Humanitarian Action." In *Humanitarianism in Question: Power, Politics, Ethics,* edited by M. Barnett and T. Weiss. Ithaca, NY: Cornell University Press: 73–97.

Fassin, Didier. 2012. *Humanitarian Reason: A Moral History of the Present.* Berkeley: University of California Press.

Foucault, Michel. 1984. "On the Genealogy of Ethics: An Overview of Work in Progress." In *The Foucault Reader,* edited by P. Rabinow. New York: Pantheon, 340–372.

Gramsci, Antonio. 1994. *Letters from Prison.* Edited by F. Rosengarten. New York: Columbia University Press.

Rieff, David. 2002. *A Bed for the Night: Humanitarianism in Crisis.* New York: Simon and Schuster.

Slim, Hugo. 1997. "Doing the Right Thing: Relief Agencies, Moral Dilemmas and Moral Responsibility in Political Emergencies and War." *Disasters* 21(3): 244–257.

Terry, Fiona. 2002. *Condemned to Repeat? The Paradox of Humanitarian Action.* Ithaca, NY: Cornell University Press.

Voltaire. 1991. *Candide.* Translated and edited by R. Adams. New York: W. W. Norton.

PAUL E. FARMER, BRUCE NIZEYE, SARA STULAC, AND SALMAAN KESHAVJEE

34 STRUCTURAL VIOLENCE AND CLINICAL MEDICINE

Many selections in this reader have shown the myriad ways that social inequalities can lead to poor health outcomes. As this book has discussed in some depth, poverty and social inequality can lead to poor health, through access to food and water (Sections 4 and 6), through environmental inequalities (Sections 4 and 5), and through the stress that accompanies social inequalities (Section 7). In this article, the physician and anthropologist Paul Farmer argues that because these social inequalities affect health so severely, they amount to a form of violence: he calls this **structural violence**.

Mundane and avoidable circumstances of poverty—especially endemic hunger, lack of clean water, unsanitary conditions, inadequate housing, unemployment, and low wages—are structural violence because they cause suffering, disease, and death. In this selection, Paul Farmer and colleagues take this observation and ask: How can awareness of structural violence be translated into better clinical care? The authors point out that most doctors and public health professionals are well aware that social factors deeply affect health, but that they are not always trained to address these important social factors when treating patients.

Then the authors offer the example of two projects that they think successfully took social factors into consideration when offering treatment for HIV/AIDS. One of the projects the authors describe was in Baltimore; the other was in rural Rwanda. In both, doctors and health staff thought hard about the social reasons for poor clinical outcomes, and did what they could to address the problems they identified.

As you read this selection, consider these questions:

- **Do you agree with Galtung and the authors that the kinds of phenomena they describe should be described as "violence"?**
- **Why do the authors argue that structural violence is often invisible compared with violence in a war?**
- **Why do you think it is the case that, as the authors argue, "medical professionals are not trained to make structural interventions"?**
- **Beyond training, why do you think more doctors don't take the kinds of steps that are described in this article?**
- **Do you think that public health practitioners do a better job than doctors do at addressing the structural determinants of health? Why or why not?**
- **What do the authors mean when they say that "distal and proximal interventions are complementary, not competing"? In the context of limited resources, do you agree with them?**
- **The authors write that when doctors and academics don't take history and social structure into account when talking about illness and disease, "structural violence is perpetrated through analytic omission." What does this mean?**
- **Why do you think some people working in global health get uncomfortable when talking about politics? Are political dimensions so complicated and thorny that they make solutions seem less possible?**

Paul E. Farmer, Bruce Nizeye, Sara Stulac, and Salmaan Keshavjee. "Structural Violence and Clinical Medicine." *PLOS Medicine*, October 2006, 3(10): e449.

CONTEXT

The authors of this article are all affiliated with Partners in Health, an organization that works to provide medical care in a number of countries, including the United States and Rwanda (the two discussed in this article). Paul Farmer, Sara Stulac, and Salmaan Keshavjee work and teach at Harvard Medical School and Brigham and Women's Hospital in Boston.

Paul Farmer is a medical anthropologist and medical doctor who specializes in the treatment of infectious diseases. When he was a medical student, Farmer founded a clinic for the treatment of AIDS and tuberculosis in a very poor rural area of Haiti. That clinic grew into a large international organization, Partners in Health, which provides health care and advocacy for poor communities throughout the world. A readable biography of Farmer, written by Tracy Kidder, is *Mountains Beyond Mountains* (New York: Random House, 2003).

Bruce Nizeye is an engineer who directs Partners in Health's (Inshuti Mu Buzima) Program on Social and Economic Rights in Rwanda—the program responsible for providing many of the services described in this article.

Because of contact with patients, physicians readily appreciate that large-scale social forces—racism, gender inequality, poverty, political violence and war, and sometimes the very policies that address them—often determine who falls ill and who has access to care. For practitioners of public health, the social determinants of disease are even harder to disregard.

Unfortunately, this awareness is seldom translated into formal frameworks that link social analysis to everyday clinical practice. One reason for this gap is that the holy grail of modern medicine remains the search for the molecular basis of disease. While the practical yield of such circumscribed inquiry has been enormous, exclusive focus on molecular-level phenomena has contributed to the increasing "desocialization" of scientific inquiry: a tendency to ask only biological questions about what are in fact *biosocial* phenomena.[1]

Biosocial understandings of medical phenomena are urgently needed. All those involved in public health sense this, especially when they serve populations living in poverty. Social analysis, however rudimentary, occurs at the bedside, in the clinic, in field sites, and in the margins of the biomedical literature. It is to be found, for example, in any significant survey of adherence to therapy for chronic diseases[2,3] and in studies of what were once termed "social diseases" such as venereal disease and tuberculosis (TB).[4–8] The emerging phenomenon of acquired resistance to antibiotics—including antibacterial, antiviral, and antiparasitic agents—is perforce a biosocial process, one which began less than a century ago as novel treatments were introduced.[9] Social analysis is heard in discussions about illnesses for which significant environmental components are believed to exist, such as asthma and lead poisoning.[10–15] Can we speak of the "natural history" of any of these diseases without addressing social forces, including racism, pollution, poor housing, and poverty, that shape their course in both individuals and populations? Does our clinical practice acknowledge what we already know—namely, that social and environmental forces will limit the effectiveness of our treatments? Asking these questions needs to be the beginning of a conversation within medicine and public health, rather than the end of one.

Defining Structural Violence

The term "structural violence" is one way of describing social arrangements that put individuals and populations in harm's way (see Box 1).[16] The arrangements are *structural* because they are embedded in the political and economic organization of our social world; they are *violent* because they cause

BOX 34.1 What Is Structural Violence?

Structural violence, a term coined by Johan Galtung and by liberation theologians during the 1960s, describes social structures—economic, political, legal, religious, and cultural—that stop individuals, groups, and societies from reaching their full potential.[57] In its general usage, the word *violence* often conveys a physical image; however, according to Galtung, it is the "avoidable impairment of fundamental human needs or . . . the impairment of human life, which lowers the actual degree to which someone is able to meet their needs below that which would otherwise be possible".[58] Structural violence is often embedded in longstanding "ubiquitous social structures, normalized by stable institutions and regular experience".[59] Because they seem so ordinary in our ways of understanding the world, they appear almost invisible. Disparate access to resources, political power, education, health care, and legal standing are just a few examples. The idea of *structural violence* is linked very closely to *social injustice* and the social machinery of oppression.[16]

injury to people (typically, not those responsible for perpetuating such inequalities). With few exceptions, clinicians are not trained to understand such social forces, nor are we trained to alter them. Yet it has long been clear that many medical and public health interventions will fail if we are unable to understand the social determinants of disease.[17,18]

The good news is that such biosocial understandings are far more "actionable" than is widely recognized. There is already a vast and growing array of diagnostic and therapeutic tools born of scientific research; it is possible to use these tools in a manner informed by an understanding of structural violence and its impact on disease distribution and on every step of the process leading from diagnosis to effective care. This means working at multiple levels, from "distal" interventions—performed late in the process, when patients are already sick—to "proximal" interventions—trying to prevent illness through efforts such as vaccination or improved water and housing quality.

As with many other concepts, structural violence has its limitations.[19] Nevertheless, we seek to apply the concept to what remain the primary tasks of clinical medicine: preventing premature death and disability and improving the lives of those we care for. Using the concept of structural violence, we intend to begin, or revive, discussions about social forces beyond the control of our patients.

These forces are not beyond the reach, however, of practitioners of medicine and public health. In this article, we describe examples of the impact of structural violence upon people living with HIV in the United States and in Rwanda. In both cases, we show that it is possible to address structural violence through structural interventions. We then draw general lessons from these examples for health professionals and policy makers worldwide.

Delivering AIDS Care Equitably in the United States

The distribution and outcome of chronic infectious diseases, such as HIV/AIDS, are so tightly linked to social arrangements that it is difficult for clinicians treating these diseases to ignore social factors. Although AIDS is often considered a "social disease," clinicians may have radically different understandings of what makes AIDS "social." Many doctors have focused on the "behaviors" or "lifestyles" that place some at risk for HIV infection.[20–23] Yet risk has never been determined solely by individual behavior: susceptibility to infection and poor outcomes is aggravated by social factors such as poverty, gender inequality, and racism.[24–26] Unsurprisingly, in less than a decade AIDS became a disease that disproportionately affected America's poor, many of whom engaged in "risk behaviors" at a far lower rate than others who were not at heightened risk of infection with sexually transmitted diseases.[27–29]

Factors Affecting Disease Course

HIV attacks the immune system in only one way, but its course and outcome are shaped by social forces having little to do with the universal pathophysiology of the disease. From the outset of acute HIV infection to the endgame of recurrent opportunistic infections, disease course is determined by, to cite but a few obvious factors: (1) whether or not postexposure prophylaxis is available; (2) whether or not the steady decline in immune function is hastened by concurrent illness or malnutrition; (3) whether or not multiple HIV infections occur; (4) whether or not TB is prevalent in the surrounding environment; (5) whether or not prophylaxis for opportunistic infections is reliably available;[30] and (6) whether or not antiretroviral therapy (ART) is offered to all those needing it.

Throughout the usually decade-long process of HIV progression, detrimental social structures and constructs—structural violence—have a profound influence on effective diagnosis, staging, and treatment of the disease and its associated pathologies. Each of these determinants of disease course and outcome is itself shaped by the very social forces that determine variable risk of infection.

Although the variability of outcomes has been especially obvious in the era of effective therapy, it was so even before ART became widely available. In Baltimore in the early 1990s, Moore et al. showed that race was associated with the timely receipt of therapeutics: among patients infected with HIV, blacks were significantly less likely than whites to have received ART or *Pneumocystis* pneumonia prophylaxis when they were first referred to an HIV clinic, regardless of disease stage at the time of presentation.[31] The timeline from HIV infection to death was further shortened in situations where TB was the leading opportunistic infection, as it is in much of the poor world.[32] These fundamentally biosocial events call into question a "natural history" of HIV infection and AIDS.

Addressing Disparities in HIV Care

In an attempt to address these ethnic disparities in care, researchers and clinicians in Baltimore reported how racism and poverty—forms of structural violence, though they did not use these specific terms—were embodied[33,34] as excess mortality among African Americans without insurance. After documenting these disparities, these clinicians and researchers asked: what would happen if race and insurance status no longer determined who had access to the standard of care?

Their subsequent interventions were decidedly proximal: in addition to removing some of the obvious economic barriers at the point of care, the clinicians and researchers considered paying for transportation costs and other incentives as well as addressing comorbid conditions ranging from drug addiction to mental illness. They also implemented improvements in community-based care, conceived to make AIDS care more convenient and socially acceptable for patients. The goal was to make sure that nothing within the medical system or the surrounding community prevented poor and otherwise marginalized patients from receiving the standard of care.

The results registered just a few years later were dramatic: racial, gender, injection-drug use, and socioeconomic disparities in outcomes largely disappeared within the study population.[35] In other words, these program improvements may not have dealt with the lack of national health insurance, and still less with the persistent problems of racism and urban poverty, but they did lessen the embodiment of social inequalities as premature death from AIDS. Similar work elsewhere has shown the ability of providers to lessen the impact of social inequalities on AIDS outcomes among the homeless, the addicted, the mentally ill, and prisoners.[36–38]

The program in Baltimore was improved in part by linking an understanding of social context to clinical services. The importance of such programs is underscored by the emergence of multidrug-resistant HIV in the United States.[39] Microbial acquisition of resistance to antibiotics, including antiretrovirals, is necessarily a biosocial phenomenon. Most microbes mutate when challenged with antibiotics; the rate of mutation may be hastened by imprudent use of antibiotics or by inadequate or interrupted therapy.[40,41] Although structural violence lessens both access and adherence to effective therapy, it is a rarely discussed contributor to epidemics of multidrug-resistant HIV. In reality, it is impossible to understand the dynamics of drug-resistant disease without understanding how structural violence is embodied at the community, individual, and microbial levels.[9,42] The lessons from Baltimore show us that by viewing access to care and adherence to treatment as structural issues requiring programmatic solutions, we can alter the very biology of HIV and the "natural history" of AIDS.

Preventing Pediatric AIDS in Rwanda: Lessons from Rural Haiti

The impact of structural violence is even more obvious in the world's poorest countries and has profound implications for those seeking to provide clinical services there. Over the past year, working with the nonprofit organization Partners In Health (PIH), we have sought to address AIDS and TB in Africa, the world's poorest and most heavily burdened continent. Specifically, we have transplanted and adapted the "PIH model" of care, which was designed in rural Haiti to prevent the embodiment of poverty and social inequalities as excess mortality due to AIDS, TB, malaria, and other diseases of poverty.[43,44]

The PIH Model

In some senses, the model is simple: clinical and community barriers to care are removed as diagnosis and treatment are declared a public good and made available free of charge to patients living in poverty. Furthermore, AIDS care is delivered not only in the conventional way at the clinic, but also within the villages in which our patients work and live.

Each patient chooses an *accompagnateur*, usually a neighbor, trained to deliver drugs and other supportive care in the patient's home. Using this model, we currently provide daily supervised ART to more than 2,200 patients in rural Haiti. This model, with conventional clinic-based (distal) services complemented by home-based (more proximal) care, is deemed by some to be the world's most effective way of removing structural barriers to quality care for AIDS and other chronic diseases. It is also a way of creating jobs in rural regions in great need of them. We have used a similar model in urban Peru,[45,46] and in Boston, Massachusetts.[37]

The Challenge of HIV in Rwanda

Rwanda presents unique challenges, but many barriers to care are quite similar to those seen in Haiti and other settings where social upheaval, poverty, and gender inequality decrease the effectiveness of distal services and of prevention efforts. Like Haiti, Rwanda is a densely populated, predominantly agrarian society. Although both countries have endured large-scale political violence, that which registered a decade ago in Rwanda due to war and genocide was unprecedented in scale. In the two rural districts of Rwanda in which the PIH model was introduced in May 2005, an estimated 60 percent of inhabitants are refugees, returning exiles, or recent settlers; not a single physician was present to serve 350,000 people.

AIDS has recently worsened this situation and is a leading cause of young adult death. In spite of the availability of significant resources to treat complications of HIV infection in Africa, almost all patients enrolled on ART live in cities or towns. Indeed, some have noted that rapid treatment scale-up is likely to occur largely in urban settings, where infrastructure, though poor, is better than in rural regions.[47] The challenge, however, is to reach rural Africa, where fewer than five percent of those who need ART receive it. Rural treatment scale-up is far from impossible: less than a year after our program began in 2005, more than 1,500 rural Rwandans with AIDS were already enrolled in care using the PIH model.

To deepen our discussion of interventions designed to counter structural violence, consider the prevention of mother-to-child transmission (MTCT) of HIV in rural Rwanda. Where clean water is unavailable and HIV prevalence is high, the policy of universal breast-feeding—driven by the desire to reduce diarrhea-related mortality—leads to increased transmission of the virus to infants, even when ART is offered. We knew from our experience in Haiti that we could reduce rates of MTCT from as high as 25 to 40 percent to as low as 2 percent. We knew that such a dramatic reduction could be made possible by: (1) providing combination ART to the mother during pregnancy; (2) enabling formula-feeding and close follow-up of infants; and (3) launching potable water projects within the catchment area—in even the most difficult regions, where electricity is scarce, food insecurity widespread, and health and sanitation infrastructure rudimentary at best.[48]

Although our pilot project in Rwanda is only a year old, its feasibility is almost certain. In the first six months of operation, we screened for HIV infection more than 31,000 persons in the two districts in which we work. Without exception, pregnant women found to be infected with HIV expressed interest in ART to prevent MTCT, and all requested assistance not only with procuring infant formula, but also with the means to boil water and to store the formula safely (Figure 1).

Medical Professionals are not Trained to Make Structural Interventions

Our distal intervention is to provide ART to all women in the catchment area with the help of *accompagnateurs*. More proximal interventions include the distribution of kerosene stoves, kerosene, bottles, and infant formula; we also provide food aid and housing assistance when possible. Already, we are seeing a lowering of HIV infection rates amongst newborns, and we believe that, as the program becomes well established and services become available earlier during the course of pregnancy, rates of MTCT will continue to decline.

Unsurprisingly, opposition to the PIH model did not come from rural Rwandan women living with HIV. Rather, we faced the most resistance to this approach from local and global health policy makers who continued to promote universal breastfeeding, a policy which made eminent sense prior to the advent of HIV. Instead of trying to overcome programmatic barriers, the experts argued that formula-feeding was simply not feasible in rural Rwanda and that HIV-related stigma would prevent women from enrolling in such projects.

The examples of Rwanda and Haiti have shown us that, to date, there is little reason to believe that thoughtful structural interventions will fail to improve HIV prevention and treatment outcomes. Any failure is more likely to be due to programmatic shortfalls than to stigma or to non-compliance on the part of the patients enrolled in the program. Structural interventions of the sort described here remove the onus of adherence from vulnerable patients and place it squarely on the health system and on providers.

Incorporating Structural Interventions in Medicine and Public Health

If structural violence is often a major determinant of the distribution and outcome of disease, why is it or a similar concept not in wider circulation in medicine and public health, especially now that our interventions can radically alter clinical outcomes? One reason is that medical professionals are not trained to make structural interventions. Physicians can rightly note that structural interventions are "not our job." Yet, since structural interventions might arguably have a greater impact on disease control than do conventional clinical interventions, we would do well to pay heed to them.

Acknowledging and addressing structural impediments, however, should never be the sole focus of our work. For decades, those who study the determinants of disease have known that social or structural forces account for most epidemic disease. But truisms such as "poverty is the root cause of tuberculosis" have not led us very far. While we do not yet have a curative prescription for poverty, we do know how to cure TB. Those who argue that focusing solely on economic development will in time wipe out tuberculosis may be correct, but en route toward this utopia the body count will remain high if care is not taken to diagnose and treat the sick. The same holds true for other diseases of poverty. Clean water and sanitation will prevent cases of typhoid fever, but those who fall ill need antibiotics; clean water comes too late for them.

The debate about whether to focus on proximal versus distal interventions, or similar debates about how best to use scarce resources, is as old as medicine itself. But there is little compelling evidence that we must make such either/or choices: distal and proximal interventions are complementary, not competing. International public health is rife with false debates along precisely these lines, and the list of impossible choices facing those who work among the destitute sick seems endless. In reality, there is no good way to tackle the health crisis in Africa when the scant resources previously available are so bitterly contested; thus is structural violence perpetuated at a time in which science and medicine continue to yield truly miraculous tools. Without an equity plan to bring these tools to bear on the health problems of the destitute, these debates will continue to waste precious time.[49]

The Lessons of Baltimore, Haiti, and Rwanda

What are the lessons that can be drawn from the examples of successful structural interventions in the diverse settings of Baltimore, rural Haiti, and rural Rwanda? First, we have seen that it is possible to decrease the extent to which social inequalities become embodied as health disparities. While some interventions are straightforward, we also have to recognize that there is an enormous flaw in the dominant model of medical care: as long as medical services are sold as commodities, they will remain available only to those who can purchase them. National health insurance and other social safety nets, including those that guarantee primary education, food security, and clean water, are important because they promise rights, rather than commodities, to citizens. The lack of these social and economic rights is fundamental to the perpetuation of structural violence.[50]

Second, we have learned that proximal interventions, seemingly quite remote from the practice of clinical medicine, can also lessen premature morbidity and mortality. To put this in sociological terms, interventions that increase the agency of the poor will lessen their risk of HIV. Similarly, it is not possible to have an honest discussion of alcoholism among Native Americans,[51] or crack cocaine addiction among African Americans,[52] without discussing the history of genocide and slavery in North America. Again, such commentary is often seen as extraneous in medical and public health circles, where discussions of substance abuse are curiously desocialized, viewed as personal and psychological problems rather than societal ones. Here, too, structural violence is perpetuated through analytic omission.

Third, we have seen that structural interventions can have an enormous impact on outcomes, even in the face of cost-effectiveness analyses and the flawed policies of international bodies. Taking the components of the distal interventions already underway in Rwanda—infant formula, clean water, fuel, and so forth—it is possible to go further and describe more proximal interventions to improve access to each component of the project. These would include, of course, legislation to promote generic medications, improved distribution networks for ART and infant formula, clean-water campaigns, and the development of alternative fuels. More proximally still, they would include enhancing agricultural production; creating new jobs outside of the agricultural sector; addressing gender inequality through legislation about land tenure and political representation;[53] and promoting adult literacy.

These are not the tasks for which clinicians were trained, but they are central to the struggle to reduce premature suffering and death. The importance of structural interventions for the future of health care means that practitioners of medicine and public health must make common cause with others who are trained to intervene more proximally. Sometimes public health crises, such as the AIDS pandemic in Africa, can lead to bold and specific interventions, such as the campaign to provide AIDS prevention and care as a public good.[54] When linked to more structural interventions, such ostensibly specific campaigns can help to trigger a "virtuous social cycle" that promises to shift the burden of pathology away from children and young adults—a major victory in the struggle to lessen structural violence.

Conclusions

Pioneers of modern public health during the nineteenth century, such as Rudolph Virchow, understood that epidemic disease and dismal life expectancies were tightly linked to social conditions.[55,56] Such leaders might not have employed the term "structural violence," but they were well aware of its toll and argued compellingly for proximal interventions: education, basic sanitation, land reform, sovereignty, and an end to political oppression. These interventions are no less needed now that we have better distal tools, including vaccines, diagnostics, and a large armamentarium of effective therapeutics.

It does not matter what we call it: structural violence remains a high-ranking cause of premature death and disability. We can begin to address this by "resocializing" our understanding of disease distribution and outcome. Even new diseases such as AIDS have quickly become diseases of the poor, and the development of effective therapies may have a perverse effect if we are unable to use them where they are needed most. By insisting that our services be delivered equitably, even physicians who work on the distal interventions characteristic of clinical medicine have much to contribute to reducing the toll of structural violence. The poor are the natural constituents of public health, and physicians, as Virchow argued, are the natural attorneys of the poor. In this struggle, equity in health care *is* our responsibility. Only when we link our efforts to those of others committed to initiating virtuous social cycles can we expect a future in which medicine attains its noblest goals.

Acknowledgments

The authors work with large teams of providers—*accompagnateurs*, social workers, nurses, physicians—in both Haiti and Rwanda. We are deeply grateful to our colleagues.

REFERENCES

1. Farmer P (2002) Social medicine and the challenge of biosocial research. In: Opolka U, Schoop H, editors. Innovative Structures in Basic Research: Ringberg-Symposium, 4–7 October 2000. Munich: Max-Planck-Gesellschaft. pp. 55–73.
2. Osterberg L, Blaschke T (2005) Adherence to medication. N Engl J Med 353: 486–497.
3. Sumartojo E (1993) When tuberculosis treatment fails: A social behavioral account of patient adherence. Am Rev Respir Dis 147: 1311–1320.
4. Brandt A (1987) No magic bullet: A social history of venereal disease in the United States since 1880. New York: Oxford University Press. 290 p.
5. Dubos R, Dubos J (1996) The white plague: Tuberculosis, man, and society. New Brunswick (NJ): Rutgers University Press. 277 p.
6. Packard R (1989) White plague, black labor: Tuberculosis and the political economy of health and disease in South Africa. Berkeley: University of California Press. 389 p.
7. Feldberg GD (1995) Disease and class: Tuberculosis and the shaping of modern North American society. New Brunswick (NJ): Rutgers University Press. 274 p.
8. Keshavjee S, Becerra M (2000) Disintegrating health services and resurgent tuberculosis in post-Soviet Tajikistan: An example of structural violence. JAMA 283: 1201.
9. Farmer PE, Becerra M (2001) Biosocial research and the TDR agenda. TDR News 66: 5–7.
10. Akinbami LJ, Schoendorf KC (2002) Trends in childhood asthma: Prevalence, health care utilization, and mortality. Pediatrics 110: 315–322.
11. McConnochie KM, Russo MJ, McBride JT, Szilagyi PG, Brooks A, et al. (1999) Socioeconomic variation in asthma hospitalization: Excess utilization or greater need? Pediatrics 103: e75.
12. Gottlieb DJ, Beiser AS, O'Connor GT (1995) Poverty, race, and medication use are correlates of asthma hospitalization rates. A small area analysis in Boston. Chest 108: 28–35.
13. Zabel EW, Castellano S (2006) Lead poisoning in Minnesota Medicaid children. Minn Med 89: 45–49.
14. Maharachpong N, Geater A, Chongsuvivatwong V (2006) Environmental and childhood lead contamination in the proximity of boat-repair yards in southern Thailand—I: Pattern and factors related to soil and household dust lead levels. Environ Res 101: 294–303.
15. Fraser B (2006) Peruvian mining town must balance health and economics. Lancet 367: 889–890.
16. Farmer P (2004) An anthropology of structural violence. Curr Anthropol 45: 305–326.
17. Mosley WH, Chen LC (1984) An analytical framework for the study of child survival in developing countries. Popul Dev Rev 10S: 25–45.
18. Lane SD, Keefe R, Rubinstein RA, Webster N, Rosenthal A, et al. (2004) Structural violence and racial disparity in heterosexual HIV infection. J Health Care Poor Underserved 15: 319–335.
19. Wacquant L (2004) Response to: Farmer PE (2004) An anthropology of structural violence. Curr Anthropol 45: 322.
20. Treichler PA (1987) AIDS, homophobia, and biomedical discourse: An epidemic of signification. In: Crimp D, editor. AIDS: Cultural analysis, cultural activism. Cambridge (MA): MIT Press. pp. 31–37.
21. Treichler PA (1988) AIDS, gender, and biomedical discourse: Current contests for meaning. In: Fee E, Fox DM, editors. AIDS: The burdens of history. Berkeley: University of California Press. pp. 190–266.
22. Oppenheimer G (1998) In the eye of the storm: The epidemiological construction of AIDS. In: Fee E, Fox

DM, editors. AIDS: The burdens of history. Berkeley: University of California Press. pp. 267–300.

23. Oppenheimer G (1992) Causes, cases, and cohorts: The role of epidemiology in the historical construction of AIDS. In: Fee E, Fox DM, editors. AIDS: The making of a chronic disease. Berkeley: University of California Press. pp. 49–83.
24. Farmer PE (2006) AIDS and accusation: Haiti and the geography of blame. 2nd edition. Berkeley: University of California Press. p. 338.
25. Farmer P, Connors M, Simmons J, editors (1996) Women, poverty, and AIDS: Sex, drugs, and structural violence. Monroe (ME): Common Courage Press. p. 473.
26. Stryker J, Jonsen AR, editors (1993) The social impact of AIDS in the United States. Washington, DC: National Academies Press. p. 336.
27. Toltzis P, Stephens RC, Adkins I, Lombardi E, Swami S, et al. (1999) Human immunodeficiency virus (HIV)-related risk-taking behaviors in women attending inner-city prenatal clinics in the mid-west. J Perinatol 19: 483–487.
28. Gottlieb SL, Douglas JM Jr, Schmid DS, Bolan G, Iatesta M, et al. (2002) Seroprevalence and correlates of herpes simplex virus type 2 infection in five sexually transmitted-disease clinics. J Infect Dis 186:1381–1389.
29. National Center for Health Statistics (1994) Annual summary of births, marriages, divorces, and deaths: United States, 1993. Hyattsville (MD): US Department of Health and Human Services, Public Health Service, CDC. pp. 18–20.
30. Wiktor SZ, Sassan-Morokro M, Grant AD, Abouya L, Karon JM, et al. (1999) Efficacy of trimethoprim-sulphamethoxazole prophylaxis to decrease morbidity and mortality in HIV-1-infected patients with tuberculosis in Abidjan, Côte d'Ivoire: A randomised controlled trial. Lancet 353: 1469–1475.
31. Moore RD, Stanton D, Gopalan R, Chaisson RE (1994) Racial differences in the use of drug therapy for HIV disease in an urban community. N Engl J Med 330: 763–768.
32. Lucas SB, Hounnou A, Peacock C, Beaumel A, Djomand G, et al. (1993) The mortality and pathology of HIV infection in a west African city. AIDS 7: 1569–1579.
33. Scheper-Hughes N, Lock M (1987) The mindful body: A prolegomenon to future work in medical anthropology. Med Anthropol Q 1: 6–41.
34. French L (1994) The political economy of injury and compassion: amputees on the Thai-Cambodian border. In: Csordas TJ, editor. Embodiment and experience: The existential ground of culture and self. Cambridge: Cambridge University Press. pp. 69–99.
35. Chaisson RE, Keruly JC, Moore RD (1995) Race, sex, drug use, and progression of human immunodeficiency virus disease. N Engl J Med 333: 751–756.
36. Bangsberg D, Tulsky JP, Hecht FM, Moss AR (1997) Protease inhibitors in the homeless. JAMA 278: 63–65.
37. Behforouz HL, Farmer PE, Mukherjee JS (2004) From directly observed therapy to *accompagnateurs*: Enhancing AIDS treatment outcomes in Haiti and in Boston. Clin Infect Dis 38: S429–S436.
38. Mitty JA, Macalino GE, Bazerman LB, Loewenthal HG, Hogan JW, et al. (2005) The use of community-based modified directly observed therapy for the treatment of HIV-infected persons. J Acquir Immune Defic Syndr 39: 545–550.
39. Little SJ, Holte S, Routy JP, Daar ES, Markowitz M, et al. (2002) Antiretroviral-drug resistance among patients recently infected with HIV. N Engl J Med 347: 385–394.
40. Neu C (1992) The crisis in antibiotic resistance. Science 257:1064–1073.
41. del Rio C, Green S, Abrams C, Lennox J (2001) From diagnosis to undetectable: The reality of HIV/AIDS care in the inner city [abstract]. 8th Annual Conference on Retroviruses and Opportunistic Infections; 2001 4–8 February; Chicago, Illinois, United States of America. Available: http://gateway.nlm.nih.gov/MeetingAbstracts/102244586.html. Accessed 20 September 2006.
42. Walton DA, Farmer PE, Dillingham R (2005) Social and cultural factors in tropical medicine: Reframing our understanding of disease. In: Guerrant RL, Walker DH, Weller PF, editors. Tropical infectious diseases: Principles, pathogens, and practice. 2nd edition. New York: Elsevier. pp. 26–35.
43. Farmer P, Léandre F, Mukherjee JS, Claude MS, Nevil P, et al. (2001) Community-based approaches to HIV treatment in resource-poor settings. Lancet 358: 404–409.
44. Walton DA, Farmer PE, Lambert W, Léandre F, Koenig SP, et al. (2004) Integrated HIV prevention and care strengthens primary health care: Lessons from rural Haiti. J Public Health Policy 25: 137–158.
45. Mitnick C, Bayona J, Palacios E, Shin S, Furin J, et al. (2003) Community-based therapy for multidrug-resistant tuberculosis in Lima, Peru. N Engl J Med 348:119–128.
46. Shin S, Furin J, Bayona J, Mate K, Kim JY, et al. (2004) Community-based treatment of multidrug-resistant tuberculosis in Lima, Peru: Seven years of experience. Soc Sci Med 59: 1529–1539.

47. Wilson DP, Kahn J, Blower SM (2006) Predicting the epidemiological impact of antiretroviral allocation strategies in KwaZulu-Natal: The effect of the urban-rural divide. Proc Nat Acad Sci 103:14228–14233.
48. Raymonville M, Léandre F, Saintard R, Colas M, Louissaint M, et al. (2004) Prevention of mother-to-child transmission of HIV in rural Haiti: The Partners In Health experience [poster]. A Multicultural Caribbean United Against HIV/AIDS; 2004 5–7 March; Santo Domingo, Dominican Republic.
49. Farmer P (2001) The major infectious diseases in the world—to treat or not to treat? N Engl J Med 345: 208–210.
50. Farmer PE (2005) Pathologies of power: Health, human rights, and the new war on the poor. 2nd edition. Berkeley: University of California Press. p. 402.
51. Shkilnyk A (1985) A poison stronger than love: The destruction of an Ojibwa community. New Haven (CT): Yale University Press. p. 276.
52. Chien A, Connors M, Fox K (2000) The drug war in perspective. In: Kim JY, Millen JV, Gershman J, Irwin A, editors. Dying for growth: Global inequalities and the health of the poor. Monroe (ME): Common Courage Press. pp. 293–327.
53. Lacey M (2005 February 26) Women's voices rise as Rwanda reinvents itself. The New York Times; Sect A: 1 (col 3). Available: http://www. peacewomen.org/news/Rwanda/Feb05/voicesrise.html. Accessed 20 September 2006.
54. Kim JY, Gilks C (2005) Scaling up treatment—why we can't wait. N Engl J Med 353: 2392–2394.
55. McKeown T (1980) The role of medicine: Dream, mirage, or nemesis? Princeton (NJ): Princeton University Press. p. 224.
56. Porter D (2006) How did social medicine evolve, and where is it heading? PLoS Med 3: e399. DOI: 10.1371/journal.pmed.0030399.
57. Galtung J (1969) Violence, peace and peace research. J Peace Res 6:167–191.
58. Galtung J (1993) Kultuerlle Gewalt. Der Burger im Staat 43: 106.
59. Gilligan J (1997) Violence: Reflections on a national epidemic. New York: Vintage Books. p. 306.

SECTION 9 CASES FOR TEACHING AND LEARNING

Visit the companion website, www.oup.com/us/brown-closser, for direct links to the featured online resources.

Emory Global Health Institute Case Writing Team, *"¡Alto a la Violencia!" Reducing Gun Violence in Honduras*

Students learn about the determinants of violence in Honduras and research and present interventions for reducing this violence.

Paula Johnson and Rachel Gordon, *Dr. Sam Thenya: A Women's Health Pioneer*

This case follows the establishment of several facilities in Kenya devoted to women's health, with particular attention to violence against women. Instructors will need to develop their own questions to pose to students about this case.

Novick et al., *Adolescent Suicide Prevention*

Students investigate the epidemiology of adolescent suicide in Onondaga County, New York, and consider prevention strategies.

Pabo et al., *HIV Voluntary Counseling and Testing in Hinche, Haiti*

This case describes a public health intervention based on Paul Farmer's analysis of structural violence (Reading 34). Students learn about voluntary counseling and testing for HIV, as well as treatment, in a program run by Partners in Health in Haiti. They consider how to sustain a broad basket of services for HIV-positive people. There is a follow-up case, *Two Years in Hinche,* online.

SECTION 9 VIDEOS AND WEB RESOURCES

Visit the companion website, www.oup.com/us/brown-closser, for direct links to the featured online resources.

Visuals: Stockholm International Peace Research Institute

This interactive website allows students to explore military spending by country over time.

Searching for Syria – UNHCR and Google

This interactive website provides an accessible and engaging introduction to Syria and illustrates the devastation caused by war. It draws on a number of personal stories and includes video of Syria and refugee camps. It is a particularly clear introduction to the current refugee crisis.

Triage: James Orbinski's Humanitarian Dilemma

This feature-length film follows the ethical dilemmas that Nobel Peace Prize winner James Orbinski faced during his work with Doctors Without Borders (see Chapter 33).

Out of Sight, Out of Mind – Pitch Interactive

This interactive website chronicles fatalities in Pakistan owing to US drone strikes through 2015. It powerfully illustrates the number of child and civilian casualties as a result of drone strikes. It can be usefully paired with Chapter 40, which discusses the impact of violence in Pakistan on polio eradication.

Futures Without Violence

This website has many resources, from videos to reports and discussion guides, dealing with issues of intimate partner and family violence. It has a section devoted to sexual assault on college campuses.

***13th* – Ava DuVernay**

A powerful feature-length film about race and mass incarceration in the United States. The film provides a particularly clear example of structural violence and is also very useful in discussions of police violence.

PART

4

Interventions to Improve Health

SECTION

10

A History of Health Institutions and Programs

Public health programs funded by high-income countries and implemented in low-income countries are not a new phenomenon. The idea of intentionally influencing the health of populations of low-income countries has been around for several hundred years. The fascinating and sometimes troubled history of these programs can shed light on many of the challenges of the present. In this section, we turn to history as a way to understand modern global health approaches and strategies.

The section begins with a chapter describing the different "root cultures" of international and global health. Some of the early institutions in colonial medicine and international health facilitated colonial military efforts, others aimed to relieve suffering created by disasters like war (see Section 9), and yet others had religious motivations. As Reading 35 describes, the philosophical legacies of these early institutions live on.

Often, considering the ethical dilemmas of the past can provide clarity on modern moral issues. The reading by Greenough (Reading 36) explores *how* the quintessential example of success in global health—the eradication of smallpox—was accomplished. This reading stands in contrast with the earlier reading on the smallpox eradication program (Reading 4) because it documents how the "disease warriors" used intimidation and coercion to get the job done in the face of local resistance. We think that considering the moral complexities of one of the great success stories in public health can help students develop a nuanced approach to global health ethics.

Finally, there is a reading by Randall Packard (Reading 37) that provides the historical context for the creation of the field of global health. He describes the historical factors that led to an emphasis on cost-effectiveness and technological solutions.

» CONCEPTUAL TOOLS «

- **Many colonial governments engaged in colonial medicine, often designed primarily to protect troops and colonizers from so-called tropical diseases.** Much of the thinking in this era of **tropical medicine** relied on racialized ideas of susceptibility to disease, which conceptualized white people as not only being more delicate and susceptible to disease but also as having superior bodies overall. In most cases, colonial public health projects did not extend broadly to the citizens of colonized countries but were mostly designed to protect colonial rulers and elites from disease.

- **The era of International Health started after World War II**, when a number of new international institutions, including the World Health Organization (WHO), were created. Around this time, many formerly colonized areas of the world became newly independent countries. The general framework of international health was that rich countries would provide money and technical assistance to improve health in poor countries. Since many of these rich countries were former colonizers and many of these poor countries were formerly colonized, there were many historical and conceptual ties to the earlier era of tropical medicine.
- **In the mid-2000s, the name of the field of international health shifted to global health.** The name "**global health**" reflected increasing attention to the fact that that health problems in one area of the world are tied to health problems in other places. But some critics say that nothing has really changed, that the name "global health" is old wine in new bottles and the same rich country–poor country power relations that characterized international health remain.

Major Players in Global Health

- There are many actors in global health. One important group is organizations affiliated with the United Nations (UN), sometimes called "multilateral organizations." Many modern UN organizations were formed shortly after World War II. **The two UN organizations with the most involvement in global health are the World Health Organization (WHO) and UNICEF.**
- The **WHO** was created immediately after World War II. The organization was based in part on the success of the **Pan American Health Organization (PAHO)**, a group of governments in the Americas (including the United States) that collaborate on health issues. **The WHO's mandate is to set norms and standards, shape the global research agenda, provide technical support to countries and monitor disease trends.** It is an organization of governments; every country on Earth gets one vote in the World Health Assembly, the governing body, no matter how large or small that country is. This means that China and Lichtenstein each get one vote!

  The WHO's budget is relatively small; much of its funding comes from dues paid by its member countries, but many member countries are behind on their payments. Recently, the WHO has been receiving money from some private donors, including the Gates Foundation, but it is still much less well-funded than many other global health organizations. Partly because of this, it has been losing influence over the last 3 decades. But it is still an important organization.
- **UNICEF** was also created right after World War II, to help displaced and refugee children in Europe in the aftermath of the war. When that crisis had passed, UNICEF turned its attention to children globally, and **in the 1980s and 1990s, UNICEF increasingly became involved in various child survival initiatives.**

Unlike WHO, UNICEF has a substantial budget that it can administer independently. This is in large part because of its extensive fundraising operation in rich countries. You may be familiar with UNICEF cards or you may have trick-or-treated for UNICEF as a child. Currently, UNICEF is particularly active in immunization programs, especially those targeting polio and measles, but it participates in a range of child survival programs.

- **The World Bank and the International Monetary Fund (IMF) are multilateral financial organizations.** They are called the "Bretton Woods organizations" because they were created at a conference at a fancy hotel in Bretton Woods, New Hampshire, in 1944. They have very different mandates.
- **The World Bank is, as its name suggests, a bank. It lends money to countries for projects that it thinks will generate a return on investment.** It is staffed by economists, not health professionals. Since the early 1990s, the World Bank has been increasingly lending to countries for health projects, because it believes that these investments will pay economic dividends. In general, the World Bank's philosophy is that the market is the best way to deliver health care—putting them at odds with people who argue for government-funded primary health care (PHC) for all (see following discussion). In the last 20 years, because of its resources, the World Bank has become an important actor in global health.

  At the World Bank, countries have voting power proportional to the size of their economy. So the World Bank's policies are driven by wealthy countries, and the United States has an effective veto.
- The **International Monetary Fund, or IMF,** is the other Bretton Woods institution. Rather than lending to countries on a routine basis, **the IMF steps in when countries are in financial crisis. Frequently, this intervention takes the form of structural adjustment programs.** Structural adjustment often includes the privatization of national industries and cutbacks in government payroll and employees. Often these steps can be devastating to government health systems, so many public health professionals are very critical of the IMF (see Reading 41).
- **Bilateral organizations are aid agencies created by governments to assist other governments.** The United States' bilateral aid organization is the United States Agency for International Development (USAID). Most major bilateral organizations give a substantial proportion of their funding to health programs.
- **Bilateral organizations often have political goals.** The US government's biggest health aid recipients, for example, include Afghanistan, Pakistan, Jordan, Ethiopia, Haiti, Kenya, and Iraq. These are not necessarily the countries that need aid the most; rather, they are the ones where the United States has strategic diplomatic or military interests.
- **Private foundations created with rich people's money have a long history of heavy involvement in global health.** The Rockefeller Foundation, for instance, founded with the oil wealth of the Rockefeller family, implemented a number of disease control programs in many countries in the early 1900s. Foundations—particularly the Bill and Melinda Gates Foundation—continue to be important.
- **Currently, the Bill and Melinda Gates Foundation has an enormous influence in global health.** With its enormous budget and thus its enormous influence, it sets many global health agendas. At least until recently, it has been focused on

technical innovation—like new vaccines or new technologies for mosquito control—as the way to solve global health problems.

- **Governments are perhaps the biggest player in health globally.** Nearly every country in the world has some kind of government health system—some are much more extensive than others, but government policy powerfully shapes health care everywhere in the world.
- **There is a dizzying array of nongovernmental organizations (NGOs) in health.** Since all that NGOs have in common is that they are not governments, it is nearly impossible to make any generalizations about them. Sometimes they are seen positively because they may be less bound by politics than governments are (though this is not always the case). At other times, they are seen negatively because they can draw resources away from government health systems. But the truth is that they are so diverse that they are nearly impossible to characterize. Many provide exceptional health services to people beyond the reach of government systems. Some effectively help people organize and advocate for the right to health. Some provide mediocre services, yet produce glossy reports to impress donors. Yet others provide few health services at all, functioning mainly to financially enrich the people who run them. It depends on the NGO!

Vertical Programs or Primary Health Care?

- **Eradication is the permanent and total obliteration of a disease from the face of the Earth.** It means that no one will ever get that disease again because the agent that causes the disease is gone forever. Smallpox is the only human disease to ever be eradicated. The smallpox virus is extinct in the wild, so nobody can contract the disease. (Unfortunately, smallpox virus still exists in labs; see Erroll Morris's video in the Web Resources of Section 1 for more on this situation.)
- **Disease eradication is extremely difficult and expensive.** It's also risky: most eradication programs in history have failed. To succeed, an eradication program has to effectively reach all populations in infected areas of the globe, from the most marginalized populations in war-torn areas, to groups that distrust the governments and affiliated organizations, to nomadic populations that live far from any organized infrastructure. And because eradication leaves no room for error, programs must reach these populations with programs of the very highest quality. This is very difficult to achieve in practice.

  Most diseases are not eradicable. To be eradicable, a disease must exist only in humans (since stopping disease in multiple species in all countries of the world simultaneously is even more difficult than stopping it just in humans), and there must be an extremely effective means of stopping the chain of transmission. In the case of smallpox, that was a very effective vaccine. In the case of guinea worm, a parasite that is close to being eradicated, clean drinking water can stop the chain of transmission completely. But for most diseases, it is difficult or impossible to completely stop transmission across the world with the tools at hand.
- **Elimination, on the other hand, means that a disease has been completely stopped in a country or a part of the world.** Polio, for example, has been eliminated from the Americas. Thanks to widespread vaccination, there is no

poliovirus transmission in North or South America at all. But because there are still cases of polio in other parts of the world (at least when this book went to press), it has not yet been eradicated.

- **The most common goal in public health is disease control.** Unlike eradication or elimination, the goal in disease control is to bring transmission down to some level deemed acceptable. Of course, what is seen as acceptable varies in different times and places!
- **Sometimes health programs use the words "eradication" and "elimination" when they are not actually trying to eradicate or eliminate a disease according to the previous definitions.** Often this is because these words sound good to donors. For example, the Stop TB program, a global control program, says it is aiming for a world "free of tuberculosis" with "zero deaths, disease, and suffering." This might sound like eradication—but, in fact, tuberculosis (TB) is not an eradicable disease because of the difficulty of preventing transmission. With existing technology, the best we can hope for is TB control: reducing TB incidences and TB deaths from their current levels.
- **Vertical programs are public health programs focused on just one disease.** The Global Polio Eradication Initiative and Stop TB are both vertical programs: they focus on cutting down polio or TB transmission globally and don't worry about other diseases. Eradication programs are all vertical programs since they are focusing on getting rid of just one disease. Vertical programs have some major strengths: they allow focus and clarity in goals, and they can be very appealing to donors. But they also have strong critics because they can ignore a community's most pressing health needs while they focus on their disease of choice.
- **Primary Health Care, or PHC, is the comprehensive provision of a broad range of basic health services**. Sometimes, other services like water and sanitation are also considered a part of PHC. PHC is conceptually the opposite of a vertical program: rather than a laser-like focus on one disease, proponents of PHC aim for integrated care that addresses a wide range of health issues. The philosophical differences between public health practitioners advocating PHC and those focused on vertical approaches are substantial and form one of the most long-standing and contentious debates in global health.
- **The concept of primary health care was most famously articulated at a conference held in 1978 in Alma-Ata, Kazakhstan.** With the slogan "Health for All by the Year 2000," the Alma-Ata conference pushed forward goals of comprehensive PHC and community participation in health. But while the Alma-Ata document laid out a lofty vision, figuring out how to actually achieve these goals proved difficult, and many donors found the fuzzy ideals less appealing than the clear objectives of vertical programs.
- **After Alma-Ata, UNICEF introduced what it called selective primary health care, which was not really PHC; rather, it was a collection of vertical programs that aimed to achieve improvements in child health in a measurable way.** The basket of services advocated by the selective PHC campaign was **GOBI-FFF**. GOBI stands for growth monitoring; oral rehydration solution in cases of diarrhea; breastfeeding; and immunization. Later, UNICEF added the Fs, which stand for family planning; female education; and food supplementation.

UNICEF selected these interventions because they are **cost-effective**: that is, they provide a big health benefit per dollar. Cost-effectiveness is a common way for global health agencies to make decisions about which programs to fund; it makes sense to try to do the most good with the money you have. But this way of thinking is also controversial: Paul Farmer, for example, argues that the logic of cost-effectiveness block expensive life-saving treatments from reaching poor people, reserving them for the rich.

Vaccination

- **Vaccination is one of the most effective and cost-effective technologies in public health**. It is a major reason for the decline in infectious disease rates throughout the world.
- **The first vaccine, for smallpox, was developed by Edward Jenner in the late 1700s.** He observed that milkmaids, who were often exposed to cowpox, generally did not get smallpox. Jenner experimented on a 9-year-old boy, infecting him with cowpox from a sore on a milkmaid's hand. Later, he repeatedly exposed the boy to smallpox, and the boy did not get sick. (Obviously, this research would not pass ethical review today.)

  Jenner was certainly a pioneer, but his work built on the longstanding practice of variolation, or deliberately infecting people with smallpox under controlled conditions so that they would develop immunity. Variolation was risky—in some settings, as many as 2% of variolated people died from the procedure—but compared with death rates from smallpox as high as 30%, it could be a very rational choice. Variolation was widely practiced in Asia and sub-Saharan Africa, but much less commonly practiced in Europe, in part because many Europeans found it hard to believe that any medical practice of Asians and Africans could be superior to their own. There were exceptions—for example, Lady Mary Wortley Montagu tried to popularize the practice in Europe, and Cotton Mather promoted it in America.

  Vaccination differs from variolation; vaccination is deliberately infecting someone with a milder or different form of the target disease that still triggers an immune response against that disease. Smallpox vaccine, derived from cowpox, was much safer than variolation. Ultimately, nearly 200 years after Jenner's first experiments, it led to the eradication of smallpox.
- All vaccines carry some risk—the specifics of the risks vary by vaccine. If you get a vaccine in the United States, you will be provided with an information sheet that details the risks of the vaccine you are receiving. But **the benefits of the vaccines that are recommended for children in the United States and around the world vastly outweigh the risks.** When high percentages of people in a population are vaccinated, morbidity and mortality from most vaccine-preventable diseases all but disappears. On the other hand, the most common side effects from a vaccine might be a sore arm or a low-grade fever.
- **For vaccination to be effective at a population level, herd immunity is necessary.** Some people with immune disorders cannot be vaccinated, and for nearly all vaccines, there is not full effectiveness—some percentage of people will still

be susceptible to disease even after being vaccinated. But, if everyone around them is vaccinated, these people will likely never be exposed to the disease in question, because everyone around them is immune and protected. Vaccination is thus a social contract—we must all participate to get the population benefit.

- **Vaccination does not cause autism.** Many high-quality studies have been done comparing vaccinated and unvaccinated children, and rates of autism are similar in both groups. Vaccination also does not cause children to become sterile—another common rumor (though not one widespread in the United States).
- **Current recommendations for routine childhood vaccinations in the United States provide protection from fourteen different infectious diseases:** chickenpox, diphtheria, Haemophilus influenza, hepatitis A, hepatitis B, influenza, measles, mumps, pertussis, pneumococcus, rotavirus, rubella, and tetanus. There are also some vaccines that are recommended for adults, including human papillomavirus virus, herpes zoster, influenza, meningococcal diseases, pneumococcal diseases, and Varicella zoster.
- **The best way to protect a child's health is to give them vaccines on schedule.** The small risks associated with vaccines are not lessened by increasing the time between shots. Spacing out vaccines over additional time actually increases a child's risk of disease, since they are less protected against vaccine-preventable diseases in the interim.
- **Fears about vaccination are common.** In part, this is because it is a medical procedure done on healthy people that carries risks (albeit small ones). Sometimes, concerns about vaccination arise because people do not have complete trust in the government or other agency providing or recommending the vaccinations—and often people have good reasons for distrust. However, receiving vaccinations recommended by the Centers for Disease Control and Prevention (CDC) and the WHO on schedule is the best decision for one's health. Methods of countering rumors and misinformation will be covered in Section 12.

PETER J. BROWN

35 THE FOUR 19TH-CENTURY CULTURAL ROOTS OF INTERNATIONAL AND GLOBAL HEALTH: A MODEL FOR UNDERSTANDING CURRENT POLICY DEBATES

Understanding the past can help us make sense of the present. This piece explains how understanding the origins of the field of "tropical medicine" in the 1800s can shed light on some controversies and tensions within the field of global health today.

There have been a few particularly important global shifts in the orientation of the field of global health. Figure 35.1, based on the work of historians Theodore Brown, Marcus Cueto, and Elizabeth Fee, shows the most important shifts: the changes in the label of this field from tropical medicine, to international health, to global health. These shifts are also described in the first reading of this book (Reading 1).

This essay covers events that happened in the first column of Figure 35.1—the period of colonialism and imperialism from around 1800 to 1950.

This piece is written by an anthropologist, not a historian, and it focuses on the idea of culture. "Culture" refers to a way of life of a particular group of people; it is everything we learn from the people around us (including parents, teachers, friends, and coworkers). From a biological point of view, all human groups are essentially the same, but the variations in cultural lifestyles—from food to religion—are enormous. Cultural differences are what make our species so interesting and successful.

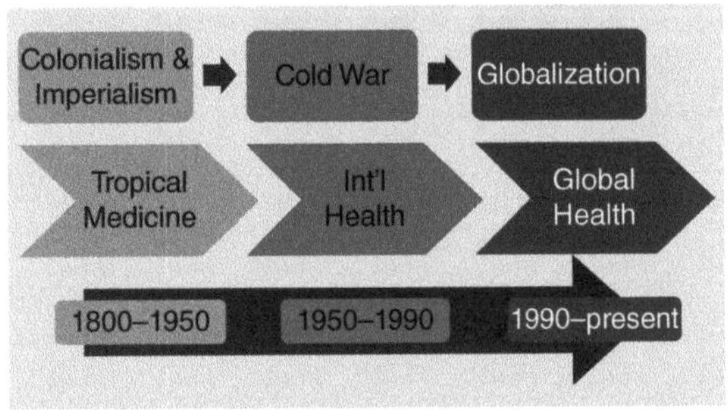

FIGURE 35.1 Important Shifts in the Field of Global Health.

Many people have more than one culture because they simultaneously live as members of more than one group. Cultural traditions are:

- ***Cherished.*** *We have emotional attachments to the foods and festivals we grew up with.*
- ***Constructed.*** *Over time, groups of people invent their own cultural beliefs and behaviors.*
- ***Changing.*** *Cultures are always changing because of the flow of generations and the necessity of adapting to shifting contexts.*
- ***Conservative.*** *Change does not come easily, because people often want to conserve their ideas and way of life.*
- ***Conflicting.*** *They say, "If it ain't broke, don't fix it," but whether the system is broken or not depends on the different points of view of individuals on different levels of a sociopolitical hierarchy. As such, conflicts within social groups over what rules people should live by are a part of being human.*

Anthropologists believe that people need to be aware of their own cultural biases; they seek to "make the strange familiar and the familiar strange." By delving deeply into the cultures of global health, this piece aims to help people who may not even be aware they are part of these cultures gain new insight into the beliefs they hold.

As you read this piece, consider the following questions:

- **Why do you think the author calls these schools of thought within global health**

This article is original to this volume.

"cultures," when they all originated in the same region of the world around the same time?

- **The author talks about the cultures he describes as being "ideal types." What does this mean? Do you think this approach is useful?**
- **Think of a disease eradication program and a primary health care program (you can refer to earlier sections of this book to jog your memory). Does each fit the organizational cultures laid out in this article?**
- **Think about a global health program you learned about earlier in the book. What organization developed this intervention? Where does the intervention fall on the continuum of "to protect" versus "to serve"? Is this what you would expect based on this article?**

CONTEXT

Peter Brown, a professor at Emory and co-editor of this volume, has extensively studied the history of malaria eradication, with a particular focus on the history of the eradication effort on the island of Sardinia, off the coast of Italy. Some of this work has focused on the cultures of the organizations, like the World Health Organization, aiming to control malaria. This piece takes a broader view, looking at patterns of culture in disease control programs since the 1800s.

Within the field of global health, nearly every health project involves a cross-cultural interaction. Culture exists on both sides of the "them"-and-"us" divide. The problem is that people are not always aware of their own cultural assumptions and beliefs. Effective cross-cultural communication requires that people be both reflexive—aware of their own biases—and empathetic. Everyone is ethnocentric in the sense that, under it all, they believe that their view of the world and ideas about how things should be done is correct.

One good way to understand the culture of Global Health is to examine its roots. In the second half of the 19th century—from about 1850 to 1900—there were four distinct cultures that eventually grew together to be called international health and then global health; these four *historical* roots of global health can be thought of as four different cultures. Over time, they became an amalgam with a single name but multiple motives and practices. By identifying these cultural roots, it is possible to better understand some current controversies and policy conflicts in the field.

While these four root cultures grew together during the 20th century, they are still the unseen foundation of essential contemporary differences. As such, the field of global health has incorporated conflicting goals, objectives, epistemologies (ways of knowing), measures of success, funding sources, and attitudes about social justice, science, political ideology, internationalism and humanitarianism. A primary dichotomy is unearthed when we dig into the roots of the field in the 1800s. That dichotomy is between a goal "to protect" and a goal "to serve." There has been a historic tension between two sides: one aiming to protect the rich from health problems and another aiming to serve the poor.

The Four Cultures

The four root cultures that sprang up in the late 1800s were International Health Regulation; Disaster and War Victim Relief; Military Biomedical Research; and Missionary Medicine. Social scientists would call these four labels "ideal types"—this model is an oversimplification that aids in the interpretation of sociocultural phenomena. Figure 35.2 shows this model: the four cultures are distinct from one another but are all part of the same larger field.

This reading describes each of the four cultures of the 1800s. Next, it compares the four cultures in terms of their economies, ideologies, and programs. Finally, it uses this model to explain some modern conflicts and patterns.

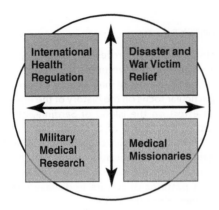

FIGURE 35.2 The Four Cultures of Global Health.

The First Culture: International Health Regulations

The biomedical science of disease causation flourished in the second half of the 19th century, when there were vigorous debates between "miasmists" and proponents of the new germ theory. Miasmists thought that disease was spread by something in the air where there were swamps or poor people lived; miasma was a stink that people living in unhygienic conditions had to breathe. For miasmists, the solution to the problem of disease was the purification of people or an area, cleaning up imbalances in the body or environment. On a metaphorical level, they were correct—considering what we know about the social determinants of health. Of course, on a less metaphorical level, they were wrong, because tiny germs are the real cause of disease.

The germ theory of disease, in contrast, posited that people become sick when small alien organisms invade their bodies. Microbiological discoveries and hospital-based medical experiments, as well as the new practice of governments collecting vital statistics, caused a revolution. Obviously, the germ theory eventually became the scientific foundation of modern Biomedicine. This new biomedical science offered the hope for the cure or prevention of disease on an individual level.

There were some famous arguments at international meetings between the two schools. The germ theorists won the arguments about the most important disease of the day—cholera. There had been a series of outbreaks starting with the pandemic of 1829. In 1851, the French government held the first International Sanitary Conferences to standardize international quarantine regulations against the spread of cholera. The issue of quarantine was one of important commercial and diplomatic interest, because the costs of quarantine were enormous and the regulations stymied international trade. British merchants, for example, felt that their ships were being held hostage in foreign ports because of quarantine. Quarantine stations involved isolation, fumigation, and the paying of taxes. The arguments of the germ theorists supported the dismantling of onerous quarantine laws.

There were eleven International Sanitary Conferences held between 1851 and 1903. Each focused on a specific disease, like plague or yellow fever. The five goals of these meetings were to: (1) remove health barriers to trade; (2) maintain epidemiological boundaries; (3) standardize health regulations, policies and best practices; (4) coordinate scientific expertise with national policies; and (5) encourage data collection with standardized surveillance measures. Primary participants in these meetings were both government officials and scientists.

Between World War I and World War II, some organizations were formed that drew on the legacy of the Sanitary Conferences. These were the *Office International d'Hygiene Publique* and the League of Nations Health Organization. The motivations, as for the Sanitary Conferences, were to advance both science and international cooperation. But the motivations were also to protect local people and property by creating and maintaining epidemiological boundaries; such borders could be maintained by quarantine, vaccination and the health inspection of foreign travelers and immigrants.

This root culture of international/global health was continued with the foundation of the World Health Organization (WHO) in 1948, after the Second World War. The WHO hosts an annual World Health Assembly and supervises the collection of epidemiological data and sets international standards for technologies and strategies. The WHO is among the most powerful of global health organizations, but it is poorly funded.

It is impossible to entirely separate agencies focusing on global health from other institutions.

Other contemporary international institutions share this historical root culture, even if their primary mission is economic; these include the World Bank and the World Trade Organization (WTO).

As an anthropologist I think that one can know something about the culture of an institution like the WHO by observing the clothes that the natives wear. If you are a man and you visit the WHO, you should wear a business suit—and of course, an official name badge is required.

The Second Culture: Humanitarian Relief

The second root culture of global health in the 19th century is humanitarian relief in war and disasters. The primary objective of humanitarian aid is to save lives, alleviate suffering and maintain human dignity. It can be distinguished from development aid, which seeks to address the underlying socioeconomic factors that may have led to a crisis or emergency.

Humanitarian aid in the 19th century began as a reaction to terrible famines and wars. The Irish Potato Famine was a period of mass starvation, disease, and emigration in Ireland between 1845 and 1852. During this period, about one million Irish died and one million emigrated—reducing the population by one quarter. British newspapers called attention to the crisis, and some charitable organizations not only donated funds but also pressured the colonial British government to act.

From 1876 to 1879, both China and India experienced terrible famines; In China alone, some 10 million people died. Emergency responses from England and other European countries were clearly insufficient, and there was the irony that these terrible famines were probably caused by colonial economic policies.

The 19th century also marked a turning point in military history and weapons technology. While wars had existed forever, the new guns and cannons of large organized armies wounded more soldiers and caused more battlefield death than ever before. In Europe, old battlefield tactics, like the charge of a brigade of horsemen armed with swords, became suicide missions against defending forces with machine guns.

In June 1859, the Swiss businessman Jean-Henri Dunant traveled to Italy to meet French emperor Napoléon III with the intention of discussing difficulties in conducting business in a French colony. When he arrived in the small town of Solferino on June 24, he toured the field of the Battle of Solferino, an engagement in the Austro-Sardinian War. In a single day, about 40,000 soldiers on both sides died or were left wounded on the field with no one to help them. Dunant was shocked by the terrible aftermath of the battle, the suffering of the wounded soldiers and the near-total lack of medical attendance and basic care. He abandoned the original intent of his trip and for several days, he devoted himself to helping with the treatment and care for the wounded. He succeeded by motivating the local villagers to provide relief without discrimination.

The needless suffering that Dunant witness inspired him to write a book, *A Memory of Solferino*, which not only described the disaster but made concrete suggestions for the formation of national voluntary relief organizations to help nurse wounded soldiers during war. In addition, he called for the development of international treaties to guarantee the protection of neutral medics and field hospitals for soldiers wounded on the battlefield. The idea was clear-cut, rational and humane. Diplomats from a large number of European countries established the International Federation of Red Cross societies. Dunant's ideas also prompted the signing of the Geneva Conventions for the ethical treatment of wounded soldiers in war. The symbol of the red cross on a white background is an inverse of the Swiss flag, and it represents humanitarian assistance and neutrality. (The red crescent was added in 1919 with the organization of national societies in majority Muslim countries.)

The 19th century also saw the rapid development of the profession of modern nursing, which combined scientific principles of bioscience with the merciful tradition of caring and the alleviation of suffering. Florence Nightingale and Clara Barton were two important leaders in this movement. The American Red Cross, founded by Barton, expanded to assist victims of natural disasters, including forest fires, floods and hurricanes. In the last decade of the century, the American Red Cross provided assistance in foreign countries. For example, in 1896 there was a 5-month mission to Constantinople to help Armenian victims of Turkish oppression.

The headquarters and museum of the International Red Cross and Red Crescent is down the street from the WHO in Geneva. It is a striking museum that describes human suffering caused by war, and to a lesser extent, suffering caused by natural disasters.

Today, the International Red Cross and Red Crescent Movement is an international humanitarian movement with about 100 million members. The ideal is charitable help in times of emergency, provided by volunteers inspired by their own moral principles. The concepts of emergency, victims, temporary help, volunteerism and charity are central to the cultural belief system. National Red Cross agencies often work in collaboration with their own country's military establishment. However, in the context of war and disaster, there is also an ethic of neutrality—victims deserve temporary relief from their suffering simply because they are fellow human beings.

There are three basic goals of the Red Cross and Red Crescent and other organizations with similar humanitarian cultures: (1) to alleviate the immediate suffering of victims of disasters, wars and displacement; (2) to decrease unnecessary morbidity and mortality in emergency situations; and (3) to assist displaced people and refugees in getting the necessities of life. Besides the Red Cross and Red Crescent, the most famous humanitarian organization is probably *Médecins Sans Frontières* (MSF, Doctors without Borders) which, besides sending teams to areas of crisis throughout the world, is also leading a global effort to increase access to essential medicines.

The culture of charity and volunteerism is reflected in the economy of modern humanitarian emergency relief institutions. They are primarily funded by individual donations, although there a few other sources of revenue like running blood banks, training courses in first aid and contracting with governments to provide some emergency assistance.

International emergency assistance is an important and huge enterprise, but in some emergencies, the many groups offering help are uncoordinated and inefficient. For example, after the Haitian earthquake of 2010, nearly one hundred different NGOs sent medical assistance teams—not counting the many national Red Cross and Red Crescent organizations—and disorganization was a problem; a similarly enormous outpouring of donations for assistance came after the 2004 Indian Ocean tsunami. Nor do the actual practices of large humanitarian aid bureaucracies always live up to the ideas that drove the founding of their organizations. Nevertheless, the culture of humanitarian relief organizations that began with Henri Dunant in the mid-19th century is a remarkable testament to human generosity and a fundamental expression of the universal value of solidarity between people.

If you are going to visit an organization doing emergency care for victims of wars or disasters, you will probably see many participants dressed in field khaki clothes or shirts with red cross symbols on them. Wear clothes that can get dirty.

The Third Culture: Military Medicine and Hygiene

There was another reaction in the second half of the 19th century to new technologies for killing. Imperial armies grew much more professional and prepared for treating wounded soldiers.

In addition to trauma surgery, military medicine focused on preventive medicine. Keeping soldiers healthy is paramount for any army, especially when they are in a new climate with unfamiliar diseases. Levels of morbidity and mortality in tropical climates were extremely high in colonial armies posted in different parts of the globe. Therefore, the military instituted a wide variety of rules, regulations and tradition that emphasize cleanliness and order. This is part of the "spit and polish" culture that is still inculcated in new recruits. Order and cleanliness in military encampments were designed to impose discipline and obedience, but they were also aimed at keeping fighting forces healthy and fit.

An early technology for preventive medicine was Edward Jenner's development of vaccination against the terrible epidemic disease of smallpox. Colonial armies required vaccination for their soldiers; in fact, Napoleon thought that Jenner's vaccine was one of the most important medical inventions in history. (Thomas Jefferson agreed.)

Governments and the military began to fund research for disease prevention. In the case of malaria, for example, pioneer scientists like Laveran and Ross developed their ideas with military funding. For them, malaria was not a domestic problem but one very important to the colonial Empire. Later, an accelerated military medical scientific research program searching for a malaria treatment during WWII was a national security priority; a parallel to the Manhattan project, this one resulted in the development of the medicine Chloroquine and the residual insecticide DDT.

On the domestic front, military medicine and hygiene were related to the 19th century Sanitary Movement. People in this movement were sometimes called "apostles of cleanliness" or sanitarians. While many today associate germs with connections between health and cleanliness, many sanitarians were convinced by miasma theory. Sanitarians were social reformers; their ideal was to clean slums, improve housing, provide clean water and sewers and advance occupational health and safety.

In Britain, the most famous leader of the Sanitary Reform Movement was Edwin Chadwick, a lawyer by training who worked for the government. He championed social planning and "social engineering" with the goal of maintaining political order. Chadwick was very conservative; he argued for investment in the public's health for reasons of political stasis and financial expediency. His solution for disease was to eliminate the sources of miasma arising from the execrable habits and filthy living conditions that he argued characterized poor neighborhoods. Garbage pick-up, installation of sewers and drainage were central.

Chadwick's famous Sanitary Report of 1842 used carefully collected statistical data to support his policy advocacy. As an administrator of the Poor Laws, he showed that improvement of working conditions resulted in men staying alive longer, and in savings to the government since fewer widows and children needed charity. Such cost-effectiveness analysis is still an essential component of the culture of Public Health.

This third root culture of international and global health emphasized medical research, especially the development of technologies for the prevention of infectious diseases. Laboratory science was an essential part of this culture, particularly the refinement of the germ theory of disease. The hygienic movement related to germ theory revolutionized the practice of medicine, especially in hospitals and surgery. The nursing profession was also associated with this culture of the military and the work to save the lives of men wounded in battle. Florence Nightingale was known to demand military precision and absolute cleanliness in her charges.

Many contemporary research institutions are descendants of the 19th century root culture of military medicine and hygiene. These include the London School of Tropical Medicine and Hygiene, Walter Reed Army Hospital, the National Institutes of Health and the United States Army Medical Research Institute for Infectious Diseases (USAMRIID). The US Centers for Disease Control and Prevention (CDC) began with a clear association with the military as an agency called Malaria Control in War Areas, whose mission was to try to prevent the reintroduction of malaria from returning servicemen into local populations of the American South. Some of these agencies still have clear military missions, like USAMRIID, and they were involved in programs for the development of biological weapons in the past. In popular mythology, like the movies "Outbreak" or "Contagion," we expect the heroes who will protect us from the ravages of infectious epidemics to come from this sector.

If you are visiting the CDC, you may see epidemiologists in Navy uniforms (members of the Commissioned Corps of the Public Health Service), white lab coats (and even more extensive protective costumes in biocontainment laboratories) or epidemiologists in business casual clothes.

The Fourth Culture: Missionary Medicine and Medical Missionaries

Religious motivations, institutions and missions have always played a central role in the history of global health programs. Christian missionaries from Europe and the United States played a major role in the colonial enterprise. Capitalist colonialism aimed to control the production and consumption of colonized populations by exploiting raw materials and encouraging the consumption of goods made in the colonial power. The point was profit. At the same time, the colonial enterprise had an ethnocentric aim of "civilizing" the people in their colonies by having them adopt Christianity and Western customs—including biomedical treatment. Colonialism and imperialism brought "modern" clinical medicine and hospitals to much of the world.

The term "mission" is used in religious, military, medical and diplomatic contexts. It involves sending a group to another place with a specific self-imposed purpose. A "missionary" is a member of a religious group sent into an area to do evangelism or service, such as health care, economic development, education or social justice. The term refers to a Christian tradition of proselytizing and converting nonbelievers, but there can be missionaries with other ideologies also. For example, there is a difference between "missionary medicine" and "medical missionaries." The latter refers to individuals whose missionary zeal is primarily to spread the ideas of science and biomedical technology.

The heyday of Protestant missionaries in South Asia and sub-Saharan Africa was in the 19th and early 20th centuries. Missionaries intended to stay indefinitely, and, therefore, they built permanent outposts to "serve the natives" in a complete way—body, mind and soul. As such, missionaries established churches, hospitals and schools. For example, in 1874, the Free Church of Scotland founded the famous mission station of Livingstonia (in contemporary Zambia). The mission was inspired by the call of David Livingstone—a heroic explorer and medical doctor—to bring "Christianity, commerce and civilization" to southeast Africa.

From the very beginning, the delivery of Western medicine was an important part of the effort of the mission movement. The doctors of the Livingstonia Mission conceived of their work as not only curative but also evangelical and educational. They saw their work as a means to relieve physical suffering among members of the local population but also as a witness to the love of God and as a demonstration of the superiority of Western Christian society, culture and science. Missionary doctors were responsible for the health of the European missionaries themselves, but they also were pioneers of biomedicine and surgery. Dr. Robert Laws, for example, did the first surgery using the anesthesia chloroform in Livingstonia in 1876, only 15 years after its discovery in Britain; in the next 20 years, he performed 7,000 surgeries. The Livingstonia mission built thirteen hospitals and sixteen dispensaries that had treated nearly 80,000 patients by the beginning of the 20th century. The ideal purpose of medicine within the context of the mission was to demonstrate Christian kindness and mercy.

The institutional descendants of these medical missionaries are the numerous Faith-Based Organizations (FBOs), as well as many other NGOs currently involved in contemporary global health and development efforts. It is difficult to know how many such organizations there are, but some have had a continuing presence in Africa for over 150 years, providing significant curative and palliative care. For example, it is estimated that 60% of health services in Kenya are provided by FBOs. Modern iterations of this root culture include organizations that are not obviously religious, but have underlying motivations that stem from ideologies of morality, mercy, human dignity and social justice. For the most part, the economies of these FBOs are based on charitable contributions from individuals in wealthier countries. Often these are charities associated with church denominations or networks.

It is often difficult to identify people from the missionary root culture by the clothes they wear: they dress like individuals working in secular settings. In the past, some people—like nuns—had distinct clothing for working in hospitals. Medical missionaries may wear white coats if they are doctors, but there might be other indications of identity, like religious symbols or the wearing of "native" garb.

Comparing the Four Root Cultures

During the 20th century, these four root cultures grew into an amalgam called international health and then global health. Even though the four cultures have merged, there remain dynamic tensions between them concerning both goals and strategies. The contemporary organizations that have evolved from these four root cultures are strikingly different in their work, economies, values and customs. While they are all part of the same Global Health universe and share basic interests, there are some fundamental contrasts between the two columns on the left and those on the right. There are three areas where these cultures differ: their health orientations, political economic constraints and ideologies.

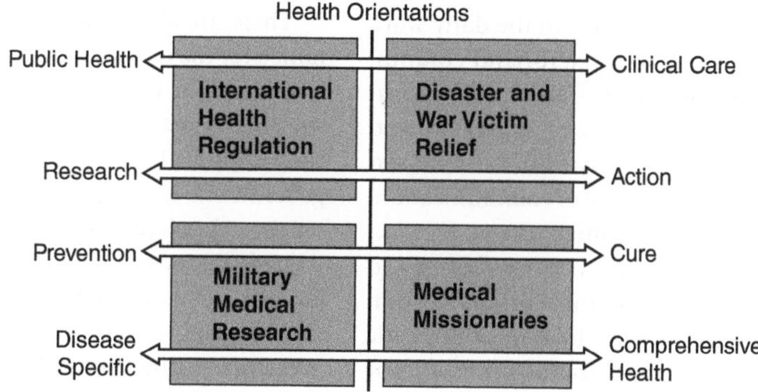

FIGURE 35.3 Health Orientations.

Health Orientations

The left-hand column in the chart of the four cultures above is oriented toward public health, while the column on the right is more oriented toward clinical care in medicine. The left side emphasizes long-term problems, while the right focuses on short-term solutions. This distinction was emphasized in the introductory essay (Reading 1).

The cultures in the column on the left, regulation and research, deal with population health in the abstract, focusing on monitoring and evaluation of preventive health measures. The fields on the left are generally disease specific—people specialize in particular single diseases, for example, malaria or polio. People working in global health research often name the disease they are working on when asked what they do. Organizations like the WHO are also subdivided by disease categories.

In contrast, the cultures in the column on the right, victim relief and missionary medicine, focus on saving individual patients, one at a time. Ideally, the column on the right hopes for medical cures, or at least a reduction in unnecessary suffering; this approach emphasizes *care*, and that is why the field of nursing is so important in those fields. Disaster relief workers and missionary medical provides must deal with whatever health problems come to them—they are not specialists, except in the sense that they are nearly always dealing with emergencies.

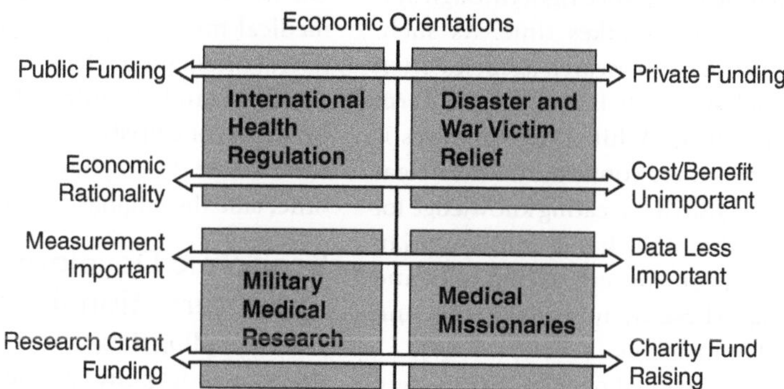

FIGURE 35.4 Economic Orientations.

Economic Orientations

Possibly the most important differences have to do with the economic orientations of these different cultures. The column on the left is dependent on public funding from the government, and thus is responsible for more accountability in their spending. Numbers are very important in the daily work and discourse of people in the left-hand column. That means that measurement—for testing hypotheses, determining morbidity and mortality and monitoring and evaluation—is of utmost importance. Statistics form a key mode of communication, and data are presented in graphic form.

On the right side of this chart, measurement and statistics are much less important. Communication often uses images of suffering children or dramatic rescue stories to prove an organization's worth. Their "data" involve narratives—a type of information that is disparaged by the other side. People from the cultures on the right side think that the other side emphasizes measurement and quantitative analysis too much; they might say "not everything that counts can be counted, and not everything that can be counted counts."

There are also differences in how money is obtained for the two sides. Militaries, governments and international organizations often rely on public funding. Most global health researchers must get their support by writing grant proposals (often to government agencies). Agencies like the Red Cross, on the other hand, require donations, and church-related missions depend on the generosity of congregations. One of the most famous of medical missionaries, Albert Schweitzer, spent six months every year raising money for his hospital in Africa by giving lectures.

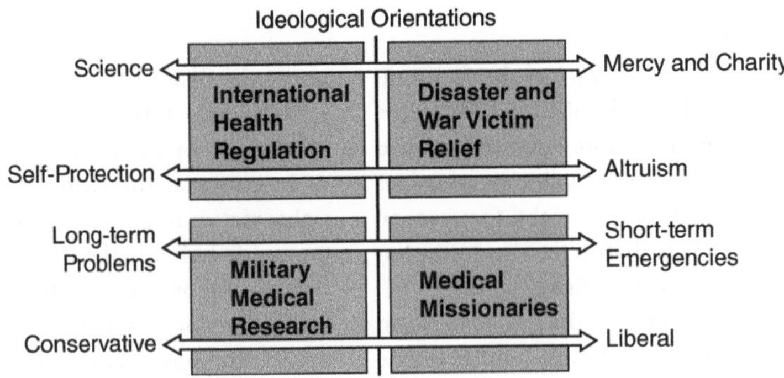

FIGURE 35.5 Ideological Orientations.

Ideological Orientations

One ideological difference between these different cultures is the level of importance placed on scientific research. Getting the science right through systematic painstaking work takes time. As such, scientists in regulation and research agencies often conceptualize global health issues as long-term problems and challenges. While their emphasis is on applied research, there continues to be a clear value put on basic research—creating knowledge for its own sake. On the other hand, humanitarian relief agencies focus on concern saving lives and reducing suffering. These are immediate, humanitarian and moral motivations.

As cultures (not individual people), health regulation agencies as well as military medical research institutions tend to have a conservative orientation, emphasizing the development of medical science for the protection of the health and welfare of society. On the other side of the aisle, the disaster relief and medical missionary types generally share a more liberal orientation where action oriented service to the poor and disenfranchised is motivated by humanist or Christian values of mercy and charity. On one side the emphasis is to "protect," and on the other side the emphasis is to "serve."

Economic Development and International Health

Understanding these four root cultures can help in thinking about policy debates in the world of Global Health. Sometimes it seems that there are temporal "fads" in policies and strategies, but the underlying historical structure of the field provides a logic to the debates and the policy transformations.

In addition to the root cultures from the 1880s, there was a new paradigm, that of "development," introduced at the end of colonialism and the beginning of the Cold War after WWII. Economic development aid was first institutionalized in the United States with the aim of post-war reconstruction, for example through the Marshall Plan. This foreign aid came in the form of financial support and "technical assistance." Such programs have always emphasized *economic* development, particularly in agricultural production and infrastructure like dams. The model that Americans designing foreign assistance programs had in mind was the economic development of the Southern United States—an area characterized by rural poverty and poor health. New technologies—like electrification and dams by the Tennessee Valley Authority—were thought to be the key to economic improvement. These ideas and programs were expanded to Latin America and then a wide variety of so-called "Third World" countries. They continue today through bilateral institutions like the United States Agency for International development (USAID) and the United Kingdom's Department for International Development (DFID).

International health programs dovetailed with these economic development programs, even though the economic development industry had much more funding. One disease that was seen to be a huge burden on the economic and population of the southern states in the United States was malaria. Malaria control, often in the form of swamp drainage and land reclamation, was publically funded work programs that had twin goals of improving population health and placing for land into agricultural production. Similarly, in Italy, a significant part of the nation-building enterprise of the late 1800s was a war against malaria. The idea that malaria was hindering "development" fueled a large focus on malaria in the era of International Health.

It should be noted that this type of foreign assistance has not always been designed as altruism. Most programs contained significant economic advantages for US businesses and technocrats. These include aspects of food-aid programs that have negative consequences for local agricultural production.

The Root Cultures and Global Health Policy Debates

The cultures of international health regulation and military medical research led to several major eradication programs in the international health era. After the introduction of DDT as a new weapon in the war against malaria, the WHO agreed to begin the global Malaria Eradication Program in 1955. This policy was influenced by anti-malaria Military Medical Research and the WHO. For a variety of reasons, malaria eradication was considered a failure and was ended in 1969. Meanwhile, the Smallpox Eradication Program began in 1966 and was successfully completed in 1980. Both programs were more difficult than anticipated, and the achievement of smallpox eradication was based on good fortune and some questionable strategies (see Readings 4 and 46).

In contrast to vertical programs like eradication, the primary health care (PHC) movement is the cultural descendant of the root cultures of missionary medicine and emergency aid. The Alma-Ata conference endorsing PHC in 1978 endorsed the slogan "Health for All by the Year 2000" (see Reading 7).

Comprehensive PHC became the stronger of the global health paradigms of the early 1980s, but it

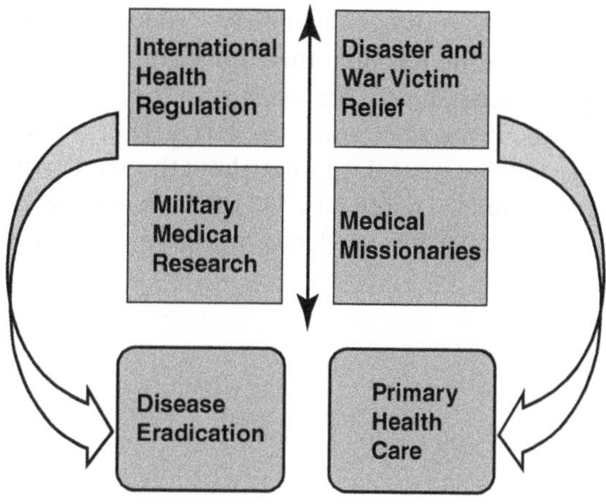

FIGURE 35.6 How the Root Cultures Influenced the Debates about Vertical and Horizontal Program Policies of International Health.

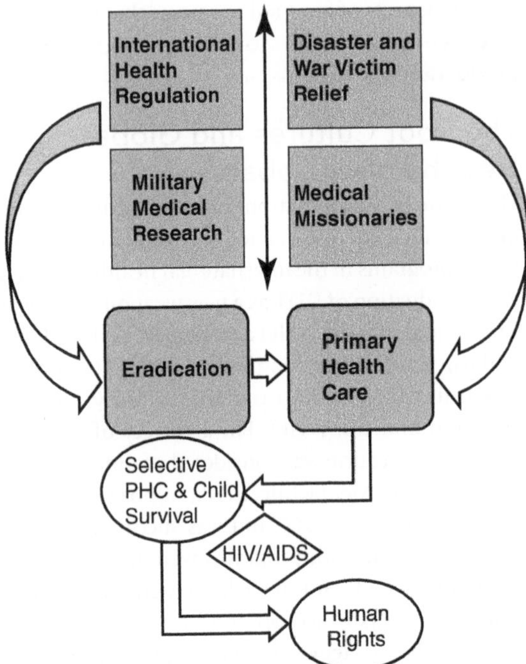

FIGURE 35.7 How the Root Culture Influenced Policy Debates during the Era of Global Health.

was immediately challenged by the cultures on the left side of the equation who argued that comprehensive PHC was vague, not measureable and medical rather than population health oriented. In its 1982 "Child Survival Revolution," UNICEF suggested an approach that they called "selective PHC"—really less PHC than a handful of measurable disease-specific programs.

About the same time, the HIV/AIDS epidemic began to be recognized throughout the world, with reports in 145 countries by 1989. Some historians say that the HIV/AIDS pandemic changed everything in the world of global health. Certainly it spurred an unparalleled research effort (although it was slow to start) to find a treatment. And, once the antiretroviral therapies (ARVs) became available, there was a huge effort to make them available to the poor of the world (see Reading 8). The argument for universal access to ARV was based ideological notions from the right side of the equation—morals, humanitarianism and the declaration of an emergency. This has been called a human rights approach to global health. At the same time, many programs providing ARVs are classic disease-specific programs, focused on research and monitoring for just one disease.

Other disease-specific programs also continue. The Global Polio Eradication Initiative (GPEI) began in 1988 and has yet to be completed (see Reading 40), and the Bill and Melinda Gates Foundation resurrected the dream of malaria eradication in 2007.

Conclusion

Contemporary global health is a field that is complex and multifaceted. The health problems of humanity are varied and extremely challenging—there are so many infectious and non-communicable diseases that need to be addressed, especially among the world's poor. The number of global health institutions is large and the diversity of their economies, ideologies and strategies can seem daunting. Understanding the past can provide a framework for understanding the essential elements that grew together to create global health today. In the final analysis, the multiplicity of strategies and institutions may be global health's strongest asset. The remarkable progress that was made in reaching the health-related Millennium Development Goals is proof of that fact. There is no single pathway into the future.

PAUL GREENOUGH

36 COERCION AND CONSENT IN SMALLPOX ERADICATION

The first section of this book introduced the US Epidemic Intelligence Service (EIS) (Chapter 9) and the successful eradication of smallpox (Chapter 4), the only successful disease eradication campaign in history. In earlier chapters, the Americans who assisted in successfully eradicating smallpox were presented in a heroic light.

This selection complicates that narrative. It describes many of the same historical events mentioned by Bill Foege in "House on Fire" (Chapter 4) but focuses on some of the troubling details of those events. Specifically, it looks at how American EIS officers sometimes intimidated and coerced people into accepting smallpox vaccination.

The argument that Paul Greenough makes in this piece is well known and somewhat controversial among those familiar with smallpox eradication. The intimidation and coercion by EIS officers that Greenough describes here actually happened. Some people who were involved in smallpox eradication, though, have argued that this account makes coercion seem more widespread and pervasive than it actually was. Others have said that even those American EIS officers who engaged in coercive practices generally learned quickly that it was counterproductive.

Why include this information in a textbook on global health? Why dredge up the troubling practices of the people who permanently ended the horrors of smallpox? The answer is that two issues discussed here in unflinching detail are extremely relevant when thinking about modern global health programs.

First, issues of coercion and resistance in vaccination programs have been around as long as there have been vaccines. And these issues are very much relevant today. Recently, for example, local governments in areas of both Nigeria and Pakistan have threatened parents who refuse polio vaccination with arrest—a controversial and arguably counterproductive response to international pressure to eradicate polio. As this selection describes, such coercive tactics can lead to increased resistance. People who work on vaccination programs should carefully consider their perspectives on coercion.

Second, power differentials between international and local staff are still very much present in global health programs. Anyone who has worked for long in global health can likely provide an example of an "aid cowboy" (or cowgirl), often from a wealthier nation, who parachutes into a setting with little understanding of it and proceeds to tell everyone how things should be run. On the flip side, anyone who has worked for long in global health can also likely provide an example of humble and intelligent people—both local and international—building strong collaborations that make the most of their different backgrounds. Both of these dynamics were present in smallpox eradication, and both are present in many modern global health programs. We think that honest discussion of these issues is, therefore, useful.

The point of this article is not to vilify those involved in smallpox eradication. Rather, understanding history can often provide helpful insight into current issues. Careful consideration of problematic or complicated behaviors in the past can be helpful in charting a path that avoids them in the future.

As you read this selection, consider these questions:

- **Is coercion ever justified in public health programs? Why or why not? If so, under what circumstances?**
- **Do you think that the practices described in this piece are human rights violations?**
- **In what ways were the problematic actions of EIS officers related to their mandate to eradicate (rather than control) a disease?**

A previous version of this article appeared in *Social Science and Medicine,* 1995, 41(5): 633–645.

- **Why do you think some of the EIS officers were sometimes very dismissive of their Indian colleagues? Is there any training or preparation that might have led to more respectful relationships?**

CONTEXT

Paul Greenough is an emeritus professor of history at the University of Iowa who holds a joint appointment at the school's College of Public Health and a position as a board member on the University's Center for Human Rights. His interest in the complexity of public health programs was first sparked when he got Hepatitis B from a cholera vaccination administered by a public health worker in India. He has written extensively about smallpox and about epidemiologists, as well as about environmental history in India.

Is it possible that health officials themselves evoke resistance simply by pressing the public too hard? In this paper I review occasions during 1973–1975 when physician-epidemiologists in South Asia, working under the auspices of the World Health Organization (WHO), intimidated local health officials and resorted to coercive vaccination in the final stages of the Smallpox Eradication Programme (SEP). Both intimidation and coercion evoked resistance and therefore interfered with the smooth functioning of public health immunization. These physician-epidemiologists were all Americans who had been recruited by the U.S. Centers for Disease Control and Prevention (CDC).

Both intimidation and coercion evoked resistance. Evidence for these statements comes from interviews, published statements and journals kept at the time. Several of these men now express regret over their participation in patterned acts of intimidation and coercion.

I am aware that in raising such issues I may be giving them undeserved prominence. The extent of intimidation, coercion and resistance in South Asia in 1973–1975 cannot be documented quantitatively and may have been negligible, although I doubt this was the case.[1,2] I might also be said to be diverting attention from the great efforts made by CDC personnel on behalf of South Asians during those years. An ancient, deadly, often blinding disease, normally prevalent in numbers measured in tens of thousands of cases per year, was eliminated as a result of SEP personnel's hard work supported by brilliant epidemiological analysis and innovative organizational measures. Hundreds of expatriates disrupted their own careers for no other reward than later to be able to say that they had helped eradicate smallpox—not only from South Asia but also from Africa, South America and Southeast Asia.[1–5] Nothing I write can detract from this remarkable record of success, and my motive here is simply to document the fact that heavy-handed methods were sometimes relied upon in the final stages of the eradication campaign in India and Bangladesh. While successful in the short-run, these methods underlined the divide between foreign and host-country health professionals and may have widened the gap between the latter and the public. Thus the long-term effects may have been negative for other health campaigns that require official, professional and popular cooperation for success.

The Smallpox Eradication Programmes in India and Bangladesh

In India a large health bureaucracy, reaching from New Delhi down to nearly 560,000 villages, carries out disease control activities. The Smallpox Eradication Programme was established inside this structure in 1962 with the goal of immunizing 80% of the population. At that time SEP managers assumed that at the 80% vaccination coverage level smallpox transmission would cease. By 1964, however, after 80% had in fact been achieved in some states, outbreaks continued to occur. It was then recognized that mass vaccination had in fact been concentrated on the most easily accessible groups, such as schoolchildren (many of whom were vaccinated repeatedly); vaccination had now to be carried to slum dwellers, migrant workers, poor fishermen and the inhabitants of numerous villages in less accessible regions. From 1964 to 1967 a mass vaccination goal of 100% coverage was set, with emphasis on the smallpox-endemic states of Bihar, Madhya Pradesh, Uttar Pradesh and West Bengal.

A review of the programme in 1967 concluded that, because of serious organizational problems, bad epidemiological data, the low productivity of poorly paid and badly supervised vaccinators, and because of technical problems with the cold storage of liquid vaccine, the incidence of smallpox was rising, not falling. It was further discovered that only 10% of the actual cases were being reported, the remaining 90% being concealed by lower-level health personnel or otherwise lost to knowledge because of a cumbersome reporting system. From 1968 to 1972, during which time the WHO global eradication campaign was inaugurated, the Indian SEP undertook a wholesale administrative shake-up; it renovated reporting, instituted the production of freeze-dried vaccine, and shifted emphasis to the detection of outbreaks and their containment by mobile vaccination teams. Numerous outbreaks occurred, however, and between 1970 and 1973 more than 130,000 cases were reported. By any measure India in 1973 was still the world's largest reservoir of smallpox (1, p. 20; 3, p. 719).

In the east of the Indian subcontinent where the Ganges and Brahmaputra rivers and their tributaries form an alluvial delta, Bengal has been an endemic focus of smallpox for centuries. Up to the time of the 1971 civil war in East Pakistan (later Bangladesh), the closely guarded border between that province and India had been an effective barrier to smallpox. In August of 1970 the East Pakistani smallpox programme, employing mass vaccination and strengthened surveillance methods, succeeded in halting transmission throughout the province, and no cases of the disease were detected during 1970–1971. After the civil war, smallpox was reintroduced in late 1971 and early 1972 into the new nation of Bangladesh (i.e. former East Pakistan) as Bengali refugees streamed back from Indian border camps. Massive outbreaks in Bangladesh followed (1, p. 86; 2, p. 24; 3, p. 807).

Beginning in mid-1973, an intensified eradication campaign was launched in both India and Bangladesh under the general guidance of the WHO, which set up technical units and appointed expatriate epidemiologists from several countries to work in close coordination with national SEP authorities. The WHO epidemiologists convinced the two health ministries to shift their investment away from routine mass vaccination toward ever more focused programs of surveillance and containment in endemic districts, especially during the cold months from October through January when smallpox always fell to its lowest incidence. Staff at all levels of the health system were pulled off other projects to support smallpox eradication. The reporting systems were improved, but it was active surveillance—aggressively seeking out cases instead of waiting for them to be reported through written notification systems—that became the key measure. Surveillance teams were equipped with jeeps and motorcycles so that they could roam near and far searching markets, schools, pilgrimage sites, tea-shops and slum settlements for cases. Repeated village-to-village and then house-to-house searches were launched in both countries. Cash rewards for pinpointing hidden cases were offered, first to the public and then to the health workers as well.

At the same time ever more rigorous containment measures were instituted. Motorized teams rushed to the scene of outbreaks to backstop local vaccination personnel. When active cases were located, the patients were either confined to their homes with guards or put into secure isolation hospitals to prevent additional contacts; local vaccinators were hired to immunize co-villagers regardless of their prior immune status. A huge monitoring effort was made to track all known cases and contacts, and supervision was exercised at every level of the SEP hierarchy. Paperwork tasks increased and required vaccinators and their supervisors to keep a variety of records and registers up to date.

Despite these much more coordinated and stringent measures, the SEP came close to collapse in India in the first six months of 1974. There was an explosion of outbreaks in Bihar and Madhya Pradesh, and the largest number of new cases anywhere in the world during the prior six years was recorded in May of 1974. There was also a serious disagreement between the WHO advisers, on the one side, and India's Director General of Health Services and the Bihar health minister, on the other; these two officials had lost faith in surveillance/containment methods and advocated a return to mass vaccination (3, p. 765). Similar high-level calls for mass vaccination came from Bangladesh early in 1975 (3, p. 835).

In response, WHO leaders made desperate efforts to bring more expatriate epidemiologists into South Asia in an effort to shore up the surveillance/containment organization. After June of 1974 the number of foreign epidemiologists in India doubled to about 100. In Bangladesh, new short-term WHO staff began to arrive from abroad in strengthened numbers early in 1975; approximately 40 expatriates were in the country throughout the year. WHO epidemiologists were equipped with jeeps, gasoline and large sums of cash to hire personnel, print leaflets, reward the discovery of outbreaks and make on-the-spot arrangements for surveillance and containment tasks (3, pp. 757, 773, 777; 2, pp. 206, 214).

The Context of Coercion and the Logic of Resistance

Most of the several hundred WHO epidemiologists who served in South Asia in the 1970s stayed for less than six months. In theory they had a merely advisory relationship with Indian and Bangladeshi SEP personnel, but in fact they assumed responsibility for most eradication activities once they were assigned to rural districts. Expatriates differed in their degree of comfort with the assignment; some had never worked in rural Asia before, while others were accustomed to the conditions and felt right at home. All were aware, however, that the global eradication effort was hanging in the balance.

Coercion arose during containment operations, when expatriate epidemiologists accompanied by vaccination teams went into villages. Initially containment simply meant vaccinating the known contacts of active smallpox cases; the names of contacts were elicited from patients by trained interviewers—classic public health contact-tracing. These interviewers also determined the immune status of the contacts, who would be excused from vaccination if they could demonstrate prior successful smallpox immunization (e.g. by showing a characteristic scar). These interviews could be slow and were obviously hampered when smallpox patients were too ill to speak or died. In time WHO epidemiologists, few of whom spoke local languages and who were dependent on others, disparaged the interview method, arguing that even when it was well done it was not foolproof. Containment was thus redefined in 1973 to mean that everyone in a village where active cases of smallpox had been detected had to be vaccinated, regardless of his or her prior immune status. This put an end to dilatory interviews-and indeed to the need to converse with villagers at all.

In the last phase of the eradication campaign, containment was again defined to mean the vaccination of everyone living within a 1-1.5 km radius of an outbreak. The actual application of this containment, however, often produced chaos in the affected villages. This was described by Stanley Music, a senior WHO physician-epidemiologist from CDC assigned to the Bangladesh SEP during 1973-1975:

> In the hit-and-run excitement of such a campaign, women and children were often pulled out from under beds, from behind doors, from within latrines, etc. People were chased and, when caught, vaccinated. Many misunderstandings arose and tempers often flared in these heated situations. Attempts were made to secure the cooperation and "blessing" of village headmen, thereby putting social pressure on the villagers to stand their ground and accept vaccination. Still, however, some form of minor chaos was the rule, as headmen's authority did not extend into individual's homes. . . . Known infected villages were revisited-often repeatedly-to check for new cases and left-outs. Almost invariably a chase or forcible vaccination ensued in such circumstances. . . . We considered the villagers to have an understandable though irrational fear of . . . . We

> just couldn't let people get smallpox and die needlessly. We went from door to door and vaccinated. When they ran, we chased. When they locked their doors, we broke down their doors and vaccinated them (6, p. 35).

Containment teams generally had their way, and sustained resistance (other than flight) was infrequent. When resistance did occur, it took various forms, ranging from mild avoidance to violent protest. The teams, always fearful that new outbreaks would undo their hard work, met resistance with coercion. The expatriate WHO advisers initiated it; they felt uniquely obliged to demonstrate to the subordinate vaccination staff that no exceptions could be allowed.

Cases of Coercion and Resistance

The following accounts document a range of coercive encounters involving American WHO advisers in Bangladesh and India between 1973 and 1975.

Case 1. Bangladesh 1973

The narrator is Music[6] and the scene is rural Bangladesh during 1973:

> [She was] an old woman who wore a dirty grey plain cotton sari over her gaunt and emaciated body. The [Sanitary Inspector] said that she wanted food and would not take vaccination unless someone gave her food. She was a beggar by "profession" but the times had been hard and she was frankly starving. I entered her house—a jute-stick and mud hut with thatch roof in poor repair—and asked her to take vaccination. She asked if I had brought her any food. I said no. She refused vaccination. I pleaded with her and took her outside to see the child two houses away only minutes from death [from smallpox]. I said that if she remained unprotected, she stood a good chance of getting smallpox. She [said she] had never been vaccinated in her life. She said that if I didn't care whether or not she died of starvation, why should I care if she got smallpox! After explaining that she was a risk to others in villages where she might beg, I told her that I had no choice but to vaccinate her with or without her consent. I promised to arrange some food for her and then vaccinated her myself. . . . I felt it was important to get 100% vaccination and drive home the point that there could be no exceptions. With an eye to how the SI [Sanitary Inspector, a local-level health worker] and his staff would regard this situation, I felt compelled to vaccinate her there and then with or without her consent (6, p. 46).

Here the woman verbalizes her reason for refusing vaccination: if you don't care whether or not I die of starvation, why should I care about smallpox? Her argument represents a common response to vertical disease campaigns among the poor. She unashamedly bargained her immune status for food, and coercion in this case lay in taking advantage of her hunger.

Music notes that "By vaccinating her first and then providing food afterwards as a personal gesture, I emphasized that there were no exceptions. Later, beggars were to be revealed as a major mode of spread, and we were to establish isolation centres for the care and feeding of these people until they would no longer be infectious" (6, p. 49).

Case 2. Bangladesh 1973

A second case based also on Music's experience in a Bangladesh village in 1973 reveals a much higher level of coercion in response to forthright resistance.

> [A man refused] to let anyone into his house or to come out to be vaccinated. When he left his house he locked the women and children inside with a padlock. When he came home he barred it from within. The [Sanitary Inspector] had tried three times to convince the family to take vaccination. I waited for the man to come home and when he did I told him that he had to take vaccination and to let his wife and children be vaccinated. He refused, went inside and barred the door. I broke the door down and vaccinated-with a struggle—every member of his family, including the man. He was very angry and told me he was going to initiate a case against me. Approximately three months later I was told by the local magistrate that a case had been registered against me but that it had been thrown out of court (6, p. 46).

Blazing anger distinguishes this response from the previous one; unlike the beggar-widow, this man felt himself empowered to resist. He not only contested the WHO adviser personally but on behalf of others, especially his female dependents (1, p. 112; 2, p. 179).

The fact that the man subsequently began a court case indicates his continuing confidence that right was on his side, and it is not clear whether the case was quashed for lack of merit or because the defendant was a powerful foreigner.

Throughout Music's narratives there are hints that local vaccinators brought WHO advisers forward like pieces of artillery to be discharged against resistant villagers whom they did not care to challenge directly.

Case 3. Bihar, India 1975

The third case refers to an unusually violent encounter in eastern India in 1975 in an aboriginal village in the Jharkhand region of Bihar. The narrator, Lawrence Brilliant, was a WHO physician-epidemiologist who had married an Indian woman and was fluent in Hindi.[7]

> In the middle of the night an intruder burst through the door of the simple adobe hut. He was a government vaccinator, under orders to break resistance against smallpox vaccination. Lakshmi Singh awoke screaming and scrambled to hide herself. Her husband leaped out of bed, grabbed an axe, and chased the intruder into the courtyard. Outside, a squad of doctors and policemen quickly overpowered Mohan Singh. The instant he was pinned to the ground, a second vaccinator jabbed smallpox vaccine into his arm. Mohan Singh, a wiry 40-year-old leader of the Ho tribe, squirmed away from the needle, causing the vaccination site to bleed. The government team held him until they had injected enough vaccine; then they seized his wife. Pausing only to suck out some vaccine, Mohan Singh pulled a bamboo pole from the roof and attacked the strangers holding his wife. While two policemen rebuffed him, the rest of the team overpowered the whole family and vaccinated each in turn. Lakshmi Singh bit deep into one doctor's hand, but to no avail.[8]

After seeing his family vaccinated, Mohan Singh addressed the medical team and his fellow villagers, who had been assembled, in the following terms:

> My *dharma* [moral duty] is to surrender to God's will. Only God can decide who gets sickness and who does not. It is my duty to resist your needles. We must resist your needles. We would die resisting if that is necessary. My family and I have not yielded. We have done our duty. We can be proud of having been firm in our faith. It is not a sin to be overpowered by so many strangers in the middle of the night. Daily you have come to me and told me it is your dharma to prevent this disease with your needles. We have sent you away. Tonight you have broken my door and used force. You say you act in accordance with your duty. I have acted according to mine. It is over. God will decide.[8]

Brilliant admits to being troubled by the attack on Mohan Singh's house.[9] At the time it was justified on epidemiological grounds. A serious outbreak of smallpox had occurred in the nearby industrial city of Jamshedpur, and one case had been traced to the Ho village. The containment rules were clear. Nonetheless, in recognition of Mohan Singh's status as chief and the obvious advantages of enlisting his authority, he had been given time to change his mind. But Mohan Singh clung to a view of disease that struck the rationalist-modernist health workers as profoundly archaic. The village was thus forcibly vaccinated in a military-style operation.

This display of force-massed policemen and jeeps at midnight-gives the account a peculiar vividness, but there is no difference in principle between this and earlier cases: local norms have no standing and are swept away. In repeating Mohan Singh's views, Brilliant said he was struck that Singh's objections were explicitly and profoundly religious. Religious opposition to vaccination is bound to give pause to Euro-Americans whose own public health traditions include special arrangements in matters of conscience.

Case 4. Bihar, India 1974

A fourth case illustrates that coercion could evoke personal violence against an expatriate WHO worker as a calculated act of retribution. The speaker here is T. Stephen Jones, who describes an incident in rural Bihar in late 1974:

> I was doing good. I was religiously fervid, I was a crusader. . . . There was a clear commitment to working on something that was for the benefit of people. . . . I became so convinced of that, that I did some very excessive things in the name of righteousness. One of the rules was that everybody gets vaccinated. I was awful in my conviction of purity of purpose—in breaking down doors and vaccinating crying women. . . .
>
> And they were very solid doors!
>
> A typical thing was, someone [a health worker] would [come to me and] say "we have someone here who refuses to be vaccinated, will you help us out?" Part of that was that I was a white man in that society, and I could do things that others couldn't do . . . and get away with it.
>
> Although I didn't always . . . in December of 1974 . . . On a full moon night I went to investigate a report of a case of possible smallpox. . . . I went into this household; there was a young child or baby with obvious chickenpox. But the rule at that time was that you vaccinated the household anyway, and for a good reason—sometimes you make a mistake in the diagnosis of chickenpox. There was a 26- or 27- or 28-year-old, chubby, somewhat effeminate man there who refused to be vaccinated. So I vaccinated him. . . . By force . . . I just held his arm and vaccinated him. He was crying and upset. Whimpering on the floor. Mean son of a bitch I am. But I knew that I was doing the right thing, of course! . . .
>
> Sometime thereafter, I'm not clear exactly how long, there was some noise outside [the just-vaccinated man's] house. I was working at that time with a PMA [physician's medical assistant] who I had found and trained and who was absolutely wonderful. So I said to him, "Are we in difficulty?" And he said, "Yes." And we went outside and there were a whole bunch of the villagers, and the story was . . . that we were reported to be robbers, thieves. And they began pushing my PMA. It was an aggressive crowd, no question. There were 20 or 30 men with bamboo sticks, *lathis*. With a brass fitting on the end of the *lathi*. So they pushed him, and I set myself between him and the people who were pushing him, for that was my experience-that I was invulnerable. And then I felt dizzy. And then I sort of crumpled down on the ground and found that I had blood in my eyes and a laceration on the top of my scalp. And my PMA was lying over me, and protecting me. Ram Chandra Pandey, a wonderful man! Then some schoolteacher appeared after a while and came in under the pile and said, "Who are you?" And I said 'Tm working with WHO." I learned a real lesson from that.[10]

Jones is remarkably candid in this account, which shows hints of racial, cultural and masculinist arrogance seeded into the epidemiological explanation of his actions. It also shows him to be aware that his psychological state at the time was one of messianic conviction; this state gave him a sense of personal invulnerability that swept away all sense of restraint.

Intimidating Host-Country Staff

Most of the American physician-epidemiologists who worked for WHO in South Asia during 1973–1975 were recruited on short-term contracts from U.S. medical and public health programs. They agreed to participate in the eradication campaign because they were idealistic and wanted to be a part of the achievement of a historically significant public health goal. Few, however, had any international health training or experience, and fewer still realized what it would mean to work side by side with South Asian colleagues seven days a week for several months under difficult field conditions. While many firm friendships were cemented between Americans and South Asians during the eradication campaign, a not uncommon pattern was for members of each group to become bitter critics of each other.

Significant cultural and professional differences divided the Americans from their South Asian counterparts. These differences became more apparent in the difficult months of 1973–1975 when financial, administrative and political problems tested the limits of the surveillance-containment approach. Foreign epidemiologists were provided with fuel and transport and given cash resources that were normally unavailable to Indian and Bangladeshi physicians, let alone lower-level health workers.

At a deeper level, the professional norms of public health work in India and Bangladesh differed sharply from those in North America. For example, the Americans defined every smallpox outbreak as a health crisis and expected their South Asian colleagues to devote themselves to SEP work with flat-out intensity, all day every day. Smallpox was the only target in their sights. In contrast, many of the South Asian SEP staff had seen outbreaks of disease for many years; they had frank doubts about eradication in general and surveillance-containment in particular. Some objected to being yanked off other local-level health programs, such as malaria control and family planning, while others appear to have been rattled by the arrival in their districts of demanding expatriates. The South Asian SEP staff members were well aware that there had been top-level disputes about the merits of surveillance/containment vs. mass vaccination.

The Experience of Joshua Pryor

A young epidemiologist named Joshua Pryor (a pseudonym) arrived in New Delhi at the end of August of 1974 after a long flight from the States. In the U.S. Pryor's training had been focused on non-infectious diseases and he had never seen a case of smallpox. Like many others recruited to India by the WHO, Pryor had served for two years in the U.S. Public Health Service as an epidemic intelligence officer of the Centers for Disease Control (4, p. 98). As he began his flight to India he began a personal diary into which he entered detailed notes throughout his tour.

Four months before Pryor's arrival, in May of 1974, smallpox in India had peaked at more than 8600 outbreaks in a single week. The fate of the whole programme seemed to be hanging in the balance in a few densely populated paddy-growing districts along the Ganges River in the state of Bihar.

On his first night in India, Pryor and other newly-arrived physician-epidemiologists stayed at the Lodhi Hotel, a modest New Delhi establishment, where the dining room served vegetarian meals only and it seemed prudent to drop Halazone tablets into the water. The following day was spent "masochistically" driving 150 miles to and from Agra to see the Taj Mahal and other sights. For the first time Pryor plunged through Indian crowds and came face to face with beggars, street venders and touts. It was warm and noisy, and strange animals—buffaloes, elephants, camels—appeared everywhere. As is usually the case with inexperienced foreigners, Pryor was overwhelmed by the Indian surface, confiding to his diary that, although it had been "touristy and tiring," it was "probably the most remarkable day I can recall."

Early in September Pryor began the first of two days of orientation at WHO headquarters in New Delhi. Dr William Foege, chief CDC epidemiologist in the country and the head of the WHO team, gave the lectures. The picture, as Pryor recorded it, was fairly simple: smallpox had been contained at last in the hugely populous state of Uttar Pradesh, but there were 2600 active outbreaks in neighboring Bihar. Each WHO epidemiologist would be assigned an affected district, where he was to strengthen the search and containment procedures, paying particular attention to record-keeping and supervising all aspects of the campaign. His role was that of adviser; he was there to backstop the work of the permanent SEP staff, mostly members of the Indian health services. The following morning Foege and others drilled the recruits in hypothetical problems that refreshed their epidemiological skills. Everything else they needed to know, they were told, would become clear on site.

On September 4th, the morning of departure, Pryor began to have stomach cramps on the way to the Delhi rail station and felt himself "pre-clinical." The sights, sounds and smells of the station oppressed him, and he later noted that "as the train pulled out precisely on time. . . . I had that sinking feeling of final self-doubt. Why am I here?"

Over the next few days, Pryor eased into his new duties in Bihar: he was taken to a village outbreak outside Patna and saw his first cases of smallpox. He met local medical officials and civil administrators. He began to learn the complex SEP recordkeeping system. His guide was another American epidemiologist who had himself been in India only three months and was slated to depart on September 7th.

Neither spoke more than a few words of the local languages, Hindi and Bihari, and Pryor stumbled in his diary when he tried to spell *chapatti*, the most ordinary form of local bread—he thought he heard *cachotee*.

On September 9th Pryor was called back from Goyal to Patna; there was to be a big monthly meeting of WHO-SEP workers throughout Bihar. Pryor's notes from this meeting suggest the mix of science, politics and affect driving the foreign team:

> It began at nine with Bill Foege giving a summary of India and the world. Now more than ever Bill thinks we can eradicate smallpox from the face of the earth . . . The epidemiologists at the meeting were from all over the world. Russia, Sweden, U.K., America, India and Burma. The unity of all these men in a common cause that transcends personal politics is refreshing and remarkable. Everyone [is] committed to the goal of Zero Smallpox by December. The multinationality and urgency that the group exudes is highly infectious atmosphere [sic]. Anyone who could sit in that meeting room and not want to have at smallpox would be strange. . . .
>
> After lunch the meeting resumed and the Indian Minister of Health came with great pomp and spoke in Hindi about instituting a mass vaccination campaign in parallel with the search and containment programme. Everyone raised opposition to such a programme. The field workers felt that to try a mass campaign would be extremely foolish. First, they thought it would fail to reach the target population, second it would not stop smallpox (as their previous campaigns had not), and third and most important it would siphon off valuable search and containment staff. After 45 minutes of debate featuring Indians and Americans and British proponents, the Minister conceded the point and left with a flourish.

The spectacle of young foreigners hammering their objections to an elected health minister's proposals must have been an uncommon sight in Bihar. Within a few days every SEP staff member in the state knew of the dispute.

Pryor's loneliness and cultural distress from this time became more palpable. He saw his first Hindu cremation, which reminded him of his own mortality. A "million" mosquitoes came through his net at night. There was no coffee. The electric pump failed, and he cut his foot while pulling water from an outdoor well. A telegram told him of his mother-in-law's death, and the letters he expected from his wife and family didn't arrive. The nearby river frequently flooded, interrupting transportation, and the local terrain was muddy. He detected his driver stealing petrol.

Despite these mishaps, worries and annoyances, Pryor settled into a routine of constant movement about the district, accompanied by his Indian medical collaborator, Dr Satyesh Majumdar. They enjoyed each other's company, and Majumdar became Pryor's guide, translator and confidante as well as his colleague in the eradication work.

Their most important task was to determine whether search and containment measures were being strictly maintained. This required them to make surprise visits to outlying health stations, and Pryor's notes record many occasions when he found Indian physicians and vaccinators shirking their duty. The following extracts contain grossly prejudiced statements that belittle the competence of Indian health personnel. Much of what Pryor asserts was written under stress, and these passages are reproduced to indicate how Pryor's critical attitudes hardened into markedly unsympathetic prejudices.

> *September 21.* In the afternoon we met with the BMOs [Block Medical Officers] from the entire district. We discussed the search, assessment of present status of outbreaks, containment, reasons for not doing mass vaccination and a host of other things. I'm afraid I was a bit rough on the BMOs who were doing their jobs poorly. Some of these guys are either incredibly lazy or they are not bright enough to hold the jobs they hold . . . The other thing that strikes me is the Jack of sense of responsibility that these BMOs show. They don't consider it negligent to wait a week before confirming a possible smallpox outbreak. It is beyond me.
>
> *September 22.* [I] returned to Haripur village and met the health worker, who was very frightened of

me (and well he might be having done a perfectly horrible job). Right under his nose I could point out 11 cases of smallpox over the past two months. It is rubbish to think that he didn't know. The villagers told my driver on the sly that the BMO [Block Medical Officer] knew very well but was too busy with his [private] practice (illegal by Centre policies) to visit his sick and dying people. What a terrible blotch on the medical profession. . . . I also met an old school dispensary doctor. He still felt that mass vaccination was the way to go, gulp! We arrived in Goyal at 9:15 tired and dirty, disgusted and disgruntled, but ready to begin again tomorrow to do the job that must be done. WHO made no mistake sending in outsiders.

October 4. Unless you are shown otherwise you can assume that everyone is corrupt and takes bribes. There is an urgency to know everyone's business every minute so that false bribes can be extracted. For example: if a clerk knew I was going to Thakji, he might tell a PMA [Primary Medical Assistant-lowest level health officer in the district] from Sompur I was coming to raise hell and that only a bribe would save my visit. The bribe would be paid and I, as planned, would be miles away. The straightforward bribe is also popular. Just like America you pay someone for silence, a favor, a lie, a lost letter, etc. The amount of unblinking lying that goes on even between men who have long been friends is astounding. Doctors frequently lie to me, to the DMOH [District Medical Office of Health] and Dr Yakub. Every time I hear it, it "blows me away."

October 7. We have fairly good evidence that the young energetic Dr Thakur is totally void of medical responsibility. More than that, he knows about outbreaks and will not go himself to see the cases. I really don't know how to express the sense of frustration. He knows the problem, knows the methods to rectify it and won't do it. . . . In Phulganj I had my first failure to vaccinate a resistant woman. She would not listen to reason. I tried all the usual techniques-that I was an American come 10,000 miles just to vaccinate her, that it was the only way to keep her well, etc., etc. Finally, her husband got very agitated, started screaming and threw me out, saying that I had insulted his house and that I had no right being there (true). I really felt bad about that one. . . . I hope I won't do that again. Dr Majumdar smoothed things over, but I left feeling rather sheepish.

I have quoted Joshua Pryor at length, because one can observe his frustration building almost day by day. His distress with Indian medical colleagues became nearly pathological, and this led him to harangue them, try to catch them in error and show his exasperation. In private he made extremely prejudiced statements about their technical knowledge, professional ethics and personal motivation. Each of these generalizations was belied by his collaborator, Dr Majumdar, who worked just as hard and was just as motivated as Pryor, but was completely at home in the setting and capable of "smoothing things over" when Pryor exploded.

It seems clear that the government physicians and subordinate vaccination staff in Pryor's district were unimpressed with surveillance/containment, and it seems probable that some of them refused to exert themselves to make it work. The fact that the most senior health officer in the state, the Bihar health minister, was openly advocating mass vaccination at the same time that Pryor was pushing hard for surveillance/containment surely played a part in determining some of the Indian staff's inaction. Whatever the precise combination of causes, Pryor felt himself surrounded by incompetents and morally anesthetized saboteurs. Nonetheless, he and his team succeeded in freeing the district from smallpox by the time he departed from India.

The Experience of Stanley Music

Stanley Music also had a series of confrontations with Bangladeshi SEP staff. Contempt for most of his Bangladeshi subordinates arose very quickly after he and four other expatriate WHO epidemiologists were given responsibility for reorganizing the country's smallpox program in the summer of 1973. As was the case with Pryor's remarks on health personnel in India, much of what Music asserts here about Bangladeshi health personnel in the following passages is strongly prejudiced.

We had no idea how much smallpox there really was at this point. Very little was being reported. . . . We had learned very quickly that we couldn't trust the

> routine claim of freedom [from] smallpox. Though we, the foreigners, tried to console one another with great displays of cynicism and dispassionate posturing, our inner emotions were quite another thing entirely. We felt hurt that we were lied to. We felt responsible for the smallpox in our areas. And we got mightily angry at the petty jealousies and red-tape mountains that occupied the health workers and left them lethargic if not totally unresponsive to the smallpox that we had to point out to them over and over again in their own villages. . . . The anger we hurled at the GHAs [Government Health Assistants], SIs [Sanitary Inspectors], etc., was anger of frustration [or] impotence. Like most angers it didn't last long (6, p. 37).

From Music's subsequent narrative, however, it appears that his anger could be tenacious. It was within his power, for example, to discipline lower-level Bangladeshi health officials. In one case he dismissed a GHA (Government Health Assistant) whom he confronted with evidence of falsifying the containment records in a rural area. The GHA "admitted that the reports were falsified, that he had done no vaccination, that he had not visited the area, and that he had been passing his time as a cultivator in order to feed his family . . . everything was fine until the surveillance team reported the outbreak; even then the GHA thought he would simply be reprimanded and never dreamed that he would lose his job." As Music notes, "the massive intervention was possible only for a foreign adviser" (6, p. 53).

From the evidence offered, expatriate American epidemiologists found eradication work in South Asia a struggle not only against disease but also against some host-country colleagues whom they found dissembling and ineffective. Active surveillance, designed to find smallpox, kept turning up lies and haziness; this led in some cases to drawn-out efforts to instill discipline in SEP cadres by making examples. Intimidation—in this case threatening to punish malfeasant South Asian colleagues—became a time-consuming concern for some Americans, who could not stand back from their immediate problems to try to grasp what was happening in India and Bangladesh as a whole.

In both countries the key difficulty was that some district- and sub-district level health workers were still not fully persuaded that arduous methods of surveillance and containment were necessary. In both countries there were officials at the highest levels who disputed the effectiveness of containment under South Asian conditions, and in fact smallpox had been eliminated from Bangladesh in 1970 by rigorous application of the familiar method of mass vaccination. Some WHO epidemiologists, arriving in the country after 1973, held Bangladeshi SEP workers personally responsible for the huge amount of smallpox present, even though the ultimate source of the disease lay in eastern India and had only re-entered Bangladesh with the return of refugees in late 1971.

In Bangladesh as in India, the WHO advisers' access to abundant extra resources, their higher-level qualifications and their single-minded focus on smallpox to the exclusion of other health issues isolated them from the concerns of their Bangladeshi colleagues. Severe administrative problems in the new nation and everyday norms that allowed government employees to manipulate their contacts in the higher bureaucracy drove American WHO workers to distraction. While some of the latter had served in health departments in the United States (Music, for example, had served in the Florida Department of Health), they nonetheless arrived with exaggerated expectations about the probity and efficiency of local-level South Asian bureaucracies. Virtually parachuted into exotic settings without knowledge of local languages, occupational norms and cultural values, it was predictable that they would react sharply to perceived failures around them. That a few would pursue malfeasant South Asian colleagues and subordinates with great tenacity and turn to coercion against vulnerable sections of the public that resented highly intrusive containment was less predictable. These developments, however, speak to the Americans' own inadequate preparation for a difficult assignment.

Legacies of Smallpox Eradication

Why raise the issues of coercion and intimidation? Hasn't smallpox eradication justified itself over and over by saving hundreds of thousands of lives and by averting blindness among nearly 5% of the survivors? Don't these results, and the substantial sums saved by dismantling a 175-year-old world-wide vaccination program, justify a limited number of obscure acts of zeal in India? By and large they do. Yet I believe there are three reasons for stirring up the embers of the South Asian eradication programme today.

In the first place the success achieved in the South Asian campaign has been highly influential and has demonstrated the technical feasibility of disease eradication as a significant public health strategy. Global coordination by professional and highly motivated disease-control units inside the WHO, large-scale fund-raising efforts for control/eradication of targeted diseases among official, multilateral and private aid agencies, all-out national mobilization of public health personnel at the expense of other disease-control and primary care programmes, outbreak-driven containment measures dependent upon surveillance efforts by expatriates—these once-novel characteristics of the Smallpox Eradication Programme are now, in various combinations, normal features of recent campaigns against, for example, polio, hepatitis B and dracunculiasis and the six EPI target diseases, as well as new vaccines against other grave diseases, such as childhood pneumonias and diarrheas.

Second, coercion can leave behind a residue of resentment that sours public attitudes toward the next vaccination campaign. The social memory of traumatic encounters with the state and its agents runs deep in South Asia. Rumors that disparage the motives or revile the conduct of government agents are as great an enemy of public health as the disease because they lead to avoidance and opposition. SEP managers themselves understood this point in retrospect, as indicated above, but in the heat of the campaign it was difficult to keep in mind. It is also worth considering whether some of the resistance that vaccinators encountered in the villages of India and Bangladesh in 1975 might not itself have been the result of prior half-completed but unsuccessful immunization campaigns in which coercion had played a role. In any case, every new health campaign requires renewed public interest and support, and coercion does not foster continuing public demand. Once public opinion turns against state-enforced measures, the task of health workers becomes much more difficult.[11]

Third and finally, it would be an ethical error to hold that consent to immunization is less important in villages of Bihar and Bangladesh than it is in Birmingham or Buffalo—unless one accepts the ethical partition of the world. No one in the WHO leadership argued for a partition in so many words, yet coercion against resistant villagers in South Asia was tacitly accepted as necessary because it "worked," it "got the job done."

Where did these rough and ready field values come from? Some might see in them a resurgence of colonial conduct, abetted by the post-colonial state. But an ultimate source probably lies in the tradition of coercive vaccination in the North during the nineteenth century. Smallpox vaccination was one of the few effective preventive measures available to European and American governments between 1800 and 1900, and a drawn out conflict between centralizing public health authorities and organized anti-vaccinationists was a notable feature of Victorian urban life. By the beginning of the twentieth century the struggle between partisans for and against vaccination in the U.S. and Britain ended in a draw; vaccination was made compulsory but the statutes allowed exemption on the basis of proven religious or conscientious objections. Ever since, the legal and political constraints on vaccination have compelled European and North American health agencies to stimulate public demand for immunization by means of persuasion. In the United States much of the success of the Centers for Disease Control and Prevention has been built upon its ability to realize the technical promise of mass immunization in a significantly anti-authoritarian political environment.[12]

Given this hard-won experience, no one in the CDC has ever argued publicly that public health in the developing world requires coercive methods. Yet CDC epidemiologists and other expatriates employed by WHO in India and Bangladesh clearly consented to coercion during the mid-l 970s. This telling contradiction requires attention.

We are thus left with the question whether expatriate epidemiologists in South Asia in the mid-1970s felt that coercion and intimidation were necessary to achieve 'victory.' In a thoughtful study of the global smallpox eradication programme, Jack W. Hopkins has drawn out ten "lessons for the future" which the international health community should absorb. Several of these lessons speak directly to the issues raised in this article. In particular, Hopkins advises organizers (lesson three) to "pick good people" to run disease eradication and control programmes, and, following Lundbeck, he suggests that "good people" are those who can "surmount obstacles such as religious beliefs, political disagreements, administrative inefficiency, indifference, personal craving for power and influence and a number of other human weaknesses".[13] At first glance Hopkins' lesson is faultless, but, as this essay has tried to show, religious belief, political disagreement, administrative inefficiency, etc., may rise up especially powerfully in local contexts where expatriate health workers parachute onto the scene with their surgically narrow agenda, brief commitments, dizzying resources and messianic impulses. Whether local difficulties are to be 'surmounted' by force and intimidation or by persuasion and education should not turn on the personal character of expatriates-on whether they are "good people"-but on a careful, site-specific consideration of the long-term and short-term consequences of working with or on the local health personnel and populace. It may be that there is a defensible case to be made for coercion and intimidation—some clearly believe these methods must be kept in reserve[14]—but let the case for strong methods at least be made openly.

REFERENCES

1. Basu R. N., Jezek Z. and Ward N. A. The Eradication of Smallpox from India. WHO Series History of International Public Health, No. 2, WHO South-east Asia Regional Office, New Delhi (1979).
2. Joarder A. K., Tarantola D. and Tulloch J. The Eradication of Smallpox from Bangladesh. WHO Regional Publication, South-east Asia Series, No. 8, WHO South-east Asia Regional Office, New Delhi (1980).
3. For CDC's role in the WHO's Smallpox Eradication Programme, see Fenner F., Henderson D. A., Arita I., Jezek Z. and Ladnyi I. D. Smallpox and Its Eradication. WHO, Geneva (1988), s.v. "Centers for Disease Control."
4. Ogden H. G. CDC and the Smallpox Crusade. HHS Publication No. (CDC) 87-8400, U.S. Government Printing Office for the U.S. Public Health Service, Washington, D.C. (1987).
5. Etheridge E. W. Sentinel for Health, A History of the Centers for Disease Control, pp. 188-210. University of California Press, Los Angeles (1992).
6. Music S. I. Smallpox eradication in Bangladesh: reflections of an epidemiologist, p. 35. Unpublished DTPH dissertation, London School of Hygiene and Tropical Medicine, June 1976.
7. Miracle of Love: Stories about Neem Karoli Baba, pp. 163-169. Arkana-Penguin, New York (1991).
8. Brilliant L. and Brilliant G. Death for a killer disease. Quest May-June (1978).
9. July 1992 telephone interview with Dr Brilliant, now associated with the SEVA Foundation, San Francisco.
10. Interview with T. Stephen Jones, M.D., Centers for Disease Control, Atlanta, GA, 27 June 1984. Author's collection, Tape 2, side B, Soundesign index 730.
11. Vicziany M. Coercion in a soft state: the family-planning programme of India. Pacific Affairs 55, 373 et seq. (1982) and Bishop M. F. Coercion in a soft state: the family planning programme of India. Pacific Affairs 56, 510 (1983).
12. Etheridge E. W. Sentinel for Health: A History of the Centers for Disease Control, Chaps 5, 10, 14, 21. University of California Press, Berkeley (1992).
13. Hopkins J. W. The Eradication of Smallpox: Organizational Learning and Innovation in International Health, pp. 126 127, note 21. Westview Press, Boulder, Colorado (1989).
14. Hussain S. A., Menezes R. G. and Nagaraja S. B. Parents in Pakistan arrested for polio vaccine refusal: a necessary step? Lancet 385, 1509 (2015).

RANDALL PACKARD

37 LOOKING BACK IN TIME FROM EBOLA: THE HISTORY OF GLOBAL HEALTH

Most Americans take many things in their lives for granted—not only drinkable water, sufficient food, showers, and toilets but also access to education and quality health care. It is the job of historians to describe and analyze those changes. The historical perspective allows us to look backward in time to understand the present. It is valuable to think deeply about how the world has become so unequal—why some have so much and some have so little. Historians help us understand the social, political and economic processes that created our current circumstances.

This article, written by the preeminent historian of global health, begins with the Ebola outbreak of 2014–2015 and examines why the healthcare infrastructure of West Africa was so weak that it took extraordinary (and expensive) international efforts to contain it (see Readings 9 and 44). Reconstructing past epidemics is difficult, whether it is Zika in 2016, Ebola in 2014, SARS in 2003, AIDS in 1981, influenza in 1918 or cholera in 1853 (see Chapters 2, 3 and 8). This article takes a broad historical perspective to understand the underlying causes of the Ebola epidemic.

As we saw in the introduction (Chapter 1), the field of global health came of age in the 1990s. You might ask: "What was going on with that name change from international to global health?" In fact, the name change was already occurring before there was a published intellectual rationale for it. The department where Peter Brown (co-editor) teaches changed its name twice in a 2-year period.

While the name change from international health to global health happened very quickly and without a great deal of discussion, there were three logical reasons for the change. First, the distinction between domestic and international health problems was misleading and anachronistic in a globalized world. Second, because of emerging and reemerging diseases, even people in wealthy countries are at risk for infectious disease—because pathogens do not recognize political boundaries. Third, political-economic policies of wealthy countries affect health conditions in low-income countries.

But there were also five unstated reasons that the name change had so much momentum: (i) "everybody's doing it"; (ii) the central topic of development studies and macroeconomics had been globalization for the past decade; (iii) the National Council for International Health had already changed its name in 1998 to the Global Health Council; (iv) historians of public health had declared that the age of international health ended in 1990; and (v) the largest single private health research funder in history—the astonishing Gates Foundation begun in 2000—was referring to its mission in terms of global health.

The previous essay about the four cultures of International Health in the 1800s (Chapter 35) described two distinct approaches—one involving scientific technologies and the other providing humanitarian assistance. This is the classic debate between vertical approaches and primary health care. This essay describes the way in which the pendulum of those approaches has swung back and forth over time—and how today it is decidedly emphasizing technological fixes rather than improvements in basic health systems and the social determinants of health. That history helps us understand how and why the Ebola outbreak of 2014 occurred.

As you read the following article, consider the following questions:

- **History is rather unimportant in the medical school curriculum and science courses in general. Do you agree with that statement? Do you think global health should be different in this regard?**
- **Paul Farmer says that the "four Ss" are required to improve health: stuff, space, staff and**

Excerpt taken from *A History of Global Health*, by Randall Packard. Baltimore: Johns Hopkins University Press, 2016, pp. 1–6, 273–278, 327.

systems. In your opinion, which of these is the most important?

- **Do you think that fear has been a factor in the sudden expansion in funding for global health? Why or why not?**
- **The previous essay argued that there are two approaches in global health—to protect and to serve. Do these reflect different moral values? How do global health institutions and program have to appeal to both sides?**

CONTEXT

Randall Packard is the William H. Welch Professor and Chair of the History of Medicine in the School of Medicine at The Johns Hopkins University, where he is also a professor of International Health in the Bloomberg School of Public Health. Previously, he taught at Emory University and Tufts University. He is the author or editor of six books. He is an expert in African history and infectious diseases like tuberculosis, malaria and dengue fever. This article is taken from sections of the book *A History of Global Health: Interventions into the Lives of Other Peoples* (2016). That volume has been described as a "brilliant and sweeping book [that] brims with new insights and provocative claims, all masterfully researched and compellingly argued . . . it is also charged with a moral force that crackles and glows from its subtitle to the last paragraph of its conclusion."

In early December 2013, a two-year-old boy named Emile Ouomuono became very ill. He had a fever and black stools and was vomiting. Emile lived in the village of Meliandou in southeast Guinea, a few miles from the country's borders with Liberia and Sierra Leone. Four days after developing these symptoms, he died. Emile was buried in his village. Soon afterward, on December 13, his mother developed similar symptoms and also died. The boy's three-year-old sister died with the same symptoms on December 29. His grandmother, in whose house Emile had stayed when he became ill, also developed symptoms of the disease. She sought the help of a male nurse who lived in the town of Guéckédou, a bustling trading hub where people converged from Liberia and Sierra Leone. The nurse tried to offer assistance but possessed neither the knowledge nor the medical supplies needed to treat her. The grandmother returned to Meliandou, where she died on January 1. In early February, the nurse who had treated Emile's grandmother also developed a fever. When the nurse's condition deteriorated, he sought help from a doctor in Macenta, in the next prefecture. The nurse stayed just one night in Macenta—sleeping in the doctor's house—and died the next day. The doctor died several days later.[1]

Whatever was killing the residents of this remote part of Guinea was on the move. But word of the outbreak did not reach health officials in Conakry until January 24, when a doctor in the town of Tekolo called a superior to report that something strange was happening in a village under his jurisdiction. It took another six weeks before a team of physicians from the humanitarian relief organization Médecins Sans Frontières (Doctors Without

[1] This narrative is based on a series of news accounts describing the beginnings of the Ebola outbreak in southeastern Guinea. We still do not know exactly what happened during those early days of the epidemic. This, as best as I can tell, is close to the events that occurred. See Holly Yan and Esprit Smith, "Ebola: Who is Patient Zero? Disease Traced Back to 2-Year-Old in Guinea," CNN, updated January 21, 2015, http://www.cnn.com/2014/10/28/health/ebola-patient-zero/index.html; Childby Bahar Gholipour, "Ebola 'Patient Zero': How Outbreak Started from Single Child," *Live Science*, October30,2014,https://www.livescience.com/48527-ebola-toddler-patient-zero.html; Jeffrey E. Stern, "Hell in the Hot Zone," *Vanity Fair*, October 2014, https://www.vanityfair.com/news/2014/10/ebola-virus-epidemic-containment.

Borders) was able to reach Guéckédou and collect samples, which were subsequently tested in a laboratory in Lyon, France. On March 20, the lab identified the condition as Ebola. By then the disease had reached Conakry and was spreading farther, into Liberia and Sierra Leone. On March 25, the US Centers for Disease Control and Prevention (CDC) confirmed that an outbreak of Ebola fever was occurring in Liberia, Guinea, and Sierra Leone.[2]

The disease continued to spread. By December 2014, there were 12,000 laboratory-confirmed cases in the three affected countries, and additional cases had occurred in Mali, Senegal, and Nigeria. More than 7,000 people had died from the disease. The outbreak was the largest since the disease first appeared in Zaire in the 1970s, and it evoked a massive emergency response from global-health organizations trying desperately to contain the outbreak before it spread across the globe.

Ebola is a terrifying disease. In its most overt form it produces horrific symptoms that include high fever, vomiting, diarrhea, and massive hemorrhaging. The majority of infected people, if not properly treated, die from the disease within days of developing symptoms. Yet Ebola often presents itself with less clear symptoms, which makes it difficult to distinguish from other diseases, including malaria and cholera. Without a laboratory test, it is impossible to make a definitive diagnosis.

Ebola does not spread easily. A person infected with the virus can remain symptomless for 10–21 days. During this time, he or she is not infectious to others. The disease only spreads through direct contact with an infected person's bodily fluids once symptoms have begun to appear. But because Ebola is a severely debilitating disease, which kills quickly, a person who develops symptoms normally has limited opportunities to infect others. Despite these constraints, Ebola spread rapidly from Guinea to neighboring countries. Why?

The answer to this question is complicated, involving a number of converging factors. At the beginning of the epidemic, much of the media's and public-health groups' attention focused on the local customs and behaviors of the population affected by the epidemic. We were told about the local consumption of "bushmeat," which may have infected the first person who contracted the disease; local aversion to using Western medical services; and burial practices that brought family and friends into close contact with diseased bodies. All of these behaviors occurred and no doubt played a role in the epidemic. But they were not why Ebola burned rapidly through these three countries. Moreover, focusing on these behaviors deflected attention from other, more fundamental causes of the epidemic and represented examples of cultural modeling and victim blaming, which have been part of how those living in the global north have often made sense of the health problems of those living in the global south.[3]

The epidemic was also fueled by the poverty both of those it affected and of the countries in which it occurred. The forest area in southeastern Guinea, where the epidemic first appeared, was one of the poorest in the world. There was no industry or electricity, and roads were nearly impassable at certain times of year. Families existed on a combination of agriculture, foraging, and hunting in the forest. Average annual earnings were less than US$1 a day, and 45 percent of the children suffered chronic malnutrition. Local resources were further depleted by the influx of thousands of refugees from the civil wars that wracked Liberia and Sierra Leone. The recent expansion of agribusiness and mining had contributed to deforestation and forced residents to forage and hunt deeper in the forest, which may have increased their exposure to the animal-borne viruses. Finally, the need for local residents to seek economic opportunities outside of this impoverished forest zone produced patterns of

[2] Centers for Disease Control and Prevention, "Initial Announcement," March 25, 2014, www.cdc.gov/vhf/ebola/outbreaks/2014-west-africa/previous-updates.html.

[3] Michael McGovern, "Bushmeat and the Politics of Disgust," *Cultural Anthropology Online*, Ebola in Perspective series, October 7, 2014, https://culanth.org/fieldsights/588-bushmeat-and-the-politics-of-disgust.

labor migration that contributed to the spread of the epidemic.

But the most immediate cause for the rapid spread of Ebola was the absence of functioning health systems. Ebola was able to go undiagnosed for three months and to spread rapidly throughout the region because the three countries in which it initially occurred lacked basic health-care services. The medical workers who first encountered the disease possessed neither the supplies nor, in some instances, the medical knowledge needed to manage Ebola cases. There is no cure for Ebola, but basic palliative care—including, most importantly, intravenous fluids for rehydrating patients—can dramatically reduce mortality; 90 percent of the patients who were transported to hospitals in Europe and the United States survived. Clinics and even hospitals in the three countries most affected by Ebola lacked these basic medical supplies. Health workers were also unprepared to control the spread of infection, lacking a basic infrastructure and the necessary protective equipment. Patients were not isolated, and health workers took few precautions to protect themselves from being infected.

Not surprisingly, health workers were among the first to contract the disease and die from it, further weakening already-stretched health systems and contributing to the spread of the disease.[4] Moreover, some health workers, especially those who had not been paid for weeks, abandoned their posts for fear of dying from the disease. As Ebola spread, clinics and hospitals became places where people with the disease went to die. The association of Ebola deaths with health services caused family caregivers to avoid these services and treat their loved ones at home. This decision contributed to the spread of the disease among family caretakers. Health services, far from containing the outbreak, often amplified it.

The epidemic spread as well because the health services that existed were not integrated into the communities they served. The early spread of the disease was linked to local burial practices. Burial activities, like burial practices everywhere, are deeply imbedded in local cultural systems. But health workers might have intervened in ways that would have limited the spread of infection from the diseased bodies of Ebola victims to mourning relatives, had the health workers been viewed as part of the community. Only after the epidemic was well under way were local efforts made to work with communities and modify their burial practices.

In addition to lacking fully prepared health services, Guinea, Liberia, and Sierra Leone did not have laboratory services to test for Ebola or epidemiological services to keep track of infected persons. The absence of a network of laboratories that could have tested for Ebola, and the difficulties of conveying samples to distant medical centers, delayed both recognition of what was killing people and efforts to mount an effective response to the disease. Lack of knowledge of the nature and seriousness of the epidemic also meant that people who were infected with Ebola but had not yet developed symptoms were able to travel to neighboring regions and, eventually, to large metropolitan areas like Conakry and Monrovia, where they succumbed to the disease, becoming foci for its farther spread. Only after it was recognized that the region faced an epidemic of Ebola were efforts begun to track patient contacts and contain the spread of the disease.

The CDC summarized the state of health service unpreparedness in Liberia in October 2014:

> Ebola emergency preparedness plans at the county and hospital level were lacking. . . . In all counties, there was insufficient personal protective equipment to care for patients with Ebola. Health care

[4] Sharon Alane Abramowitz, "How the Liberia Health Sector Became a Vector for Ebola," *Cultural Anthropology Online*, Ebola in Perspective series, October 7, 2014, https://culanth.org/fieldsights/598-how-the-liberian-health-sector-became-a-vector-for-ebola. Abramowitz noted that in Guinea, the government invested only 1.8% of the GDP in health care. Liberia's public health sector, even before the Ebola crisis, was virtually nonexistent. What health services were available were provided largely by NGOs, which ran three-quarters of the government-owned health facilities. The costs of this reliance were laid bare when, in 2006-2007, Medicins Sans Frontieres (MSF) withdrew its branches from Liberia in order to move its resources to other areas deemed to be in greater need of MSF's emergency services. This resulted in the closure of critical regional and urban hospitals, and the abrupt closure of 30 World Vision clinics in Monrovia.

> providers had not received training on the donning and removal of personal protective equipment. No training on case investigation, case management, contact tracing, or safe burial practices had been provided at either the county or hospital level. No Ebola surveillance systems were in place.[5]

As Anthony Fauci of the National Institutes of Health noted in December 2014, "if the West African countries stricken by the current Ebola outbreak had a reasonable health-care infrastructure, the outbreak would not have gotten out of control."[6]

The health systems in the rural areas of Guinea, Liberia, and Sierra Leone were among the weakest in the world. Thousands of children died every year from malaria and respiratory and diarrheal diseases, due to a lack of available medical care. The three countries also had some of the highest infant mortality rates in the world. Yet their medical systems shared characteristics with rural health services in many countries in Africa and other parts of the global south in terms of their lack of trained medical personnel, supplies, and infrastructure. In India, for example, 66 percent of the rural population do not have access to preventive medicines and 33 percent have to travel over 30 kilometers to get needed medical treatments. Also, 3660 of that country's primary health centers lack either an operating theater or a lab, or both. The poor condition of state-run health services has led 80 percent of the patients to seek care from private-sector health providers. In the rural areas, however, medically trained physicians provide few of these private services.[7] A survey in rural Madhya Pradesh found that 67 percent of health-care providers had no medical qualifications at all.[8] The poor quality of rural health services has contributed to major health disparities between urban health and rural health. The infant mortality, neonatal mortality, and prenatal mortality rates in India's rural areas are nearly double those in urban areas.[9] In many places, urban health services, while possessing more facilities, are also plagued by limitations in supplies, infrastructure, and medical personnel.

The Ebola epidemic that occurred in West Africa in 2014 and 2015 was a symptom of a larger, global health-care crisis. At the best of times in many countries in Africa, Asia, and Latin America, clinical coverage is inadequate, forcing patients to travel long distances for treatment. Once they get to medical facilities, they find drug shortages or outages of basic medicines to treat common health problems. Basic equipment, such as disposable gloves and syringes, rehydration fluids, and bandages, is unavailable. Patients or their family caretakers are required to purchase what is needed outside the hospital. Staff are underpaid or not paid for months on end, encouraging them to set up parallel private services on the side instead of attending to public-sector patients. The ties between local health services and the communities they serve are often tenuous, at best. It is not surprising that local populations have little faith in these services. Health systems also lack the surveillance capabilities, including testing laboratories, necessary to track and report emerging epidemics in a timely manner. In short, health services in many parts of the world lack what Partners In Health cofounder Paul Farmer refers to as the four S's: "Staff, Stuff, Space, and Systems."[10]

[5] Joseph D. Forester, Satish K. Pillai, Karlyn D. Beer, Adam Bjork, John Neatherlin, Moses Massaquoi, Tolbert G. Nysenwah, Joel M. Montgomery, and Kevin de Cock, "Assessment of Ebola Virus Disease, Health Care Infrastructure, and Preparedness—Four Countries, Southeastern Liberia, August 2014," *Morbidity and Mortality Weekly Report* 63, 40 (2014): 891-900.

[6] Anthony Fauci, "Lessons from the Outbreak," *Atlantic*, December 17, 2014.

[7] See Rashmi Kumar, Vijay Jaiswal, Sandeep Tripathi, Akshay Kumar, and M.Z. Idris, "Inequality in Health Care Delivery in India: The Problem of Rural Medical Practitioners," *Health Care Analysis* 15, 3 (2007): 223-233.

[8] See Jishnu Das, Alaka Holla, Venna Das, Manoj Mohanan, Diana Tabak, and Brian Chan, "In Urban and Rural India, a Standardized Patient Study Showed Low Levels of Provider Training and Huge Quality Gaps," *Health Affairs* 31, 12 (2012): 2774-2784.

[9] Parthajit Dasgupta, "The Shameful Frailty of the Rural Healthcare System in India," *Future Challenges*, February 2, 2013, https://futurechallenges.org/local/the-frailty-of-rural-healthcare-system-in-india/.

[10] Paul Farmer, Arthur Kleinman, Jim Yong Kim, and Matthew Basilico, *Reimagining Global Health: An Introduction* (Berkeley: University of California Press, 2013).

These conditions tend to be viewed by those in the global north as just the natural state of affairs in so-called underdeveloped parts of the world: "It's Africa or India, after all. What do you expect?" Yet these conditions have a history. They are the product of the unwillingness or inability of governments to fund health services, particularly in rural areas. Health systems have also been weakened by civil wars, such as those that occurred in Sierra Leone and Liberia before the Ebola outbreak, that continue to disrupt large areas of the globe. But they are also the product of a long history of neglect on the part of multinational and bilateral aid donors, including the United States. It needs to be pointed out that over the 10 years preceding the Ebola epidemic, Liberia, Guinea, and Sierra Leone received nearly US$1 billion—directed toward improving health conditions—from the President's Emergency Plan for AIDS Relief; the President's Malaria Initiative; the World Bank; and the Global Fund to Fight AIDS, Tuberculosis and Malaria. Yet very little of this aid was directed toward training health workers or building a health-care infrastructure.

Little attention has been given, as well, to the underlying determinants of ill health. Many rural regions may have access to clinics but lack basic sanitation or a clean water supply. Sewage, contaminated water, overcrowded housing, and unhealthy diets also haunt the populations of many low-income countries. These conditions continue to undermine the health of millions of people across the globe.

Investments in efforts to improve the health of peoples living in resource-poor countries (what we now call global health) by governments and organizations situated in the global north have focused primarily on the application of biomedical technologies—vaccines, antiretroviral drugs, insecticide-treated bed nets, vitamin A capsules—to eliminate specific health problems through vertically organized programs. Yet these programs are only loosely connected to the recipients' national health systems, which struggle to provide even the most basic forms of care.

Global health emerged as a set of practices, organizations, and ideas in the early 1990s, as the world's health community faced new disease threats. The most important of these was HIV/AIDS. From the early 1980s to the 1990s, AIDS went from being a rare wasting disease, seen among groups of gay men in Europe and the United States, to a disease that affected growing numbers of men and women in sub-Saharan Africa, to a threat to all humanity. Linked to the growing AIDS epidemic, though initially independent of it, was an emerging epidemic of multidrug-resistant TB, produced by the failure of health systems around the globe to adequately treat TB patients. By the early 1990s, these new plagues were joined by epidemics of emerging diseases that spread rapidly across the globe. Dengue hemorrhagic fever, severe acute respiratory syndrome (SARS), and various deadly forms of influenza traveled along transportation routes that were the product of globalization: the increasing integration of the world's population into a single, global, economic system.

These events connected the health (and sickness) of people in Baltimore and Chicago with that of people in Nairobi and Delhi and led to a new awareness of the interconnectedness of global health. Plagues were no longer limited to the populations of underdeveloped countries. As a *Time* magazine article on the SARS epidemic noted in 2003: "It is becoming clear that what is taking place in Asia threatens the entire world. Epidemiologists have long worried about a highly contagious, fatal disease that could spread quickly around the globe, and SARS might end up confirming their worst fears. Microbes can go wherever jet airliners do these days, so it is a very real possibility that the disease has not yet shown its full fury."[11]

These fears were heightened after the 2001 terrorist attack on the World Trade Center in New York City, and the subsequent release of anthrax in the nation's capital. Fears that terrorists might employ biological weapons to attack the United States contributed to concerns about traveling microbes and the need for improved global-health surveillance and intervention. It also sparked a massive increase in the funding of emergency-preparedness measures, aimed in part at preventing infectious-disease disasters. For example, the Centers for Disease Control and

[11] Michael D. Lemonick and Alice Park, "The Truth About SARS," *Time*, April 27, 2003.

Prevention's annual budget increased from US$2.1 billion in 1998 to US$7.7 billion in 2002. These fears also led to fresh outpourings of support for health programs in developing countries, aimed at heading off future plagues. Total funding for global-health activities rose from US$5.8 billion in 1990, to US$27.7 billion in 2011, to over US$30 billion in 2013.

Neither the fears nor the efforts to attack diseases overseas were new. The US invasion of Cuba in the nineteenth century was stimulated in large measure by the need to prevent yellow fever from spreading to cities in the southern United States. The *Time* magazine article's reference to jet airlines carrying infectious agents across the globe reminds us of the airline map and the 1932 Cape Town conference's concerns about the global extension of yellow fever. Yet the speed with which microbes could travel across the globe had increased dramatically, as seen in the spread of SARS. The first case was reported in China on February 15, 2003. Less than a month later, on March 5, a patient had died from the disease in Toronto, Canada.

These fears were increased by the near-instantaneous speed with which information about epidemics traveled across the globe. The experiences of individuals in the middle of a major outbreak of dengue fever in Rio de Janeiro in 2010 were broadcast globally, via thousands of Twitter messages. Sitting at home in Baltimore, I could share the alarms and anxieties of people living thousands of miles away, as well as their occasional sense of humor: "If it makes you hot and takes you to bed it is dengue, not love." I could also view real-time reports of dengue cases occurring in Singapore on my iPhone, via a government-supported app called Dengue X.

Dread of the global spread of epidemic diseases was only one of the forces defining global health in the early 1990s. A second was a growing belief among international donor agencies and governments that diseases like AIDS and malaria were a major drain on the economic development of resource-poor countries. The idea that disease undermines development was not new. It had been a central argument used by public-health authorities to justify investments in health going back to the beginning of the twentieth century and earlier. Yet these arguments gained wider acceptance in the 1990s. Central to this new popularity was a recognition of health as an economic variable, both by economists at the World Bank and by the work of WHO's Commission on Macroeconomics and Health, established in 2000.

The landscape of global health was also defined by the conditionalities set by the organizations providing the bulk of global-health funding during the 1990s and early 2000s. These stipulations reflected the concerns of donor countries and organizations in the global north about the ineffectiveness and inefficiency of existing patterns of development aid for health. Critics of this aid, particularly in the United States, argued that too much aid money was being wasted on programs that were unable to demonstrate impact. Other saw resources being lost within bloated and corrupt governmental bureaucracies, which were unable to effectively deploy the resources they received or, worse, channeled them into private bank accounts. Critiques of how aid monies were being spent also flowed from neoliberal economists and politicians who sought to reduce the role of governments in the provision of health services for their citizens. These critics called for more privatized health systems, in which patients bore a larger share of their health costs, and for development assistance to be funneled through nongovernmental organizations. Neoliberal ideas, which had gained ascendancy during the Reagan and Thatcher years, had a much wider influence during the 1990s. The breakup of the Soviet Union and the decline of socialism as a counterweight to capitalist/free-market ideologies in the late 1980s were viewed as validating neoliberal policies, at the same time that they eliminated alternative sources of bilateral aid from socialist countries. These changes increased the hegemony of neoliberalism in the world of global development.[12]

In line with neoliberal efforts to reduce the role of governments in health and avoid funding inefficient governments, the 1990s saw an explosion of both locally based and international NGOs. According to

[12] See Randall Packard, Will Dychman, Leo Ryan, Eric Sarriott, and Peter Winch, "The Global Fund: Historical Antecedents and First Five Years of Operation," in *Evaluation of the Organizational Effectiveness and Efficiency of the Global Fund to Fight AIDS, Tuberculosis, and Malaria*, Annex 2, Technical Evaluation Reference Group, 265-274.

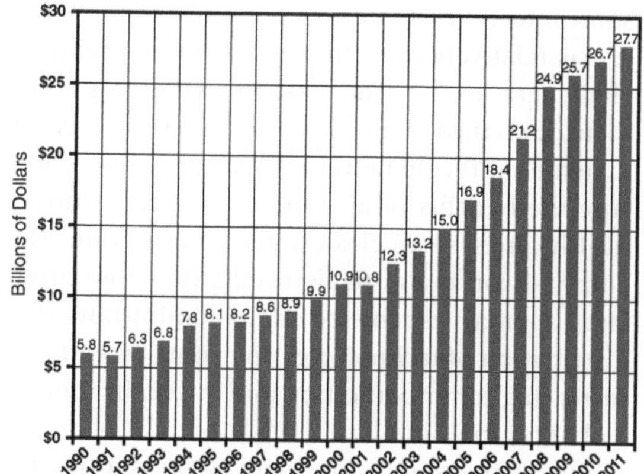

FIGURE 37.1 The Growth of Global-Health Funding. *Source:* Institute for Health Metrics and Evaluation. (2012). *Financing Global Health 2012: End of the Golden Age?* Seattle: University of Washington, 13.

UNESCO, the number of NGOs linked to UN agencies rose from just over 9000 in 1980, to 17,419 by 1990, and then to nearly 28,000 by 2006.[13] But this was only the tip of the iceberg. The numbers did not include thousands of local NGOs, run by individuals in small storefronts or with only a briefcase, that operated locally in various countries across the globe. There were an estimated 100,000 NGOs in South Africa; 300,000 in Brazil; and over a million in India by 2005.[14]

NGOs came in all flavors. Some, such as Partners In Health and Doctors Without Borders, worked independently to bring improvements in health to peoples living in resource-poor settings, though they operated in very different ways. Others were dedicated to raising funds to support ongoing health interventions or research. Beginning in the mid-1980s with the Ethiopian famine, the number of organizations dedicated to raising charitable contributions to help particularly hard-hit populations in the global south grew dramatically. Still others, including thousands of local-stakeholder organizations, worked at the local level, providing partners to implement policies designed by bilateral and multilateral organizations.

Many NGOs were a source of creativity, developing innovative grass-roots programs that supplemented, and sometimes replaced, health services that were not furnished by the public sector in resource-poor countries. In many rural areas in Africa, the interventions provided by NGO-run health programs were often the only health services available. Yet NGO programs seldom replaced the need for a well-developed, government-run health system. NGO-operated health programs often targeted specific health problems and did not provide the basic infrastructure and medical personnel needed to sustain health care. NGO-based care also failed to provide systems for surveillance and case reporting that would prevent disease out-breaks from getting out of hand. Finally, NGO programs were most often supported by outside sources with funding that could be reduced or disappear completely. In short, reliance on NGO health programs could be a double-edged sword.

Donors concerns about the ineffectiveness of existing UN agencies, particularly WHO, in managing global-health funding also defined global health in the 1990s. For many involved in trying to initiate and manage global-health programs, the bureaucratic inefficiencies and internal politics of WHO had made it part of the problem, not the solution. They viewed WHO as a place where good ideas went to die. If the world was going to dedicate vast amounts of new financial resources to improving global health, different mechanisms had to be found for distributing these resources. This led to the creation of new organizations, such as the Global Fund to Fight AIDS, Tuberculosis and Malaria; new public/private partnerships, like the Global Alliance for Vaccines and Immunizations; and private foundations, including the Bill & Melinda Gates Foundation. These organizations demanded accountability. Funded programs needed to both keep careful track of the funds they received and demonstrate impact.

For its part, the World Health Organization, buffeted by the winds of neoliberalism, adapted to the

[13] UNESCO, "Non-Governmental Organizations Accredited to Provide Advisory Services to the Committee," http://www.unesco.org/culture/ich/en/accredited-ngos-00331.

[14] Jim Igoe and Tim Kelsall (eds.), *Between a Rock and a Hard Place: African NGOs, Donors, and the State* (Durham, NC: Carolina Academic Press, 2005), 7.

times. It encouraged programs aimed at promoting economic growth, moved from primary health care to supporting disease-specific interventions, employed cost-effective calculations as a basis for policy choices, and supported market-driven solutions. Many of WHO's programs were designated as partnerships that included private foundations and multinational companies. WHO attempted to maintain some of its commitments to universalism and to serving the needs of the poor. It also made chronic noncommunicable diseases, including cardiovascular disease and mental illness—problems receiving little attention from other global-health organizations—a central concern. In addition, it launched campaigns against the bottlefeeding of infants and tobacco use. Yet WHO's limited financial resources prevented it from developing an effective counterbalance to the emerging neoliberal approach to global health that was promoted by the World Bank, the Global Fund, and major bilateral aid initiatives.[15]

Finally, the need for accountability led to an increased reliance on evidence-based interventions. Randomized controlled trials, long the gold standard for measuring efficacy within the pharmaceutical industry, became a central tool for evaluating the effectiveness of global-health interventions. Yet some interventions were easier to test than others. It was relatively easy, though clearly not without challenges, to test a new vaccine, vitamin supplement, insecticide-treated bed net, or TB drug. It was extremely difficult, however, to set up a trial to measure the benefits of a community-based primary health care system, clean water, or sanitation. The emphasis on quantifiable results therefore privileged approaches centered on the administration or distribution of technologies and contributed to an increasing commodification and medicalization of global health.

Under pressure from donor organizations for measurable-impact programs, from neoliberal economic strategies that encourage the commodification of health, and from the changing landscape of public-health training, with its growing reliance on funding tied to scientific discovery, global health has become centered on developing, deploying, and measuring the impact of technologies. During the course of the twentieth century, the pendulum, which has swung between narrow technological approaches to eliminating diseases and broader-based efforts to build health systems and address the underlying structural causes of health, has moved decidedly toward the former. The consequences of this shift were visible in 2014 in the villages and urban slums of Liberia, Sierra Leone, and Guinea.

[15] Nitsan Chorev, *The World Health Organization between North and South* (Ithaca, NY: Cornell University Press, 2012), 8-9.

SECTION 10 CASES FOR TEACHING AND LEARNING

There is unfortunately a dearth of teaching cases with a historical perspective. However, students can deepen their understandings of global health history by applying historical lessons to modern global health projects. For the cases listed here, we suggest prompts that can be used to encourage students to apply historical thinking to modern case studies. These prompts assume that students have read the selections in this section of the book.

Visit the companion website, **www.oup.com/us/brown-closser**, for direct links to the featured online resources.

Brooks et al., *The Global Trachoma Mapping Project*
In this case, students learn about the global effort to control trachoma.

Suggested prompt: Design two projects to control trachoma: one that takes the form of a vertical program, and one based on primary health care. Which approach is closer to the one adopted by the Global Trachoma Mapping Project? What lessons might those running this project take from history?

R. Dhillon and J. Rhatigan. *The Measles Initiative*
This case describes the Measles Initiative, a global effort to control (and perhaps ultimately eradicate) measles through vaccination campaigns.

Suggested prompt: Create a policy brief for the Measles Initiative on historical lessons for modern measles control and elimination efforts. You should cover three historical lessons that modern planners should keep in mind.

SECTION 10 VIDEOS AND WEB RESOURCES

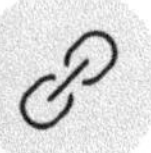

Visit the companion website, www.oup.com/us/brown-closser, for direct links to the featured online resources.

Historical Materials

The following websites provide a wealth of interesting resources, with varying amounts of contextual information. A paper assignment asking students to investigate the historical context of an image or collection of images can be a useful way to engage with this material.

US National Library of Medicine Digital Collections
A fascinating collection of posters, images and videos from the history of public health and medicine in the United States. It also includes material from US health programs abroad. For a starting point with a connection to the Peter Brown reading, students can take a look at the cartoon *Private Snafu vs. Malaria Mike.*

Public Health Image Library – Centers for Disease Control and Prevention
The Centers for Disease Control and Prevention's image library includes a wealth of historical and current images. Students can search by topic or disease to find images relevant to their interests.

The History of Vaccines
This website's image gallery of drawings and photos from the history of vaccination is an especially useful resource.

Smallpox Warriors

Quest for the Killers: The Last Wild Virus

This 1985 hour-long TV program is hard to find, but it contains striking footage of the Smallpox Eradication Program in Bangladesh, including instances of coercion. It provides an excellent companion to the Greenough piece if it is available through your university library.

***Stamping Out Smallpox Is Just One Chapter of His Brilliant Life Story* – PBS NewsHour**

A short (6 min) piece on the fascinating life of Larry Brilliant, who is featured in Greenough's chapter on smallpox eradication.

SECTION

11

Health Systems and Aid

Local health systems that supply preventive and curative health services are a key aspect of global health. They need to be effective, equitable, efficient, and sustainable.

Successful health interventions need the four Ss: systems, staff, space and stuff. All of these things require money. Global health financing is complicated because of the wide variety of organizations involved—from governments to worldwide World Health Organization (WHO) programs to small charity-driven nongovernmental organizations (NGOs). The conceptual tools below describe some of the different kinds of global health funding, including bilateral (government to government) systems and special multinational funding systems aimed at more coordinated efforts (e.g., the Global Fund to Fight HIV/AIDS, TB and Malaria).

Local governments and local health care providers, obviously, are the key players in an effective health system. Readings 38 and 40 provide a look at two very different groups of health workers. Reading 38 explores the experiences of medical students in Malawi, illustrating the challenges they face and exploring some of the factors that cause **brain drain** of trained health staff from poor countries to rich ones. Reading 40 describes what is happening to Lady Health Workers in Pakistan who are targeted with lethal violence while working on polio campaigns.

In Reading 43, Vikram Patel, a leader in the field of global mental health, describes an approach to providing quality care in the context of brain drain and low resources. He argues that **community health workers** (CHWs) can provide mental health care in places where there are almost no psychiatrists.

These and other local health workers are parts of larger health systems, and many of these larger health systems are funded in part by international aid. Readings 39 and 41 take a critical look at the power dynamics of the international aid system. Reading 41, by James Pfeiffer, describes the relationships between donors, NGOs and the government in Mozambique and explains why the international aid system can be counterproductive. Reading 39, by Nigel Crisp, also starts with the situation in Mozambique and suggests a way forward from some of the problems of the aid system: to "turn the world upside down," so that the world benefits from the knowledge and expertise of everyone, not just people from rich countries.

Yet even as there are very real problems with the international aid system, Reading 42 explains why aid is important. Sten Vermund and Ann Kurth provide readers with a number of arguments that are very useful when talking to people who might say that international aid is "money down the drain." They argue that aid benefits both the recipients and the donors.

Finally, the section ends with a reminder that no health system exists in isolation, and that understanding the treatment choices that people have in this multicultural world is important. Reading 44 describes traditional medical systems—what anthropologists call ethnomedical systems—and how it is necessary for biomedical health systems to understand and sometimes accommodate and cooperate with local medical practitioners.

» CONCEPTUAL TOOLS «

- **The vast majority of countries in the world have a government health system that provides health services to citizens.** These systems vary widely in quality, funding and approach, but they generally share a common goal: to ensure that all citizens of a given country have access to basic health services (and sometimes quite complex and expensive treatments as well). The governments of most countries have a **Ministry of Health (MOH)** that runs the government health system.

  The United States is very unusual in its lack of such a government health system. In the United States, even when the government funds health care for civilians (e.g., for citizens over the age of 65 through the Medicare program), that care is provided through the private sector, not by government-employed health professionals. Government funding for health care is very controversial in the United States, as is illustrated by the arguments over the Affordable Care Act aka "Obamacare". But it is not controversial in most countries in the world.
- **In addition to government health systems, people in most areas of the world also have other sources of health care available, provided through the private sector or through NGOs.** Often the private sector is only available to people who can afford to pay for their health care.
- **Many health systems use mechanisms of health insurance.** Universal access to health insurance is currently a global health priority, but with the exception of a few innovative programs, the majority of the world's poor are uninsured.

Health Aid

- **The governments of many poor countries rely on donor funding for a large portion of their Ministry of Health budgets.** This includes bilateral aid provided by the governments of individual wealthy countries (like the United States' USAID or the Japan International Cooperation Agency). It also includes multilateral aid from the World Bank and United Nations organizations like the WHO and UNICEF. Some countries also get substantial funding from private **foundations** like the Gates Foundation.
- **The result of all of this donor funding is that governments can find it very difficult to set priorities for their own health programs.** Since donors decide what to fund and what not to fund, they often dictate the health agenda,

including what health issues will be targeted and how they will be addressed. People often say that many health programs are "donor-driven."

Donor funding tends to be relatively short-term (often it runs on a 2- or 3-year cycle), which can make it hard for Ministries of Health to make long-term plans. Also, donor funding can sometimes follow global fads that may not fit the needs of a particular country. Many Ministries of Health in low-income countries accept a relative lack of control as a necessary side effect of accepting funding. But in recent years, some Ministries of Health (like those of India, Ethiopia, and Rwanda) have taken steps to ensure that donor funding better fits the long-term plan of the recipient country rather than the desires of the donor.

International Goals

- **The Millennium Development Goals (MDGs) marked an important stage in the history of global health.** Through the UN, all of the countries of the world agreed upon eight ambitious goals aimed at improving lives on the planet over the period 2000 to 2015. The goals had specific targets and measures for health, poverty reduction, gender equality, education, ecology, and global political cooperation. The MDGs attracted significant funding for a wide variety of projects, and these goals focused attention, political capital, and money on achieving these specified targets. During this period, remarkable progress was achieved toward the ambitious targets in many areas, although there is still much to do.
- **The Sustainable Development Goals (SDGs) set new targets for global improvements in people for the period 2015 to 2030. Building on the success of the MDGs, stakeholders reconvened to articulate a new set of goals.** The SDGs are much broader and more ambitious than the MDGs; there are seventeen goals, 169 proposed targets for these goals and 304 proposed indicators to show compliance. The goals are ambitious—perhaps to the point of being more aspirational than actually being a planning document: the SDG list starts with ending poverty by 2030.

The Building Blocks of a Health System

- The WHO conceptualizes health systems as made up of six **building blocks**. Health systems are complex, and the building blocks are a simplification. But they can be a useful way of thinking about the kinds of resources that a health system needs. Without all of these building blocks in place, there can be delivery bottlenecks that keep the entire system from functioning—for example, a state-of-the-art diagnostic lab for tuberculosis is of little use if there are no trained staff to run it or there are no treatments available. The building blocks are:
  - **Leadership/governance.** Good management is a critical part of an effective health system.
  - **Health-care financing.** All of these building blocks cost money!
  - **Health workforce.** This building block is discussed in detail in the following paragraphs—health workforce shortages are a major problem in many health systems around the world.
  - **Medical products and technologies.** Not only do products like drugs, vaccines and test kits have to be purchased, they have to be delivered to the people who need them. This is very important and very complicated—stock outs of

essential drugs are common in many health systems without enough funding. Thus, both ample supplies and logisticians to keep those supplies flowing where they need to go are keys to a well-functioning health system. As just one example, health systems need a **cold chain** that keeps heat-sensitive drugs and vaccines cold all the way from their point of manufacture to the people who need them—people who may live in places without reliable electricity. A functioning cold chain, then, may need to include fridges, freezers, refrigerated transport, generators, fuel for the generators and more.

- **Information and research.** Understanding what is going on is a key part of solving problems. This building block includes disease **surveillance**.
- **Service delivery.** This is the most obvious and visible part of a health system: the actual provision of health services to the people who need it.

The Health Workforce

- **There is a global shortage of doctors and other trained health staff.** The WHO estimates that to achieve global coverage of essential health interventions, we would need more than 2 million more health workers in the world—an increase of about 70% from what we have now.
- **The staff that exists are concentrated in high-income countries.** Figure CT11.1, from www.worldmapper.org, shows countries sized by the number of doctors they have. As you can see, many countries, particularly in sub-Saharan Africa, with great health needs have extremely small numbers of doctors to meet those needs.
- **Wealthy countries hire health staff trained in low-income countries, a process known as "brain drain."** Many doctors trained in sub-Saharan Africa are working in wealthy countries. This means that the money that low-income countries

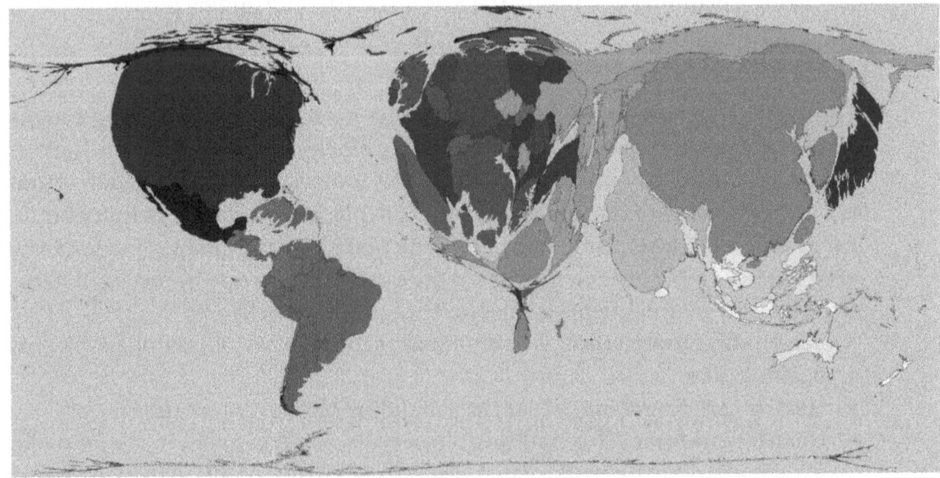

FIGURE CT11.1 Territory Size Shows the Proportion of All Physicians (Doctors) that Work in that Territory.
Source: http://www.worldmapper.org.

spend to educate a health workforce is often lost as skilled doctors and nurses leave for wealthy countries. The WHO estimates that around 20–25% of the doctors trained in many sub-Saharan African countries are working in high-income, OECD countries. As is described in Reading 38 by Claire Wendland, health workers migrate for good reasons: like all of us, they want safe, healthy environments for themselves and their families. They also want to work in settings where they can effectively serve their patients.

- More than one-fourth of the doctors and nurses in the United States were trained abroad. We do not train enough doctors and nurses to serve our population, but we solve our health workforce problems by issuing visas. This means that rural areas of the United States that would otherwise be underserved have enough doctors, but it also makes workforce shortages worse in many "sending" countries. The solution to the brain drain lies in the policies of wealthy countries more than the policies of low-income countries.
- Short-term medical missions, where rich-country doctors go to low-income countries for a week or two, can make minor inroads on specific problems but cannot solve the health workforce crisis. Doctors attracted by the promise of medical missions could potentially make a much bigger impact on health workforce issues by pushing the United States to meet the WHO's goal of halving our dependency on foreign-trained health professionals by 2030. This will require big increases in the numbers of doctors, nurses, and other staff we train domestically.
- Many diseases that are major causes of morbidity and mortality for people living in poverty—like diarrhea, malaria and pneumonia—are reasonably straightforward to diagnose and treat. Lay workers can be trained to identify, prevent, and treat uncomplicated cases of these diseases in a few months. Also, many essential health services like family planning don't necessarily require a doctor's level of training to understand and distribute. Many countries are increasingly looking to Community Health Workers (CHWs) as one potential solution to the human resource crisis. **Moving care responsibilities from highly-trained workers like doctors to competent and more available workers with less training, like nurses and CHWs, is known as task shifting.**

  Ideally, because they serve the communities they are from, CHWs can be advocates for those communities. However, because they are often minimally paid and at the bottom rung of health systems, in practice CHWs are often exploited workers, given many responsibilities but few opportunities to shape policy.

Ethnomedicine

- **All societies have a medical system as part as their culture.** Sometimes these are called "traditional medicine," but "ethnomedicine" is a better label because most medical systems are constantly changing and modernizing. In the simplest sense, all ethnomedical systems have three parts: (i) a way to explain how and why people get sick, (ii) techniques for diagnosis and (iii) practices of appropriate therapy.
- **Biomedicine is an ethnomedicine.** Most of the tools of global health come from biomedicine—the tradition of scientific, biologically oriented methods of

diagnosis and cure. Biomedicine is a relatively recent tradition that is technologically sophisticated and often extremely successful in curing. Biomedicine is international, cosmopolitan, dominant and hegemonic. (This means that its ideas shape the way people think around the world.)

Biomedicine is not culture-free. There are significant and fascinating national and regional differences in the practice of biomedicine. For example, in different parts of the world, there are significant differences in the interpretation of schizophrenia or low blood pressure. Between European countries and the United States, there are very different rates and styles of surgery.

- **In nearly all societies, people may choose between one or more medical systems (or use them at the same time).** For example, in North American and European societies, in addition to biomedicine, people also seek out complementary and alternative medicine, such as herbalism, homeopathy or acupuncture.

The Private Sector

- **Beyond governments and NGOs, there are many private companies involved in health.** These range from multinational pharmaceutical companies to for-profit hospitals to start-ups trying to develop innovative solutions to health problems. Depending on the setting, private actors can have positive or disruptive impacts on health systems.
- **Social entrepreneurship**, the idea that start-ups should be developing good ideas for global health much the same way that they innovate for technology, is currently a popular trend. Good ideas are necessary in global health! But, as Michael Hobbs argues in Reading 48, good ideas are not enough to improve people's lives without a consideration of how innovative ideas might fit into systems that already exist.
- **Multinational and national pharmaceutical companies play important roles in global health.** Sometimes that role is positive: for example, the Carter Center's program to control river blindness, which is caused by a parasite, is driven by drug donations from pharmaceutical companies. But often, the role of pharmaceutical companies is more complicated. For example, in part as a result of US government lobbying, international patent protections (in particular those under an agreement called TRIPS) can mean that many medicines are too expensive to use in low-income countries. There are ways that governments can get around these trade rules if they are working for public health (under another agreement called the Doha Declaration), but, in practice, this can make things difficult for many low-income countries.
- **Sometimes, too much medical care is bad for you.** The United States has by far the highest per capita spending in the world on health care but does not have very good health outcomes compared with many other countries that spend far less. In fact, the expensive medical care we obtain may in some cases be hurting our health, because our capitalist system sometimes financially rewards providers for overtreatment. The Dartmouth Institute website listed in the Web Resources for this section has much more information on this complex problem.

38 A HEART FOR THE WORK

This reading describes the experiences of medical students in Malawi, a small landlocked country between Tanzania and Mozambique. In Malawi, as in many countries in the world, there is a shortage of doctors and other trained health staff. In fact, in the mid-2000s, Malawi's Ministry of Health felt that their health system was "near collapse" because there were so few trained health staff available and so much demand for health care. In 2004, Malawi had just one doctor per 100,000 people (compared with nine in Ghana, seventy in South Africa, and 230 in the USA, Malawi had one of the world's most acute human resource shortages for health problems.

The problem of brain drain hit Malawi particularly hard, but the country is not alone in facing this problem. Many doctors trained in sub-Saharan Africa and Asia are working in wealthy countries. This means that the money that low-income countries spend to educate a health workforce—like the money spent to run the medical school that the students described in this selection attended—is often lost as skilled doctors and nurses leave for wealthy countries.

The solutions to this problem are often beyond the power of Ministries of Health of countries like Malawi. More than one-fourth of the doctors and nurses in the United States, for example, were trained abroad. We don't train enough doctors and nurses to serve our population, but we solve our health workforce problems by issuing visas. The solution to the brain drain lies in the policies of wealthy countries more than the policies of poor countries.

Yet, even as they cannot solve these problems themselves, countries like Malawi are doing their best. Starting in 2004, the Malawian Ministry of Health implemented an Emergency Human Resources Program aimed at training and retaining more doctors and other health workers. The students described in this piece were one part of that program.

The program had some significant successes. For example, when the Emergency Human Resources Program started, there were only forty-three physicians working in government health facilities in the country. By 2009, there were 265 physicians. There were also increases in numbers of lab techs, pharmacy techs, nurses and surveillance officers—all critical staff positions for ensuring public health. The Ministry of Health did this through a combination of expanding training, giving salary "top-ups" or bonuses for staff who chose to stay in Malawi, creating positions for foreign "volunteer" health staff (who were actually given incentive packages more valuable than the salaries of Malawian staff), and improving management structures.

As you read this selection, consider these questions:

- **Why might medical students choose to migrate to a wealthier country once they finish their medical training? If you were in their situation, what would you do?**
- **Why did medical students feel that they were pressured to "be saints"? Do you think American doctors feel this way? Is this fair?**
- **Why do you think expatriate doctors were given higher salaries than Malawian doctors?**
- **What could countries like the United States do to solve these problems?**

CONTEXT

Claire Wendland first went to Malawi as a medical student and was struck by the disparity in resources there compared with to what she was used to in her training in the United States. After getting her MD, she worked as an obstetrician and gynecologist for the Navajo Area

continued

Excerpt from *A Heart for the Work*, by Claire Wendland. Chicago: University of Chicago Press, 2010, pp. 2–4, 120–133, 157–163.

Indian Health Service. Later, when Malawi opened its medical school and Dr. Wendland was getting her PhD in anthropology, she went back to do research on the experiences of medical students in Malawi. That research led to the selection here, which is taken from the book *A Heart for the Work* (2010). Today, Wendland is an associate professor and assistant chair of the Anthropology Department at the University of Wisconsin–Madison

I am in Malawi, walking to Queens Hospital in the cool early-morning shade of the blue gum trees. A Malawian medical student walks by my side. She is slim and tidy in appearance, braids pulled into a neat knot at her nape, white coat covering her simple dress. She is in her third year of school, and she is telling me about her studies. This year is a real challenge, she says (pronouncing the word in the Malawian way: "chah-*lenj*"). You have to move back and forth from the microscopes and textbooks to the hospital, learning pathology in the classroom block and then seeing it in real life—and death—among the patients at Queens. But it is fascinating, too. When yet another thin man with a high fever and a cough walks into the outpatient department, she can "zoom into his body" with her mind. She can actually picture what the inside of his lungs would look like under magnification and how the processes she could see there would cause his symptoms. She doesn't yet know how to treat the problem, but at least she knows what's causing it. I ask if she feels like a doctor yet. She laughs. "Maybe almost."

At the junction with Chipatala Road, streetside vendors hawk hard candies and Fanta, fruit and groundnuts, dried fish dusted with orange pepper, and giant yellow bread rolls that taste a little like sawdust (and are rumored to contain it).

My student companion stops for a moment to make a purchase. She's good at bargaining, and the vendor gives her two tangerines for her five *kwacha*, about a third of what I would pay. She begins peeling a tangerine, telling me that she's missed breakfast to study. Back at the medical-school complex behind us, students get breakfast free in the noisy and chaotic cafeteria—"the caf"—but then you sacrifice what she's found is the best time to hit the library. Over fifty students are sharing two textbooks and half a dozen microscopes. There is no way to avoid the line at the microscope, which stays locked in the lab, but during mealtime there is much less competition for the books.

Her small book stipend for the year wouldn't buy even the one text she was reading this morning, the fat fifteen hundred–page guide to the pathologic basis of disease. All the Malawians she knows have very good memories, she tells me, but even among them her memory is exceptional, praise God, and she can make do without photocopies. I wonder whether, like many of her fellow students, she is trying to save the book stipend to help out with school fees for her siblings or other family obligations, but I don't feel I know her well enough yet to ask.

I'm walking on to the obstetrics and gynecology ward, but my student companion is headed for the main hospital block, and we say our good-byes as she turns off toward the big double doors. She quickly peels her tangerine and pops the cool, juicy pieces in her mouth before she reaches the entrance. It's always tough to leave behind the smoky, faintly eucalyptus-scented air of Chipatala Road for the bloody, bleachy, sweaty smell of the hospital; the residual fragrance of tangerine helps, I know. My watch says it's a couple of minutes before half seven. It will be time for her to find the other students and the consultant for morning rounds. Time to stand quietly at the edge of the group and try to soak up the knowledge she will need soon when she's sent out to run a district hospital, time to figure out how to make a diagnosis without most of the laboratory tests in the pathology textbook and to treat an illness without most of the drugs in the pharmacology book. Time to learn to be a doctor. I watch her square her shoulders inside her white coat, pull open the door, and walk in to begin the day.

Entering the Hospital

Students beginning their clinical training encountered a hospital that did not much resemble the idealized one in their textbooks. At the turn of the millennium, on the medical and surgical wards of Queens, an estimated 80 to 90 percent of the patients were hospitalized for complications of HIV/AIDS: estimated, because the public sector rarely had the money to buy reagents for HIV testing. It was not just reagents that were unavailable. On a Ministry of Health spot check, the pharmacy stocked only 46 percent of the country's already quite limited list of "essential drugs." Intermittently in 2003, the operating theater had no iodine or "spirits" (methyl alcohol), so surgical site preparation was done without benefit of antiseptics. In 2007, we had spirits and sometimes iodine, but the entire country ran out of suture for a period of several weeks. Sutures well past their expiration dates that had been saved to teach students surgical knot-tying, emergency donations shipped in by the Red Cross, and sterilized fishing line stretched the supply chain at Queens, but at more than one outlying hospital, patients died because they could not get necessary operations or have traumatic injuries repaired. At times, barely adequate equipment could be patchworked together from donors, government stores, and various multinational research projects. Sometimes we were flush with odd bits of equipment: ostomy bags, for instance, or donated disposable surgical gowns. At other times, the hospital was without soap, water, "plaster" (surgical tape), or gauze. When I worked there in 2002 and 2003, the labor and delivery ward rarely had a thermometer and never had a scissors, although ten to twelve thousand births took place there in a year. Midwives sometimes conducted deliveries using as their tools only a bare scalpel blade—without the handle—and two pieces of string, at the largest tertiary-care referral center in Malawi.

Staff was stretched just as thin. The pediatrics special care unit, on the day I spoke with an intern there, had twenty-eight beds, 106 patients, and one nurse. On wards so poorly staffed, if a nurse failed to show up for work, there might be no trained clinical staff at all, only students and cleaners.

When I started working at Queens, first as a medical student many years ago, then returning as a volunteer staff member, I thought the poverty, chaos, and sadness I saw there were products of my Northern vision, that of a doctor used to abundance, order, and the systematic concealment of suffering and death in hospital settings. Again and again, my journal recorded a plaintive question: "What kind of a hospital is this?" During this research, I struggled—mostly successfully, I believe—not to let my shock and dismay at the clinical conditions leak into the interview setting, lest they compromise the data. After many interviews and many informal conversations with patients and staff, I came to believe that most Malawians, including clinicians, also found the hospital overwhelming. As a young Malawian man who had come from the village to visit a dying friend told me, "He had TB, and he was on 3B [the male medical ward], and I went to see him. It was awful. I went in, and I thought—it will be a miracle if *anyone* in this ward survives and goes home." Such comments about Malawi's public hospitals were common even in casual conversation.

Other than the privileged few, sick people in Malawi faced difficult choices. The patterns of resort varied, but typically people tried home remedies, often proceeding next to various local healers and choosing hospitals or clinics either simultaneously or as a last hope (Chokani 1998). Wealthier Malawians seeking biomedical care could afford to go to the better-equipped private hospitals, and the richest could fly to South Africa for top-notch private care. The rest faced a choice between defunded, decrepit, and demoralized public hospitals and health centers, medium-quality mission hospitals, or small and minimally regulated private clinics. The public settings were nominally free, while either of the latter options involved potentially crippling payments. Even a minor illness could plunge a family living on the edge into desperate poverty.

The student doctor assigned to a medical, surgical, or pediatrics ward in a public hospital (for students did not rotate through missions or private hospitals) typically faced sixty to a hundred patients daily, some with relatively minor illnesses and most with very serious ones. In all but a few wards, the great majority were HIV-positive. For each of these patients, the illness represented a complex set of social and economic problems that reached well beyond the sick individual into a web of family and other connections. For the students, there was little if any time to address such complexities and little to be done about many of the problems that brought patients in to the hospital.

An ethical and emotional crisis engulfed many trainees when they reached these wards and encountered their first living patients, when the professional identity and expectations they had taken on during preclinical education came up against the realities of patient suffering and physician helplessness in this extraordinarily resource-poor setting. These students had come to envision themselves as scientist-doctors whose knowledge of pathophysiology would enable them to heal using global medical technologies. For two years, like the Northern students studied by others, Malawian physicians-in-training had been anticipating this moment with a mixture of attraction and dread: wearing their white coats among patients instead of cadavers; laying hands on the sick; diagnosing and curing; cutting and stitching live flesh. Malawi's medical students faced a clinical reality far different from that of their Northern counterparts, however. "Most of the time we have had to meet patients where you have *zero* thing to offer," fifth-year student Itai Chilenga reflected. "Oh, you are thinking, now that's it—I have nothing to offer them. That hurts a lot." Lacking access to many of the medical tools and technologies their textbooks assumed to be available, faced with the realities of risk, poverty, and an apparently endless workload, they struggled with this transition in ways that ultimately forced many to reevaluate their roles as doctors.

Workload and Compromised Ideals

"There is too much to be done, but you can't do it all," a tired intern explained at the end of a day in which he had seen 150 patients in the outpatient department. "All these patients require time in order to be treated, that by the end of the day you can say, 'I have *worked* with the patient.' But sometimes that time is not there. So, you see, sometimes you feel that what you might offer you don't offer, simply because you're alone." Compromise could also involve treating patients with a detachment students had not described earlier in their training. One intern remarked that the workload could produce a dehumanizing effect that he characterized as the hallmark of bad medicine. When I asked him to tell me about a bad doctor, Zaithwa Mthindi described himself on a busy day.

> When I'm doing ward rounds, you know. Sometimes you are so immersed in the—you are so concerned about finishing the ward rounds, so you don't really—treat *people*. You are just treating diseases. You are examining bodies, not examining people. For all your good intentions, you get so consumed with the bulk of work, and you lose your human face. And you realize that you have done ten, fifteen patients without even smiling at patients. Without even just giving a kind greeting. . . . I wish I could do better. I wish I could do better.

Fifth-year students, who often worked side by side with the interns, knew both the workload they already faced and what they would be expected to face soon. An intern might be expected to staff a clinic alone, or to round on an entire ward in a half day, making decisions on treatment plans, conducting bedside exams, performing minor diagnostic or therapeutic procedures. Patients had to be seen in two minutes or less, barely enough time to explain what the problem was. Sometimes students and interns just copied the diagnosis from the previous note without reinvestigating. Zaithwa, who described "losing your human face," also told me of a patient who had been admitted for unexplained muteness, a diagnosis repeated in his file for days until one morning a medical student finally greeted him—and he responded.

Students and interns agreed that it was impossible to do an adequate job under these circumstances, but they felt they had no other choice. Many spoke about the work in language that made a generic reality of their individual experiences by using the second person, and that evoked helplessness in the face of inevitable reality: "You have no option." "You must do it." "You get consumed." Intern Brian Msukwa's framing was typical: "You see all the patients that come through the doorway. . . . You forge ahead. You just do it. We don't—we don't have another option, just do it." When students talked about the wards and the clinics, rather than using the battleground metaphors so common in the North, they evoked floundering, wandering, drowning: the wards were "the deep end," "the forest."

At the time I conducted the bulk of the initial interviews, roughly twenty-nine million people in sub-Saharan Africa were estimated to be living with HIV/AIDS (UNAIDS 2003). Malawi was neither the hardest- nor the lightest-hit of African countries, but the impact of the epidemic, visible if insidious elsewhere, was enormous in the hospitals.

> You are very aware now that we have—apart from the many curable diseases—that we have the HIV/AIDS. And this alone is a very big challenge. A very big challenge in the sense that it has actually added to the influx of patients to the hospitals. . . . And at the same time, you talk of the risk of being a physician. If you have to work at a district hospital, you cannot run away from the knife, you know? You have to do some surgeries and those kind of things. And not only surgeries but even in the ward itself. Interacting with HIV/AIDS in your patients is not quite a simple thing. (preclinical student and experienced clinician Joe Phoya)

Their risk of infection was exacerbated by the poverty of Malawi's health sector. Students were not immunized against the few preventable contagions, such as hepatitis B, because there was not enough money. Postexposure prophylaxis for preventing viral disease was unheard of, and reliable protective equipment (such as gloves, masks, sharps-disposal containers) was often unavailable. (By 2007, short-course antiretroviral medications were available for Ministry of Health employees who had "blood-borne exposures" to HIV while at work. They were not offered to students.)

The interaction of poverty-related factors could be synergistic. In the seventy surgical cases I did at Queens in 2002–3, I had five blood-borne exposures, or needle-sticks as clinicians more commonly call them. It was a small number but a high rate, more than twice what would be predicted, and several factors contributed. First, the operating theater usually lacked a working suction machine. When too much blood welled up to see the point of the needle or scalpel—not uncommon in surgery—it had to be dabbed away from the surgical site by hand with sterilized cloths rather than sucked away with a plastic catheter, a catheter that would have kept my fingers far from the needle. Second, there was only one overhead light, instead of the three customary in American operating rooms, further impairing visibility. Third, our needle holders were either used donations from abroad or old Ministry of Health relics. The gripping teeth that should hold a needle in place had worn down long ago, but there were no new replacements, so we kept using them. Fourth, we used the needles that were cheapest for the Ministry of Health to purchase in bulk: round in cross section, these needles were less expensive than the three-sided "cutting" suture needles I often use in the United States, but they were prone to slipping. With a toothless needle holder grasping a round-bodied needle, no matter where one put the needle into the tissue, one couldn't be sure where it would come out as it twisted and torqued in its holder. The interns spoke of them resignedly as "dancing needles," and all of them had plenty of needle-sticks or scalpel lacerations, too. In fact, blood-borne exposures were so common that students and staff often shrugged them off fatalistically. Clinicians saw their exposure as inevitable and were more inclined to worry about their posthumous reputations, as a graduate of the College of Medicine working a public-sector job with a heavy surgical case-load explained:

> It's a very challenging job, because we are being hand in hand with the fluids of the patient, which are contaminated with HIV. But it's part of the job we have. So that is hard. And in the end, when you die of HIV yourself, people may think otherwise. They can't think, "Oh, she is a doctor, she might have had it from a patient." But they think, "No, she was going some other—going outside [having an affair]." I don't know. I think there will be more and more infectious conditions which when—maybe by the time they have been identified, most of us doctors will have acquired them. It will be too late for us. (Ellen Mchenga, graduate)

Did occupational exposure really increase the risk for doctors, nurses, hospital cleaners, and other personnel? The consensus among Malawian students and doctors, all of whom knew colleagues lost to HIV/AIDS, was "of course." However, very little research has been conducted on occupational exposure to HIV in Africa (Akeroyd 2004), except among sex workers. Epidemiologic research in Africa, in marked contrast to studies in Europe or North America, consistently shows that increased levels of education and socioeconomic status are associated with *increased* risk of HIV/AIDS among the general public. (The theory, which fits well with Western assumptions about African sexuality, is that mobility and income increase opportunities for sexual exposure. See World Bank 1999 for a good overview of the data, much of it unpublished.) This pattern makes it very difficult to sort out how much additional risk might be due to occupational exposure.

Some researchers believe occupational exposure to be a negligible risk factor. It is true that, if they were representative of their age and geographical cohorts, two or three in ten of the students should have already been HIV-positive when they began their training. It is also true, however, as Ellen's comment suggests, that Africans have been fairly consistently assumed—by researchers as well as by gossiping relatives—to be victims of their own promiscuity. A recent review (Gisselquist et al. 2002) attributing up to a fifth of African HIV cases to faulty medical procedures and supplies drew enormous criticism, in large part because health policymakers and others feared it would detract from the consensus on behavior change. The fracas over this report suggests that supporting good-quality studies on occupational exposure to HIV was simply not a priority for the major research funders. Malawian doctors and students I knew typically assumed that substantial health care transmission was likely, for both health care workers and patients. I agreed with them. But whether exposure was actually a major risk for students or only a major fear, it affected clinical students and interns negatively.

In 2002 and 2003, students for the most part appeared uninterested in HIV testing, either for themselves or for their patients. Rumor had it that only one College of Medicine graduate applied for a prestigious scholarship for postgraduate education in a country that mandated HIV testing as part of the application process. One preclinical interviewee told me she was appalled when she saw a doctor recommend an HIV test to a patient:

> I was actually shocked. This doctor was seeing a patient and just said plainly, "I think you should get an HIV test." Just like that! Telling someone basically, "I think you have HIV. You should lose all hope." I think that is wrong. One thing people need to have is hope. (Thokozani Sokela, preclinical student)

This situation was very different when I spoke again with students and hospital staff four years later. Many knew their own status, some were on antiretrovirals (although few were open about this with their colleagues), and all whom I asked recommended HIV testing for patients. In 2004, Malawi had begun a public-sector program of antiretroviral therapy that, although it had reached only a fraction of those who needed treatment, was expanding quickly and functioning fairly well. An HIV diagnosis no longer meant "you should lose all hope."

Poverty and Frustration

The numbers and riskiness of patients were sources of concern, then, but a more significant problem for most students was the lack of resources available to help their patients. Patients came in too late to be treated because they lacked funds for transport; once they did arrive, there might be little with which to treat them. Nearly all the textbooks the College of Medicine used came from First World settings and were oriented toward First World technomedicine; many were the same classics—in updated editions—over which I had pored in medical school in Michigan many years earlier. The students' textbook concepts of technological medicine, acquired in preclinical training, crashed headlong into a clinical world of understaffed, under-equipped hospitals that frequently lacked basic supplies, not to mention magnetic resonance imaging, fluoroscopy, mechanical ventilator support, or other technologies of "global" biomedicine.

The hospital day in every clinical department began with "handover rounds," in which the overnight on-call team (typically, an intern, a third-year student, a fifth-year student, and the night nurse or nurses) handed over responsibility to the incoming group. Handover rounds nearly always featured tensions between what students and doctors thought should have been possible and what had actually happened. The report began with summary numbers of patients admitted, discharged, transferred, absconded, and died; the ward nurse would read from her report book a summary of any surgical cases, complex problems, or deaths—marked in the report book with a red ink cross and "RIP." These reports were typically very brief: "Chimwemwe Chisale, 22-year-old gravida one para zero admitted with septic abortion around 1 a.m. At 3:30 a.m. patient found to be gasping. At 4:10 a.m. returned to see patient, who was found to have died. Very sorry." Faculty members could then make inquiries into any of these cases, and the team would defend management. Handover had both practical and pedagogical purposes: students and interns were expected to have read up on complex cases in their textbooks to assure faculty they had mastered the knowledge assumed to be important for every doctor. Yet the discrepancy between textbook and ward was often glaring, and available options shaped or foreclosed therapeutic choices.

One steamy morning in the early rainy season, fifth-year student Catherine Gunya gave the handover report; the pied crows squawked through the open hospital windows as they picked at detritus in the courtyards, nearly drowning out her quiet voice. Emergent Cesarean section for fetal distress following a failed forceps extraction had led to a neonatal death, Catherine reported. The infant had come out pink but then breathed in thick meconium, a tarry stool passed in situations of distress that should be promptly suctioned from the newborn's trachea at birth. "Was the infant suctioned?" "No, sir." "Why not?" "The suction machine was not working. We intended to suction manually, but the batteries were stolen from the laryngoscope [a lighted tool used to see the trachea properly], and there were no replacements. We tried to suction without seeing, but the infant died in the operating theater." That same night a twenty-six-year-old woman had died on the gynecology ward of a malignancy that had spread to her lungs. Catherine explained that she had made the diagnosis—the pregnancy-related tumor called choriocarcinoma—a week earlier by seeing the classic round "cannonball lesions" on chest X-ray. A biopsy or blood test would have confirmed it, but there was no histopathologist in the country to read the biopsy, and the appropriate blood test was unavailable. "What is the proper treatment for choriocarcinoma?" "First, you must give methotrexate, but we do not have any. We just gave her oxygen therapy." And so a disease that Catherine's textbook reported to be 95 percent curable with a low-cost drug remained 100 percent fatal for her patients.

In this context, the new would-be doctors often felt they saw little return on their learning and hard work, because they had little to offer patients. Fifth-year student Itai Chilenga had had "a very bad time" on his pediatrics attachment: "Almost all the patients who I was able to see, three-quarters of them passed away, and it—it became stressful." He described fighting the urge to skip his on-call shifts. "It becomes demoralizing. And at times, you always get discouraged. Why should I go to work at night, when obviously the patient maybe who I might see may die two or three days later? But if there were something I could have given the patient—ah." Young doctors often commented on the disjuncture between textbook and clinic: "Sometimes you just read in order to pass your exams, but you can't be able to meet such situations in real life, and that—that, that is quite difficult. . . . So, really, what you learn in medical school is not exactly applicable when you start working." Students learned about diseases of the elderly but had almost no elderly patients. They learned about neuroimaging and fluoroscopy and care of the extremely premature neonate, but had access to none of the equipment necessary.

HIV/AIDS complicated this picture further, for in 2002 and 2003, there was little to offer HIV-positive patients. Many students talked about a sort of helplessness-induced fatigue that set in on the medical wards, where so many of their patients could not be treated effectively: "It's been useless all these years. Studying from first year to third year, fourth year, and, and at the end of the day, people still die."

Third-year student Mirriam Kamanga had entered medicine to "make a difference in the suffering of children." She found pediatrics particularly hard: it was "difficult for me to watch these mothers sit there and pray and hope that their child will be all right, yet I know myself that it's—you know, it's going to be really difficult, and that's not gonna be the case." Students and interns quickly grew sick of feeling useless, and bored with the frequency of AIDS-related illnesses they could do little or nothing about.

> You know, you want to help someone, but you can't see a positive result. You don't have enough drugs to offer. Most of your patients are terminally ill, and not everyone is cut out to do that kind of work, working with terminal cases all the time. And then there are the dangers you have with it as well—you know, blood everywhere, exposure. But also in some ways it's hard to see the same things all the time. Someone comes in with a problem, and you know exactly what's going to happen next. There are no surprises. (Diana Kondowe, intern)

> Medicine will not be very much interesting, because all your focus will be on HIV. . . . Really, there's very little that a doctor in a developing country can do in such cases. (Zebron Ching'amba, fourth-year student)

Readers may wonder why their conditions of work were so demoralizing for these young doctors. They were Malawians: had they not seen plenty of death, plenty of HIV, plenty of poverty before? Did they truly not know what to expect? The answer to these questions varied somewhat with the social situation of the entering medical student. It was very common for the most privileged students to report that medical school gave them their first inkling of what life was really like for most Malawians. The group of previously trained clinicians, on the other hand, seemed to be somewhat inoculated against this particular shock. Experienced clinical officers were the only students who spoke about Queen Elizabeth Central Hospital as a site of relative abundance (compared to the smaller Malawi district hospitals in which they had worked). The majority of the students fit neither of these categories, however. For most members of the class, it seemed to be the experience of their own powerlessness in the face of medical need and systemwide breakdown that was demoralizing. They were already aware of the magnitude of poverty and suffering in their country, but they were not used to facing it as those charged to heal yet unable to do so.

Flight Plans

Emigration figured prominently in students' talk, in interview settings and casual discussion, from their premedical years through internship. Salaries were a major issue and an especially sore point, but brain drain was about much more than money. Students were very aware that medicine in Malawi was not what it could be elsewhere, and neither was the life of the doctor. They made these distinctions clear from the beginning of training.

> Mkume Lifa: Another frustration will be the working conditions themselves. You know we have a lot of HIV/AIDS and TB here. The chance of contracting disease is high. The working environment is nasty, unhygienic, not clean. You don't have even basic equipment and drugs. . . .
>
> Phillip Tembenu: What you earn is not the only thing pushing doctors out of the country. If you are a doctor who wants to operate on complex cases but there is no equipment, if it is a cancer, there is no chemotherapy—it's difficult. (first-year focus group)

When I asked them specifically, one in three medical students and nearly all the interns thought they would be gone from Malawi within ten years.

The question of where graduates actually ended up working was a contentious one. College of Medicine faculty and administrators often told me that nearly all graduates stayed in Malawi and worked in the public health sector. Students, on the other hand, commonly claimed that most graduates either had already emigrated or were attempting to leave. People who saw the College of Medicine as an expensive white elephant, including many expatriate doctors, tended to share the students' view. Physician brain drain, some contended, was one reason the school should be seen as an inappropriate investment for Malawi.

In a retrospective of the first ten years of the University of Malawi College of Medicine, two faculty members took on the critics by reporting that two-thirds of graduates were actually working in Malawi, with another quarter about to return from postgraduate specialty training (Muula and Broadhead 2001). The numbers they provided are summarized in Table 38.1. Several students and interns brought up this article when talking about their own futures, but none believed the data presented there. They usually questioned whether the graduates listed as receiving postgraduate training abroad had any intention of coming back to Malawi, as it was far easier for a specialist to find work abroad than for a general practitioner. Many wondered where the thirty-one "other" graduates actually were. Interns and students were well aware both that the college was under pressure to make it appear that graduates stayed in the country and that physician shortages remained acute. Joe Phoya was one of the skeptics: "Honestly speaking, on paper it can be made to look that way, but practically, I don't think that is right. Because right now you talk of some districts in Malawi who don't have doctors. So, what, what are we talking about? Where *are* those people?"

Although my own inquiries tended on the whole to corroborate the results given in Muula and Broadhead's article, many trainees and some faculty strongly believed that most graduates of their college either had already gone abroad or were waiting for the earliest opportunity to do so. Students and interns consistently alluded to large numbers of graduates abroad, but none could name more than a few. The émigré-doctor archetype seemed to acquire an importance for students out of proportion to the actual number of doctors who had left the country for good.

TABLE 38.1 Disposition of College of Medicine Graduates.

Work Status	Number	(%)
Specialists		
In postgraduate training abroad	38	(28)
In Malawi after postgraduate training abroad	19	(14)
Generalists		
In internship in Malawi	20	(15)
In district or mission hospitals	18	(13)
Left Malawi	4	(3)
Died	4	(3)
Other: "either working in COM or other government or NGOs"	31	(23)
Total graduates 1992–2001	134	

Source: A. Muula, and Broadhead, R. "The First Decade of the Malawi College of Medicine: A Critical Appraisal." *Tropical Medicine and International Health*, 2001, 6, 155–159.

Conditions of practice and other obligations—to family, to community, to nation—preyed on trainees' minds and came up in their conversations as they imagined emigration. I found no demographic differences that correlated reliably with plans to leave Malawi. Other differences surfaced, however. Students who said they hoped to stay in Malawi were more likely than their peers to express nationalist sentiments, were more impressed with the social status of doctors, and were more likely to describe medicine as a calling. Students likely to want to emigrate, in contrast, expressed more strongly a desire for jobs in which the tools and technologies of medicine would be available to them. In addition, for this group, the issue of work-life balance sometimes did come up. Although no one actually used the word *balance*, students who wanted to emigrate were more concerned about being able to set limits on working hours and more desirous of private lives.

Whether they planned to get out of Malawi as soon as possible or hoped to stay, those discussing it very often characterized emigration as "human nature" or "only human." The tendency to characterize emigration as inevitable, a natural human desire, may explain why students insisted that "most" doctors had left the country even when evidence suggested otherwise. This characterization allowed those who wished to leave to feel normal and highlighted the sacrifice of those who chose (or had) to stay. Their choice of words suggested that many saw patient care in Malawi as a superhuman—or perhaps inhuman—endeavor.

Indeed, *most* students felt that they were being held to high standards of self-sacrifice by donor countries, by the college administration, and by their own government: they were expected to practice in very poor conditions, for long hours, and with little remuneration. Some accepted this call to altruism as part of the job, describing it as a sacrifice but voicing no complaint. Others expressed resentment at the expectation that they would "be saints." One student asked me to take a message to Americans who believed a medical school was the solution to Malawi's health problems:

> Tell them what you really deal with, what you really have. 'Cause that's like—in developed countries, what they have, they are *advanced*. They have advanced medicines. All we have are basics. We don't even *have* the basics sometimes. And maybe they should try to imagine if they were in this place, where they don't have many opportunities, many medications—what would *they* do? Would they still follow the same path? Because they say, "Train doctors, train doctors." Yes! Train doctors. But if *they* had to come here and they'd do this, would they go through with it? Or would they choose other careers? (Bridget Nyasulu, clinical student)

The bitterness of Bridget's comment, like those of others, had much to do with the anticipated frustrations of medical work. The clinical poverty, personal risk, and heavy workload discussed in the previous chapter remained central concerns, but they were not the only issues. As students graduated and became doctors, other features of their working lives also daunted them.

Money and Sacrifice

No subject was as ubiquitous when students and interns discussed actual practice as money, and no subject elicited as much agreement in interviews and on questionnaires. Their comments did not demonstrate the increasing focus on money with the passage of years in training that is often noted in the North; even Malawians in their first year at medical school often brought up physicians' pay. Students and interns agreed that doctors' pay was scandalously low: *peanuts*, to use the word many favored. Poor salaries added insult to the injuries of heavy workload and limited clinical resources.

Brian Msukwa had initially wanted to go into medicine "to help the nation." At the time I interviewed him, halfway through his internship, he was embittered, tired, and angry.

> One thing that I would say is that in Malawi, now that I am in the system, the government doesn't care what we need here. You present your problems, they do nothing about it. It's like really *slavery*, the work. It's no wonder most of the doctors just leave the government. . . . You may have that heart in you to work—but, I mean, you need *some* money to support yourself!

Brian planned to use some American connections to arrange for postgraduate training there and expressed doubt about whether he would ever return to Malawi to work.

Whether the financial situation for these doctors was really that bad depended on one's vantage point. New doctors in Malawi earned much more than the average citizen—eighteen times as much, in fact. But students rarely compared themselves to ordinary Malawians, who were among the poorest people in the world: "too poor to buy soap," as the students often put it. They compared themselves to college classmates who went on to become lawyers or accountants (each requiring fewer years of training than medicine), or to the politicians who determined their pay. They compared themselves to peers who owned cars, lived in houses with plumbing, and sent their children to school without worrying about the cost. They also compared themselves to the trainee doctors who came from abroad, showed up intermittently on the wards for a few weeks, then disappeared on safari or to the expensive lakeside resorts. In these comparisons, Malawian doctors' salaries fell scandalously short (see Table 38.2).

In fact, the salary figures presented here may be too optimistic. Salary packages were supposed to include housing near the hospital, but few places were available, and most interns had to seek their own rentals. Their housing allowance was not enough to rent even a fairly basic place to live; minibus transport back and forth to the hospital further ate into their take-home pay. Salaries also all too often went unpaid for months at a stretch. The nurses and interns working at Queens Hospital got no paychecks in November or December of 2002 due to "computer problems" at the Ministry of Health. At the end of January, they began receiving monthly pay-checks again but six months later were still waiting for their back pay. Similar "computer

TABLE 38.2 Pay Scales.

	Annual Pay in 2003 US$ (PPP-Adjusted)	
	Malawi	United States
Putting wages in perspective		
Per capita GNP	160 (570)	35,277 (34,320)
Population living on less than $1 per day (%)	41.7	<1
Typical starting salaries		
Secondary school teacher	696 (2,479)	27,989 (27,229)
Intern	2,148 (7,652)	38,000 (36,969)
General practitioner	2,904 (10,346)	130,000 (126,473)
Accountant	6,312 (22,487)	39,397 (38,328)

Sources: General economic data are from UNDP 2003. Malawi salaries were taken from my field notes, where I recorded civil service wage scales for 2003; they include housing and other special allowances, which could be quite a high proportion of salary, and have been converted to US dollars using the average 2002–2003 exchange rate of MK95/US$. United States figures (except intern salaries) are from the Occupational Outlook Handbook, 2002–2003 edition, published by the Bureau of Labor Statistics (bulletin 2540). United States intern salaries were averages found in a 2003 online search of positions advertised.

problems" kept some interns working for months without pay in 2007.

Doctors' feeling of being underpaid was exacerbated by several perceived injustices. First, most were aware that pay scales for other public-sector employees had been upgraded in recent years. Junior lawyers earned considerably more, for instance, despite being civil servants at the same level as junior doctors; the government had found improvements in pay essential to ensure an impartial judiciary. In contrast, the possibility of upgrading pay scales for doctors had been "under study" for some years, but the only change that had actually occurred was to make the housing subsidy taxable starting in 2002, representing a real decrease in total income of about 18 percent.

A second injustice was more specific to the College of Medicine: the Ministry of Education, through which faculty salaries were paid, used different pay scales for expatriates and Malawians. Faculty from outside Malawi not only took home substantially larger paychecks but were allocated better-quality housing and had their children's school fees paid, unlike their Malawian counterparts. Junior faculty, some of them College of Medicine graduates, felt the dual salary structure doomed any efforts to "Malawianize" the College of Medicine. Dr. Arthur Gumbo, one of the first Malawian faculty members I interviewed, responded with a dismissive wave of the hand when I asked him how he thought things would change as the teaching staff became more heavily Malawian:

> This college is not going to be Malawian. That is a theory, but it will never happen. . . . Why would Malawians want to come here? The more Malawians we train, the more will just go outside, to the UK or other places. The salary is too low. You go outside, you see what else is available. Or you stay here and you see that expatriates are paid much more than Malawians. . . . If I get the opportunity, I will go, sure. So I don't see this place being Malawianized.

When I challenged him, saying that faculty I had spoken with predicted otherwise, his retort was brusque. "Who are the others? If they are Malawians, they are afraid. They are being political. And the other ones—well, it's in their interest to say that they are going to Malawianize the school. It is a nice theory." The dual wage structure meant that expatriates could keep their well-paid jobs, he held, even while imagining themselves as agents of African development and deploring the insufficient patriotism of Malawians who emigrated.

Whether the expatriate faculty were speaking cynically or simply under-estimating the effects of pay discrimination on their Malawian colleagues, Dr. Gumbo was right. Only expatriates predicted the Malawianization of the school. The College of

Medicine, championed by Dr. John Chiphangwi, started as a Malawian project, but it risked becoming an expatriate one. Many students initially talked about wanting to teach "even here at this college," but plans to teach in Malawi diminished with years in training, and by internship, several doctors specifically mentioned the pay disparity as a factor in their loss of enthusiasm. It is difficult to overestimate how embittered young physicians felt about unequal pay for equal work, and how much it contributed to a desire to emigrate among those who had wanted to teach. As a registrar who had recently found out about the differing pay scales said, "I won't stay in that world. I wanted to stay here, but now I am preparing for my exam. I have to get out of here unless the conditions are to change."

New Malawian doctors perceived the sharpest injustices in the public excesses of national politicians. Discrepancies between politicians' and doctors' lives, in terms of workload, responsibilities, pay, and perks, came up in conversation and interviews more than any other comparison. Politicians would line their own pockets at the expense of the public in any way they could, even treating hospital budgets as sources of personal revenue, students and interns complained. Although no one I spoke with espoused the return of dictatorship, many linked increasing rapacity among the political class to democracy. "Ever since we have had democracy," one young graduate explained, "it has been a matter of get rich any way you can."

Lawyers, politicians, foreign teachers, doctors traveling in from other countries, all could live luxuriously while they exhorted their Malawian medical colleagues to greater sacrifice for the sake of national development. The new graduates wanted to help their country, but they did not want to be fools or pawns. Few graduates saw any reason they as doctors should be the only ones expected to give up a decent living for Malawi.

REFERENCES

Ackeroyd, Anne V. 2004. Coercion, constraints, and "cultural entrapments": A further look at gendered and occupational factors pertinent to the transmission of HIV in Africa. In *HIV and AIDS in Africa: Beyond epidemiology,* ed. Ezekiel Kalipeni, Susan Craddock, Joseph R. Oppong, and Jayati Ghosh, 89–103. Malden, MA: Blackwell Publishing.

Chokani, Angela C. V. 1998. Local medicines audit: Reasons for going to the *sing'anga* first. MBBS Year IV project, on file with the Department of Community Health, College of Medicine, University of Malawi.

Gisselquist, David, Richard Rothenberg, John Potterat, and Ernest Drucker. 2002. HIV infections in sub-Saharan Africa not explained by sexual or vertical transmission. *International Journal of STD and AIDS* 13 (10): 657–66.

Muula, Adamson S., and Robert L. Broadhead. 2001. The first decade of the Malawi College of Medicine: A critical appraisal. *Tropical Medicine and International Health* 6 (2): 155–59.

UNAIDS (Joint United Nations Programme on HIV/AIDS). 2003. Report on the global HIV/AIDS epidemic 2002. http://data.unaids.org/pub/Report/2002/brglobal_aids_report_en_pdf_red_en.pdf

UNDP (United Nations Development Program). 2003. *Human development report 2003.* New York: Oxford University Press for the United Nations Development Program.

World Bank. 1999. *Confronting AIDS: Public priorities in a global epidemic.* New York: Oxford University Press for the World Bank.

39 TURNING THE WORLD UPSIDE DOWN

The author of this piece, Nigel Crisp, argues that there are two flows of "unfair trade" in global health. The first part of the unfair trade is the **brain drain**, *discussed in the previous selection (Reading 38) by Claire Wendland. In this flow of unfair trade, doctors and other health professionals flow away from the poorest communities that need them most and toward wealthier communities with fewer health problems.*

The second flow of "unfair trade" is discussed in this selection. As health workers are flowing from poor to rich countries, something else is flowing from rich to poor countries: ideas. *Ideas are not, of course, a bad thing in and of themselves. The problem arises when Ministries of Health must navigate a cacophony of ideas from a wide variety of donors, all becoming less ideas than mandates when they are tied to funding. Sometimes, rather than focusing on building a cohesive, coherent health system, Ministries of Health must try to manage the expectations of donors that want specific vertical programs, want to meet specified targets in maternal survival or have other specific ideas and aims.*

As just one example, James Pfeiffer explains in Reading 41 that in the late 1990s, so many donors wanted to support Traditional Birth Attendants in Mozambique that the Traditional Birth Attendants had more support than nurses attending births in hospitals. But 20 years later, the pendulum has swung the other way: many donors prefer to support births in health facilities, and in many countries, Traditional Birth Attendants are discouraged from practicing at all (see Reading 13).

In addition to navigating a multitude of conflicting ideas and mandates from donors, Ministries of Health must also attempt to make long-term plans when most donor projects are on 2- to 3-year cycles. With political changes in donor countries or shifts in development fads, funding priorities can change.

The problem with ideas flowing from rich countries into poor countries—and not vice versa—is that it implies that outsiders know better than the people who are from a given area how best to address health problems. Nigel Crisp doesn't argue against idea exchange, but he insists that it should not be a one-way street: the United States, for example, which has the highest health-care costs (but not the best health outcomes) in the world, might have a lot to learn from less wealthy countries when it comes to effective ways of delivering care. This is what Crisp means by "turning the world upside down."

As you read this selection, consider these questions:

- **What did the former Health Minister of Mozambique mean when he said that he was really the minister for health projects that were run by foreigners?**
- **How do former colonial relationships affect the flow of ideas?**
- **What do you think it would actually mean for people from wealthy countries to "listen better" to people from low-income countries? How could this be institutionalized? Is it realistic?**
- **What does Crisp mean when he says that problems with health systems are "our crisis too"?**
- **What are the reasons that wealthy donors sometimes have power over the governments of low-income countries?**

CONTEXT

Nigel Crisp was the chief executive of the United Kingdom's National Health Service in the early 2000s. He has also worked with the Global Health Workforce Alliance and as a consultant to the World Health Organization and the Gates Foundation. He was knighted in 2003. The selection here is from his book, *Turning the World Upside Down* (2010).

I was the wrong person with the wrong question at the wrong time.

As the Mozambique Minister of Health entered the small committee room with his officials in tow I could see immediately that he was cross, very cross. We were at the World Health Assembly in Geneva in 2006 and I had requested an interview in order to ask him what more the UK should be doing to help improve health in Africa.

I don't know where he had just come from. I now wonder if he had been sitting all morning in meetings where he and his African colleagues had felt patronised by people from rich donor countries telling them what they should be doing; perhaps he was merely suffering from too many hours of long speeches and the interminable time wasting of that great Assembly.

Upright, smartly dressed and very articulate, he let me know from the outset that he was fed up with being told what to do by foreigners. He understood his own country very well, thank you. He knew what his priorities were. Did I understand that the international agencies providing pills for immunisation were only doing part of the job? What use was a pill if a child didn't have any clean water to swallow it with? He didn't care if immunisation was their priority. He wanted help with infrastructure, water, roads, schooling and employment. He didn't want to be told what he should be doing.

This, my first meeting with Minister Paulo Ivo Garrido, reminded me of the story I had heard about one of his predecessors as Health Minister for Mozambique, who had naturally assumed that on taking office he would be responsible for the health of his population. He discovered, however, that he was really the Minister for health projects which, he paused for effect, were run by foreigners.

It also underscored very clearly what it felt like to be a recipient of foreign aid. Mozambique, in common with other countries, received aid from many individual countries, including the UK, from international agencies and from many NGOs, small and large. All of them gave aid on their own terms and all of them wanted it monitored against their own criteria. It is only a small step from here to telling people what to do.

This problem is not unique to Africa. Many countries receive more than 100 separate monitoring visits a year, two or more per week, and have to write reports for all their donors. Some countries need to devote half the precious manpower of their ministries of health to dealing with foreigners and "projects run by foreigners."

It must have been very galling for the Minister. I learned, as I got to know and respect him at later meetings, about the passion and energy he brought to the role. Unlike many, he was in the post for the long term and, as a surgeon, understood healthcare well.

For my part I got far more from the interview with the Minister than I had expected, being, as I was, forcefully reminded that aid and development are also about power and about who sets the agenda and, of course, about who is accountable to whom.

This story sets the scene for a chapter in which I describe some of the ways in which ideas and ideologies are imported from richer to poorer countries alongside aid, trade and other relationships. It is very important to stress at the outset that very many of these ideas are extremely beneficial: scientific knowledge, technical knowhow, commercial and governmental understanding are all immensely valuable. However, like all good things, they bring their own problems, some of which get in the way of progress. This chapter concentrates on this darker side.

In health, as Minister Garrido understands too well, power sets the agenda. Ideas and ideology come with the money. It is no surprise that donor countries impose explicit conditions on how money is spent. In 2005, for example, the UK required Malawi to make basic health services free to all its citizens as a condition of a massive investment in staffing and health infrastructure.

It shouldn't come as a surprise either to know that donor countries don't all want the same things. The USA, by contrast, promotes health insurance and, by implication, wants users to pay some of the cost of their own healthcare. Each country it seems, exports its own beliefs about how health services should be run, regardless apparently of the success or failure of those policies in their home countries.

This is not in itself a new trend. Former British Colonies from Hong Kong to Jamaica have health services modelled on the British NHS and for a long period their medical and nursing schools had many expatriates on their staffs. This legacy lives on in the thousands of young professionals who have come to the UK for their training and who still aspire to membership of one of the UK Royal Colleges.

Medical staff from former French Colonies can tell a similar story and exhibit the same high level of pride in their graduation from a French University and their years of training in Paris or Lyon or Marseilles. They, just like the South Americans or Filipinos trained in the US system, take home with them a share in the experience and worldview of their teachers and mentors.

More problematically, we have seen the intrusion of current domestic politics into international development. Two linked issues, birth control and abortion, have heavily influenced American policy, provoked a split with many other donors and slowed progress on improving death rates amongst women and children as well as on AIDS.

Domestic American politics meant for years that US aid officials were unable to embrace the full ABC of AIDS prevention, where A stands for abstinence, B for be faithful and C for use a condom if the other two do not apply. They have in many cases been forbidden to promote condom use or other forms of contraception outside marriage because to do so has been considered to be condoning or even encouraging immoral behaviour.

There are meetings, conferences, assemblies, planning sessions, reviews, monitoring visits and liaison between donors and recipients, between donors and donors and between regional and national groupings. It is the domain of economists and policymakers who mix politics with their professional analysis as they dispense vast sums of public money.

There is waste, there is bureaucracy and both must be tackled; but there is also a wider problem embedded in the very notion of international development. This is the implication it so often carries of people doing things for other people, of knowing better, and of there being somehow a clear distinction between developed and developing countries.

We could start by listening to individuals. There are many outstanding people in poor countries and many outstanding leaders. We could invite more of them to our meetings. We could listen better. We could find better ways to listen to the voices of the poor and try to understand why so many poor people "define poverty as the inability to exercise control over their lives."[1]

We could also try to listen out for and understand better the implications of the far-reaching changes underway in many countries. I have concentrated in this chapter on Africa and the poorest countries in the world and presented a relatively simple picture of the relationship between two groups, the rich and the poor. The reality is much more complex and far messier.

Power and influence are shifting and what, even 10 years ago, looked to the West like a fairly simple picture of high-, low- and middle-income countries with a one-way flow of aid and development, is now much more differentiated and complex. There are different power groupings, different flows of aid, different influences and different identities being forged.

Our relationship with poorer countries is not just about them and their needs. It is also about us and our needs. We are at a point when many people in rich countries are beginning to recognise the problems we have in sustaining and growing our health systems. We are reaching the limit with our current model. It needs major attention. This is our crisis too.

Recognising our own weakness in this way should make us more open to new ideas. It should also help us to support the development of poor countries better. It could, even, break down some of the barriers between developed and developing countries and help us as equal partners to learn and develop together.

Just as the idea of international health—the health of others—has been replaced by a shared notion of global health, co-development or global development, the development of equals, needs to replace the idea of international development.

We must also free our minds from some of the ingrained assumptions associated with western scientific medicine. These are very powerful, deep seated and difficult to challenge. This is nowhere better illustrated than by the current debate about "task shifting." This expression is used to describe the way in which some tasks previously done by one group of professionals such as doctors are shifted to another group such as nurses. Similarly, some tasks done by nurses might be shifted to other less well-trained groups.

It is often argued that poor countries can't afford to have many doctors and nurses and therefore every effort should be made to find ways to shift as many tasks as safely as possible to cheaper groups. Many people seem to see this as a purely temporary solution to be used only until the countries can afford the desirable level of staff. Nevertheless, a great deal of effort is now going into devising training courses and protocols to put this in place.

I remember discussing this in a meeting in Kampala when one by one the Africans in the room ridiculed the notion. Their complaint was not about unskilled people taking on these tasks, but about seeing the world purely in terms of the established professions. Why were we starting with the professions and deciding what would be done? Shouldn't it be the other way up? Shouldn't we decide what needs to be done and then decide who is best placed to do it? Or as they put it rather more forcefully, who do they think has been doing these tasks all along? Let them send us some doctors and nurses and we will gladly shift some tasks to them.

In unfreezing our minds, we need to look at what is happening elsewhere and think about how it applies to the rich world as well. BRAC, the massive Bangladesh NGO, is doing just that and is applying its learning in its home country to projects it is establishing in Africa, but also in the USA.

This chapter has been about what we import into poor countries from the rich. What if it were the other way round? What might we learn?

Ultimately it is the coming together of ideas from rich and poor countries that will have the most effect.

REFERENCE

1. Narayan D. *Poverty is Powerlessness and Voicelessness.* Finance and Development, International Monetary Fund. 2000. Available at: www.imf.org/external/pubs/ft/fandd/2000/12/narayan.htm.

SVEA CLOSSER AND RASHID JOOMA

40 WHY WE MUST PROVIDE BETTER SUPPORT FOR PAKISTAN'S FEMALE FRONTLINE HEALTH WORKERS

In the early 20th century, polio was one of the most feared diseases in industrialized countries. Soon after the discovery and introduction of effective vaccines in the 1950s and 1960s, polio was brought under control in high-income nations.

The Global Polio Eradication Initiative (GPEI) is the largest and most expensive Global Health program in history; it has involved huge vaccination campaigns, millions of workers and billions of doses of oral polio vaccine. The last case of polio caused by a wild virus in the western hemisphere was in 1991. Nevertheless, success in total eradication seems elusive.

In 1988, when the GPEI began, polio paralyzed more than 1,000 children worldwide every day. Since then, more than 2.5 billion children have been immunized against the disease. The program itself has involved the cooperation of more than 200 countries and an international investment of more than US$11 billion. The global incidence of polio cases has decreased by 99%, and, as of 2017, there are only three countries where polio transmission has never been stopped. Pakistan, the topic of this article, is one of those countries.

The story starts with an account of murders of Lady Health Workers (LHWs) who were distributing polio vaccine in Pakistan. Starting in December 2012, antigovernment militants began murdering local health staff while going door-to-door delivering polio vaccine. The campaign workers—mostly women—are not highly paid aid workers nor do they have ties to international interests. They are earning just a few dollars a day to support their families and vaccinate their neighbors' children. How could this possibly happen?

LHWs have become an attractive target for insurgents in Pakistan because polio eradication is an obvious priority of international actors and the Pakistani government. International agencies and the government have loudly announced their commitment to the eradication of polio. So, attacking polio workers is a symbolic attack on both the government and foreign donors. LHWs are easy targets, and their deaths attract international attention.

Making things worse, the CIA used a fake hepatitis vaccination campaign in their hunt for the Al-Qaeda leader Osama Bin Laden in 2011. The CIA hired local staff to pretend to give hepatitis vaccinations, and instead, they took blood from children to be tested for their relationship to Osama bin Laden. This terrible program has of course led to increased suspicion of all vaccination campaigns in Pakistan.

As ***task shifting*** *becomes more common, community health workers (CHWs) like LHWs are increasingly asked to take on a wide variety of health tasks (including but going beyond activities like vaccination campaigns). The key to successful primary health care programs often depends on people like LHWs. CHWs are often seen as* ***cost-effective*** *because they can be paid very little. However, as this article argues, paying CHWs the least amount possible is often exploitative.*

As you read this article, consider the following questions:

- **When it was first launched, GPEI leaders predicted that the disease would be eradicated in less than 10 years, but the target date has been extended, and now it has been twice that long. Do you think that financial donors will get frustrated and withdraw their support? Why or why not?**
- **There are criticisms of the strategy of disease eradication because it focuses incredible efforts on a single disease that may not be highly important for local people. Do you agree with this critique?**

Svea Closser and Rashid Jooma, "Why We Must Provide Better Support." *PLOS Medicine,* 2013, 10(10): e1001528.

- **Immunity to polio in the hygienic conditions of places like Pakistan requires multiple doses of vaccine, and this is a reason why the GPEI must conduct multiple community-wide "vaccination days" every year. This is different from the smallpox vaccine, which only requires one dose. Do you think it was the right decision to focus on eradicating a disease when the biomedical tools were not as strong as the ones used against smallpox?**
- **Do you think that CHWs, many of whom may have less than a high school education, should have opportunities for "career advancement" as the authors suggest? Is this realistic?**
- **Do you think that the arguments here about the importance of pay and career advancement only apply because the LHWs' lives are in danger? Or, should these issues be important for all CHWs?**
- **If you were a LHW involved in polio eradication, would you quit that work because of the danger?**

CONTEXT

Svea Closser is a co-editor of this book. She is an associate professor in the Department of Sociology and Anthropology at Middlebury College in Vermont. She earned a PhD in anthropology and a MPH in global health from Emory University. She is author of the book *Chasing Polio in Pakistan: Why the World's Largest Public Health Initiative May Fail* (Nashville, TN: Vanderbilt University Press, 2010); this book won the Norman L. and Roselea J. Goldberg Prize for the best project in the area of medicine. The interviews described in this article were part of a project supported by UNICEF (although they are not responsible for the conclusions drawn here). Rashid Jooma is the former Director-General of Health for the country of Pakistan. He is now a professor of neurosurgery in the Department of Surgery at Aga Khan University in Karachi, Pakistan. His medical training was in Pakistan, Scotland and England.

Polio is a crippling and deadly viral disease. Through an impressive effort involving millions of people and billions of doses of oral polio vaccine, the Global Polio Eradication Initiative (GPEI) has interrupted polio transmission in all but three countries: Pakistan, Afghanistan, and Nigeria.[1]

In Pakistan, weak health systems are a key reason that polio elimination is so difficult.[2–4] Rates of routine immunization, which would provide a population-wide firewall against polio, remain low.[5]

Critical to the eradication effort in Pakistan are the country's 106,000 Lady Health Workers (LHWs), government health staff who work on vaccination teams in special door-to-door immunization campaigns. But militant groups have begun to target these workers, breaking down the front line of defense against polio.

Why Are Lady Health Workers Being Killed?

In December 2012, militants murdered 9 polio campaign workers in Pakistan, and the killing has continued into 2013 with the death toll now nearing 20. Workers going door-to-door delivering polio vaccine have been shot, and Lady Health Workers have been the targets of bombings at health centers.[6–13]

Aid programs generally, and vaccination programs specifically, have become associated with CIA and Western interests in Pakistan. The CIA's tactic of employing a fake vaccination campaign to search for Osama Bin Laden damaged health workers' credibility.[14] The Taliban have targeted LHWs in the Swat Valley, ostensibly for promoting contraceptives and representing Western interests.[15]

In this context, polio eradication's high political profile contributed to making the program a militant target. In the past few years, the leadership of the GPEI made a strategic decision to intensely and publicly engage national leaders in the hope of leveraging their perceived authority and oversight for the polio program.[16–21] The resulting greater political involvement has increased commitment and accountability.[1,22,23] Many observers see this development as wholly positive. However, we believe that the much-publicized importance of polio eradication to national leaders and international organizations helped to make polio eradication workers, including Lady Health Workers, targets of anti-government and anti-state elements.[24,25]

Deep-seated ideological opposition to polio eradication by militants is unlikely: the Taliban, for example, actively support polio vaccination campaigns when it is politically advantageous.[26,27] Militants might be killing polio workers for political reasons: attacking polio eradication is a way to attack national and international interests.

Here, we argue that achieving polio eradication and strengthening Pakistan's health system depend on a shift in the center of gravity of international engagement, away from high-profile engagement with federal leaders and towards supportive partnerships with Lady Health Workers and other ground-level staff.

Lady Health Workers Are Needed to Improve Pakistan's Health System

Each Lady Health Worker acts as the interface between around 150 urban slum or rural households and the health system. In addition to polio campaigns, she visits families monthly to promote family planning; advise on nutrition and hygiene; and create demand for antenatal care, childhood immunization, and use of skilled birth attendants. While the program is not perfect, independent evaluations have consistently shown improved health outcomes on a range of primary healthcare measures in populations with LHW coverage. The households served by LHWs are 15 percentage points more likely to have children under 3 years old fully immunized. Over 90% of communities served by LHWs report that they benefit from her services.[28,29]

Lady Health Workers Are Needed for Polio Eradication

Pakistan's current polio eradication Emergency Action Plan[22] mandates that each of the approximately 80,000 mobile teams deployed in polio campaigns include a female. As there are few other women in the government health system, Lady Health Workers (LHWs) are an essential part of the polio workforce—more than 85% of the total number of LHWs are engaged in each campaign. They contribute to polio eradication through health education and door-to-door delivery of polio vaccine. Most importantly, because most are locally known women, their presence increases access to conservative households and decreases refusals.

Pakistan has decided not to suspend polio campaigns even in the face of danger to LHWs and other workers. This decision has received international approval because halting campaigns would probably mean a resurgence of polio, including possible reinfection of countries like India and China.[30] Decades of painstaking progress might slide away.

In many parts of Pakistan, UN staff who work on polio campaigns have been pulled from the field for their safety. At the same time, LHWs continue to put their lives at risk.[31,32]

Without UN staff in the field, polio eradication needs LHWs more than ever. If eradication is to succeed, particularly in conflict-torn areas, LHWs' full support is essential.

Lady Health Workers Risk Their Lives, But Do Not Receive a Living Wage

While media accounts of the killings commonly depict female vaccinators as "aid workers" heroically working for the health of others, the reality is more complicated.[8,33–35] LHWs are often in desperate financial straits and work for pay of under US$5 per day because there are few other jobs available to women (Box 1). Financial insecurity is a serious problem for LHWs. It is also a major issue for other women who are hired temporarily a few days a month for polio vaccination campaigns. Married women often become LHWs because their husbands are absent, drug addicts, disabled, or underemployed; unmarried women often take on the work because their father is dead or unemployed and any brothers are unable to financially support the family.[36–38]

In 2011, SC conducted semi-structured interviews with more than 60 frontline polio workers and supervisors, a sample drawn from all provinces of Pakistan. Detailed information on this study was presented in a report for UNICEF.[36] In these interviews, the vast majority of LHWs and other frontline polio workers said their income was insufficient for basic needs: food, transport, and housing. Most were in families with a rate of income around—or well below—US$2 a day per person. Female polio workers said that low pay dampened their motivation. "When after working so hard you get so little money, your heart breaks," one woman explained. "And you don't want to do that work. It's the truth".[36]

As many female health workers in Pakistan are the sole or primary source of income for their families, a living wage to ensure food security and availability of school fees for their children is a necessary first step towards engaging them as strong partners. The GPEI, which has an annual budget of over US$1 billion, should prioritize funding for this purpose.[39] At a minimum, workers should receive Rs. 1000 (a little under US$10) per day for the three days a month they work on polio campaigns, and both regular and polio pay should be delivered on time.

A living wage can be the linchpin of a stronger policymaker–LHW partnership, and can have positive effects beyond polio eradication. One analysis of routine immunization coverage in Pakistan recommended changing incentives for health workers and better engaging LHWs.[40]

Building Stronger Partnerships with LHWs Will Lead to True Health System Strengthening and Help Eradicate Polio

Contribute to Security by Lessening the Visible Involvement of Political Leaders

The induction of a new government in Islamabad after the recent elections presents an opportunity for partners in polio eradication to shift their focus from a "leader-centric" model to one that focuses on gaining the true support and advocacy of grassroots health workers. To contribute to secure conditions for these workers, national engagement must visibly shift away from the federal level. The international stakeholders of the GPEI should, in the near term, restrict high-profile involvement with government functionaries and focus on a new strategy that values, supports, and engages its critical frontline workers.

Such a program could be at once far-reaching and low-profile, building on the existing system for training polio workers to communicate their crucial role in this historic project. This strategy should complement a program of empowerment and career development for these workers.

Build Capacity by Providing More Opportunities for LHWs

Limited opportunity for career advancement is a real problem for LHWs.[36,41–44] Many LHWs and other polio campaign workers desire more education and the opportunity to advance within the health

BOX 40.1 Financial Need and Health Work: A Lady Health Worker's Story

I became an LHW because of problems at home. I have no choice. I get paid for my blood and my sweat, but there's relief in the work too. . . . Everything is so expensive now, so expensive—but I can scrape by. Thank God.

When I became an LHW, I was responsible for my son. I was living with my parents. My husband had left. He came back after three years, after I'd figured out how to take care of myself, how to take care of my son. And I'm very satisfied that I didn't have to beg from anyone. Sure, my salary was very small, but it was my own money. With that money I took care of myself, I took care of my son, I'm sending him to school. I'm very satisfied with that. My son is seven, *mashallah*, and he's in second grade . . .

It doesn't matter what your family background is, standing on your own two feet is the most important thing. . . . It's just the first step that someone has to take by themselves. When someone tries, Allah surely will give them rewards for their work, and Allah builds courage in that person.

[Interview conducted by SC in June 2011.]

BOX 40.2 **Job Advancement: The Experience of One Lady Health Worker**

I became an LHW when I was very young . . . I had such desire to become a doctor! There was a dentist here, and I used to go to her office and follow her around and work for her, just out of interest, I wanted to know more about how I could become a doctor. . . . I've been thinking of further study, because really, I want to move up. But I look, and there really aren't any ways for me to advance. There's no chance, absolutely no way. All of my dreams, I've left them all behind. What I wanted to do.

[Interview conducted by SC in June 2011.]

system, but feel that opportunities to do so are not available (Box 2).

Pakistan's Expanded Program on Immunization has recently started training LHWs to administer injectable vaccines in an effort to bolster lagging national immunization rates and augment the efforts of facility-based vaccinators. This promising start could be deepened and expanded by making the LHW responsible for routine vaccinations in her area and making her home, the "Health House" of the community, the vaccination center for her neighborhood.[29] Studies in a variety of settings show that such community-centered vaccination is effective in strengthening routine immunization.[45–47] The health establishment of Pakistan should be assisted in gradually increasing the number of LHWs to cover the 40% of rural and urban slum populations presently outside the ambit of the program. Such steps could improve Pakistan's weak routine immunization rates, which would also further the eradication of polio.[5]

To make such changes empowering and not exploitative they must be built on improved wages and enhanced support for LHWs from supervisors and district health officers. Problems in the pharmaceutical supply chain and payment provision must be addressed.[29,36,48] The recent "regularization" of LHWs, which extends to them the same job security and benefits that other government employees enjoy, along with an increase in regular salary to Rs. 9,000 (about $90) a month, is a major step in the right direction.[49] A program truly engaging LHWs as partners would build on this promising start to craft a program of collaborative engagement that listens to LHWs and takes their needs seriously.

A critical part of supporting LHWs is providing effective security. Some LHWs are refusing the police escorts provided to them, apparently because they make LHWs more visible.[12] This suggests that current security strategies are suboptimal, and that the government machinery alone cannot provide secure conditions for vaccination outreach. Complicating the issue is the fact that the threat to health workers is multidirectional and includes local players in many troubled districts. The GPEI currently employs experts in epidemiology, virology, and communications. Now it is critical that, in addition, the program engage security experts to develop district-wise strategies for providing world-class security to LHWs. These local solutions should be incorporated into the polio campaign plan.

To provide broader support for LHWs, formal opportunities for job advancement should be provided. Pakistan has an acute shortage of nurses.[50–53] Opportunities for midwifery, nursing, and other advanced training for Pakistan's most experienced and conscientious LHWs would open doors for hardworking women and add cadres of skilled health staff to Pakistan's health system. Studies have identified opportunities for career advancement and professional development as two important contributors to vibrant community health worker programs.[54–56] Tying such opportunities to clearly communicated performance targets would give talented women struggling to support their families fresh reason for commitment.

Pakistan's LHWs have the potential to achieve universal immunization and polio eradication in the country. In fact, both of these goals are probably impossible without their full support. Achieving them depends on a shift from treating frontline female health staff as disposable labor to truly engaging them as well-supported, active partners in achieving a healthier Pakistan.

REFERENCES

1. Independent Monitoring Board of the Global Polio Eradication Initiative (2013) Seventh Report. London.
2. Ahmad K (2007) Pakistan struggles to eradicate polio. Lancet Infect Dis 7: 247. doi:10.1016/S1473-3099(07)70066-X.
3. Mushtaq MU, Majrooh MA, Ullah MZS, Akram J, Siddiqui AM, et al. (2010) Are we doing enough? Evaluation of the Polio Eradication Initiative in a district of Pakistan's Punjab province: a LQAS study. BMC Public Health 10: 60. doi:10.1186/1471-2458-10-60.
4. Nishtar S (2010) Pakistan, politics and polio. Bull World Health Organ 88: 159–160. doi:10.1590/S0042-96862010000200018.
5. Hasan Q, Bosan AH, Bile KM (2010) A review of EPI progress in Pakistan towards achieving coverage targets: present situation and the way forward. East Mediterr Heal J Rev Santé Méditerranée Orient Al-Majallah Al-Ṣiḥḥīiyah Li-Sharq Al-Mutawassiṭ 16 Suppl: S31–38.
6. IED blast injures lady health worker (2013). Express Trib. Available: http://tribune.com.pk/story/516158/ied-blast-injures-lady-health-worker/. Accessed 22 March 2013.
7. Khan S (2013) Polio workers come under fresh attack in Pakistan. CNN. Available: http://www.cnn.com/2013/02/26/world/asia/pakistan-polio-workers-attack/index.html. Accessed 22 March 2013.
8. Polio vaccination workers shot dead in Pakistan (2012). The Guardian. Available: http://www.guardian.co.uk/world/2012/dec/18/polio-vaccination-workers-shot-pakistan. Accessed 15 March 2013.
9. Gunmen kill police officer protecting polio workers in Pakistan (2013). The Guardian. Available: http://www.guardian.co.uk/world/2013/jan/29/pakistan-polio-vaccines-gunmen-shooting. Accessed 22 March 2013.
10. Walsh D, Khan I (2013) 2 Pakistani Polio Workers Killed in Blast. New York. Available: http://www.nytimes.com/2013/02/01/world/asia/two-more-pakistani-polio-workers-killed.html. Accessed 25 March 2013.
11. Polio Eradication Initiative Pakistan (2013) Background Document for the Independent Monitoring Board. Available: http://www.polioeradication.org/Portals/0/Document/Aboutus/Governance/IMB/8IMBMeeting/5.2_8IMB.pdf. Accessed 27 June 2013.
12. Khan I (2013) 2 Polio Workers Killed in Pakistan. New York. Available: http://www.nytimes.com/2013/06/17/world/middleeast/2-polio-workers-killed-in-pakistan.html. Accessed 29 June 2013.
13. Tank Killing: Lady Health Worker Shot Dead (2013). Express Trib. Available: http://tribune.com.pk/story/572624/tank-killing-lady-health-worker-shot-dead/. Accessed 5 July 2013.
14. McNeil D (2012) C.I.A. Vaccine Ruse in Pakistan May Have Harmed Polio Fight. New York. Available: http://www.nytimes.com/2012/07/10/health/cia-vaccine-ruse-in-pakistan-may-have-harmed-polio-fight.html. Accessed 28 June 2013.
15. Ud Din I, Mumtaz Z, Ataullahjan A (2012) How the Taliban undermined community healthcare in Swat, Pakistan. BMJ 344: e2093. doi:10.1136/bmj.e2093.
16. Niles C (2012) United Nations Secretary-General hosts high-level polio meeting. UNICEF. Available: http://www.unicef.org/health/index_65979.html. Accessed 26 June 2013.
17. Spotlight on: Pakistan (2012). Polio News. Available: http://us2.campaign-archive2.com/?u=1519be1cd815ed6195660c2c&id=2b312fa956&e=#Spotlight. Accessed 26 June 2013.
18. Aseefa decorated for fight against polio (2013). The News.Available:http://www.thenews.com.pk/Todays-News-2-182550-Aseefa-decorated-for-fight-against-polio. Accessed 26 June 2013.
19. McNeil D (2011) Gates Calls for a Final Push to Eradicate Polio. New York. Available: http://www.nytimes.com/2011/02/01/health/01polio.html. Accessed 29 June 2013.
20. Governments of Nigeria, Pakistan, and Afghanistan (2012) Global Polio Emergency Action Plan 2012–13. Geneva: WHO.
21. Zardari seeks people's help to eradicate polio (2010). News Int Pak. Available: http://www.thenews.com.pk/Todays-News-6-14443-Zardari-seeks-people's-help-to-eradicate-polio. Accessed 30 July 2013.
22. Government of Islamic Republic of Pakistan (2013) National Emergency Action Plan 2013 For Polio Eradication. Islamabad: GoP.
23. Roberts L (2012) Fighting Polio in Pakistan. Science 337: 517–521. doi:10.1126/science.337.6094.517.
24. Wilkinson I, Yusufzai A (2009) Taliban blocks UN polio treatment in Pakistan. The Telegraph. Available: http://www.telegraph.co.uk/news/worldnews/asia/pakistan/5057026/Taliban-blocks-UN-polio-treatment-in-Pakistan.html. Accessed 30 July 2013.

25. Nizza M (2008) Pakistan's Polio Problem Continues. The Lede. Available: http://thelede.blogs.nytimes.com/2008/07/28/pakistans-polio-problem-continues/. Accessed 30 July 2013.

26. Kingman S (2001) For Afghan polio eradication the show goes on. Bull World Health Organ 79: 1088.

27. Trofimov Y (2010) Risky Ally in War on Polio: the Taliban. Wall Str J. Available: http://online.wsj.com/article/SB126298998237022117.html. Accessed 29 June 2013.

28. Oxford Policy Management (2009) Lady Health Worker Programme: Third party Evaluation of Performance. Available: http://www.opml.co.uk/projects/lady-health-worker-programme-third-party-evaluation-performance.

29. Hafeez A, Mohamud BK, Shiekh MR, Shah SAI, Jooma R (2011) Lady health workers programme in Pakistan: challenges, achievements and the way forward. J Pak Med Assoc 61: 210–215.

30. Donaldson L (2013) Open Letter to Margaret Chan. Independent Monitoring Board of the Global Polio Eradication Initiative. Available: http://www.polioeradication.org/Aboutus/Governance/IndependentMonitoringBoard/Reports.aspx. Accessed 17 February 2013.

31. Wasif S (2012) Polio campaign: Distressed with security and monetary concerns, LHWs camp outside PM Secretariat. Express Trib. Available: http://tribune.com.pk/story/483148/polio-campaign-distressed-with-security-and-monetary-concerns-lhws-camp-outside-pm-secretariat/. Accessed 11 February 2013.

32. Lady health workers in a fix about threats (2013). Dawn.Available:http://dawn.com/2013/01/08/lady-health-workers-in-a-fix-about-threats/. Accessed 8 February 2013.

33. Walsh D, McNeil DG (2012) Female Vaccination Workers, Essential in Pakistan, Become Prey. New York. Available: http://www.nytimes.com/2012/12/21/world/asia/un-halts-vaccine-work-in-pakistan-after-more-killings.html. Accessed 5 February 2013.

34. Khazan O (2012) Where it's most dangerous to be an aid worker. WorldViews. Available: http://www.washingtonpost.com/blogs/worldviews/wp/2012/12/26/heres-where-its-most-dangerous-to-be-an-aid-worker/. Accessed 5 February 2013.

35. Chatterjee S (2012) As Deaths Mount In Pakistan, Ending Polio Becomes An Act Of Courage. Forbes. Available: http://www.forbes.com/sites/realspin/2012/12/27/as-deaths-mount-in-pakistan-ending-polio-becomes-an-act-of-courage/. Accessed 25 March 2013.

36. Closser S (2011) Experiences and Motivations of Polio Eradication's Front-Line Workers in Pakistan. UNICEF. Available: http://www.comminit.com/polio/content/experiences-and-motivations-polio-eradications-front-line-workers-pakistan.

37. Khan A (2008) Women's Empowerment and the Lady Health Worker Programme in Pakistan. Karachi: Collective for Social Science Research.

38. Khan A (2011) Lady Health Workers and Social Change in Pakistan. Econ Polit Wkly 46: 28–31.

39. Polio Global Eradication Initiative (2012) Financial Resource Requirements 2012–2013 (as of 1 May 2012). Geneva. Available: http://www.polioeradication.org/Portals/0/Document/FRR/FRR_ENG.pdf.

40. Loevinsohn B, Hong R, Gauri V (2006) Will more inputs improve the delivery of health services? Analysis of district vaccination coverage in Pakistan. Int J Health Plann Manage 21: 45–54.

41. Haq Z, Iqbal Z, Rahman A (2008) Job stress among community health workers: a multi-method study from Pakistan. Int J Ment Health Syst 2: 15. doi:10.1186/1752-4458-2-15.

42. Afsar HA, Younus M (2005) Recommendations to Strengthen the Role of Lady Health Workers in the National Program for Family Planning and Primary Health Care in Pakistan: The Health Workers Perspective. J Ayub Med Coll Abbottabad 17. Available: http://www.ayubmed.edu.pk/JAMC/PAST/17-1/HabibYounus.htm.

43. Mumtaz Z, Salway S, Waseem M, Umer N (2003) Gender-based barriers to primary health care provision in Pakistan: the experience of female providers. Health Policy Plan 18: 261–269. doi:10.1093/heapol/czg032.

44. Closser S (2010) Chasing Polio in Pakistan: Why the World's Largest Public Health Initiative May Fail. Vanderbilt University Press. 256 p.

45. Fields R, Kanagat N, LaFond A (2012) Notes from the Field #3: Bringing Immunization Closer to Communities: Community-Centered Health Workers. Arlington, VA: JSI Research & Training Institute, Inc., ARISE Project for the Bill & Melinda Gates Foundation.

46. Ryman TK, Dietz V, Cairns KL (2008) Too little but not too late: Results of a literature review to improve routine immunization programs in developing countries. BMC Health Serv Res 8: 134. doi:10.1186/1472-6963-8-134.

47. Patel AR, Nowalk MP (2010) Expanding immunization coverage in rural India: A review of evidence for the role of community health workers. Vaccine 28: 604–613. doi:10.1016/j.vaccine.2009.10.108.

48. Haines A, Sanders D, Lehmann U, Rowe AK, Lawn JE, et al. (2007) Achieving child survival goals: potential contribution of community health workers. Lancet 369: 2121–2131. doi:10.1016/S0140-6736(07)60325-0.

49. Junaidi I (2013) 100,000 lady health workers get their service regularised. Dawn. Available: http://dawn.com/2013/01/21/100000-lady-health-workers-get-their-service-regularised/. Accessed 11 February 2013.

50. Bile KM, Hafeez A, Jooma R, Khan Z, Sheikh M (2010) Pakistan human resources for health assessment, 2009/Evaluation des ressources humaines pour la sante au Pakistan en 2009. East Mediterr Health J 16: S145+.

51. Global Health Workforce Alliance, World Health Organization, GIZ (2011) Pakistan: WHO Global Code of Practice on International Recruitment of Health Personnel - Implementation Strategy Report. Available: http://www.who.int/workforcealliance/knowledge/resources/PAK_ImmigrationReport.pdf.

52. World Health Organization (2013) Global Health Atlas. Available: http://apps.who.int/globalatlas/.

53. Global Health Workforce Alliance (2011) Progress report on the Kampala Declaration and Agenda for Global Action. Global Health Work-force Alliance. Available: http://www.who.int/workforcealliance/knowledge/resources/kdagaprogressreport/en/.

54. Witmer A, Seifer SD, Finocchio L, Leslie J, O'Neil EH (1995) Community health workers: integral members of the health care work force. Am J Public Health 85: 1055–1058.

55. Willis-Shattuck M, Bidwell P, Thomas S, Wyness L, Blaauw D, et al. (2008) Motivation and retention of health workers in developing countries: a systematic review. BMC Health Serv Res 8: 247. doi:10.1186/1472-6963-8-247.

56. Manongi RN, Marchant TC, Bygbjerg IC (2006) Improving motivation among primary health care workers in Tanzania: a health worker perspective. Hum Resour Heal 4: 6. doi:10.1186/1478-4491-4-6.

JAMES PFEIFFER

41 ARE NGOs UNDERMINING HEALTH SYSTEMS IN MOZAMBIQUE?

The last few selections have described government health systems, government health workers, and international donors. The hospital doctors in Malawi (Reading 38), the health officials in Mozambique (Reading 39), and the Lady Health Workers in Pakistan (Reading 40) are all employees of their governments' Ministries of Health, and they provide health care to their fellow citizens.

This article, also about Mozambique, describes two other groups of workers. These are representatives of donor institutions, and the foreign and local employees of nongovernmental organizations (NGOs). In this reading, it becomes obvious that government, NGO, and donor staff all have different aims, because they are rewarded for doing different things. The resulting conflicts can be a serious problem.

In low-income countries, donor money for health projects is often channeled either through Ministries of Health or through ***NGOs****. As the name implies, the NGO label can apply to any organization that is not a government—so NGOs are diverse and hard to characterize as a group. A few of the largest and most famous ones are described in this book: see Reading 5 for a discussion of the pioneering work of the Bangladesh Rural Advancement Committee (BRAC) in oral rehydration therapy, Reading 33 for an exploration of the moral dilemmas faced by Doctors Without Borders (MSF), and Reading 34 for a description of Partners in Health's approach to AIDS care. We included these organizations in this book because they are among the most well-known and respected health NGOs in the world—and because each has very different aims. But there are many millions of big and small NGOs throughout the world—some, obviously, better than others.*

There are many reasons that donors might choose to give funds to NGOs rather than to local government agencies. Depending on the NGO, there may be more transparency and accountability for donor dollars. Some government health systems may be inefficient or corrupt. Sometimes the goals of a particular NGO fit with a donor's value system and aims better than the goals of a government. Or, some donors may be reluctant to give money to repressive or autocratic governments or to governments whose politics they don't like.

But the shift to NGOs is not just about donor preferences. It has happened in the context of World Bank and International Monetary Fund economic policies called ***structural adjustment programs****. Structural adjustment is a set of reforms often pushed by international banks as a condition for receiving economic aid, often in the form of loans. In general, structural adjustment programs require that governments slash public services—including health services—in an effort to balance budgets. After a structural adjustment program, private services often expand to fill the gaps created by government cuts. The problem is that such private services are only available to those who are able to pay. As is the case in this selection about Mozambique, the poor may be left without quality health services. In other words, these outside global forces weaken the health system by requiring that governmenst abandon their mandate to provide health services to all citizens.*

In Mozambique, the country described in this selection, structural adjustment placed limits on government health system spending. Even if donors wanted to channel funding to the government system, they could not. Instead, they had to channel the funds through NGOs. Many European donors would have preferred to finance the government health system in the 1990s, but could no longer do so. Instead, they gave funds to NGOs and then tried to coordinate these NGO activities with government

Revised from James Pfeiffer, "International NGOs and Primary Health Care in Mozambique: The Need for a New Model of Collaboration." *Social Science & Medicine*, February 2003, 56(4): 725–738.

health services. This led to the development of the sector-wide approach to planning (SWAP) strategy in Mozambique that is described here.

In this selection, James Pfeiffer examines the impacts of the shift toward NGOs in Mozambique. Decisions to fund NGOs rather than governments can have far-reaching unintended consequences, as this selection describes. In particular, it can mean that government services end up underresourced, understaffed and dependent on outsiders.

As you read this selection, consider the following questions:

- **Why does it matter that the expatriates lived in compounds, isolated from their Mozambican colleagues?**
- **What are "aid cowboys" and "aid mercenaries"? If you are interested in going into global health, do you think that either of these labels might in some way apply to you?**
- **Why might that the short-term, results-oriented way of working of many expatriate NGO workers undermine the longer-term goals of the health system?**
- **What underlying factors led to pay being so much better in NGOs than in the government health system?**
- **Why did meetings aimed at "coordination" turn into deal-making and turf wars?**
- **Do you think that the payments described at the end of the article, like per diems for training and salary top-offs, are instances of corruption? Why do you think expatriates and locals engaged in these practices?**
- **Why do you think Pfeiffer argues for a "frank discussion" of the issues he describes? Do you think this would change the situation?**

CONTEXT

James Pfeiffer is a professor of global health and anthropology at the University of Washington. He is executive director of Health Alliance International, an NGO affiliated with the University of Washington Department of Global Health that works in Timor-Leste, Mozambique, and Cote D'Ivoire, where it conducts research and advocacy to help strengthen government-provided primary health care. In addition to research on health systems, Pfeiffer has also done research on HIV/AIDS, nutrition and Pentecostalism in Mozambique.

In 1999, Doctors without Borders (*Medecins Sans Frontieres*) was awarded the Nobel Peace Prize. This award demonstrated the extent to which international nongovernmental organizations (NGOs) and their expatriate aid workers have become key players in health promotion in the developing world. Over the last 20 years, the major donors in international health, including the United States Agency for International Development (USAID) and the World Bank, have increasingly channeled aid to the health sector in poor countries through NGOs (USAID, 1995; World Bank, 1993, 1997; Buse & Walt, 1997; Green & Matthias, 1997).

The ostensible rationale for this shift rests on the largely unexamined assumption that NGOs have a "comparative advantage" since they can often reach poor communities more effectively, compassionately, and efficiently than public services (Edwards & Hulme, 1996b; World Bank, 2000; Turshen, 1999). However, the choice to shift aid to NGOs has been ideologically driven, intimately bound up with the neo-liberal emphasis on free markets and privatization (Edwards & Hulme, 1996a; Chabal & Daloz, 1999; Turshen, 1999).

Across much of the world, government health services have been deeply affected by World Bank/International Monetary Fund-promoted structural adjustment programs (SAPs) that normally slash government health spending to pay back international debt (Turshen, 1999; Laurell & Arellano, 1996). In Africa, USAID and the World Bank have been the most aggressive proponents of SAPs and have recruited NGOs to provide the social safety nets for the poor as public services were scaled back (Anang, 1994; Ndengwa, 1996; Okuonzi & Macrae, 1995). In the new climate of privatization, international NGOs have been promoted to fill the gaps.

However, based on findings from a case study in central Mozambique, this paper argues that the inundation of the health sector by international NGOs since the late 1980s may have in fact damaged the Primary Health Care (PHC) system. Rather than redistributing resources to promote greater equity and help alleviate poverty, the flood of NGOs and their expatriate personnel has fragmented the health system and contributed to intensifying social inequality in local communities. A new model for collaboration between foreign technical experts, national providers, and local communities is urgently needed to maintain equity-oriented primary health care.

The NGO Phenomenon in the Health Sector

A familiar mix, or what some have called an "unruly melange" (Buse & Walt, 1997), of international donors (bilateral and multilateral) and the health agencies they support, such as Save the Children, Doctors without Borders, Africare, Care, World Vision, Oxfam, Concern, Food for the Hungry International, Family Health International, Pathfinder, Population Services International, and myriad others can be found in many developing countries where they have become key players in financing and implementing primary health care programs. Western NGOs have become central fixtures across the Third World.

There is an unusual social interface between highly educated technicians from rich countries and communities in extreme poverty, where relationships of power and inequality are enacted in ways that profoundly shape primary health care policies and programs. Expatriate NGO workers can be found at all levels of many developing world health sectors; from Ministry of Health offices in capital cities to remote villages where they are involved in health program implementation. These NGOs' activities may be integrated into government Ministry programs or conducted completely outside the public system. In addition to their expatriate staff, NGOs usually employ small armies of "nationals," from trained health professionals and office workers to drivers and guards. Usually these workers are paid far more than their counterparts in the government health system. In Mozambique, the manner in which expatriate agency workers engaged both their Mozambican counterparts, and the larger communities where they resided, had an enormous and often negative impact on many PHC programs.

This paper provides a brief ethnographic sketch of these relationships in a province in central Mozambique from 1993 to 1998. The vignette seeks to provide a case study of the social cost to primary health care and the poor populations it serves, of donor policies that channel aid through foreign NGOs at the expense of the public sector.

Background

The Health System in Mozambique

After independence from Portugal in 1975, Mozambique established a primary health care system that was eventually cited by the WHO as a model for other developing countries (Walt & Melamed, 1983). By 1978, over 90% of the population had received routine immunizations, and by the early 1980s 1200 rural health posts had been constructed and staffed. Over 8000 health workers were trained and placed in service. During this period about 11% of the government budget was committed to healthcare (Gloyd, 1996). A war initiated by the Rhodesia and apartheid South Africa-backed Mozambique National Resistance, known by their Portuguese acronym RENAMO, targeted infrastructure and personnel in the government services from 1980 to 1992. By 1988, hundreds of health posts were destroyed and many health workers killed, injured, and terrorized.

During this period, in 1987, Mozambique initiated an IMF-promoted structural adjustment program in which currency was devalued and government services cut back. By 1990, state per capita spending on health was half of its 1980 level (Cliff, 1993). In that year, the IMF pressed Mozambique to intensify economic reform and privatization (Hanlon, 1996). After over a decade of adjustment, government spending on health care declined to only 2% of the national budget, reflecting constraints placed on public spending and a shift away from health demanded by the structural adjustment programs (Gloyd, 1996). Much of the foreign funding to the health sector was directed away from the health system toward vertical project aid to address specific donor-identified objectives. By 1996, there were 405 individual projects managed by these agencies (Hanlon, 1996). The findings reported here derive from three-and-a half years of fieldwork spread over two periods, 1993–1995 and 1998, when the author was program coordinator and country representative for a US health agency working in the health sector in the province.

Findings

Research Setting and the Primary Health Care System

The majority of the population in the province (about one million people) was rural and very poor with an estimated annual per capita income under US$100. Basic health indicators reflected this severe impoverishment; cumulative under-five mortality was estimated at 200/1000, with maternal mortality perhaps as high as 1500/100,000 (Mozambique Ministry of Health, 1997). The primary health care system had been extended into isolated rural areas through construction of health posts and centers that offer basic maternal-child health, immunization, nutrition, first aid, and referral services. After several years of rebuilding after the war, the provincial health sector consisted of nearly 70 rural health posts and 500 health workers, including 10 Mozambican doctors and 200 nurses distributed throughout ten districts. The Provincial Health Directorate, or DPS (*Direção Provincial de Saúde*), managed the health system from its offices in the capital city.

Expatriates in the Community

International aid agencies arrived with large budgets and US dollars to pay out. Three health organizations in the province had budgets of over one million US dollars each to spend in the health sector per year, compared to the DPS budget of only $US 750,000. Dozens of expatriate health and development workers and their families set up their homes in the provincial capital in the early 1990s. Two agencies built walled compounds, one with armed guards and a swimming pool, to house their European staff. If not compound bound, most expatriate workers lived in the larger and better kept homes in the "cement city"; the label given to the central areas of Mozambican cities inhabited by the Portuguese during the colonial period.

The foreign compounds became centers for expatriate social activity. Only a select few Mozambicans could make it past the armed guards at the gates. The construction of one of the compounds in the city by a European agency to house its foreign staff generated great resentment among Mozambican health workers and the general community. The agency had also constructed several much smaller houses for top-level Mozambican health workers outside the compound walls. The Mozambicans jokingly referred to the walled-in European area as "Pretoria" and the Mozambican area as "Soweto". The compound provided perhaps the most visible representation of the new environment of exclusion created by the arrival of aid in the province.

Many of the new group were aid professionals who moved from contract to contract throughout the Third World and expressed no particular interest in Mozambique itself. Most of the new aid set were middle or upper-middle class Europeans and Americans with at least a university education, and some had advanced degrees in medicine, public health, or international studies. Nearly all had career aspirations in international aid, academia, or public health and many were working their way up the ladder in their respective organizations. Some were younger Europeans who viewed their experiences in Africa as an adventure that alleviated pre-career ennui. While most had contracts ranging from1 to 4 years, a regular stream of European and American consultants flowed through town to conduct baseline studies and program evaluations on short-term contracts.

During this period, two new social figures emerged that were emblematic of the new aid culture. These were self-described "aid cowboys" and "aid mercenaries". The former term was often used to describe the foreign worker who derived a thrill from working in dangerous conditions and told aid "war stories" from postings in such places as Sudan, Cambodia, Angola, or Sierra Leone. Aid mercenaries, and there were several in the province who referred to themselves as such, admitted very frankly that their only real interest in working in Mozambique was the money.

Most aid workers expressed good intentions, but a majority described themselves in discussions as non-ideological technical specialists and professionals not particularly interested in Mozambican political history, culture, the context of international aid, or philosophical concerns with "development." Several expatriates privately expressed contempt for Mozambique and eagerly awaited their transfer out of the country. Many had little if any understanding of the recent conflict or colonial history of the country. They simply wanted to fulfill their contracts and implement their projects.

Their main concerns centered on perceived Mozambican ineptitude and the corruption of their counterparts in the government—corruption that had clearly been fed and nurtured by the arrival of loosely managed foreign aid. With the exception of two NGOs, expatriates were paid from US$1000 to US$6000 per month, usually tax-free. Most agencies provided housing, private access to project cars, and funding for personal vacations. One engineer working for a European agency calculated that at the end of his four-year contract he would have saved nearly US$300,000. Many in the new aid set regularly left Mozambique whenever possible to countries in the region with better tourist infrastructures.

The Professional Culture of Aid Workers

Many hardworking and committed foreign health professionals engaged in harmful organizational practices because their positions demanded it. Appropriate planning, coordination, and concern for maintaining the integrity of existing public programs was often not rewarded by the agencies and donors active in the province. In fact, adherence to the principles of good coordination and planning could lead to poor evaluations and the loss of a job in some cases if project targets were not met as a result. In the prevailing aid culture, the tireless, dedicated, "results-oriented" project coordinator that stopped at nothing to meet his or her output objectives often produced uncompromising, short-term thinking and planning that undermined the broader goals of the health system.

Many donors such as USAID that funneled much of their aid to the health sector through grants to NGOs increasingly emphasized the need to show short-term results: that is, measurable improvements in health outputs, such as under-five mortality or nutritional indicators, over short project periods (1–2 years in some cases). This directive was captured in the slogan "managing for results" promoted during annual meetings of USAID-funded NGOs in Maputo.

The short-term orientation fit well with the general aid experience of most expatriates who moved from country to country and contract to contract. One European worker stated, "If you stay longer than two or three years, people start wondering "what's wrong with him?" Mozambican counterparts in the health system in general were acutely aware that expatriates would only be there for a year or two at best. One Mozambican planner remarked, "Just when they finally know how things work here, and they finally can speak Portuguese, they leave." As a result of this orientation and professional imperative, the province was inundated with fast moving project coordinators who worked 6 to 7 days per week setting up offices, administrative systems, baseline studies, interventions and evaluations.

Coordinators had to be competitive and driven to promote both their own specific project goals and the public images of their organizations on the national stage. For many organizations it was important to become well-known for working a given area, such as nutrition, reproductive health, or AIDS prevention. This self-promotional ethos contributed to the notion among some expatriates that the government was an obstacle to their important, well planned projects, and to their individual careers. Successful projects for many, usually measured by achievement of narrowly defined project outcomes, also meant the potential for promotion within their organizations. The frenetic pace of expatriate professional lives starkly contrasted with the inertia felt within provincial health offices where poorly paid health staff often found little motivation to show up, let alone invest significant energy in their work (although many did). Many expatriate workers expressed frustration at the perceived slower pace of their government counterparts who were seen as barriers to project implementation and success.

Foreign Aid, Social Inequality, and Structural Adjustment

This international aid culture, with its well-resourced and driven foreign professional class, engaged a society experiencing its own rapid class formation in the privatizing economy. The new free market had stimulated the growth of the local merchant sector, and city stores began filling with gleaming commodities, in contrast to the years of war and socialism when consumer products were difficult to find.

The rapid social differentiation was visible throughout the town. New cars here and there, fancier clothes and shoes on some, and roof tops in the cement city bristling with new TV antennae and satellite dishes where several years earlier there had been none, contrasted with the deteriorating conditions in the poor bairros that ringed the city, where most of the population did not share in the new bounty. The removal of price subsidies had made it more difficult for many to gain access to adequate food (UNDP, 1998; Fauvet, 2000). The government's own Poverty Alleviation Unit estimated that the percentage of the population under the poverty line increased during this period around the country (World Bank, 1995; Hanlon, 1996; Fauvet, 2000).

Health workers were among those whose incomes dropped drastically. From 1991 to 1996, nurses' monthly salaries dropped from US$110 to US$40; doctors' salaries dropped from US$350 to US$100 (Hanlon, 1996). Because of constraints on budget expenditures mandated by the Structural Adjustment Program, staff salaries could not be increased with foreign aid. In spite of the influx of aid dollars, most of the funds were project-specific and were not used to increase staff salaries or benefits.

The drop in salaries was matched by mounting material shortages, pharmaceutical deficits, equipment failures, and vehicle breakdowns in the midst of the millions of aid dollars that landed in the province. There were frequent reports that pharmaceuticals were being stolen from the health service and sold to market vendors or administered on a fee-for-service basis at the private homes of health service workers. For example, one survey of health post supplies conducted by the author's organization found that over half the health posts in one district had no chloroquine tablets for malaria treatment even though abundant supplies had been delivered to the province. Health workers asserted that much of the chloroquine had been diverted to private practice or sold to private vendors in the open markets. Fuel shortages and lack of vehicle spare parts reduced the number of mobile motorcycle vaccination brigades into remote areas in some districts. In an unpublished assessment of district health center labs, the author's organization discovered that most of the electric agitators needed to conduct RPR syphilis tests for prenatal care patients were not functioning in the province due to lack of spare parts. These kinds of shortages and the unpredictability of medical supplies fed the increasing demoralization of health system workers.

Brain Drain

The drop in salaries and attendant demoralization amidst a growing aquisitive and competitive culture in the towns made many health workers vulnerable to the financial temptations offered by the private sector and foreign agencies. By 1998, a private clinic had opened up in the city that provided fee for service treatment at prices that were unaffordable to the majority of the population. Health system workers, including some physicians and nurses, occasionally left their posts to treat patients at the clinic, or worked there during off hours. It was widely reported that medical supplies were being diverted from the government system to the private practices of health staff.

The demoralization took its toll on feelings of loyalty to the health service reportedly felt by many Mozambicans in the system's early years. Some Mozambican health workers in the province were lured out of the government system by high salaries to work for NGOs. NGO salaries for trained health professionals ranged from US$500 to US$1500 per month, compared to the US$50 monthly wage for mid-level staff in the government health system. To get a job with an NGO was like winning the lottery.

In one year of work for an NGO, one could potentially earn the equivalent of 20 years' salary in a government job. At these rates, not even retirement benefits and job security could motivate government workers to stay. Jealousy and conflict within the government system surrounded any speculation that a worker was being wooed for an NGO position. The author was contacted discreetly on many occasions by counterparts in the provincial health directorate seeking work. As a culture of individual promotion crept into the government system, lower-level staff privately expressed frustration at perceived corrupt practices on the part of higher-level program chiefs. For many talented staff, the provincial health directorate seemed to offer few chances for professional advancement. This fed the pervasive demoralization. One Mozambican nurse who had left a government post to work with an NGO for a two-year period spoke angrily about returning to the provincial system. "What future do I have there? They want to control me. And you know how the *chefes* [the head officers] are. They just take everything for themselves. I don't have a future there". Careers in the government system paled in comparison to a professional life within the well-maintained offices, new cars, high salaries, and social status associated with NGO employment.

Coordinating Aid to the Health Sector

The most popular of the government programs chosen for support by donors were those in maternal-child health, such as traditional birth attendant (TBA) training and prenatal care, mobile immunization brigades, nutrition and growth monitoring, AIDS prevention, and health education. In order to manage the confusing array of aid program interests in the province, the government called an annual meeting each January of all foreign agencies with interests in funding specific programs, usually primary health care-oriented, in the province's annual plan. The special annual meeting with NGOs and agencies provided an opportunity for all the provincial players in the health sector to sort out who would support which programs. Support could be rationally allocated during the meeting to different districts to avoid overlap.

This process appeared very sound superficially, but, in practice, most foreign agencies arrived at the meeting with programs and pet projects approved by their donors or head offices with very specific objectives and targets that would be evaluated to ensure their own continued funding. This pressure drove individual coordinators, including this author, to promote their own agendas and interventions, whether or not they made sense in the overall provincial plan. For example, so many organizations wanted to support the Traditional Birth Attendant training that some Traditional Birth Attendants received more support than their counterpart maternal-child health nurses in the health posts, who suffered supply shortages (Gloyd, 1998).

Behind-the-scenes deal-making and turf struggles among foreign agencies actually dominated the coordination process. The deal-making nearly always hinged on the provision of extra financial benefits to health service workers. These strategies were generally considered temporary alternative ways to augment salaries that nearly everyone in the aid community and the health system acknowledged were far too low. However, special benefits were also used to sway provincial health system program heads to support one NGO's program over another in disruptive turf conflicts. Government health workers could play NGOs off one another and bargain for better deals, while NGO coordinators placed greater emphasis on achieving their own program targets than supporting vaguely defined ideals of agency coordination.

These processes of deal-making, patronage and foreign agency influence often hinged on the use of several key financial incentives: (1) per diem payments for travel, (2) seminar training with per diem payments attached, (3) extra contracts for work tasks such as surveys conducted during off-hours, and (4) temporary topping off of salaries and travel opportunities for higher-level staff to neighboring African countries and even to Europe. Direct incentives were often complemented by smaller favors such as rides to work provided by foreign agency vehicles, and support for personal home construction. Many of these favors and benefits were provided by foreign workers in a spirit of support and compassion for Mozambican colleagues who could barely feed their families on their formal salaries. However, such favors and benefits were also frequently used for leverage in gaining support for agency programs and securing positive responses from health workers when projects were evaluated by donors.

Per diem travel payments, virtually never used during the earlier years of the national health system, gradually became necessary components of all field-based project work. Competition among agencies for access to health system workers contributed to inflationary pressures on the per diem rates. From 1992 to 1998, the average overnight per diem increased from about US$3 to nearly US$15 for mid-level health workers. By 1998, this meant that one week of per diems, on average, yielded higher pay than a month's salary for workers at most levels in the health system. Government and agency regulation was weak. Projects that included per diems for numerous field visits away from home were often favored in annual planning.

The per diem phenomenon had immediate detrimental effects on some routine community health programs. In the early post-independence period, mobile vaccination brigades initially relied on local communities to provide food and lodging to visiting vaccination teams. However, by the early 1990s, as salaries plummeted, large per diems were routinely paid to the mobile brigades. Unneeded district personnel often accompanied brigades in order to receive the per diem payments. Much of the funding for per diems was distributed per NGO by district. However, if an NGO decided to stop funding the brigades because its project cycle ended or it changed its program, the per diems would dry up and health workers would then often refuse to make the trips. The provincial head of immunizations became exasperated, "Nothing gets done without per diems anymore. People won't even show up for a training at their own health post if there isn't a per diem attached."

The per diem problem was intensified by a proliferation of seminars and training for health workers in the annual provincial plan; training was usually designed to upgrade skills for involvement in foreign agency projects. Health workers eagerly supported seminars that required travel since one week of per diems at a seminar was worth more than a month's salary. This proliferation of seminars was jokingly referred to by planners as *seminarite* in Portuguese (or seminaritis). There was little incentive to reduce the number of training sessions since seminars allowed agencies to claim that they were "capacity building," while the per diems provided crucial salary augmentation for local workers. The seminars also pulled workers away from their routine duties, leading to major gaps in key activities such as patient consultation, data collection, supervision visits, and reporting.

Most foreign projects included baseline studies, surveys of target communities, evaluations, and additional project activities outside the scope of normal health worker duties. Foreign agencies regularly hired key health system staff to work on these extra activities, offering lucrative contracts. A standard payment in 1998 for one day's work on a survey was US$25, almost equivalent to an entire month's salary for mid-level workers. While these contracts sometimes provided valuable experience and training to the workers, they also drew health staff away from their routine duties. At least one organization that worked within the provincial health system made additional contributions to the salaries of higher-level health workers, ostensibly to compensate them for the extra work they would have to do to participate in the foreign agency's activities. One agency provided travel to Europe for top provincial personnel to visit the home offices of the donor organization. Travel opportunities outside the province, or to neighboring African countries, ostensibly for work purposes, were extended to higher-level provincial personnel who could accumulate significant per diem income from the trips.

In themselves these favors and incentives could be seen as providing valuable experiences and important salary supports. But in the context of foreign agency competition and health worker competition for benefits, these practices were often part of endless negotiations and power plays around health project promotion. And as Pavignani and Durão state, "The variety of topping-up, subsidies, incentives, part time private practice, grants, per diems has reached enormous proportions, and one may wonder if the global cost of these transactions is not approaching, even surpassing, the bill that would be paid by the treasury if the salary levels were adjusted to acceptable levels" (1997, p. 12). As a result of participation in NGO-sponsored seminars, travel, surveys, evaluations and other activities, the DPS offices began to empty out. By 1998, there were week-long periods in which no community health program heads were conducting routine health system work; all were either conducting NGO-sponsored surveys, or attending training seminars put on by NGOs to prepare for NGO projects.

Discussion

Examples of harmful practices on the part of foreign aid agencies abound in Mozambique and elsewhere in Africa. Recent attempts to confront these kinds of problems signal growing and widespread recognition of the need for change. Local voluntary "codes of conduct" generated by NGO consortiums have appeared in a number of other African settings in recent years including Namibia, South Africa, Ethiopia, and Botswana indicating an increasing concern within the NGO community itself over these issues (Namibian,1999; SANGOCO, 2001; The Reporter, 1999; BOCONGO,2001).

Perhaps the first step toward a new approach is to overcome the reluctance of policy-makers, health researchers, and others in the NGO world to admit the abuses and failures of the current model. One potential point of departure for generating discussion could be the development of an industrywide international code of conduct for NGO activities in the health sector. While local voluntary codes of conduct are unlikely to be very effective, a broad-based discussion focused on an international code among key actors in international health including major NGOs, donors, and host countries would focus attention on the shortcomings of current approaches. Perhaps most importantly, the process of generating an international code of conduct would provide a forum for a badly needed and more fundamental discussion on new approaches to collaboration in the health sector. The Mozambique case suggests that a new model centered on building relationships and coordinating with public sector systems and health workers, rather than achieving short-term project outputs, could help prevent abuses and restore some measure of self-determination to national health systems. An international code of conduct embraced by donors, NGOs, and ministries of health could help provide a broad-based mutual understanding of what constitutes appropriate NGO activity, thus creating a better foundation for building trust between expatriates and local counterparts.

Significant change in the NGO approach to health sector support will be enormously difficult to achieve under current conditions. The ongoing promotion of privatization both within the health sector and through the wider economy in Africa threatens to reinforce a two-tiered provision of services that siphons off resources and personnel from a poorly funded public system further undermining morale, commitment, and organizational capacity. The current NGO model of cooperation and participation exacerbates the degradation of public primary health care programs in this environment. Nevertheless, growing disquiet among concerned fieldworkers, donors, and host nations may provide an opportunity to bring these troubling dynamics into full view in the development community. A frank discussion is long overdue.

REFERENCES

Anang, F. T. (1994). Evaluating the role and impact of foreign NGOs in Ghana. In E. Sandberg (Ed.), The changing politics of non-governmental organizations and African states (pp. 101–120). Westport: Praeger.

BOCONGO (Botswana Council of Non-Governmental Organizations) (2001). NGO code of conduct. Botswana: BOCONGO.

Buse, K., & Walt, G. (1997). An unruly melange? Coordinating external resources to the health sector: A review. Social Science & Medicine, 45(3), 449–463.

Chabal, P., & Daloz, J. (1999). Africa works: Disorder as political instrument. Oxford: James Currey.

Cliff, J. (1993). Donor dependence or donor control?: The case of Mozambique. Community Development Journal, 28(3), 237–244.

Edwards, M., & Hulme, D. (1996a). Too close for comfort? The impact of official aid on non-governmental organizations. World Development, 24(6), 961–973.

Edwards, M., & Hulme, D. (1996b). Introduction. In M. Edwards, & D. Hulme (Eds.), Beyond the magic bullet: NGO performance and accountability in the post-cold war world. West Hartford: Kumarian.

Fauvet, P. (2000). Mozambique: Growth with poverty, a difficult transition from prolonged war to peace and development. Africa Recovery, 14(3), 12–19.

Gloyd, S. (1996). NGOs and the "SAP"ing of health care in rural Mozambique. Hesperian foundation news, spring. Berkeley: The Hesperian Foundation.

Gloyd, S. (1998). Personal communication.

Green, A., & Matthias, A. (1997). Non-governmental organizations and health in developing countries. New York: St. Martin's Press Inc.

Hanlon, J. (1996). Peace without profit: How the IMF blocks rebuilding in Mozambique. Portsmouth, NH: Heinemann.

Laurell, A. C., & Arellano, O. L. (1996). Market commodities and poor relief: The world bank proposal for health. International Journal of Health Services, 26(1), 1–18.

Mozambique Ministry of Health (1997). Mozambique demographic and health survey. Maputo: Mozambique Ministry of Healthand Macro International.

Namibian (1999). NGO code to pushethical conduct. In G. Lister (Ed.) The Namibian (October 25). Windhoek: The Namibian.

Ndengwa, S. N. (1996). The two faces of civil society: NGOs and politics in Africa. West Hartford: Kumarian.

Okuonzi, S., & Macrae, J. (1995). Whose policy is it anyway? International and national influences on health policy development in Uganda. Health Policy and Planning, 10(2), 122–132.

Pavignani, E., & Durao, J. R. (1997). * Aid, change, and second thoughts: Coordinating external resources to the health sector in Mozambique. Working paper. London: HealthPolicy Unit of the London School of Hygiene and Tropical Medicine.

SANGOCO (SouthAfrican National NGO Coalition) (2001). SANGOCO code of ethics for NGOs. Braamfontein: SANGOCO.

The Reporter (Addis Ababa) (1999). Non-governable organizations? The Reporter (May 19, 1999). Addis Ababa: The Reporter.

Turshen, M. (1999). Privatizing health services in Africa. New Brunswick: Rutgers.

UNDP (United Nations Development Programme) (1998). National human development report on Mozambique. Oxford: Oxford University Press.

USAID (1995). Policy guidance: USAID—US PVO partnership. Washington, DC: USAID.

Walt, G., & Melamed, A. (1983). Toward a people's health service. London: Zed Books.

World Bank (1993). World development report: Investing in health. Washington, DC: World Bank.

World Bank (1995). Country assistance strategy. Report 15067-MOZ. Washington, DC: World Bank.

World Bank (1997). Health, nutrition, and population sector strategy paper. Washington, DC: World Bank.

World Bank (2000a). The World Bank-civil society relations: Fiscal 1999 progress report. Washington, DC: World Bank.

World Bank (2000b). World development report 2000/2001. Oxford: Oxford University Press.

STEN H. VERMUND AND ANN KURTH

42 THE VITAL CASE FOR GLOBAL HEALTH INVESTMENTS

With the surprising election of President Trump in 2016, many people working in global health began to worry about their field. Would the United States remain a leader in efforts to improve global health and well-being through programming like the President's Emergency Plan for AIDS Relief (PEPFAR) or the President's Malaria Initiative? Would funding for the United States Agency for International Development (USAID) be cut drastically? Would a massive shift in US foreign policy slow the progress in global health that has been made over the past quarter century?

Strengthening of health-care systems requires long-term collaborative government investment and not merely "charity." Practitioners and proponents of global health argue that investments in health and development programs throughout the world are in the best interests of the United States.

This succinct article was written soon after the 2016 election. The authors present a persuasive case demonstrating that continued investments in global health are in the self-interest of the United States. As stated in this book's introduction, global health has goals that individuals both on the conservative right and on the liberal left can agree on. For example, investments in global health are important for national security and the protection of US citizens when one considers the risks of a global pandemic of a novel emerging disease. Pathogens do not recognize national borders; germs spread very quickly because of air travel.

The Ebola outbreak in West Africa from 2013 to 2016 was a terrible epidemic that killed over 10,000 people, including one American citizen. International response to the epidemic was significant but uncoordinated and inefficient. As we saw in Reading 37, the fundamental problem with the international response was that the health-care infrastructure of the West African countries was so weak. As this article demonstrates, this inefficient response was costly, in terms of both money and social panic. Protection of US citizens requires global health preparation and skilled personnel—and those necessitate continued investment.

This article also describes the function of global health investments as a diplomatic tool. There is a long history of this idea in international relations dating to the 1800s (see Reading 35). Most Americans vastly overestimate the percentage of the federal budget that goes to foreign aid. In one survey, Americans thought it might be one quarter of the national budget, while in reality it is less than 1%. The United States spends a huge portion of its budget on the military, and President Trump campaigned on promises to increase military spending a great deal. But no weapon system will be able to protect Americans when a plague arrives.

As you read this article, consider the following questions:

- **Do you think the argument that global health investments are in the self-interest of the United States is persuasive? Why or why not?**
- **What do the authors mean when they refer to health and development aid by the United States as "soft power?" What's "hard power" then?**
- **How might funding global health research and programs be considered an *investment* rather than charity?**
- **Which of the four points that the authors make do you think is the most important? Why?**
- **Many students of global health do not like this type of argument. Why do you think they do not? Does this type of logic make you feel uncomfortable? Are there any problematic implications of advocating for global health funding in this way, or is it a win–win?**

The article is original to this volume.

CONTEXT

Dr. Sten Vermund is the dean of the School of Public Health at Yale University. He is a pediatrician who focuses on infectious disease in low- and middle-income countries. Dr. Ann Kurth is the dean and Linda Koch Lorimer Professor of the School of Nursing at Yale University. She is a nurse–midwife interested in sexual and reproductive health; she is currently a vice chair of the Consortium of Universities for Global Health.

At the end of the 20th century and the beginning of the new millennium, there was increasing recognition of the health-related interconnectedness of human populations, pathogens, the environment and life-sustaining ecosystems, and economies. In the United States, there was bipartisan support for HIV funding through the President's Emergency Plan for AIDS Relief (PEPFAR), begun in 2003 and carried forward through this writing (April 2017). New players including the Bill and Melinda Gates Foundation, Clinton Foundation, and others began to invest heavily in global health. The Sustainable Development Goals (SDGs), signed by 150 countries in 2015, provided a defining framework for work in global health.

The Clinton, Bush, and Obama administrations emphasized the soft power of the US government, including health and development. In the second decade of the 21st century, however, anti-globalization backlash was evident in many Western countries, including the US. In the US, for example, the Trump administration campaigned on an "America First" ideology that denied the soft power achievable through health diplomacy and development support. As of April 2017, key government science and public health positions remain unfilled and the full agenda of the Trump administration towards global health is hostile. Massive cuts are proposed for the State Department and the National Institutes of Health, for example, including the complete elimination of the Fogarty International Center.

The US Congress may not go along with these draconian shifts from soft power to hard power (the military), perhaps motivated by the very strong case to be made for US government investment in global health work.[1,2] Global health investments represent a major opportunity to advance core interests of the US and, at the same time, to improve the lives of millions around the world. At least four central tenets are at the heart of this global health engagement perspective.

1. Rapid Response and Capacity Building to Control Disease at Its Source

Time and time again, microbes have emerged or re-emerged in impoverished parts of the globe, threatening all countries, including the US, through travelers to our continent or the round-trip travel of Americans overseas. The severe acute respiratory syndrome (SARS) epidemic of 2002–2004 entered Canada from Asia, for example,[3] incurring global costs of the pandemic estimated at US$30-100 billion. Had the condition been identified early in 2002 and controlled in Hong Kong and Guangdong Province, China, massive economic savings would have accrued both in Asia and around the world; lives would have been saved, including in North America in 2003. To protect Americans, emerging infections should be controlled at their source.

Similarly, from 2013–2016 the Ebola virus epidemic in West Africa killed well over 11,000 persons, including the death of an American in Texas in October 2014.[4] While Ebola virus was not widespread in North America, direct costs for core Ebola Treatment Centers in the US alone was at least $54 million,[5] with total costs likely many times this for health department expenditures, screening and quarantine, and travel restrictions. In the three most afflicted nations themselves (Liberia, Sierra Leone, and Guinea), Ebola virus costs may have been from $82 to 356 million, a vast cost for those low-income nations and for the international donor community. Other estimates confirm that the US, in total, spent well over $1 billion on the entire Ebola response, perhaps more than $3 billion; these costs were so high because setting up emergency response in the US was a massive effort and the health infrastructures of the three afflicted West African nations were so weak that foundational prevention and care investments were needed.

Health systems strengthening consists of making health systems ready for, responsive and resilient to disease outbreaks, disease burden shifts, population displacements, and both prevalent and emerging health needs. Health systems strengthening has long term benefits for the US by helping countries better respond to chronic and emergent health challenges. In 2016, Zika virus emerged in the US, most notably in Puerto Rico; costs for Zika virus prevention for the mainland are mounting through maternal and child screening, vector control, protection of the blood supply, and epidemic preparedness.[7–10] Infectious disease experts are of one mind that prevention at root sources is, in the long run, more effective and ultimately cost-efficient than coping with pandemic spread, while addressing fundamental humanitarian concerns. A bipartisan consensus should acknowledge that waiting until the US is directly affected to deal with emerging or imported diseases guarantees that the ultimate costs balloon with increased complexity of disease control.

2. Protection of the Citizenry

The field of tropical medicine was grounded in colonial traditions designed to protect expatriates and local workers in colonies of Western nations. In the 21st century, travelers from many nations, including high income countries like the US, go abroad for business, pleasure, mission work, diplomatic, or military purposes. American expatriates serve our government, non-governmental organizations, universities, businesses, religious institutions, and overseas interests. American businesses employ overseas workers and depend on their good health to maintain productivity and local goodwill. Whether for prevention, disease control, or medical care, global health investments protect these transient and long-term overseas denizens. Hence, prevention with vaccines, insect repellents, prophylactic or curative drugs, and travel advice are all helpful, but even more impact accrues with control of diseases themselves in the countries being visited, benefiting our citizens and the local inhabitants at the same time.

Beyond protecting the health of individuals is a need to protect the environment. Water-borne, food-borne, and respiratory diseases caused by microbial or toxic sources affect everyone, though often it is the most vulnerable population in a community that is disproportionately impacted. There is increasing recognition, not only from scientists but also the American public, that climate change and other ecosystem strain is worrisome. Recent survey data reported by the Yale Center on Climate Change Communication notes that 70% of Americans think climate change will harm health. Climate change and other ecosystem strains such as air pollution, ozone depletion, water and fertilizer overuse, and deforestation impact health directly and indirectly, and indicators to date are adverse for a wide variety of conditions.

The impacts of climate change on health have been a focus of John Holdren, the longest-serving Presidential Science Adviser in US history (2009–2017). In mid-2016, Dr. Holdren observed the following: "The United States would become a pariah if we backed out of the Paris [climate] agreement."[6] President Trump selected Scott Pruitt, a climate change denier, to head the Environmental Protection Agency,[7] while Secretary of State Rex Tillerson, former Exxon Mobile Chairman and CEO, had previously supported the Paris climate accords and acknowledged that climate change is occurring due to human activity. Isolationism and withdrawal from global environmental initiatives will hurt the US. Such diseases as Zika virus, neonatal syndrome, and crisis circumstances dramatized in movies such as *Contagion* are likely to become more common.

3. Need for Research into Global Health Issues

Global health research is a good investment for the US public sector for several reasons. No microbe selects only certain human groups, and walls cannot keep out diseases, given the interconnectedness of human societies and populations. Working collaboratively with colleagues around the world is prudent as well as efficient. A given disease or condition may be more common overseas, such that the research can be done more quickly and cheaply than it could be done in the US, as was the case for the development of vaccines and prevention strategies for human immunodeficiency virus (HIV), dengue virus, Ebola virus, Zika virus, or respiratory syncytial virus (a bad respiratory disease common in infants).

Even if a disease does not occur in the US, its study may be of importance to US interests—for example, malaria is important to the US military, travelers, or expatriates. An additional argument for global health research is that discovery related to one disease may lead to fundamental scientific insights into other diseases, as was the case in the discovery of HIV after insights derived from HTLV-1 and feline leukemia virus retrovirus research. We still do not know all the factors that cause certain cancers, neuromuscular diseases, brain disorders like Alzheimer's disease, and even diabetes and cardiovascular diseases, some of which may be triggered by infectious agents. Global competitive pressures in the biotechnology, pharmacology, and biomedical engineering arenas also demand a compelling research presence in international settings, given the need to improve the efficiencies and generalizability of clinical trials and product development.

4. "Soft Power" Diplomacy to Address Humanitarian Crises

Journalists, photographers, novelists, and filmmakers alike have documented the hopelessness, desperation, and sometimes homicidal anger generated by the preventable loss of a loved one to disease, disaster, or accident. The perception of the US, the world's wealthiest nation, failing to respond to the challenges of global disability, disease, and death can fuel anti-US sentiments and complicate foreign affairs in economic, business, or political realms. The US can win friends and influence governments by providing technical and concrete financial support for disease control and prevention, enabling healthy pregnancies through birth spacing and contraception, and reducing environmental hazards, to name but a few contributions now made through the Agency for International Development (USAID).

Nelson Mandela stated in January 2009, "Amidst all of the human progress made over the last century, the world in which we live remains one of great divisions, conflict, inequality, poverty and injustice. Amongst many around the world a sense of hopelessness had set in as so many problems remain unresolved and seemingly incapable of being resolved. . . . we can in fact change the world and make of it a better place."[9] It is not in the US character to ignore humanitarian crises, whether fueled by drought, famine, war and civil unrest, global climate change, pestilence, or natural disaster. Strengthening overseas health systems helps economies and thus, ultimately weans nations from donor-nation dependencies. Global trainees supported by the US are typically friends and collaborators-for-life of US universities and agencies such as the NIH, CDC, and USAID. Enlightened policies to help prevent and/or to rapidly respond to such emergencies can enable US leadership in low and middle income nations whose support the US needs for a wide swath of diplomatic, military, and business relationships. Withdrawing from leadership in, and financial contribution to, humanitarian support will lead to a decline in US standing worldwide.

Improved health can lead to greater political stability within and across countries, which can in turn result in greater economic development, local buying power, and opportunities for US business and trade. Control of global disease threats mandates the training of a cadre of US and international researchers, surveillance and disease control experts, and specialists from a wide array of health management, communications, social and behavioral science, biomedical, human rights, and policy areas; such trainees are every bit as important to national security as are our future leaders in military, diplomatic, international business, security, and other spheres.

Walls do not keep microbes out, no matter how much we would like to create epidemiological boundaries. Historically, threats to public health have been used as an excuse for anti-immigrant and racist policies. There are no communicable diseases that "belong" to a certain group; that is why we call them "communicable." Overseas risks are best tackled in the countries where they emerge, protecting

US travelers and expatriates even as the local population benefits.

Positive health engagement can enable other critical interactions by building the good will essential for effective competition or cooperation (as the case may be) on a world stage. Confronting global health challenges is not just good for the soul of America but is good for US business and diplomacy at the same time. Finally, abrogating our obligations to the human family by reducing support for global health work is not likely to save money in the short term, and most certainly can have longer term unintended consequences directly for the health of our citizens as well as those around the world. At less than 1% of the US government budget,[10] global health and development assistance is money well spent, improving health around the globe and protecting the US.[11]

REFERENCES

1. The Center for Global Health Policy; http://www.idsaglobalhealth.org/home.aspx, accessed April 15, 2017.
2. Consortium of Universities for Global Health; http://www.cugh.org/announcements/proposed-budget-cuts-threaten-us-global-health-activities-cugh-press-release, accessed April 15, 2017.
3. Wenzel RP, Bearman G, Edmond MB. Lessons from severe acute respiratory syndrome (SARS): implications for infection control. *Arch Med Res* 2005;36:610-616.
4. Climate change maps; https://www.nytimes.com/interactive/2017/03/21/climate/how-americans-think-about-climate-change-in-six-maps.html, accessed April 15, 2017.
5. Whitmee S, Haines A, Beyrer C, et al. Safeguarding human health in the Anthropocene epoch: report of the Rockefeller Foundation–*Lancet* Commission on planetary health. *Lancet* 2015;386(10007):1973-2028. DOI: 10.1016/S0140-6736(15)60901-1.
6. Reardon S, Tollefson J. Obama's top scientist talks shrinking budgets, Donald Trump, and his biggest regret. *Nature* 2016;535:15-6. doi: 10.1038/535015a.
7. New York Times. https://www.nytimes.com/2017/03/09/us/politics/epa-scott-pruitt-global-warming.html?_r=0, accessed April 15, 2017.
8. The Atlantic. https://www.theatlantic.com/science/archive/2017/01/rex-tillerson-climate-change/512843/, accessed April 15, 2017.
9. Great thoughts Treasury. Nelson Mandela, fully Nelson Rolihlahla Mandela. http://www.greatthoughtstreasury.com/author/nelson-mandela-fully-nelson-rolihlahla- mandela?page=40: January 2009. Acessed April 15, 2017.
10. Center for Global Development. https://www.cgdev.org/page/foreign-assistance-and-us-budget, accessed April 15, 2017.
11. Chapter is an expanded and modified version of a prior editorial: Vermund SH. The vital case for global health investments by the US Government. *Clin Infect Dis* 2017;64(6): 707-710. DOI: https://doi.org/10.1093/cid/cix048.

43 TREATING DEPRESSION WHERE THERE ARE NO MENTAL HEALTH PROFESSIONALS

Studies assessing the burden of disease in the world using disability-adjusted life years (DALYs; see Section 3) have revealed some surprising health challenges. For example, one surprising finding is the seriousness of road traffic safety. From a public health perspective, car crashes are not "accidents," since most traffic deaths and injuries are preventable. In low-income countries, the people most at risk of dying are pedestrians and cyclists. Most victims of motor vehicles are injured rather than killed, and those injuries can affect people for the rest of their lives. Although having access to ambulances and emergency treatment facilities are important measures, the solution to the challenge of road traffic safety in developing countries is not merely medical. Solutions must be multisectorial, involving not only emergency medicine but also automobile design, road engineering, infrastructure maintenance, law enforcement and driver education.

Another topic that rose toward the top of the global health priority list after the introduction of the DALY is mental health. These health challenges include psychoses like schizophrenia, as well as more common disorders like debilitating depression, severe anxiety and alcohol or drug dependency. While severe depression can result in death through suicide, the reason why mental health carries such a large DALY burden is that the common mental disorders (CMDs) are so widespread. Chronic depression and anxiety (also known as affective disorders) are a common source of suffering and disability. People who suffer with CMDs do not live in "a state of psychological and social well-being" that is an essential part of the World Health Organization's definition of health.

There are many other common mental health issues with serious population health impacts. For example, alcohol abuse is a serious problem throughout the world, particularly among men, strongly linked to violence. As another example, dementia among the elderly requires a significant amount of care, often supplied by families.

Possibly the most serious problem in addressing global mental health is providing mental health services when there is such a short supply of psychiatrists and other mental health professionals. This is called the "treatment gap." The World Health Organization estimates that one in four people throughout the world suffer from a CMD at some point in their lives and that about 450 million people currently need mental health care. Roughly half of the world's population lives in places where there is only one psychiatrist for every 100,000 people.

This article describes the remarkable innovations that are being designed and implemented to address these challenges. Many of these innovations involve ***task shifting*** *to community mental health workers with basic training in cognitive behavioral therapy. There are some mental health disorders that require medication, but community-based mental health care for CMDs and post-traumatic stress disorder is very promising. Examples of projects include group therapy sessions and the installation of "grandmother benches" (where elderly women trained in basic counseling techniques sit to provide free sessions) outside health clinics. Finally, many advocates are pushing the idea that it may not be necessary to use complex psychiatric terminologies or techniques. Drawing on local understandings of illness may be the most culturally appropriate way to deliver primary mental health care.*

As you read the following article, consider the following questions:

- **In the past, some people in global health thought that low- and middle-income countries**

Vikram Patel. "Treating Depression Where There Are No Mental Health Professionals." *Bulletin of the World Health Organization*, 2017, 95(3): 172–173.

could not afford mental health care, given their challenges in child survival and infectious disease. Do you think that mental health care should be a lower priority for those countries? Is mental health care a luxury or necessity?

- **Some people say that CMDs, like depression and anxiety disorders, are really just reflective of personal distress caused by the challenges of living and that they are not "real" health problems. What do you think of this?**
- **Do you think it is appropriate to give community members a little training in counseling and then having them treat people? In your opinion, is task shifting just a way to deliver second-rate care?**
- **Many cultures view mental health problems as spiritual issues rather than medical ones. Therefore, they may view interventions like exorcism as appropriate therapies. Should therapies like this be supported by global health agencies?**

CONTEXT

Vikram Patel is an Indian psychiatrist and a leader in the field of global mental health, particularly through the Movement for Global Mental Health. Author of many scientific articles, he has also written a book for community health workers entitled *Where There Is No Psychiatrist* (London: Royal College of Psychiatrists, 2012). He is best known for his work on child development and mental disability in low-resource settings. He is the co-founder of the Centre for Global Mental Health at the London School of Hygiene and Tropical Medicine, co-director of the Centre for Control of Chronic Conditions at the Public Health Foundation of India and the co-founder of Sangath, an Indian nongovernmental organization dedicated to research in the areas of child development, adolescent health and mental health. In April 2015, he was listed as one of the world's 100 most influential people by *TIME* magazine.

Many people with depression and other mental health problems can be treated successfully by community health workers, but so far no country has scaled up this approach. Vikram Patel talks to Fiona Fleck.

Q: Why did you become interested in mental health?
A: I went into psychiatry at a time when it was an extremely unattractive field and far more stigmatized than it is today. Having ranked at the top of the final university medical examinations in Mumbai, I could have chosen any specialty. At first I was interested in neurology, fascinated by the brain and its mysteries. But during my medical studies it struck me that in neurology the symptoms and signs of the condition were all important. Psychiatry was the only field where the person was central. Also, psychiatry presented a unique bridge between medicine and society.

Q: This year's World Health Day is devoted to addressing depression, can you tell us about the burden and causes of this condition?
A: Depression is probably the most well researched mental disorder globally. A 2013 systematic review for the Global Burden of Disease project identified more than 100 studies from around the world estimating the prevalence of the condition. It found that 4–5% of adults might meet diagnostic criteria for depression, which we could extrapolate to hundreds of millions of people worldwide. The global literature on depression shows that common risk factors associated with depression are related to social disadvantage and deprivation, such as low level of education, job loss, indebtedness, social exclusion or marginalization and violence. Women are also at higher risk of having depression, this is partly related to interpersonal violence and other consequences of gender inequity.

Q: What does that mean for societies?
A: Depression not only affects an individual. In a mother, it affects her child's growth and development. Depression affects a person's ability to work, making that person less productive. This not only affects households but the entire economy. A group of economists recently modelled the overall cost of depression for the World Economic Forum and came up with estimates that ran into trillions of dollars.

In addition, let's not forget suicide. While this is classified as a health outcome in its own right and not as a consequence of a mental health problem, many people who attempt suicide are depressed.

Q: Is depression curable? What treatment is needed for this condition?
A: Globally, the strongest evidence is for brief psychological treatments based on cognitive, behavioural and interpersonal mechanisms. We recently conducted a systematic review of studies of psychological treatments delivered by non-specialist providers and identified 27 randomized controlled trials from low- and middle-income countries. Since our review, the findings of at least two major trials have been published, including our own study on the Healthy Activity Program in India in the *Lancet* in January. Most of these trials testify to the effectiveness of these treatments in promoting remission and recovery. There is a smaller evidence base for antidepressants. Both talking treatment and drugs are most effective in people with severe depression. For a significant proportion of people with mild to moderate depressive symptoms, self-care and low-intensity care provided by community members are just as effective as more structured clinical interventions such as psychotherapy.

Q: The World Health Day theme "depression: let's talk" is about seeking help. How can we counter the stigma that often prevents people from seeking help?
A: Stigma is a major challenge and there is no simple solution. A recent review showed limited evidence for many strategies to address stigma. For example, promoting the concept of depression as a biological brain disorder actually led to more negative attitudes, as it suggested that the condition was an immutable aspect of the person's biology. What I think does work is disclosure: people coming out and talking about their experience of depression. In this respect, the World Health Day message is spot on. In addition, even if it's hard to change people's attitudes, we can enforce laws that reduce discrimination, for example removing barriers to education and employment for people with mental health problems. Addressing discrimination is perhaps more valuable and feasible than trying to address stigma. Many people may have a negative attitude to people with mental health problems, but what matters most is that they do not deny them a job or education.

Q: How can we encourage people to seek care for mental health conditions?
A: We recently published a paper in *Lancet Psychiatry* describing a programme in rural India where, over an 18-month period, we brought about a six-fold increase in the proportion of people with depression seeking care. Our approach emphasized a grassroots approach in which local people raised awareness using language understood by the community, avoided reference to depression as a psychiatric problem, discussed issues such as being in debt and domestic violence, championed self-care as a first-level intervention, and used culturally appropriate media such as clips from Bollywood films. We only referred to depression as a biomedical problem when it was severe and clinical interventions were needed. The awareness raising interventions were provided by community-based workers and lay counsellors, meanwhile evidence-based interventions for depression and alcohol-use disorders were made more readily available in both community settings and primary health-care centres.

Q: What do you do in communities without mental health professionals?
A: Empower people for self-care and deploy people in the community to care for others, both with the appropriate training and support. As mentioned, we just completed a review of this approach and found that six to 10 brief treatment sessions of 30 to 40 minutes for patients with severe depression, typically delivered in people's homes or primary health centres, are effective in promoting remission and recovery. One of the most important findings of this review is that it debunks the myth that patients in developing countries prefer medication to talking treatments. If talking treatments are provided in a contextually sensitive and affordable manner, their acceptability and feasibility is very high.

Q: Has this approach been scaled up?
A: Despite the robust evidence for the acceptability and effectiveness of using community workers to deliver psychosocial interventions, I cannot think

of one country or region where this approach has been taken to scale. For example, in India there are many small-scale projects delivering mental health care in places where there are no psychiatrists but what we really need is the full integration of this approach into government health-care systems, for delivery at the primary care level. This is what the PRIME (programme to reduce the treatment gap for mental disorders) consortium funded by the British government, in five low- and middle-income countries, is trying to achieve.

Q: How would the approach work if scaled up?
A: The idea is to train millions of community health workers and people in communities worldwide to deliver evidence-based psychosocial interventions. This approach can not only address mental health problems in low- and middle-income countries, but also in high-income countries where the treatment gap is high in spite of substantial specialist resources. Where mental health professionals are available, they need to provide training, quality assurance and referral pathways for complex mental health problems that do not readily respond to treatment. Digital technologies can play a role in the promotion of self-care, and in training and supervision of community workers.

Q: Why do developed countries rely heavily on medicines to treat depression when talking treatment is highly effective?
A: Mental health care has become heavily medicalized, dominated by a psychiatric profession in which the prescription of medications is customary. However, people in developed countries are increasingly seeking non-pharmacological options for their recovery, ranging from biomedical psychological treatments to spiritual and traditional approaches, such as yoga. The idea of using lay people in the delivery of mental health care is often resisted by mental health professionals, including clinical psychologists, who argue that it is not safe or effective, in spite of evidence to the contrary. Perhaps they see this as a threat to their professional authority and control over these treatments and health conditions.

Q: How did you start the Sangath nongovernmental mental health organization in Goa? What was new about it?
A: I founded Sangath with six colleagues in 1996. Today it ranks among India's leading public health research institutions. Sangath started primarily as a centre for children with developmental and mental health problems that later broadened to providing care for all population groups. There was a huge demand for such care and we were inundated with referrals. However, many families could not afford the long-term specialist care and were often unable to come to our facility regularly. So we started delivering care in community and primary-care settings by non-specialist workers and evaluating the effects. Sangath pioneered this approach in collaboration with academic and government partners for a range of different mental health conditions, from autism and alcohol dependence to depression and schizophrenia.

Q: What would you say to governments that assign mental health care low priority?
A: There has to be a fundamental value that we place on mental health. Mental health is a global public good in and of itself. We must strive to deliver whatever works to those who need it: our goal as implementation scientists is to develop effective ways to achieve this goal while maximizing acceptability to patients, their families and those who ultimately have to pay for these services. One thing is for sure: mental health is just as important as physical health, and as with physical health, we cannot deliver mental health care for free.

OBIJIOFOR AGINAM

44 BEYOND SHAMANISM: THE RELEVANCE OF AFRICAN TRADITIONAL MEDICINE IN GLOBAL HEALTH POLICY

This section of the book has described government- and donor-funded health systems in some depth. But it is important to remember that these health systems do not exist in a vacuum. In every part of the world, government and nongovernmental organization health systems coexist with a wide range of other health services. People may use government health services, private doctors and healers from other medical traditions concurrently or in succession.

All societies have a medical system—or many medical systems—as part as their culture. These are often called traditional medicine—though as this selection argues, these systems of thought are always changing, so "ethnomedicine" is a better title. In some ethnomedical systems, the explanation for illness might be witchcraft; in others, that humors within the body have fallen out of balance; in yet others, that undetectable things that we cannot see (sometimes called germs) are attacking a person's body. But in all of these medical systems, there are methods for diagnosing and treating disease.

This selection notes that medical systems in Africa are pluralistic—people have a range of systems to choose from in seeking care and may use more than one. In fact, this is the case globally. For example, in the United States, many people distrust contemporary biomedicine and seek alternative pathways to cure, like herbal remedies, fitness routines or dietary changes. The medical system of North America, like most of the world, is pluralistic. We can think of biomedicine as being a kind of ethnomedicine.

Throughout the world, many people rely on ethnomedical healers as their first stop in seeking medical care; this may be because they trust those local healers, because they are conveniently accessible or because they are perceived to be less expensive. Frequently, people in resource-poor settings would prefer biomedicine in addition to or instead of other ethnomedicines, but biomedical facilities and treatment are inaccessible or unaffordable. This lack of availability might be considered a form of structural violence because it is so often linked to poverty.

Given the severe shortage of trained medical personnel in places like rural Africa, many people have suggested incorporating traditional healers into health-care delivery and health education. But this idea has been controversial. The World Health Organization cautiously endorsed the use of traditional healers in efforts to improve health, but so far, the results of such projects have been somewhat disappointing, in part because biomedical doctors are often resistant to working with ethnomedical practitioners.

It is helpful to remember a few things about ethnomedical treatments: They often work, they are not necessarily cheaper, they are usually considered culturally appropriate, they can do harm or delay other treatments and they are often not "traditional" in the sense that they are constantly changing and often incorporate elements of biomedicine.

As this selection argues, because ethnomedicine is such an important part of treatment for people across the globe, global health professionals should take ethnomedicine seriously. Understanding how and why people use ethnomedicine is an important part of understanding the full picture of people's health-care options, particularly in the world's most marginalized communities.

As you read this selection, consider the following questions:

- **Why have biomedicine and ethnomedicine so often had a hostile relationship?**
- **Why might people choose other ethnomedical treatments, even when biomedical treatments are available?**

Obijiofor Aginam, "Beyond Shamanism." *Medicine and Law*, 2007, 26: 191–201. Reprinted with compliments to and permission of the journal.

- **How might global health practitioners benefit from better understanding ethnomedical systems?**
- **Why does the author think that current global health policy is "discriminatory" toward ethnomedicine?**

CONTEXT

Obijiofor Aginam is a lawyer and dual citizen of Canada and Nigeria. He worked as a lawyer in Nigeria on environmental and civil rights issues in the 1990s. He has worked with African civil society organizations, the World Health Organization and the Food and Agriculture Organization of the United Nations on global health, environmental governance and human rights. Currently, he is a senior research fellow at the United Nations University Institute for Global Health and an adjunct assistant professor at Carleton University in Ottawa, Canada.

Introduction

This article explores the relevance of African "ethnomedicine,"[1] "traditional medicine"[2] or "ethnopharmacology"[3] in global health policy. Although, in most of the literature, the terms *ethnomedicine and traditional medicine* are used interchangeably as being synonymous, this article prefers the use of ethnomedicine because, as Iwu argued, "ethnomedicine encompasses the use of several health-promoting cultural practices and the use of minimally processed naturally occurring products for the prevention and treatment of diseases, as well as for the maintenance of optimal

[1] *Ethnomedicine* is defined as "the study of different ways in which people of various cultures perceive and cope with illness, including making a diagnosis and obtaining therapy," *see* H. Fabrega, "The Need for an Ethnomedical Science," (1975) Vol. 189 Science No.4207 at 969.

[2] The World Health Organization defines *traditional medicine* as including "diverse health practices, approaches, knowledge and beliefs incorporating plant, animal, and/or mineral based medicines, spiritual therapies, manual techniques and exercises applied singularly or in combination to maintain well-being, as well as to treat, diagnose or prevent illness." *See* WHO, *WHO Traditional Medicine Strategy 2002-2005* (Geneva: WHO, 2002) at 7. *See* also WHO, "WHO General Guidelines for Methodologies on Research and Evaluation of Traditional Medicine" (Geneva: WHO/EDM/TRM, 2000) (defining traditional medicine as the "sum total of the knowledge, skills, and practices based on the theories, beliefs and experiences, indigenous to different cultures, whether explicable or not, used in the maintenance of health as well as in the prevention, diagnosis, improvement or treatment of physical and mental illnesses"). The terms complementary, alternative and non-conventional medicine are used interchangeably with traditional medicine in many countries. For a discussion of complementary and alternative medicine specifically, *see* David Eisenberg, "Exploring Complementary and Alternative Medicine," The Richard and Hinda Rosenthal Lectures, 2001 (Washington, D.C., Institute of Medicine).

[3] Reacting to the question, what is ethnopharmacology?, Peter A.G.M. De Smet, in his famous work *Herbs, Health and Healers: Africa as Ethnopharmacological Treasury* (Berg en Dal, The Netherlands: Afrika Museum, 1999) p11 states that; "from time immemorial, man has valued the plant kingdom and animal kingdom as sources of bioactive products. . . . Some of these traditional plant and animal substances are purely magical. They have no relevant pharmacological (i.e. drug-like) effects, which can be produced in a laboratory setting. Many substances have a measurable pharmacological action, however, which corresponds well to their traditional application. The scientific discipline, which explores this pharmacological basis of traditional drugs and poisons is called ethnopharmacology. Its focus ranges from the first-hand observation of native drug practices (by early travellers and anthropologists) through the identification of crude ingredients and their constituents (by botanists, zoologists and chemists) to the evaluation of wanted and unwanted drug effects (by pharmacologists and toxicologists)."

physical and emotional health. These indigenous or culturally based forms of medicine have their origin in antiquity, but they are not ancient medicine, so the use of the term 'traditional' to describe ethnomedicine may be misleading."[4] The term 'traditional' may therefore erroneously imply an inter-generational repetition of a fixed body of data or the gradual unsystematic accumulation of data which is hardly the case with ethnomedicine that is based on "careful observation by healers in a given generation of indigenous people."[5] Ethnomedicine is extremely controversial. Science has been the centre-point of this controversy as Western scientific discourses dismiss these ethnomedical therapies as magic, shamanism, superstition, faith healing, spiritism, ritual, barbarism, witchcraft, or sorcery. Iwu observed that spiritual healing, as a component of ethnomedicine, for instance, has remained difficult to understand in Western medicine due to the differences in the concepts of health, diseases and healing between Western societies and traditional cultures.[6] This article assesses the relevance of African ethnomedicine in global health policy by focusing on the relationship and interaction between traditional medical therapies and orthodox medicine. In this endeavour, the article argues for the recognition of the scientific worth of traditional medicine, especially herbalism, based on the age-long medicinal uses of plants across societies in Africa.

Ethnomedicine versus Western Medicine: Complementarity or Hostility?

Throughout history, the interaction of peoples and cultures, and the complexity of the manoeuvres in these interactions driven by colonialism versus self-determination, civilization versus primitivity, and modernity versus savagery has led to two systematic responses to ill-health and disease; one based on a Hippocratic modern system of medicine, and the other based on traditional therapies.[7] From ancient times, the two systems have co-existed with hostility. Staugard states that modern medicine has often demonstrated its hostility towards traditional medicine by categorizing it either as "quackery" or "witchcraft."[8] Based on some form of imperialistic paradigm, this categorization arises from an often mistaken Western epistemological conception of ethnomedicine in most of the Third World that sees herbalism, divination, magic, and faith healing as belonging to one indivisible health delivery compartment devoid of analytical Western scientific investigation. Western epistemological, anthropological and epidemiological seminal accounts of African traditional medicine have often linked it with beliefs, superstition, and rituals. In this mainstream scholarship, African disease aetiologies were devoid of any scientific insights and epistemological assessment.[9] As De Smet observed, "many Western doctors and pharmacologists believe that ethnopharmacology yields nothing but armchair amusement."[10]

The World Health Organization, since 1972, in pursuance of its global health mandate, has passed a series of resolutions on the integration of traditional medicine into the national health care systems of

[4] Maurice M. Iwu, "Introduction: Therapeutic Agents from Ethnomedicine," in M. M. Iwu & J. C. Wootton, eds., *Advances in Phytomedicine, Volume 1: Ethnomedicine and Drug Discovery* (Amsetrdam: Elsevier, 2002) 1.

[5] *Ibid.*

[6] *Ibid* at 3.

[7] *See* F. Staugard, *Traditional Medicine in Botswana* (Gaborone: Ipelegeng Publishers, 1985) 5; U. Wassermann, "Traditional Medicine and the Law" (1984) 18 *Journal of World Trade Law* 155 (asserting that "Europeans and North Americans are often inclined to think of traditional medicine only in terms of witchcraft, spiritism, laying on of hands, or with a slightly less condescending attitude of homeopathy and such more embracing systems as India's *ayurveda* or Moslem *Unani* medicine")

[8] Staugard, *Ibid* at 5. See generally, A. Mire, "The Genealogy of Witchcraft: Colonialism and Modern Science," in Z. Magubane, ed., *Postmodernism, Postcoloniality, and African Studies* (Trenton, NJ: Africa World Press, Inc, 2005) 81.

[9] *See* Isaac Sindiga, "African Ethnomedicine and Other Medi al Systems," in I. Sindiga, *et al.*, (eds.), *Traditional Medicine in Africa* (Nairobi: East African Publishers, 1995) 16.

[10] De Smet, *Herbs, Health and Healers: Africa as Ethnopharmacological Treasury*, note 3 at 11.

Member States.[11] Notwithstanding the WHO resolutions, however, there are still tensions between traditional medicine and orthodox medicine.[12]

Relevance of Ethnomedicine: Myth or Reality?

The relevance of ethnomedicine is founded on two major reasons: the first is global multiculturalism and its implications for the health of populations in radically divergent Western and non-Western cultures, and the second reason relates to the cost and affordability of health care in Africa where ethnomedical therapies may be readily available at a cost the community can afford while orthodox (Western) medical therapies are not.[13] In a multicultural world, every society, in the developing world and elsewhere, deals with illness and disease in a variety of ways. Ethno-medicine has no unifying theme across societies; thus the therapies it provides vary from one society or culture to another. Traditional medicine, according to Akerele, comprises those practices based on beliefs that were in existence for years before the development and spread of modern medicine.[14] Ethno-medical knowledge of plants by indigenous people across societies and cultures has, "long served" as crucial sources of medicines either directly as therapeutic agents, as starting points for the elaboration of more complex semi-synthetic compounds or as synthetic compounds.[15]

In most African societies, multiculturalism has given rise to what some scholars call "medical pluralism"; the existence in a single society of differently designed and conceived medical systems.[16] Such systems exist together, and may either compete with, or complement, one another.[17] Populations in

[11] The 1972 World Health Assembly Resolution WHA29.72 noted the huge manpower reserve constituted by traditional medical practitioners. The 1977 World Health Assembly Resolution WHA30.49 called on Member States to explore the utilization of traditional medicine in their health care systems. The 1978 the World Health Assembly Resolution WHA31.33 noted the medicinal value of medicinal plants in the health systems of many developing countries.

[12] For a discourse of the challenges of the legal protection of traditional medicine, *See* Richard Wilder, "Protection of Traditional Medicine," Commission on Macroeconomics and Health, Working Paper Series No.4, July 2001; Ursula Wassermann, "Traditional Medicine and the Law," supra at note 7; O. Akerele, "The Best of Both Worlds: Bringing Traditional Medicine up to Date" (1987) Vol. 24 No.2 *Social Science & Medicine* 117; Chioma Obijiofor, "Integrating African Ethnomedicine into primary Healthcare: A Framework for South-eastern Nigeria," in M. Iwu & J. Wootton, eds., supra note 4 pp 71–80; P. Omonzejele, "Current Ethical and Other Problems in the Practice of African Traditional Medicine" (2003) 22 *Medicine and Law* 29–38; David P. Fidler "Neither Science nor Shamans: Globalization of Markets and Health in the Developing World" (1999) *Indiana Journal of Global Legal Studies* 191–224. I have explored the challenges of integrating traditional medical therapies into the global malaria control strategy. *See* Obijiofor Aginam, "From the Core to the Peripheries: Multilateral Governance of Malaria in a Multi-Cultural World" (2002) Vol. 3 No. 1 *Chicago Journal of International Law* 87.

[13] For a recent global strategy on the interaction of traditional, alternative and complementary medicine and the formal health care system, *See* WHO, "WHO Traditional Medicine Strategy 2002–2005" (Geneva: WHO, 2002).

[14] O. Akerele, supra, note 12. For a study of ethno-medicine across various societies in the developing world, *see* K. Appiah-Kubi, *Man Cures, God Heals: Religion and Medical Practice Among the Akans of Ghana* (USA: Allanheld & Osmun & Co, 1981); C. Leslie & A Young, *Paths to Asian Medical Knowledge* (Berkeley/Los Angeles/Oxford: University of California Press, 1992); T. Dummer, *Tibetan Medicine and Other Holistic Health-Care Systems* (London/New York: Routledge, 1988); H.M Said, *Medicine in China* (Karachi: Hanidard Academy, 1965); G.E Simpson, *Yoruba Religion and Medicine in Ibadan*, (Ibadan: Ibadan University Press, 1980)

[15] Edith Brown Weiss, *In Fairness to Future Generations: International Law, Common Patrimony, and Intergenerational Equity* (New York: The United Nations University/Transnational Publishers, 1989) 266. On this topic, *see* generally, Maurice M. Iwu & Jacquline C. Wootton, *Advances in PhytoMedicine* Vol. 1, note 4; Ikechi Mgbeoji, "Patents and Traditional Knowledge of the Uses of Plants: Is a Communal Patent Regime Part of the Solution to the Scourge of Bio Piracy?" (2001) Vol. 9 *Indiana Journal of Global Legal Studies* 163-186

[16] David Phillips, *Health and Health Care in the Third World* (New York: Youngman, 1990) 75 defines medical pluralism as "the existence and use of a wide range of sources of medical care, traditional and modern, static and evolving."

[17] J.M Janzen, *The Quest for Therapy: Medical Pluralism in Lower Zaire* (Berkeley, CA: University of California, 1978).

the developing world resort to both traditional medicine and Western medicine simultaneously for the same illness or at different times for different illnesses. Juxtaposing ethno-medicine with Western medicine, it is often argued that the holistic approach of ethnomedicine to the art of healing is one important factor that has continued to endear it to many of its followers and adherents: a sizeable eighty percent of the population in most African rural areas. As argued by Iwu,

[T]he holistic concept in traditional medicine is commendable, in that the patient's mind and soul as well as body are considered together during treatment. . . . One increasingly important aspect of the African worldview is the belief that human beings cannot be separated from nature. There is therefore no overwhelming desire to conquer the natural world or dominate it . . . African worldview is eco-centric . . . It binds humans and the rest of nature together with the same umbilical cord.[18]

Focusing on African religious and philosophical cosmology, Mbiti argued that diseases and misfortunes are regarded as having social and religious foundations. The treatment process must therefore go beyond merely addressing their symptoms but also their social implications as well as strategies to prevent their reoccurrence.[19] Some scholars dismiss the holistic nature of traditional medicine as falsehood. David Phillips argued that,

[S]tereo-types suggest, for example, that traditional medicine is holistic, whilst modern medicine sees only the disease. This might be true in relatively isolated, small-scale societies, but in large Asian and African villages and towns, there is probably almost as much impersonal treatment by traditional healers as there is by practitioners of modern medicine. The holistic appeal of traditional medicine—that it considers the patient as a whole person, in his or her domestic and social setting—may in fact be perpetuating a false image.[20]

The holistic appeal of traditional medicine is a culture-related phenomenon just as ethno-medical therapies differ across societies and cultures. There may be instances where the relationship between the traditional healer and patient is impersonal. Nonetheless, it needs to be pointed out that, for instance in Africa, the dominant world-views as well as the concept of personhood as proffered by scholars like Mbiti[21] favour the holistic flavour of traditional medicine.[22] Linked to the holistic nature of ethno-medical therapies in the developing world, is the prohibitive cost of orthodox Western medicines, and the disinterestedness of global pharmaceutical companies to research affordable drugs for tropical (neglected) disease because of the poor return on investment.[23] A combination of these factors makes ethnomedicine popular and relevant in most developing countries.

The Scientific Value of African Ethnomedical Therapies and the Charge of Bio-Piracy

Most of the herbs used as therapies for ailments in most of the Third World have now been universally acclaimed as medicinally valid and scientifically effective.[24] As Roht-Arriaza observed,

Indigenous and local communities have a long history of using plants for almost all needs, including food, shelter, clothing, and medicine. Common remedies used today were often first developed by healers prior to contact with industrial societies. Yet, although many of today's drugs and cosmetics originated from the stewardship and knowledge of

[18] Maurice M. Iwu, "Preface," in Peter A.G.M De Smet, *Herbs, Health and Healers: Africa as Ethnopharmacological Treasury* note 3 at 9.

[19] J.S Mbiti, *African Religions and Philosophy* (London: Heinemann, 1969) 169.

[20] D.R Phillips, note 16 p81.

[21] In Africa, according to Mbiti, the individual's needs, rights, joys and sorrows are woven into a social tapestry that denies singular individuality. Traditional medical practitioners symbolize the hopes of society; hopes of good health, protection and security from evil forces, prosperity and good fortune, and ritual cleansing when harm or impurities have been contracted. *See* Mbiti, *op cit.* pp 141 & 171.

[22] On this theme generally, *see* P.H. Coetzee & A.P.J. Roux, *The African Philosophy Reader* (London: Routledge, 1998).

[23] On this theme, focusing on malaria drugs, *see* Obijiofor Aginam, "From the Core to the Peripheries: Multilateral Governance of Malaria in a Multi-Cultural World" (2002) Vol. 3 No. 1 *Chicago Journal of International Law* 87–102.

[24] See generally Iwu & Wootton, note 4.

indigenous and local communities, that knowledge remains unrecognized and unvalued until appropriated from those communities by Western corporations or institutions.[25]

Roht-Arriaza cites many examples of appropriation of indigenous scientific knowledge including quinine, a well-known and universally acclaimed cure for malaria, which comes from the bark of the Peruvian cinchona tree.[26] Andean indigenous populations used quinine as a cure for fevers, supposedly learning of its medical efficacy by observing feverish jaguars eating it.[27] Other notorious examples include the rosy periwinkle plant, unique to Madagascar, which contains properties that combat certain cancers. The anti-cancer drugs *vincristine* and *vinblastine* have been developed from the periwinkle, resulting in over $100 million in annual sales for Eli Lilly and virtually nothing for Madagascar.[28] In the same fashion, a barley gene that resists the yellow-dwarf virus has been the product of breeding and cultivation by Ethiopian farmers for centuries. Scientists and farmers in the United States patented the barley variety and now receive huge financial profits from the patent while the local Ethiopian farmers that originally developed the variety are not remunerated.[29]

Although *biopiracy* is a hotly contested term, it is necessary that the global intellectual property regime be relaxed to effectively offer legal protection and remuneration to local communities who are custodians of age old ethnomedical-herbal remedies that have proven medicinal value.[30] In this endeavour, we need to re-configure the contours and parameters of knowledge and invention to reflect both Western and non Western ideals. The debate over the patentability of traditional medical therapies based on the uses of herbs and plants has been exceedingly complex in intellectual property law. Based on mainstream intellectual property law, it has been argued that traditional medicine is not novel, and because these therapies do not entail "a new invention," they do not meet the requirements for a patent.[31] For instance, to meet the requirements of patentability under Article 27 of the World Trade Organization's Agreement on Trade-Related Aspects of Intellectual Property Rights ("TRIPS"), an inventor must prove that his invention is new (novelty), shows an "inventive step" that was non-obvious, and that the invention is industrially applicable. Based on these requirements that developed from a predominantly Western notion of patent law, Wilder has identified three impediments to patentability of traditional medical therapies. First, most traditional medicine is ancient. They are not new, and therefore do not meet the requirement of novelty. Second, traditional medical knowledge is held collectively by local communities. It is therefore difficult to identify an "inventor." Third, the cost and complexity of patent application are often beyond the reach of custodians of traditional medicine.[32] Notwithstanding the provisions of WTO's TRIPS Agreement, a more flexible legal and normative provision on patents that is protective of ethno-medical therapies seems to be occurring in other organizations and norms outside the WTO and TRIPS, especially the World Intellectual Property Organization ("WIPO"), and the United Nations Convention on Biological Diversity (CBD). Article 8(j) of the Convention on

[25] Naomi Roht-Arriaza, "Of Seeds and Shamans: The Appropriation of the Scientific and Technical Knowledge of Indigenous and Local Communities" (1996) 17 *Michigan J. of Int'l Law* 919 at 921. For an insightful discussion of bio-piracy, *see* Ikechi Mgbeoji, "Patents and Traditional Knowledge of the Uses of Plants: Is Communal Patent Regime Part of the Solution to the Scourge of Bio Piracy?" (2001) 9 *Indiana J. of Global Legal Studies* 163; Ikechi Mgbeoji, *Global Biopiracy: Patents, Plants and Indigenous Knowledge* (Vancouver: UBC Press, 2006).

[26] Roht-Arriaza, "Of Seeds and Shamns," *Ibid.*

[27] *Ibid.*

[28] *Ibid.*

[29] *Ibid.*

[30] See the solutions proffered by Mgbeoji, *Global Biopiracy*, supra, note 25.

[31] For some works that summarize this argument, *see* Carlos Correa, *Integrating Public Health Concerns into Patent Legislation in Developing Countries* (Geneva: South Centre, 2000); I. Mgbeoji, *Global Biopiracy*, supra note 25; Eugenio Da Costa E. Silva, "The Protection of Intellectual Property for Local and Indigenous Communities" (1995) 17 *European Intellectual Property Review* 546; Allan S. Gutterman, "The North-South Debate Regarding the Protection of Intellectual Property Rights" (1993) 23 *Wake Forest Law Review* 89.

[32] Richard Wilder, "Protection of Traditional Medicine," Commission on Macroeconomics and Health, CMH Working Paper Series, Paper No. WG 4: 4, July 2001 p21.

Biological Diversity provides that each contracting party shall, as far as possible and appropriate, [S] ubject to its national legislation, respect, preserve and maintain knowledge, innovations and practices of indigenous and local communities embodying traditional lifestyles relevant for the conservation and sustainable use of biological diversity and promote their wider application with the approval and involvement of the holders of such knowledge, innovations, and practices and encourage the equitable sharing of the benefits arising from the utilization of such knowledge, innovations and practices.

While this provision favours the patentability of traditional medical knowledge, it appears to be inconsistent with the requirements of "novelty," "inventive steps," and meaning of invention as codified in Article 27 of TRIPS. How then should the tension between Article 27 of TRIPS and Article 8(j) of the Convention on Biological Diversity be reconciled in order to offer intellectual property protection to ethno-medical therapies? Scholars like Correa have called for a *sui generis* system of intellectual property protection for traditional medicine.[33] While this proposal is laudable, some intellectual property law experts suggest that it is still premature to proceed with international negotiations of an international *sui generis* system because of the present state of understanding of traditional medicine.[34] Some developing countries like Panama, the Philippines, and Thailand have introduced laws to protect the rights of custodians of traditional medicine. In Africa, the Organization of African Unity (now "African Union") adopted the *African Model Law Legislation for the Protection of the Rights of Local Communities, Farmers and Breeders, and the for the Regulation of Access to Biological Resources* in 2000.[35] Legal initiatives that seek to offer intellectual property protection to traditional medicine outside of the strict TRIPS requirements of "novelty" have been supported in various ways by the World Intellectual Property Organization (WIPO), and the Secretariat of the Convention on Biological Diversity. However, because most African countries are members of both WIPO and the WTO, and also signatories to the Convention on Biological Diversity, it seems that any conflict or inconsistency between TRIPS and the Convention of Biological Diversity (both international treaties) should be resolved in accordance with the relevant provisions of the Vienna Convention on the Law of Treaties 1969, especially Article 30. In all of this, given that traditional medicine remains the major source of therapies for a sizeable percentage of populations in Africa and other parts of the developing world, it is imperative that these countries maximize the provisions of Article 8(j) of the CBD to promote and protect the health of millions of their populations.

Beyond Shamanism: A Postscript

In a multicultural world polarised by divergent determinants of health, the challenge of reconciling the tension between African traditional medicine and global health policy has become important in contemporary global health discourse. We live in a medically pluralistic world, a global policy universe, where public health presents variegated and complex challenges in culturally divergent societies. The relevance of traditional medicine in global health policy, recognising the existing tension between Western medicine and African ethnomedicine, must be built on two useful approaches: the *scientification* of ethnomedical therapies, especially the medicinal herbs, in the developing world. Traditional medicine is not just magic, superstition or shamanism, but an age-old health delivery system widely used by a sizeable percentage of African populations. Because alternative medical therapies are either unaffordable to, or unpopular among these populations, the continued relegation of African ethnomedicine to the peripheries of global health policy is intensely "discriminatory." This would make global health policy unresponsive to the health needs of vulnerable constituencies and indigenous African

[33] Carlos Correa, *Integrating Public Health Concerns into Patent Legislation in Developing Countries, supra* note 31 p28

[34] Wilder, *supra* note 32

[35] For a discussion of the African Model Law in the context of legal protection of genetic resources in Africa, *see* K. Nnadozie, *et al*, eds., *African Perspectives on Genetic Resources: A Handbook on Laws, Policies and Institutions* (Washington, DC: Environmental Law Institute, 2003). This study covers the legal framework in 12 African countries: Cameroun, Egypt, Ethiopia, Ivory Coast, Kenya, Madagascar, Nigeria, Senegal, The Seychelles, South Africa, Uganda, and Zambia.

communities where the mortality and morbidity burdens of communicable and non-communicable diseases are heavy. Innovative approaches to global health problems must strive to harmonize the tensions between African traditional medical therapies and orthodox medicine in a way that projects globalization of public health as a humane, fair and equitable enterprise.

SECTION 11 CASES FOR TEACHING AND LEARNING

Visit the companion website, www.oup.com/us/brown-closser, for direct links to the online resources featured below.

Juma et al., *Brain Drain of Health Professionals in Tanzania*
This excellent case outlines the issues surrounding brain drain globally, with a particular focus on Tanzania. It works very well paired with the Wendland selection (Reading 38). It could also be used paired with the Sue et al. case on medical education in Tanzania listed below.

Kleinman et al., *The AIDS Support Organization (TASO) of Uganda*
Students learn about community health work through the successful Ugandan nongovernmental organization (NGO) TASO. The case covers issues of NGO–government coordination, as well as funding and management.

Kristen Lundberg, *Credible Voice: WHO-Beijing and the SARS Crisis*
In this case study, students consider the political complexities that a World Health Organization (WHO) representative in Beijing must navigate when deciding what action to take at the beginning of the severe acute respiratory syndrome (SARS) crisis. This case can help students understand the role of the WHO in global health and the importance of politics in disease control efforts.

Madore et al., *Political Leadership in South Africa: National Health Insurance*
Students learn about the political complexities surrounding the rollout of national health insurance in South Africa. This program had the goal of achieving universal health coverage. This case can be particularly useful for American students, who may not be familiar with the concept of national health insurance programs.

May and Rhatigan, *BRAC's Tuberculosis Program: Pioneering DOTS Treatment for TB in Rural Bangladesh*
In this case, students learn about BRAC's groundbreaking Directly Observed Therapy, Short-Course (DOTS) program, including female community health workers delivering DOTS treatment. They also learn about other BRAC programs, including microfinance. Students consider how to adapt the program to significantly different contexts in sub-Saharan Africa. There is a follow-up case on BRAC's urban TB program in Dhaka online.

Eric Smalley, *Swaziland, HIV and Option B+: What Can We Afford?*
In this case, students take the perspective of the Swaziland Ministry of Health, weighing options for HIV control with limited resources. Students learn about issues of relationships with donors and of adapting international guidelines to local realities.

Sue et al., *Addressing Tanzania's Health Workforce Crisis Through a Public-Private Partnership: The Case of TTCIH*
This case examines the Tanzanian Training Center for International Health, a model designed to alleviate health workforce problems in Tanzania. Students consider issues of funding, sustainability and health workforce training.

Talbot et al., *Iran's Triangular Clinic*
This case describes the Iranian health system and a clinic that addresses the linked issues of HIV and drug use in marginalized populations. Students consider how the clinic could be integrated into the national primary health care system.

SECTION 11 VIDEOS AND WEB RESOURCES

Visit the companion website, www.oup.com/us/brown-closser, for direct links to the featured online resources.

Health Systems

***This Won't Hurt a Bit* – We the Economy**
This humorous and engaging video starring many famous faces illustrates the economic distortions in the American health system. (10 min)

Interactive Maps and Data – The Commonwealth Fund
This website has a variety of interactive maps focused on the United States, particularly regarding state-by-state variations in the Affordable Care Act.

The Dartmouth Atlas of Health Care
This interactive website allows students to investigate variations in spending and care provision across the United States. While students will likely need some guidance in interpreting this information, it is an excellent supplement to instructor lectures on the US health care system.

Donka: X-Ray of an African Hospital
This feature-length documentary explores the challenges facing Donka Hospital in Conakry, Guinea.

Human Resources for Health

***Africa: House Calls and Health Care* – NOW on PBS**
This documentary explores Partners in Health's *Accompagnateur* (Community Health Worker) program in Rwanda. This video is a good, basic introduction to the theory and practice of community health worker programs. (25 min)

***Nurses and Doctors* – Global Health Workforce Alliance**
This introduction to brain drain and task shifting focuses on compelling examples from Malawi and Pakistan. (8 min)

Liberia after Ebola: Turning Midwives into Surgeons
This case study in task-shifting describes a program in Liberia training midwives in Caesarean sections. (14 min)

***No One Should Die Because They Live Too Far from a Doctor* – Raj Panjabi**
In this Ted Talk, Raj Panjabi talks about his project, Last Mile Health, which trains, supports and pays community health workers. (20 min)

Medical Doctors Per 1,000 People – DataMarket
This interactive website allows students to compare the availability of doctors between different countries and over time.

Human Resources for Health: The Cuban Solution

***Debt-Free Doctors Part of Cuba's Foreign Policy Strategy* – PBS NewsHour**
This news report explains the methods and motivation behind Cuba's innovative strategy to train doctors to reach underserved populations globally. (8 min)

Salud
This feature-length documentary explores Cuba's medical schools.

Medical Brigades
This short documentary follows Cuban doctors in Haiti. (25 min)

Polio Eradication in Pakistan

***Every Last Child* – Tom Robbins**
This excellent feature-length documentary explores the difficulties in eradicating polio in Pakistan.

International Aid

Radi-Aid for Norway
In this funny and perceptive music video, Africans band together to provide aid for freezing Norwegians. (4 min)

***The Foreign Aid Paradox* – We the Economy**
This short film explores the history and present of American foreign aid. It engagingly describes the start of USAID after World Wart II, and clearly illustrates the political motivations behind aid. It also introduces some of the complicated consequences of food aid. (10 min)

Case Studies for Global Health
These short case studies, a few pages each, highlight a range of successful collaborations in global health. They are excellent resources for students interested in success stories in the field.

Poverty, Inc.

This feature-length film examines some striking negative consequences of the "aid industry" and argues for supporting entrepreneurism rather than aid. While the film presents them in a positive light, such market-based "solutions" are also controversial, since expanding the reach of capitalism often does not lead to increased equity.

***Good Fortune* – POV on PBS**

This feature-length film looks at the unintended consequences of development projects in sub-Saharan Africa. Focusing on Kenya, it tells the story of large-scale development projects from the point of view of those who suffer as a result of those projects.

SECTION

12

Health Communication

This section is about one of the most important processes for improving people's health—the transfer of knowledge that can help people choose to live in healthy ways. Global health professionals use health communication methods to promote handwashing, using condoms, wearing bike helmets, following occupational safety practices and many other behaviors. **Health communication** is not technological, but it can be extremely difficult to accomplish. Knowledge is necessary for people to change their behaviors, but it is often not sufficient to do it, especially for the long term.

In this section, the readings provide examples of the potential and challenges of effective health communication. Health communication can involve a wide variety of media: from posters to street plays to movies to social media. Chapter 45 describes an edutainment program in India that combined entertainment and education. This program successfully used a radio soap opera combined with neighborhood discussion groups.

Changing people's behavior can be difficult, especially when communities distrust public authorities. The two articles in Reading 46 focus on the West African Ebola outbreak. They discuss the challenges posed by misinformation and gossip and describe different approaches to dealing with this issue.

» CONCEPTUAL TOOLS «

- **Knowledge is a necessary but not sufficient element for people to change their behavior.** Other factors, such as structural violence, complicate the situation so that an individual's agency (their ability to make independent choices) is constrained.
- **Cigarette smoking is a good example that shows health knowledge is not enough to change everyone's behavior.** As we saw in Readings 6 and 18, the battle of public health practitioners against cigarette smoking is difficult. First, the epidemiological knowledge that cigarettes cause cancer needed to be discovered, and then the public needed to be convinced to stop or never start smoking. The communication of the facts about cigarettes did result in a significant decline of smoking.

These behavior change efforts were hampered by three factors: (i) the tobacco industry fought the dissemination of the truth; (ii) the tobacco industry used aggressive advertising to recruit smokers, including children; and (iii) cigarettes are addictive and can be pleasurable, so quitting is very difficult. In some countries like Poland, where the government depended on earnings from taxes on tobacco, the public never learned about cancer causation until the 1990s. More than 60 years after the negative health effects of cigarette smoking were identified, about 15% of American adults continue to smoke, and smoking is related to about one in five deaths.

- **The goal of public health is often to get people to do things that they do not want to do, even though it is good for their own health**. Scientific facts do not convince some people to do the right thing, especially if they distrust the sources of those facts. Understanding human behavior is important in health communication because people may need to be "nudged" in particular directions through indirect means, like making an elevator in a building difficult to find while making the stairs brightly colored and easy to use. New laws and regulations can also change behaviors, such as seatbelt laws in the United States.
- The traditional model of education is based on the assumption that the teacher has all of the knowledge and the students simply absorb and store that knowledge. Traditional health education sometimes had an authoritarian "finger wagging" tone to it. Humans do behave in ways that are bad for their health, but those behaviors are not simply because they do not have the correct information, and so health communication efforts with this assumption are often ineffective.
- **Education is empowerment**. Paolo Freire, in a famous book called *Pedagogy of the Oppressed* (1968), demonstrated that although traditional education systems like schools may create and reinforce existing power structures, adult education can be a source of empowerment for individuals and communities. He was a critic of the traditional education system (see the box "Paolo Freire"), particularly with the unequal knowledge/power relationship between teacher and students. He saw adult education for the poor as an important mechanism of increased community agency and individual self-awareness—but only if it worked against the traditional model where the teacher knows everything and the students know nothing. Health education where members of a community work together to come up with solutions to health problems is a good example of this idea.
- **Female literacy improves the health of everyone in a family.** There is solid evidence that women who have been educated and are literate have more biomedical knowledge and are more empowered to utilize available health resources. As such, female education can have an impact on child mortality rates.
- **Health communication is aimed at more than the simple transfer of information; it aims to change people's health behaviors.** There are many theories and models of behavior change, many of which center on Bandura's concept of self-efficacy—a person's belief in their own ability to succeed in specific situations or accomplish a task. There are many different theories of behavior change that are used in health education, as well as in criminology, psychology and other fields.

PAULO FREIRE, FROM *PEDAGOGY OF THE OPPRESSED*

A careful analysis of the teacher–student relationship at any level, inside or outside the school, reveals its fundamentally narrative character. This relationship involves a narrating Subject (the teacher) and patient listening objects (the students). . . . The teacher talks about reality as if it were motionless, static, compartmentalized, and predictable. Or else he expounds on a topic completely alien to the existential experience of the students. His task is to "fill" the students with the contents of his narration—contents which are detached from reality, disconnected from the totality that engendered them and could give them significance. Words are emptied of their concreteness and become a hollow, alienated, and alienating verbosity.

. . .

Narration (with the teacher as narrator) leads the students to memorize mechanically the narrated account. Worse yet, it turns them into "containers," into "receptacles" to be "filled" by the teachers. . . . Instead of communicating, the teacher issues communiques and makes deposits which the students patiently receive, memorize, and repeat.

. . .

In the banking concept of education, knowledge is a gift bestowed by those who consider themselves knowledgeable upon those whom they consider to know nothing. Projecting an absolute ignorance onto others, a characteristic of the ideology of oppression, negates education and knowledge as processes of inquiry. . . .

. . .

The capability of banking education to minimize or annul the student's creative power and to stimulate their credulity serves the interests of the oppressors, who care neither to have the world revealed nor to see it transformed. The oppressors use their "humanitarianism" to preserve a profitable situation. . . . Indeed, the interests of the oppressors lie in "changing the consciousness of the oppressed, not the situation which oppresses them," for the more the oppressed can be led to adapt to that situation, the more easily they can be dominated. . . .

But sooner or later, these contradictions may lead formerly passive students to turn against their domestication and the attempt to domesticate reality. They may discover through existential experience that their present way of life is irreconcilable with their vocation to become fully human. . . . If men and women are searchers and their ontological vocation is humanization, sooner or later they may perceive the contradiction in which banking education seeks to maintain them, and then engage themselves in the struggle for their liberation.

. . .

But the humanist revolutionary educator cannot wait for this possibility to materialize. From the outset, her efforts must coincide with those of the students to engage in critical thinking and the quest for mutual humanization. His efforts must be imbued with a profound trust in people and their creative power. To achieve this, they must be partners of the students in their relations with them.

. . .

The teacher cannot think for her students, nor can she impose her thought on them. Authentic thinking, thinking that is concerned about reality, does not take place in ivory tower isolation, but only in communication.

This reading is excerpted from *Pedagogy of the Oppressed*. London: Bloomsbury, 2014, Chapter 2.

The model most commonly used in health education is the Stages of Change model, depicted in Figures CT12.1 and CT12.2.

These two models are quite similar, except the circular figure refers to a longer cycle of behavior change that includes relapse. As most people know, changing behavior, especially habitual behavior, is a very difficult thing to do. A realistic health education program will focus on getting people just one stage beyond where they currently are.

A criticism of theories of behavior change is that they focus on the individual and exaggerate individual agency by ignoring socioeconomic constraints.

- **Social media has become a new frontier in health communication,** but misinformation and rumors are also spread on social media. For example, the falsehood that there is a correlation between vaccination and risk of autism spread

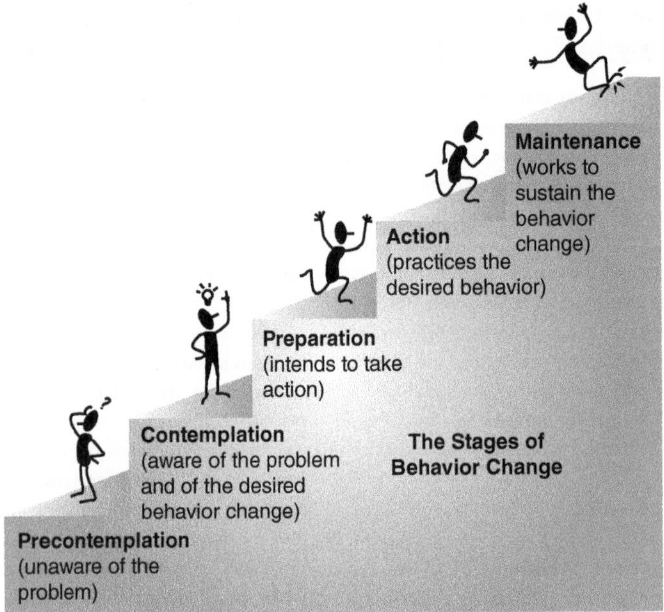

FIGURE CT12.1 The Stages of Behavior Change.
Sources: Prochaska J, Velicer WF (1997) The transtheoretical model of health behavior change. American Journal of Health Promotion 12:48 and Prochaska 1992 (148).

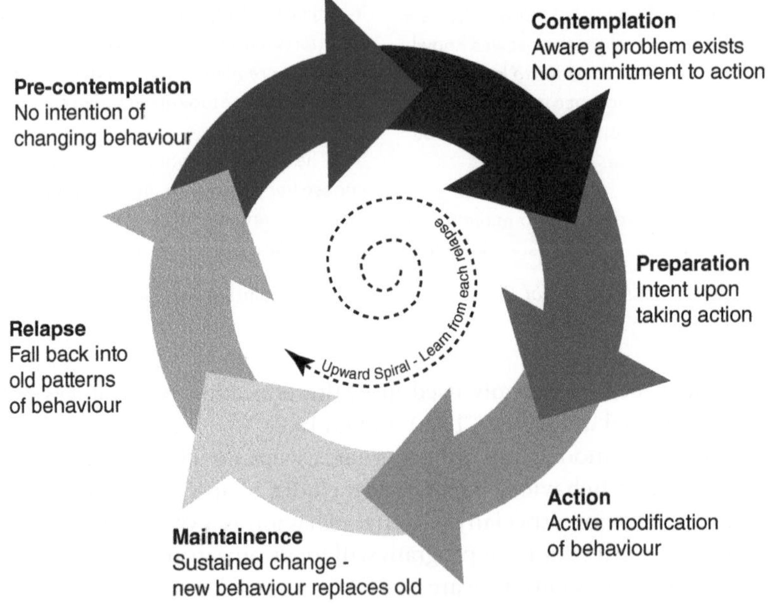

FIGURE CT12.2 *Transtheoretical* Model of Change.
Source: J. O. Prochaska, and DiClemente, C. C. (1984). *The Transtheoretical Approach: Crossing Traditional Boundaries of Therapy*. Homewood, IL: Dow Jones Irwin.

rapidly on social media, motivating an antivaccination movement that adds greatly to the risk of a measles epidemic in the United States. Rumors and misinformation have been around as long as humans, but social media sometimes accelerates their spread. On the plus side, new technologies also present new opportunities to reach people with essential health information.

- **The "fallacy of empty vessels" is that people in other societies do not have any health knowledge or beliefs.** Rather, they are "empty vessels," waiting to be filled with the knowledge of scientific medicine developed in rich countries. The fallacy implies that as soon as people are educated about new scientific knowledge for prevention and treatment, they will change their behaviors or accept the medical innovations. In reality, however, all people already have their own ethnomedical beliefs and practices, and these preexisting beliefs influence how new ideas are accepted. When one pours different liquid into already-filled vessels, a new mixture results, and when new biomedical ideas are introduced to people who already have an ethnomedical system, they are more likely to accept those ideas that fit with the preexisting system and reject those that do not. Such problems can be overcome, but only if one is aware of the fallacy of empty vessels. Understanding that people receive health messages within the context of their own beliefs is essential to achieve effective communication between health promoters and the public.
- **Trust in the person or organization delivering the information is essential in health communication.** People remember what has happened in the past, and often they have good reason not to trust governments or other agencies presenting them with health information.
- **In the end, correct biomedical information must available for everyone.** The Internet has made such information easier to access and disseminate. One important NGO doing this work is the Hesperian Health Foundation, which publishes more than forty books and health guides in thirteen languages.

Approaches to Health Communication

- **Social marketing is a method of health communication that markets health behaviors and products,** in the same way you would soft drinks or cars. **Social marketing** adapts commercial marketing techniques for health goals. Major health programs often spend a lot of time and energy creating a "brand" that is appealing to their target audience. Often social marketing efforts go beyond simple advertising, with attention to how to make health-related products available and affordable to low-income people.
- **Entertainment education programming is effective.** Behavior change information and "nudges" are appropriately communicated through media like films, TV soap operas, radio, street theater and so forth. When communication is enjoyable and entertaining, it simply works better. A good example of this is Global Dialogues (see box "Global Dialogues") and its collaborative film program for African youth, which focuses on HIV/AIDS.
- **Social mobilization is an approach that focuses on interpersonal communication as the central element in changing people's health behavior.** Social

HESPERIAN HEALTH GUIDES

Hesperian is a well-known provider of health education information. Their first book was the ground breaking *Where There is No Doctor* by David Werner. It is the most widely used manual for health workers, educators, and others involved in primary care and health promotion around the world and has been translated into more than 80 languages and used in more 200 countries. Other health guides are available for dentistry, women's health midwifery, psychiatry, community organization, and so forth.

Here is what Hesperian has to say about their work. You can read more and download many of their publications at Hesperian.org.

> Hesperian strives for a world in which people and communities are equipped to achieve health for all. Our mission is to provide information and educational tools that help all people take greater control over their health and work to eliminate the underlying causes of poor health.
>
> Hesperian produces and shares easy-to-understand health information for people worldwide. Throughout our history, Hesperian has joined together with others around the world to promote health justice, and has been a leader in the People's Health Movement, both in the US and internationally.
>
> Our work began in the 1970s in Ajoya, Mexico. There, an expanding group of volunteers working with villagers created a simple manual to use medically accurate knowledge in a culturally appropriate way to address community health needs. The Hesperian Foundation was established to publish this manual in 1973 as *Donde No Hay Doctor*. In 1977, to share it with the world, Hesperian published the English language version *Where There Is No Doctor*, now the most widely used health book in the world.
>
> Over the years, we have partnered with community health workers, villagers, medical professionals, and others to develop, publish and share information. We publish 20 titles, spanning community health, women's health, children with disabilities, HIV, and environmental health, and distribute many others. The global spread of our materials is a result of these partnerships and our common commitment to improving health conditions for those most in need.
>
> We also launched our new digital resource center in 2011 as part of our Digital Commons Initiative, an extension of our pioneering "open copyright" policy. This landmark digital platform enables global users to search, translate, customize and download our content. (http://hesperian.org/about/mission/)

mobilization programs often include social marketing and entertainment education elements, but they focus on providing direct, person-to-person health education delivered by trusted peers. This approach is very labor-intensive, but people are most likely to change their health behaviors when they are encouraged and supported by a peer that they trust.

- **Positive deviance is an approach to health education that builds on what people are already doing that is working well.** It assumes that the people living in a given situation are more likely to have figured out good solutions to their problems than outsiders. Health professionals using the **positive deviance** approach first look for people who have figured out how to do something that seems very difficult, like a mother who feeds her children sufficient and healthy food with very little money, or a sex worker who consistently gets her clients to use condoms. Then the health educators create opportunities for these people to teach others in their communities how they achieve these difficult tasks.

GLOBAL DIALOGUES

Global Dialogues is an entertainment-education program focusing on HIV/AIDS prevention. The program begins with a competition for short film scripts written by young people. The winning scripts are made into films in collaboration with professional filmmakers from Africa. The films are then made freely available in local languages for TV stations to use as public service announcements or in health education efforts by community health workers, Peace Corps volunteers, and NGOs. The idea is for the films to stimulate discussions, so most films are funny or entertaining. There is good evidence that this process works on many different levels, from improving health messaging to encouraging discussions that fight stigma.

You can watch many of these films on the Global Dialogues website at http://globaldialogues.org

The process is more than just the making of the films. There are a lot of steps in the Global Dialogues process, and all of them contribute to their goal of improving health communication and policy. Here is how the program describes what they do:

> The Global Dialogues process, steadily expanded and enhanced since the project began in 1997, includes five interconnected, mutually reinforcing components.
>
> **Youth voice & social mobilization.** Global Dialogues outreach teams operating at community level and online engage young people in innovative, participatory activities designed to stimulate and amplify youth voice. In international contests, young people express themselves by creating stories, or narratives, on global public health issues and other topics of crucial importance to our world.
>
> **Social media for change.** Through creative collaboration—or, as we like to say, intercreativity—young people's stories are brought to life as Global Dialogues films or theatre presentations, made available in numerous languages, and distributed freely at community level, on the Internet and on television, reaching hundreds of millions of people every year.
>
> **The generation of new knowledge on youth perspectives through narrative inquiry.** The stories created by young people in Global Dialogues activities are systematically studied to gain new insights into youths' thoughts and feelings, concerns and dreams, challenges and solutions.
>
> **Local and global activism.** The Global Dialogues artistic productions, as well as the new knowledge generated through narrative analysis, are applied to improve policy and programs at multiple levels.
>
> **Rigorous monitoring and evaluation and open sharing of lessons and outputs.**

ARVIND SINGHAL

45 RIDING HIGH ON TARU FEVER: ENTERTAINMENT-EDUCATION BROADCASTS, GROUND MOBILIZATION AND SERVICE DELIVERY IN RURAL INDIA

It is possible that the worst kind of health education is when there is an older person standing in the front of the room and wagging his or her finger at you. Even if the teacher knows a great deal of information—things that you were not aware of—this style of delivery can make students not want to listen to the message. In Global Health, effective communication must be more than the delivery of biomedical information.

When Kate Winskell and Dan Enger first started Scenarios from Africa (see the Box in Conceptual Tools), they found that some young people in the areas where they were working only knew about the HIV virus as this "round spikey thing," and they thought that a person could have unsafe sex one night and develop full-blown AIDS the next day. Misinformation and rumors abound in low-resource settings, where factual material may not be easily accessible—as well as in high-resource settings, where misinformation is promoted, for example, on social media.

The goal of Health Communication is to encourage behavior change—for individuals, as well as communities. This is not easy to accomplish. It might be impossible to change someone else's behavior totally, but you can move them to the next stage in a pathway to change (see Figures CT12.1 and CT12.2 in Conceptual Tools). Nudges from the right people can be helpful, like an inspirational role model or the enthusiastic support of a group of peers. Conversely, it is possible to encourage people to avoid certain behavioral decisions, like engaging in unprotected sex, by providing clear stories about the actual consequences; a good example is the reality series 16 and Pregnant *on MTV, which actually reduced teen pregnancy.*

This article is about a health communication project conducted in Bihar, the poorest state in India. The approach is called entertainment-education. The aim of the program was to change social norms around gender—a very complex and difficult task. The strategy was to develop a fictional weekly radio show aimed at rural poor communities. The storyline of the show—one might call it a soap opera—focuses on the adventures of a girl named Taru and her friend Shashikant. Taru is the star, and she is designed to be a role model for young women. Embedded within Taru's adventures and interactions with her family and members of the community are nudging messages for change in behavior and attitudes.

Sometimes, fictive behaviors from entertainment-education storylines become reality. The birthday party described at the beginning of this article is just one example, but there are many more examples from entertainment-education programs around the world.

The entertainment-education package described in this article goes beyond the simple radio drama to include the organization of Taru clubs, where women and girls can chat about the stories. In a rural village where life can be rather boring, the Taru radio show became a smash hit; there was so much excitement that it was called "Taru fever." The goal of the show and clubs is to encourage discussion within communities about topics that are seldom discussed. This is similar to the process of Scenarios for Africa in that group screenings of the short films are designed to open discussions.

As you read the following article, consider the following questions:

- **Do people in Global Health have the right to try to change other cultures?**
- **In the weekly drama, Taru never makes an actual speech or lecture. In your opinion, what might be the advantage of this type of indirect messaging?**

Excerpt from *Riding High on Taru Fever,* by Arvind Singha. Oxford: Oxfam, 2010.

- **In the United States, certain television shows have been credited with helping change cultural attitudes about homosexuality, race and women's rights. Can you think of any specific examples? How do entertaining stories nudge people to think or act in a different way?**
- **What do you think of Bandura's famous experiment with children and the videos of Bobo the clown? Do you think that watching violent shows (or video games) causes violent behavior?**
- **Just watching a program or movie is a rather passive experience. What do you think might be the advantages of conducting organized discussion groups for encouraging social change?**

CONTEXT

Arvind Singhal is a professor of Communication and the director of the Social Justice Initiative at the University of Texas, El Paso. He is the editor or co-author of twelve books in the areas of the diffusion of innovations, the positive deviance approach, organizing for social change, the entertainment-education strategy and liberating interactional structures. This article was written for OxFam Netherlands as part of a "wisdom series" on Entertainment-Education and Social Change.

Taru, A Radio Soap Opera, Rewrites Gender Roles

In the second year of the 21st century, 2002 to be precise, in India's Bihar state, in village Madhopur, while listening to their favorite radio soap opera, *Taru*, a couple in their late-20s, hears about the celebration of a young girl's birthday in the fictional rural community of Suhagpur. A girl's birthday celebration—in rural Bihar? While a son's birthday is a cause for celebration, a daughter's birthday is a date not remembered. Boys and girls receive differential treatment in Bihar's rural society. Relative to girls, boys receive better education, nutrition, and care; they have better mobility outside of homes; and are more pampered by parents, grandparents, and community elders.

Inspired by a fictional radio soap opera, the couple decides to celebrate their daughter's birthday. The invitation is sent to all households in village Madhopur, akin to what happened in the fictional drama. As the cake is cut, many young girls in Madhopur tug their mothers' saris, asking when will they celebrate their birthday? The practice spreads. The actions of this couple in Madhopur led to a string of birthday celebrations for girls in Madhopur, complete with balloons, music, sweets, and cakes. This practice then spread to several neighboring villages of Madhopur, where *Taru* was equally popular.

Taru, broadcast by All India Radio (AIR), the Indian national radio network, during 2002-2003, was an entertainment-education radio soap opera. *Entertainment-education* is the process of purposely designing and implementing a media message to both entertain and educate in order to increase audience members' knowledge about an issue, create favorable attitudes, shift social norms, and change the overt behavior of individuals and communities. *Taru's* purpose was to promote gender equality, reproductive health, caste and communal harmony, and community development.

Each episode of *Taru* began with a theme song and a brief summary of the previous episode. Each episode ended with an epilogue that posed a

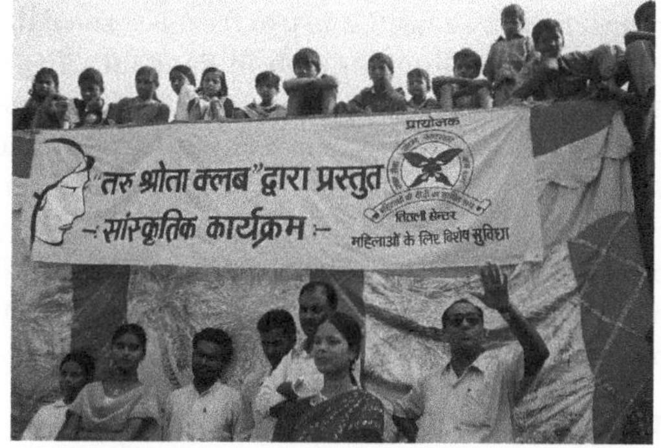

FIGURE 45.1 A *Taru* Fever Raged in Bihar's Villages before, during, and after Its Year-Long Broadcasts. Members of *Taru* listening clubs organized a wide variety of village events, including theater performances (as shown). *Photo credit:* Devendra Sharma.

question to the listeners, inviting them to write-in their responses to AIR. Thousands of audience letters were received in response.

Located a couple of miles from village Madhopur, on the other side of the main highway, is village Kamtaul where Vandana Kumari, a 17 year-old member of village Kamtaul's *Taru* listening club, also regularly listened to *Taru*. She noted: "We listen to each episode of *Taru* and discuss the episode's content in our listeners' club. After listening to this serial, we have taken decisions to wipe out caste discrimination, teach *dalit* (lower caste) children, and to pursue higher education."

In several selected villages in Bihar state, folk performances dramatizing the *Taru* storyline were carried out a week prior to the radio serial's broadcasts to prime the message reception environment. Shailendra Singh's Kamtaul village was one such site for the folk performances. Singh and his wife Sunita spread word-of-mouth messages about the folk performance, encouraging hundreds of people to attend.

Transistor radios with a sticker of *Taru's* logo were provided to groups who correctly answered questions based on the folk performance. These groups were formalized as *Taru* listening clubs. Each group received an attractive notebook (with a *Taru* logo), and were encouraged urged to discuss the social themes addressed in *Taru*, relate them to their personal circumstances, and record any decisions, or actions, they took as a result of listening to *Taru*.

RHP Shailendra Singh's daughter, Vandana, her younger sister, a cousin, and two friends formed the young women's listening club in Kamtaul village. A *Taru* fever raged in the Singh household. Discussions of *Taru* inspired the Singh family to undertake several new initiatives: They stopped a child marriage in Kamtaul village, launched an adult literacy program for *dalit* (low-caste) village women, and have facilitated the participation of *dalits* in community events, including in a wedding.

The *Taru* Narrative, Modeling New Possibilities

Taru was a 52-episode entertainment-education radio soap opera, broadcast from February, 2002 to February, 2003. The story of the radio serial revolves around Taru, a young, educated woman who works in Suhagpur village's Sheetal Center, an organization that provides reproductive health care services and carries out village self-help activities. Taru is idealistic, intelligent, and polite, and works to empower rural women. Taru is a close friend of Shashikant, who like Taru, is educated, intelligent, and involved in social work at the Sheetal Center. Shashikant is a the *dalit* (lower-caste), and is subject to discrimination by the high caste people in the village. Taru likes him for his sincerity, and he, in turn, is supportive of Taru's ameliorative efforts. While there is an undercurrent of romance between the two, they have not yet explicitly expressed it, given that Shashikant is mindful of his lower caste status (Taru belongs to an upper caste family).

Taru's mother, Yashoda, is highly supportive of Taru, whom she sees as an embodiment of her own unaccomplished dreams. On the other hand, Mangla, Taru's rogue brother, derides Taru's social work, and ridicules her friendship with the lower-caste Shashikant. With the help of Aloni Baba (a village saint) and Guruji (a teacher), Taru and Shashikant fight multiple social evils in a series of intersecting storylines, including preventing a child marriage, and encouraging girls to be treated on par with boys. In one episode, Taru and Shashikant organize a community-wide birthday celebration of a young girl, a practice hitherto unprecedented.

A subplot involves Neha, a close friend of Taru, who is newly married to Kapileshwar, the son of the local *zamindar* (landlord). Kapileshwar starts out as a controlling husband, restricting Neha's mobility outside of the home. But Neha wants to lead a meaningful life and begins a school for *dalit* (low-caste) children.

Taru, patterned after a long tradition of entertainment-education soap operas in Latin America, strategically employed media role models to promote socially-desirable behaviors, and to dissuade socially-undesirable behaviors.

The principles of media role-modeling were distilled by Professor Albert Bandura at Stanford University, who in the early-1960s conducted the famed Bobo doll experiments.[1] Young children watched a film of an adult role model beating a plastic Bobo doll, weighted at its base. The model punched, kicked, and hit the Bobo doll with his fists and a mallet. When hit, a Bobo doll falls backward and immediately springs upright as if offering a counter punch.

Children were let into a play room with several attractive toys including a Bobo doll. Interestingly, children who watched the film imitated the media model's behavior: They punched, kicked, and hit the Bobo doll. Bandura suggested that when exposed to a violent televised model, children were likely to exhibit the aggressive behavior they had observed.

Bandura's experiments also showed that audience members learn models of behavior as effectively from televised models as from ones in real-life.[3] If media models could promote aggression and other anti-social behaviors, there was no reason their power could not be tapped for pro-social purposes. Bandura's principles of role-modeling were creatively employed in the mid-1970s by Miguel Sabido, a creative writer-director-producer at Televisa, the Mexican national television network, to produce a series of entertainment-education *telenovelas* (television novels or soap operas). Between 1975 and 1982, Sabido incorporated Bandura's principles of role-modeling in seven entertainment-education *telenovela* productions.

All of Sabido's *telenovelas* were ratings hits, and evaluations suggested that they were effective in meeting their educational goals. Sabido's work in Mexico provided a systematic and codified methodology to produce entertainment-education soap operas, both for television and radio. This method then spread rapidly to other nations in Africa, Asia, and Latin America where it was adapted to local needs and conditions. Further, several home grown entertainment-education initiatives got underway (e.g. *Soul City* in South Africa, *Sexto Sentido* in Nicaragua, and Breakthrough programs in the U.S. and India), informed by on-site sensibilities and championed by local writers, producers, and directors.

Taru's Impacts

Parasocial Interaction with *Taru*

Parasocial relationships are the seemingly face-to-face interpersonal relationships that can develop between a viewer and a mass media personality.[2] The media consumer forms a relationship with a performer that is analogous to a real interpersonal relationship. When a parasocial relationship is established, the media consumer appreciates the values and motives of the media character, often viewing him or her as a counselor, comforter, and model.

Incredibly, some audience members even talk to their favorite characters (that is, to their TV or radio set) as if the characters were real people. Soni, an avid listener, in village Abirpur exemplified this intense involvement and identification: "I love Taru. She is so nice. I also like Shashikant. When Taru is sad, Shashikant makes her laugh. When Taru is sad, I am sad. When Mangla asks her to not see Shashikant, and Taru feels bad, I feel bad." Audience members view their favorite characters as close personal friends, and become emotionally upset when certain characters face difficult personal situations.

In village Kamtaul, Sunita Singh, the wife of Shailendra Singh, the village rural health practitioner, greatly admired Neha, a friend of Taru in the radio serial, who establishes a school to educate *dalit* (low-caste) children. Inspired by Neha, Sunita launched adult literacy classes for 20 lower caste women in Kamtaul's Harijan Tola (lower-caste settlement).

It is highly uncommon in an Indian rural setting for a high-caste woman to interact with women of lower castes. "If Neha could do it, so could I," Sunita Singh noted.

Parasocial interaction may be so strong that audience members adjust their daily schedules to listen to the radio program to maintain an ongoing relationship with their favorite characters. As Dhurandhar Maharaj, a male listener in Abirpur village, noted: "Every Friday at 8 p.m. I have to be close to my radio. They come into my home. It's like meeting friends."

Conversations and Sense-Making

Our research in Bihar provides numerous examples of how *Taru* stimulated conversations among listeners, creating a social learning environment for social change.

Soni Kumari, a member of the young women's listening club in Kamtaul village noted: "Almost 50 percent of the girls in our High School [out of a total of

300] listen to *Taru*. In fact, we have even painted a wall in our school to promote the listening of *Taru*. Every Monday in School, during the break, we meet to discuss the episode broadcast the previous day."

Kumari Neha, a listening group member in Abirpur village, noted: "Our discussions of *Taru* have given us strength and confidence. Now I am not shy of speaking in front of my parents. Taru taught us that one should always speak sweetly and politely. When you mean well, who can oppose you? Even the devil will melt. We have all told our parents that we will like to go to college, and we will not marry in a household which demands dowry."

Collective Efficacy Stimulated by *Taru*

Discussions, dialogue, and conversations among audience members regarding the content of a media program can clarify doubts, overcome inhibitions, and provide a sense of collective efficacy to act. *Collective efficacy* is the degree to which individuals in a system believe that they can organize and execute courses of action required to achieve collective goals. Collective efficacy helps to promote meaningful social change because such change is embedded within a network of social influences.

There were dozens of instances of *Taru* inspiring collective efficacy and community action to solve social problems. In Abirpur village, young female and male members of *Taru* listeners' groups, after seven months of discussion and deliberation, started an open-air school for underprivileged children, inspired by the character of Neha in the radio serial. Some 50 children regularly attended school, meeting six days a week, from 4 to 6 p.m. by the village well.

Four young women, all avid listeners of *Taru*, teach these children. Young men helped convince the parents to send their children to school and help with the operational logistics. Establishing the school was a collective act of both young men and women in Abirpur. Such mixed-sex collaboration is highly uncommon in Indian villages.

Power and Resistance in Social Change

While there was clear evidence that exposure to *Taru* stimulated interpersonal discussions about educational issues and motivated some listeners to engage in collective action to solve community problems, our data also suggested, consistent with our previous findings of the effects of E-E soap operas, that social change seldom flows directly and immediately from exposure to an entertainment-education media program that prompts parasocial interaction.

Instead, audience individuals who are exposed to the program may create a social learning environment in which new behavior options are considered but they discover that change often proceeds in a circuitous manner.

What works for a media character may not work so easily in real-life situations in which there is community resistance to new behaviors. Certain community members may develop a sense of collective efficacy in solving a social problem, but the solution they devise may not be effective. Although a person may say that they believe in performing a certain action, these beliefs may not reflect his or her actions.

One may argue that all such intentions in support of behavior change are important, even if that talk is not always supported by subsequent action. Thus, a mother who talks to her daughter about gender equality may influence her daughter to further her formal education, even though the mother still acts under patriarchal dominance. Neeraj Kumari, a family listeners' group member in Abirpur village, who plays the role of a traditional *bahu* (daughter-in-law), tending to the needs of her in-laws, husband, and two young children, noted: "My life is the way it is. But my children will marry whom they want. ...we will not give or take dowry."

Gudiya, a young listener in Madhopur said: "I don't know how life will turn out for me, but I will definitely make my daughter like Taru."

Participatory Theater

A few months after the *Taru* broadcasts were over, our project team members[3] returned to Bihar to organize participatory theater workshops for members of *Taru* listening clubs from four villages.

The week-long workshops were designed to empower each group and its members to develop participatory theatrical performances to capture their individual and group listening experiences in relation to *Taru* and their concomitant attempts to

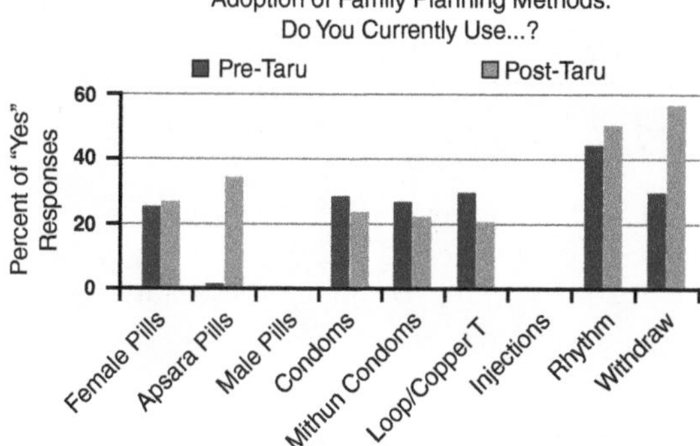

FIGURE 45.2 Adoption of Family Planning Methods: Do You Currently Use . . . ?

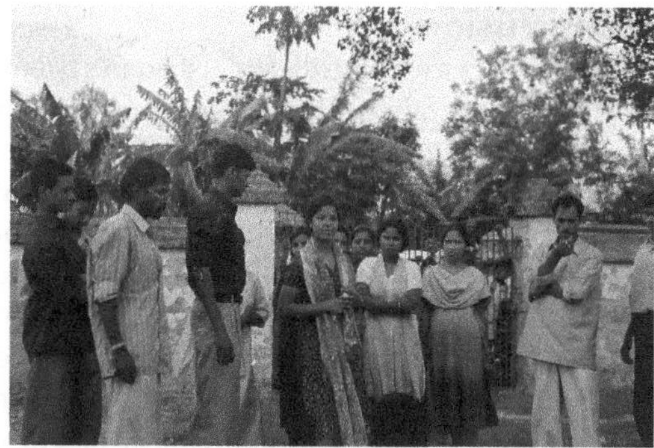

FIGURE 45.4 Rehearsals during the Participatory Theater Workshop with *Taru* Listeners.

Photo credit: Devendra Sharma.

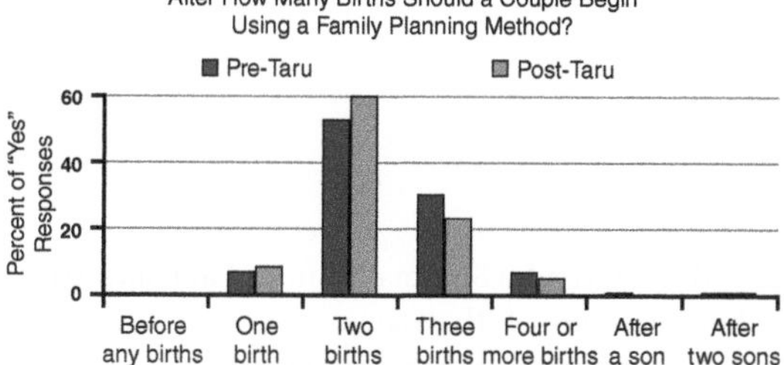

FIGURE 45.3 After How Many Births Should a Couple Begin Using a Family Planning Method?

secure political and social reform in their respective villages. These folk performances were then staged for village members to bring participants' narratives into the realm of public discourse. Participants were encouraged to use the tools of theater to acquire new ways of knowing reality and sharing that knowledge with others.

Our participatory theater efforts were in the same mold as Augusto Boal's Theater of the Oppressed, where theater is a form of "rehearsal" for people who want to give voice to their experiences and discover new ways of fighting against oppression in their daily lives. By rehearsing, and potentially accepting or rejecting, solutions to articulated problems, participants have opportunities to "try out" counter-narratives.

During the theater workshops, participants developed skills in script writing, character development, costume and set design, voice projection and body control, and acting and singing. The workshops were followed by two days of public performances. No professional actors were used in the performances; instead, participants served as cast members and as directors and set managers. Performances were promoted in advance through word-of-mouth, capitalizing on the contacts of the local RHPs, as well as family members and friends of the workshops participants. Live folk and popular songs were played on the loudspeaker to bring people to the performance site.

Each play was publicly performed in each of the four villages for audiences that ranged in numbers from 300-500 people. Interspersed with the plays were a folk dance, some songs, and a poem—all initiated and created by the participants. In each village, we situated the performance site in an open area that was easily accessible to residents. We strategically positioned women at the front of the audience, with men clustered behind them, and, in so doing, subverted the dominance usually exerted by men on such occasions. Many women who were not allowed to leave their home (e.g., young married women) watched from the terrace of their home. When space ran short, onlookers perched themselves on trees or terraces to view the performances.

Strong social networks were created among participants through this participatory theater project, networks that have remained intact and grown stronger since we left Bihar.

In Conclusion

The *Taru* project represented a watershed in systematically and strategically integrating on-air entertainment-education broadcasts with on-the-ground mobilization of opinion leaders and local service delivery. It provided an unprecedented opportunity to triangulate various quantitative and qualitative research methods to more deeply understand the effects that E-E programs have, and also the mechanisms through which such effects occur, are maintained, and can be enhanced. The *Taru* project experimented with a variety of interactive and participatory research approaches, including use of video testimony, photography, and theater. By handing over the means of producing knowledge to respondents, a deeper, richer, and more nuanced audience-centered perspective emerged in our sense-making of E-E interventions.

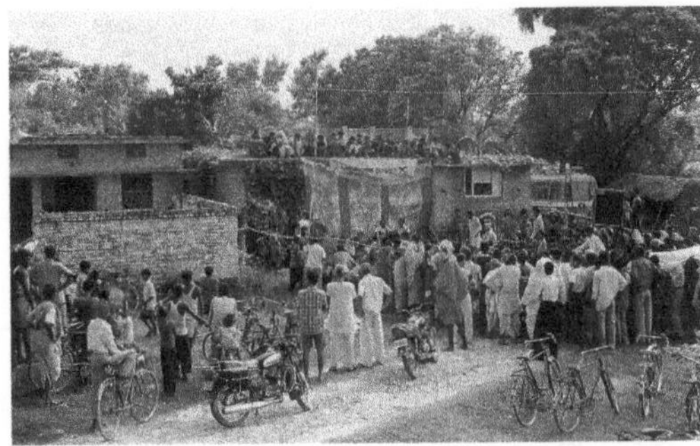

FIGURE 45.5 A *Taru* Participatory Theater Performance in a Bihar Village Where Dozens of Spectators Were Perched on Bicycles, Rooftops and Even Trees.

Photo credit: Devendra Sharma.

REFERENCES

1. Albert Bandura (1977). *Social Learning Theory.* Englewood Cliffs, NJ: Prentice-Hall.
2. D. Horton and R. R. Wohl (1956). Mass communication and para-social interaction. *Psychiatry*, 19, 215–229.
3. Led by Devendra Sharma, Saumya Pant, and Yogita Sharma—all, at that time, doctoral students in communication at Ohio University.

AMZATH FASSASSI

and

CLARE CHANDLER, JAMES FAIRHEAD, ANN KELLY, MELISSA LEACH, FREDERICK MARTINEAU, ESTHER MOKUWA, MELISSA PARKER, PAUL RICHARDS AND ANNIE WILKINSON, FOR THE EBOLA RESPONSE ANTHROPOLOGY PLATFORM

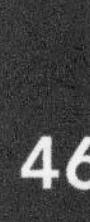

46 MANAGING RUMORS AND MISINFORMATION IN WEST AFRICA *and* EBOLA: LIMITATIONS OF CORRECTING MISINFORMATION

In 2014, the worst outbreak of Ebola in history happened in West Africa. From a few initial cases in Guinea, the disease spread to around 28,000 people, and more than 11,000 people died. Health workers, who did not always have the necessary protective equipment to keep them from contacting the disease, were at particular risk. People across the world panicked.

Communicating accurate information to help people protect themselves from infection and to minimize stigma against those who did not have the disease or had recovered were very important health goals. These two articles discuss the communication response to the Ebola outbreak.

We almost did not include the first of these articles in this reader. We were concerned that when students read about the kinds of rumors that were flying around during the Ebola epidemic some readers might reach the incorrect conclusion that poor people in Africa (or even rich people in Africa) were somehow uniquely susceptible to disease rumors.

In the end, we decided to include it, because wherever epidemics occur, fear and rumors are often not far behind. Ebola rumors were not confined to West Africa. In the United States, for example, fear and rumors ran wild during the Ebola epidemic—despite the fact that we had only a handful of cases of the disease. Politicians rushed to put quarantines into place (even as most public health professionals pointed out that they would do no good—and might discourage health professionals from going to West Africa to help with the outbreak). Nightmare scenarios that the Ebola virus might "go airborne" were repeated on the media. Antivaccine sites on the Internet spread fake news that Ebola was being spread deliberately just to create a market for a vaccine (despite the fact that a life-saving vaccine didn't yet exist). These fears and rumors created stigma that made things difficult for people coming back from West Africa, as well as for West African communities in the United States.

If these distant threats scared Americans thousands of miles away, just imagine the fear of the people living in the center of the epidemic. As described in Packard's history of Global Health (Reading #37), the primary reasons for the spread of Ebola (a disease that had been known for decades) was the weakness of the health care system. But instead of emphasizing the impoverished conditions of the health system, mass media sources from the wealthy North chose to emphasize the role of traditional cultural practices and a lack of cooperation by local people. This was one type of ethnocentric miscommunication associated with the epidemic that blamed the victims of the disease.

In thinking about how best to communicate information to people that they need to keep themselves healthy, there are a few concepts that can be useful to keep in mind.

Amzath Fassassi, "Managing Rumours and Misinformation in West Africa," April 29, 2015. http://www.scidev.net/global/ebola/feature/ebola-rumours-misinformation-west-africa.html. Clare Chandler, James Fairhead, Ann Kelly et al. "Ebola: Limitations of Correcting Misinformation." *The Lancet*, 2015, 385(9975): 1275–1277.

*First, the **fallacy of empty vessels** is that people in other societies (so-called target populations) do not have any health knowledge or beliefs. In reality, however, all people already have their own ethnomedical beliefs and practices, and these preexisting beliefs influence how new ideas are accepted. Understanding that people receive health messages within the context of their own beliefs is essential to achieve effective communication between health promoters and the public.*

Second, people's behavior is almost always understandable and logical within their own social and cultural context. The challenge, therefore, is to understand the "other's" point of view when developing health communication programs. People's behavior is not just about beliefs but is also shaped by their particular conditions of social class and their access to resources.

Third, questions of compliance or adherence are linked to issues of power. There are power differentials between the givers and receivers of health messages. Health-care providers are in a more powerful position, and they may expect their suggestions to be followed simply because of these power differences. Health-care providers sometimes perceive patient noncompliance as a problem of disobedience, and they expect the receivers of health messages to comply like obedient and powerless children. This attitude does not fit well with a model of partnership.

Fourth, many people's responses to epidemics, across the world, will be religious. Anthropologists argue that religion, defined in its broadest sense, is a universal aspect of all cultures. Religion includes beliefs that help people make sense of the world in times of crisis—like the crises of disease and death. Religion also involves rituals and practices that are associated with the belief system. Some of these practices are aimed at keeping people healthy by reducing risk of divine retribution, while other can be requests for divine healing. Religious responses to disease are not exotic or primitive—they are human.

Fifth, beyond religion, the meaning people ascribe to an illness in a particular setting is reflective of larger social, political, economic or moral concerns. When faced with a new and frightening disease, people make sense of it in larger moral terms. In a world of gross economic inequalities, there are significant moral elements reflected in the illness experience of individuals.

Sixth, stigma is a very important factor to consider in health communication programs. Stigma is the negative social attribution placed on people because a disability or illness makes her or him different or "not normal" according to local social rules. Stigma is often the result of fear, and it leads to long-lasting suffering.

Global Health efforts to stop the spread of Ebola were large, expensive, and required the courage of many health care workers who risked their lives to treat the sick. Yet, these health care workers were shunned and stigmatized.

Seventh, the illness experience may include social and psychological dimensions—like stigma—that cannot be cured with medicine. Attention to the human aspects of the illness experience is not a strength of biomedicine. In fact, many see that this major failing of biomedicine is the reason more and more people in the United States use alternative health-care systems. The human suffering of some illnesses may be in the form of discrimination, stigma, damaged self-concept and social ostracism. Suffering related to the social and psychological dimensions of illness may be worse and last longer than the disease itself; this is especially the case with chronic illnesses and highly feared illnesses like Ebola. The social meanings of illnesses can also vary from culture to culture.

Finally, trust is important. Widespread fear in social groups, as in the case of an epidemic disease like Ebola, can result not simply in scapegoating and discrimination against individuals but also in violence and forced displacement of large groups of people. Social tensions between groups can lead to a lack of trust and cooperation in times of emergency. Fear of new diseases or fear of government entities can hamper the reporting of disease outbreaks. Combating new emerging diseases, which can spread rapidly throughout the world because of airline travel, requires mutual trust and international cooperation.

As you read these pieces, consider these questions, posed by the authors of the second piece. They are relevant far beyond Ebola to nearly all health communication programs.

- **Will improving people's biomedical knowledge lead to behavior change?**
- **Should local activities be regarded as "exotic behavior"?**
- **How helpful is the message that biomedicine is the most effective way to understand and respond to disease?**
- **Are messages and modes of delivery for public health information that are standardized across contexts appropriate?**

CONTEXT

Amzath Fassassi, the author of the first article, is a reporter for the website SciDev.net. The authors of the second article, which appeared in the influential journal *The Lancet*, all contributed to the Ebola Response Anthropology Platform (http://www.ebola-anthropology.net/), a website designed to share information and analysis on how to understand political and cultural dimensions of the Ebola epidemic. The emphasis of the website is on practical information that people designing communication programs or interventions during the epidemic could use.

At the height of the Ebola epidemic, when hundreds of people died every day in West Africa, panic spread. In radio broadcasts and stories spread by word of mouth, Ebola was portrayed as an inescapable, apocalyptic threat. Jérôme Mouton, head of the Médecins Sans Frontières (MSF) response team in Guinea, said that Ebola was used as a source of horror in literature and movies across West Africa, turning the disease into a "big scarecrow." "The first messages that were broadcast portrayed Ebola as a disease that kills almost every time and one that has no cure," he said. "With such messages, to obtain a rational and thoughtful response from the population was obviously not easy. Instead of appeasing, rescue teams, in some situations, reinforced fear."

Meanwhile, misinformation was also spreading over the Internet. From the onset of the crisis, health authorities tried to use social networks such as Twitter and Facebook to distribute information on Ebola and gather hints on where their response teams might be needed next. But although social networks reach many people, it soon became clear they were not always an appropriate forum in which to discuss complex issues. Information about Ebola's spread and prevention got muddled, warped and hyped. Social media users spread half-truths and rumours in an environment already gripped by a general panic, propagating misinformation quickly.

This was exacerbated by the lack of reliable conventional media channels to broadcast reliable information. In fact, in the rush for sensational news, some traditional media outlets repeated ridiculous rumors that Ebola was a "Zombie disease" sent by God to punish atheists. Some news channels blatantly harnessed misconceptions to further their own goals, for example by playing on existing political and ethnic rivalries in the country, said Charles Vieira Sanches, the senior program manager for West Africa's branch of Article 19, an NGO working to defend freedom of speech. For instance, in Guinea the leader of the opposition party claimed that the ruling party were selectively spreading Ebola to the forested regions of the nation. Sanches and his team initiated a number of awareness campaigns on social networks, and tried to limit the political damage and social unrest this rumor and others like it were doing.

According to Sanches, the Ebola crisis flagged up the health services' inability to maintain clear information channels when faced with an epidemic. The lack of trust between the general public and the region's political and social elite only increased the problem. Sanches thinks this explains why Ebola even broke out in communities that were already under the care of health workers.

Mystical Explanations

In West Africa, many people responded to the disease by seeking out traditional healing, despite government efforts to discourage such practices. And sometimes, the witchcraft remedies would appear to work.

Sylvain Faye, a social anthropologist working with the WHO in Guinea, reported a case where a patient tested positive for Ebola and went to see a traditional healer. He was later tested again, and that time declared Ebola-free. Regardless of whether the test or the man's initial symptoms were misinterpreted, Faye and his team feared that such incidents increased beliefs that the disease was being deliberately spread by international organizations.

The idea that Ebola was a supernatural evil also meant that those who got infected often doubted their ability to recover. SaaSabasse Tèmèsadouno, a health worker at Guéckédou hospital in Guinea, was infected with Ebola while caring for other victims. As a medical assistant, Tèmèsadouno had some basic knowledge about the virus. But he still doubted his own ability to recover due to persistent rumours that Ebola was caused by witchcraft. "After I got infected many people kept saying I had no chance of surviving because there was no cure for Ebola and I started to fear the worst." Fortunately, he did recover.

Transparency Strategy

It took a long time for response teams and international health agencies to take misinformation on Ebola and its effect on local people seriously. Keita admits that the disease's social effects were "initially put aside in our technical planning." It was not until the height of the epidemic, around July 2014, that response teams realised how the social constraints generated by misinformation prevented them from stopping the epidemic. "We therefore had to take these parameters into consideration," adds Keita.

To address rumors, health authorities called in social anthropologists for advice, and used information relays such as radio and newspapers, artists, and religious and community leaders. One essential part of the strategy, according to MSF's Jérôme Mouton, was to make treatment centers and what goes on inside them more transparent to the general population. From the start, health workers had experienced problems related to these centers. Since Ebola patients need to be strictly isolated and will, for a time, only come in contact with people in strange-looking protection coats, the experience of being taken away to a center is traumatizing both for patients and their relatives.

Mouton said that this "isolation aspect" of the disease fed the rumors. "When people do not know what's going on, they imagine all sorts of terrible things," he says. "For instance, there were rumors that the centers were used for organ trafficking. No one, under such circumstances, would want to be treated in our centers." MSF decided to be clearer about how Ebola treatments work and to let healthy people look around into freshly opening health stations. He said that once are convinced of the value for their communities to temporarily suspend certain traditions in the interest of public health, communication with the population became much easier. When MSF inaugurated new centers, they would ask the population to visit them and understand what they were all about. Stressing the need for better communication, the response teams persuaded religious and community leaders to speak to the population so they understood the ins and outs of the disease.

Surmountable Challenge

The communication problems were not an insurmountable clash between tradition and modernity. MSF found that patiently and sensitively distributing accurate information about Ebola treatment and prevention did work—and it was more effective than trying to debunk witchcraft and traditional medicine. Mouton said that "Once people are convinced of the value for their communities to temporarily suspend certain traditions in the interest of public health, communication with the population becomes much easier." But such information campaigns are complicated and time-consuming, especially in the midst of an all-out health crisis. "These are things that can only be addressed at the community level through talking directly to the population."

While MSF took communication down to the micro level, The Article 19 NGO, devoted to free speech in Africa, focused on relaying information and fighting Ebola stereotypes online. The Article 19 team had to battle distrust of health workers and international aid agencies among local people and the authorities. Sanches, the leader of the team said "There was some distrust in organizations perceived as the invisible hands of the West." Putting out reassuring messages on social media helped counter such ideas, but it was only through a mix of information channels, including broadcasting and word of mouth, that opinions on Ebola were finally changed.

Article 19 used its #SenStopEbola (Senegal Stop Ebola) initiative to convince popular bloggers to focus their writing on the disease. They asked the writers to prioritize posts that addressed and cleared up rumors and misunderstandings. The organization also worked with popular artists, including

Ivory Coast reggae music star Tiken Jah Fakoly, to give its messages more clout.

As of April 2015, a year after the height of the outbreak, Ebola is abating and life in West Africa is slowly returning to normal. Nonetheless, the epidemic killed more than 10,000 people and devastated families, villages and communities. It is difficult to know whether the disease might have progressed differently if misinformation had been addressed sooner. But it is clear to all those who experienced the outbreak that addressing fears and rumors head-on was crucial to getting on top of the virus. Mouton, head of the MSF Ebola mission said that the panic caused by the epidemic explains why even the most outlandish Ebola rumors were so easily believed. "Fear is an important part of all problems we had to face while dealing with the Ebola epidemic. Fear has never helped people to think in a sensible manner. When we are scared, we no longer act rationally."

Communication and social mobilisation strategies to raise awareness about Ebola virus disease and the risk factors for its transmission are central elements in the response to the current Ebola outbreak in west Africa.[1] A principle underpinning these efforts is to change risky "behaviour" related to "traditional" practices and "misinformation." Populations at risk of contracting Ebola virus disease have been exhorted to "put aside, tradition, culture and whatever family rites they have and do the right thing."[2] Messages designed to correct perceived misunderstandings[3] include: "Ebola is caused by a virus. Ebola is not caused by a curse or by withcraft";[4] "science and medicine are our only hope";[5] and "traditions kill."[5]

Such messages follow logically from clinical and epidemiological framings of contagion. They pay little attention, however, to the historical, political, economic, and social contexts in which they are delivered. Furthermore, they reinforce external perceptions that local beliefs and practices are barriers to be overcome through persuasion or counterbalanced with incentives.[6] Such characterisations have been counterproductive in previous Ebola outbreaks.[7] We propose four questions to scrutinise some of the assumptions about current Ebola social mobilisation strategies.

First, will improving people's biomedical knowledge of Ebola lead to desired behaviour changes? Efforts to change what people do through biomedical information alone can be ineffective. Communicating knowledge about why people should wash their hands with soap, sleep under a bednet, or change their sexual practices is known to be insufficient to induce behavioural changes in practice,[8,9] usually because of people's other priorities. The situation with regard to Ebola seems to be following suit.[10] Biomedical information on risk might hold limited relevance to people when trying to care for sick loved ones or attend to the dead. Other approaches that start by addressing people's priorities need to be considered when attempting to influence health-related activities.

Second, should local activities be regarded as "exotic behaviour"? Caring for the sick is an intensely practical endeavour. Public health framings of Ebola, however, often portray caring practices as irrational and immutable traditions.[11] This perception reflects a lack of genuine engagement in the material, social, or spiritual implications of changing social practices. In many parts of Sierra Leone, Liberia, and Guinea, burial practices often incorporate procedures to distribute inheritance and ensure the deceased an afterlife. Failing to conduct funerals appropriately may cast family members as negligent, or foster suspicion of malicious causes of death; these concerns can override health considerations.[12] To disregard such concerns and take an inflexible stance in negotiating mutually acceptable courses of action precludes any genuine demonstration of respect or empathy for that person's situation.

Third, how helpful is the message that biomedicine is the most effective way to understand and respond to Ebola? The idea of trying to shift people's framings away from so-called traditional beliefs is embedded in the public health view of biomedicine as the only valid way to understand and respond to illness. From the perspective of afflicted people, however, the evidence that biomedicine is helping communities affected by Ebola can be hard to discern. Health facilities have been sources of Ebola transmission[13] and many patients admitted to treatment centres do not survive. How can trust be established or collaboration developed if local people are expected to accept ideas and practices that do not accord with their own observations and experiences? In the context of a general willingness to adopt multiple modalities to achieve care and wellbeing, safer practices can be adopted without changing people's core beliefs.[14]

Fourth, are standardised messages and modes of delivery for public health information about Ebola appropriate? Public health framings generally assume that standardised protocols that deliver "correct" health information through the "right" medium are needed to change behaviour. Protocols are typically developed at national or international levels rather than collaboratively with the people who are expected to change their behaviour. When rolled out rapidly at scale, the standardisation of messages is treated as paramount in country plans; an operational logic that hinges on the use of mass media and rote training of community liaison workers. Such a standardised approach discourages adaptation, prohibits engagement with local social realities, and ignores how people will interpret public health messages according to specific local political and social circumstances.

Engagement across communities with flexible protocols that communicate problems, request help in developing local solutions, and enable their implementation are likely to be more effective in changing high risk practices than standardised approaches. As households and communities have made clear when given the chance, what they would like is practical information about risk factors for Ebola transmission and, crucially, how to reduce risks when caring for the sick and burying the dead, as well as the material resources necessary to put this advice into practice.[7, 15]

As members of the Ebola Response Anthropology Platform, we call on all organisations involved in the response to the Ebola outbreak to question the assumption that biomedicine must correct local logics and concerns, and the effectiveness of using standardised advice for non-standardised situations. Those tasked with asking people to change practices and activities associated with Ebola transmission should be allowed the time and flexibility to negotiate mutually agreed changes that are locally practical, socially acceptable, as well as epidemiologically appropriate. Resulting approaches to managing the crisis are likely to be diverse but locally sustainable, provided they are developed with respect for local people and their priorities and resourced appropriately. Otherwise, we warn that a focus on correcting "misinformation" could do more harm than good.

REFERENCES

1. WHO, The Governments of Guinea, Liberia, and Sierra Leone. Ebola virus disease outbreak response plan in West Africa, July–December, 2014. Geneva: World Health Organization, 2014.
2. McMahon B. Sierra Leone News: Sierra Leoneans should lead the Ebola fight. *Awoko* Oct 13, 2014.
3. Oyeyemi SO, Gabarron E, Wynn R. Ebola, Twitter, and misinformation: a dangerous combination? *BMJ* 2014; **349**: g6178.
4. Centers for Disease Control and Prevention. Together we can prevent Ebola. 2014. http://www.cdc.gov/vhf/ebola/pdf/bannerforebolasierraleonev2.pdf (accessed Dec 11, 2014).
5. The Communication Initiative. Ebola: a poem for the living—video. Oct 21, 2014. http://www.comminit.com/ci-ebola/content/ebola-poem-living-video (accessed Dec 11, 2014).
6. Piot P, Muyembe JJ, Edmunds WJ. Ebola in west Africa: from disease outbreak to humanitarian crisis. *Lancet Infect Dis* 2014; **14**: 1034–35.
7. Hewlett B, Hewlett B. Ebola, culture and politics: the anthropology of an emerging disease. Belmont, CA: Wadsworth, 2007.
8. Yoder PS. Negotiating relevance: belief, knowledge, and practice in international health projects. *Med Anthropol Q* 1997; **11**: 131–46.

9. Aboud FE. Virtual special issue introduction: health behaviour change. *Soc Sci Med* 2010; **71:** 1897–900.
10. Fischer M, Kletzing M. Is sensitisation effective in changing behaviour to prevent Ebola transmission? Start Fund Project Case Study. 2014. http://www.start-network.org/wp-content/uploads/2014/09/Start-Fund-SLE-case-study.pdf (accessed Dec 15, 2014).
11. Jones J. Ebola, emerging: the limitations of culturalist discourses in epidemiology. *J Glob Health* 2011; **1:** 1–6.
12. Richards P, Amara J, Ferme MC, et al. Social pathways for Ebola virus disease in rural Sierra Leone, and some implications for containment. *PLoS Neglected Tropical Diseases Blog* Oct 31, 2014. http://blogs.plos.org/speakingofmedicine/2014/10/31/social-pathways-ebola-virus-disease-rural-sierra-leone-implications-containment/(accessed Dec 15, 2014).
13. Forrester JD, Hunter JC, Pillai SK, et al. Cluster of Ebola cases among Liberian and US health care workers in an ebola treatment unit and adjacent hospital—Liberia, 2014. *MMWR Morb Mortal Wkly Rep* 2014; **63:** 925–29.
14. Leach MA, Fairhead JR, Millimouno D, Diallo AA. New therapeutic landscapes in Africa: parental categories and practices in seeking infant health in the Republic of Guinea. *Soc Sci Med* 2008; **66:** 2157–67.
15. Anoko JN. Communication with rebellious communities during an outbreak of Ebola virus disease in Guinea: an anthropological approach. 2014. http://www.ebola-anthropology.net/case_studies/communication-with-rebellious-communities-during-an-outbreak-of-ebola-virus-disease-in-guinea-an-anthropological-approach/ (accessed Dec 11, 2014).

SECTION 12 CASES FOR TEACHING AND LEARNING

Visit the companion website, www.oup.com/us/brown-closser, for direct links to the featured online resources.

S. Arnquist and R. Weintraub, *loveLife: Preventing HIV Among South African Youth*
This case explores the HIV prevention program loveLife in South Africa. Students learn about the messaging and social mobilization strategies of the program and consider what to do when the program loses a funding source. There is a follow-up case online.

Castens et al., *Alcohol Abuse in Urban Moshi, Tanzania*
In this case, students must consider options to decrease alcohol use, which is a major cause of traumatic brain injury, at a hospital in Moshi, Tanzania. Students weigh a range of policy options including legislation restricting alcohol sales and increasing punishments for drunk driving, as well as tax policies and health education.

Leigh Gantner, *Food Advertising Policy in the United States*
This case explores the US industry of marketing food to children and its impacts on health. Students learn about the regulatory agencies involved in the United States and propose a policy for regulating food marketing aimed at children. It could be used with the following case focusing on childhood obesity prevention in California.

Lindsey Cox McDermid and Nancy M. Kane, *Childhood Obesity Prevention in California*
In this case, students take the perspective of California public health officials during the Schwarzenegger administration. Students consider a range of policy options to prevent childhood obesity, including (but not limited to) education campaigns.

Napolitano et al., *Cervical Cancer and its Impact on the Burden of Disease*
Students are tasked with presenting a cervical cancer prevention program to the Tanzanian Ministry of Health, including determining how best to educate the public about the use of Pap smears. This case, written in 2012, does not consider HPV vaccination.

SECTION 12 VIDEOS AND WEB RESOURCES

Visit the companion website, www.oup.com/us/brown-closser, for direct links to the featured online resources.

Examples of Entertainment Education

Scenarios from Africa
This organization, featured in the text, develops short films about HIV/AIDS. The films, along with information on how they are made, are available on their website. More information on this program is in the Conceptual Tools for this section (see box "Global Dialogues").

Dumb Ways to Die
This video promoting safety on Australian trains was a global sensation, with over 150 million views on YouTube. Students can discuss how this video may be different than what they think of as a public health campaign, and consider the characteristics of this video that made it so popular.

Steps for the Future
This website features a series of short films around issues of human rights and social justice in southern Africa.

Educational Resources

Hesperian Foundation
This website includes free downloads of a wealth of educational books, including the classic *Where There Is No Doctor,* in a variety of languages. This organization is also featured in this section's Conceptual Tools (see box "Hesperian Health Guides").

Ebola

***In the Shadow of Ebola* – Independent Lens**
This compelling documentary explores issues of infrastructure and communication during the Ebola outbreak in Liberia. (23 min)

Body Team 12
This Oscar-nominated short film follows a team tasked with taking the bodies of Ebola victims in Liberia away from their families. This moving documentary would pair well with the readings in this section. (13 min)

Vaccination

Vaccines – *Last Week Tonight with John Oliver*
Comedian John Oliver delivers a funny, raunchy, flame-throwing and scientifically accurate discussion of the controversy over the connection between vaccines and autism in the United States. The piece is an entertaining primer on why the public health community strongly supports vaccination. (27 min)

Vaccines: Calling the Shots – *NOVA*
This NOVA episode clearly explains the science behind how vaccines work. It includes discussion of vaccine fears in the United States, including interviews with public health experts on vaccine refusals. (53 min)

SECTION

13

Ethics, Projects and Human Rights: The Future of Global Health

This section of the book is designed to help you think about ethical issues involved in Global Health programs and research. Usually, in professional graduate training there is relatively little discussion of ethics, except in terms of the ethical conduct of research. But Global Health is much more than just research projects, because the implementation of projects can have unintended negative consequences. Some projects fail, even though the failures might have been anticipated, and waste a lot of money and resources. Is a naïve project an ethical failure? Maybe that depends on whose money is being spent.

This section starts with a discussion of "health as a human right." Philosophically, the claim that health is a human right makes a great deal of sense, but there is a large gap between the ideals and the practical realities—especially when it is necessary to ration clinical healthcare because there are not enough resources for everyone everywhere. For students interested in international law, the topic of human rights should be an interesting one.

The next reading emphasizes the need for humility in global health. The idea of "quit trying to save the world" is really a useful one to think about. Undergraduates sometimes tell us that they want to "give back." However, we have to answer the question with a question—give back *what* to *whom*? We don't mean to be flippant here—what we mean is that identifying a true need and developing the skills to contribute to addressing it is a complex and long-term project.

In the final chapter of the book, we provide a lot of advice. We also include thoughts about careers in Global Health from professionals working in the field—we think what they have to say is interesting, at times profound, and definitely worth paying attention to.

Everyone, every profession and every discipline can contribute to Global Health. None of us can save the world; progress must be incremental. But, there are ways that each of us can work toward a healthier world in the future.

» CONCEPTUAL TOOLS «

- **Ethics and morals both deal with the differences between right and wrong.** In the simplest sense, "morals" refer to individual decisions, whereas "ethics" refer to the agreed norms of behavior for an institution or organization. Universities and other entities have codes of ethics for the responsible conduct of research with human subjects; Institutional Review Boards oversee these. The three primary ethical principles for biomedical research, codified in the Belmont report, are *respect for persons, beneficence* and *justice.*
- **The core statement of the Universal Declaration of Human Rights is "All human beings are born free and equal in dignity and rights."** This was adopted in 1948 at the establishment of the United Nations. All human rights include (i) civil and political rights (e.g., the right to life, equality before the law, and freedom of expression; (ii) economic, social and cultural rights (e.g., right to work, as well as social security, health and education; and (iii) collective rights (e.g., rights to development and self-determination. Universal human rights are often guaranteed by law in the forms of treaties, international law and other places. International human rights agreements identify obligations of governments to act in certain ways or to refrain from certain acts to promote and protect individuals or groups.
- **Human Rights are often most visible in their breach**. Violations of human rights, often by governments against their own people, occur discouragingly often. The most egregious violation is genocide. Sometimes, though, it is difficult to precisely define what is a right in a positive way; all humans have a right to water, but how much and what quality? Human rights violations caused by structural violence can often be invisible. But health disparities between groups can be an indicator of human rights problems caused by discrimination.
- The preamble of the WHO's constitution states **"The enjoyment of the highest attainable standard of health is one of the fundamental rights of every human being."** The right to health is *not* the right to be healthy. Rather it means that states must generate the conditions in which everyone can be as healthy as possible. Some illness is inevitable, but easily preventable illness is a human rights violation. This means it is the obligation of the State to provide some level of preventive and curative health care. But the determinants of health are broader than just access to medical care.
- **About two-thirds of the world's states recognize the right to health and health protection in their national constitutions; the United States is not one of them.** The right to health includes not only timely and appropriate health care but also having access to the underlying determinants of health, including security, safe water, adequate sanitation, adequate supply of food, housing, safe occupational and environmental conditions and access to accurate health-related education and information.
- **Private companies in the pharmaceutical industry need to be held accountable to international ethical principles.** The costs of drug development and testing are significant, but how do you balance the need of a company to make profit and the availability and cost of treatment for people? This is especially acute

for "neglected tropical diseases," which often affect the very poor. Because their decisions directly affect the lives and deaths of large numbers of people, the ethical obligations of pharmaceutical companies are different than those of other for-profit corporations.

- **Communication during an infectious disease outbreak can make or break public health efforts.** During health emergencies like a disease outbreak, the dual challenges of effective communication of correct scientific information while simultaneously attempting to counter panic and social overreaction raise ethical questions. People who are most affected by the disease may find that their rights are violated in the face of efforts to stem an outbreak (for a historical example, see Chapter 36). In 2017, the WHO published a detailed document called "Guidance for Managing Ethical Issues in Infectious Disease Outbreaks," which was based on lessons learned from the West African Ebola epidemic of 2015. Decisions during an outbreak need to be made on an urgent basis, often in the context of scientific uncertainty, social and institutional disruption and an overall climate of fear and distrust, and sometimes ethical considerations end up being neglected.
- **Complex humanitarian emergencies raise a wide variety of ethical issues.** The phrase "complex humanitarian emergencies" refers to widespread disruption of lives, such as civil disturbances and war. The countries most affected by such disasters generally have limited resources, underdeveloped legal and regulatory structures and health systems that lack the resilience to deal with crisis situations. In a complex, political and often dangerous environment, workers are constantly confronting often difficult ethical decisions. These issues are discussed in Chapter 33.
- **The question of how much one should help others in their time of need is a moral one.** Many people offer help in the short term when media attention is highest, but needs are often long-term ones. Part of being a genuine world citizen is accumulating knowledge about conditions in the rest of the world. There may be international agreements about what nations should *not* do, but we also need to understand our obligations to each other. Discussions of ethical issues in Global Health may appear to be only rhetorical, but they are necessary to transform moral principles into action.

47 THE RIGHT TO HEALTH

As human beings, our health and the health of those we care about is a matter of daily concern. Regardless of our age, gender, socioeconomic or ethnic background, we consider our health to be our most basic and essential asset. Ill health, on the other hand, can keep us from going to school or to work, from attending to our family responsibilities or from participating fully in the activities of our community. By the same token, we are willing to make many sacrifices if only that would guarantee us and our families a longer and healthier life. In short, when we talk about well-being, health is often what we have in mind.

The right to health is a fundamental part of our human rights and of our understanding of a life in dignity. The right to the enjoyment of the highest attainable standard of physical and mental health, *to give it its full name, is not new. Internationally, it was first articulated in the 1946 Constitution of the World Health Organization (WHO), whose preamble defines health as "a state of complete physical, mental and social well-being and not merely the absence of disease or infirmity." The preamble further states that "the enjoyment of the highest attainable standard of health is one of the fundamental rights of every human being without distinction of race, religion, political belief, economic or social condition."*

The 1948 Universal Declaration of Human Rights also mentioned health as part of the right to an adequate standard of living (art. 25). The right to health was again recognized as a human right in the 1966 International Covenant on Economic, Social and Cultural Rights.

Since then, other international human rights treaties have recognized or referred to the right to health or to elements of it, such as the right to medical care. The right to health is relevant to all States: every State has ratified at least one international human rights treaty recognizing the right to health. Moreover, States have committed themselves to protecting this right through international declarations, domestic legislation and policies and at international conferences.

This fact sheet aims to shed light on the right to health in international human rights law as it currently stands, amid the plethora of initiatives and proposals as to what the right to health may or should be. *Consequently, it does not purport to provide an exhaustive list of relevant issues or to identify specific standards in relation to them.*

The fact sheet starts by explaining what the right to health is and illustrating its implications for specific individuals and groups and then elaborates upon States' obligations with respect to the right. It ends with an overview of national, regional and international accountability and monitoring mechanisms.

As you read this selection, consider the following questions:

- **What do the authors mean by saying the "right to health" is not the same as the "right to be healthy"? What is the difference? Why is this important?**
- **Name some examples of other human rights the right to health is connected to. How are exactly are they connected, in both biological and socioeconomic terms?**
- **The articles outline three obligations of the state. Choose one and, using either your knowledge, research or examples from this book, list different programs or policies that represent this obligation.**
- **Some countries have not adopted or signed treaties that agree their citizenry have a "right to health." Why do you think this might be?**

CONTEXT

This document is a "fact sheet" released by the UN agency for human rights and the WHO. It thus represents the positions of the two UN agencies most concerned with health and human rights. This summary draws on a number of international agreements. Unlike the other selections in this book, which have introductory sections that we the co-editors wrote ourselves, the introduction to this selection (aside from the study questions) comes directly from the document itself.

Key Aspects of the Right to Health

- **The right to health is an inclusive right.** We frequently associate the right to health with access to health care and the building of hospitals. This is correct, but the right to health extends further. It includes a wide range of factors that can help us lead a healthy life. The Committee on Economic, Social and Cultural Rights, the body responsible for monitoring the International Covenant on Economic, Social and Cultural Rights, calls these the "underlying determinants of health." They include:
    - Safe drinking water and adequate sanitation;
    - Safe food;
    - Adequate nutrition and housing;
    - Healthy working and environmental conditions;
    - Health-related education and information;
    - Gender equality
- **The right to health contains freedoms.** These *freedoms* include the right to be free from non-consensual medical treatment, such as medical experiments and research or forced sterilization, and to be free from torture and other cruel, inhuman or degrading treatment or punishment.
- **The right to health contains entitlements.** These *entitlements* include:
    - The right to a system of health protection providing equality of opportunity for everyone to enjoy the highest attainable level of health;
    - The right to prevention, treatment and control of diseases;
    - Access to essential medicines;
    - Maternal, child and reproductive health;
    - Equal and timely access to basic health services;
    - The provision of health-related education and information;
    - Participation of the population in health-related decision-making at the national and community levels.
- **Health services, goods and facilities must be provided to all without any discrimination.** Non-discrimination is a key principle in human rights and is crucial to the enjoyment of the right to the highest attainable standard of health (see section on non-discrimination below).
- **All services, goods and facilities must be available, accessible, acceptable and of good quality.**
    - Functioning public health and health care facilities, goods and services must be *available* in sufficient quantity within a State.
    - They must be *accessible* physically (in safe reach for all sections of the population, including children, adolescents, older persons, persons with disabilities and other vulnerable groups) as well as financially and on the basis of non-discrimination. *Accessibility* also implies the right to seek, receive and impart health-related information in an accessible format (for all, including persons with disabilities), but does not impair the right to have personal health data treated confidentially.
    - The facilities, goods and services should also respect medical ethics and be gender-sensitive and culturally appropriate. In other words, they should be medically and culturally *acceptable*.
    - Finally, they must be scientifically and medically appropriate and of *good quality*. This

requires, in particular, trained health professionals, scientifically approved and unexpired drugs and hospital equipment, adequate sanitation and safe drinking water.

Common Misconceptions about the Right to Health

- **The right to health is NOT the same as the *right to be healthy*.** A common misconception is that the State has to guarantee us good health. However, good health is influenced by several factors that are outside the direct control of States, such as an individual's biological make-up and socioeconomic conditions. Rather, the right to health refers to the right to the enjoyment of a variety of goods, facilities, services and conditions necessary for its realization. This is why it is more accurate to describe it as the right to the *highest attainable standard* of physical and mental health, rather than an unconditional right to be healthy.
- **The right to health is NOT only a *programmatic goal* to be attained in the long term.** The fact that the right to health should be a tangible programmatic goal does not mean that no immediate obligations on States arise from it. In fact, States must make every possible effort, within available resources, to realize the right to health and to take steps in that direction without delay. Notwithstanding resource constraints, some obligations have an immediate effect, such as the undertaking to guarantee the right to health in a non-discriminatory manner, to develop specific legislation and plans of action, or other similar steps towards the full realization of this right, as is the case with any other human right. States also have to ensure a minimum level of access to the essential material components of the right to health, such as the provision of essential drugs and maternal and child health services.
- **A country's difficult financial situation does NOT absolve it from having to take action to realize the right to health.** It is often argued that States that cannot afford it are not obliged to take steps to realize this right or may delay their obligations indefinitely. When considering the level of implementation of this right in a particular State, the availability of resources at that time and the development context are taken into account. Nonetheless, no State can justify a failure to respect its obligations because of a lack of resources. States must guarantee the right to health to the maximum of their available resources, even if these are tight. While steps may depend on the specific context, all States must move towards meeting their obligations to respect, protect and fulfil.

The Link between the Right to Health and Other Human Rights

Human rights are interdependent, indivisible and interrelated. This means that violating the right to health may often impair the enjoyment of other human rights, such as the rights to education or work, and vice versa.

The importance given to the "underlying determinants of health," that is, the factors and conditions which protect and promote the right to health beyond health services, goods and facilities, shows that the right to health is dependent on, and contributes to, the realization of many other human rights. These include the rights to food, to water, to an adequate standard of living, to adequate housing, to freedom from discrimination, to privacy, to access to information, to participation, and the right to benefit from scientific progress and its applications.

It is easy to see interdependence of rights in the context of poverty. For people living in poverty, their health may be the only asset on which they can draw for the exercise of other economic and social rights, such as the right to work or the right to education. Physical health and mental health enable adults to work and children to learn, whereas ill health is a liability to the individuals themselves and to those who must care for them. Conversely, individuals' right to health cannot be realized without realizing their other rights, the violations of which are at the root of poverty, such as the rights to work, food, housing and education, and the principle of non-discrimination.

LINKS BETWEEN THE RIGHT TO HEALTH AND THE RIGHT TO WATER

Ill health is associated with the ingestion of or contact with unsafe water, lack of clean water (linked to inadequate hygiene), lack of sanitation, and poor management of water resources and systems, including in agriculture.

Most diarrhoeal disease in the world is attributable to unsafe water, sanitation and hygiene. In 2002, diarrhoea attributable to these three factors caused approximately 2.7 per cent of deaths (1.5 million) worldwide.

Core Minimum Obligation

The Committee on Economic, Social and Cultural Rights has also stressed that States have a core minimum obligation to ensure the satisfaction of minimum essential levels of each of the rights under the Covenant. While these essential levels are, to some extent, resource-dependent, they should be given priority by the State in its efforts to realize the rights under the Covenant. With respect to the right to health, the Committee has underlined that States must ensure:

- The right of access to health facilities, goods and services on a non-discriminatory basis, especially for vulnerable or marginalized groups;
- Access to the minimum essential food which is nutritionally adequate and safe;
- Access to shelter, housing and sanitation and an adequate supply of safe drinking water;
- The provision of essential drugs;
- Equitable distribution of all health facilities, goods and services.

Three Types of Obligations

State obligations fall into three categories, namely the obligations to *respect*, *protect* and *fulfil*.

The Obligation to Respect

The obligation to respect requires States to refrain from interfering directly or indirectly with the right to health.

For example, States should refrain from denying or limiting access to health-care services; from marketing unsafe drugs; from imposing discriminatory practices relating to women's health status and needs; from limiting access to contraceptives and other means of maintaining sexual and reproductive health; from withholding, censoring or misrepresenting health information; and from infringing on the right to privacy (e.g., of persons living with HIV/AIDS).

In addition, the Committee on Economic, Social and Cultural Rights underlined in its general comment N° 14 that States parties have to respect the enjoyment of the right to health in other countries.

The Obligation to Protect

The obligation to protect requires States to prevent third parties from interfering with the right to health.

States should adopt legislation or other measures to ensure that private actors conform with human rights standards when providing health care or other services (such as regulating the composition of food products); control the marketing of medical equipment and medicines by private actors; ensure that privatization does not constitute a threat to the availability, accessibility, acceptability and quality of health-care facilities, goods and services; protect individuals from acts by third parties that may be harmful to their right to health—e.g., prevent women from undergoing harmful traditional practices or third parties from coercing them to do so (by, for example, enacting laws that specifically prohibit female genital mutilation); ensure that third parties do not limit people's access to health-related information and services, including environmental health; and ensure that health professionals provide care to persons with disabilities with their free and informed consent.

In its general comment N° 14, the Committee on Economic, Social and Cultural Rights also stressed

PROTECTING THE RIGHT TO HEALTH: PATENTS AND ACCESS TO MEDICINES

The Ministerial Conference of the World Trade Organization (WTO) adopted a landmark declaration in 2001 in Doha, on the Agreement on Trade-Related Aspects of Intellectual Property Rights (TRIPS) and public health. The Doha Declaration affirms that the TRIPS Agreement should not prevent member States from taking measures to protect public health. A related decision was passed in 2003 to clarify paragraph 6 of the Doha Declaration: this decision functions as a waiver to allow, in specific circumstances, countries producing generic pharmaceutical products made under compulsory licences to export the products to importing countries that are unable to manufacture the medicines themselves. States may use these clauses to ensure medicines are accessible and affordable to their own populations.

NATIONAL HEALTH SYSTEMS

The Special Rapporteur on the right to the highest standard of health has stressed that from a right-to-health perspective, a national health system should have several components: it should include an adequate system for the collection of health data to monitor the realization of the right to health; the data must be disaggregated on certain grounds, such as sex, age and urban/rural; it should include a national capacity to produce a sufficient number of well- trained health workers who enjoy good terms and conditions of employment; a process for the preparation of right-to-health impact assessments before major health-related policies are finalized; arrangements for ensuring participation in the formulation of health policies; effective, transparent and accessible mechanisms of accountability.

In addition, the Declaration of Alma-Ata highlighted the central function played by primary health care in a country's health system (art. VI). Hence, it stressed that States must formulate national policies, strategies and plans of action to launch and sustain primary health care as part of a comprehensive national health system (art. VIII).

that States parties should prevent third parties from violating the right to health in other countries. It further noted that, when negotiating international or multilateral agreements, States parties should take steps to ensure that these instruments do not have an adverse impact on the right to health.

The Obligation to Fulfil

The obligation to fulfil requires States to adopt appropriate legislative, administrative, budgetary, judicial, promotional and other measures to fully realize the right to health.

States must, for instance, adopt a national health policy or a national health plan covering the public and private sectors; ensure the provision of health care, including immunization programmes against infectious diseases and services designed to minimize and prevent further disabilities; ensure equal access for all to the underlying determinants of health, such as safe and nutritious food, sanitation and clean water; ensure that public health infrastructures provide for sexual and reproductive services and that doctors and other medical staff are sufficient and properly trained; and provide information and counselling on health-related issues, such as HIV/AIDS, domestic violence or the abuse of alcohol, drugs and other harmful substances.

Effective and integrated health systems, encompassing health care and the underlying determinants of health, are also key to ensuring the right to the highest attainable standard of health (see National Health Systems box).

MICHAEL HOBBS

48 STOP TRYING TO SAVE THE WORLD: BIG IDEAS ARE DESTROYING INTERNATIONAL DEVELOPMENT

This article tells the stories of some big innovative ideas that were funded and initiated, and failed. They illustrate that well-meaning projects can have severe unintended consequences. They also show that programs that are scaled up with great enthusiasm can fail because they lack sufficient preliminary research or ongoing evaluations. The moral of the stories in this article is that working in Global Health and related disciplines demands humility.

Some young people want to start their own NGO, because they are inspired by people like Paul Farmer and disturbed by the gross inequalities in today's world. Unfortunately, they can overestimate their own skills while underestimating the complexity of the problems and capabilities of local people.

The old saying is that "If you want to go fast, walk alone. If you want to go far, walk together." The point is about true partnerships. Socioeconomic change that benefits everyone in a society is a long process. It cannot be achieved simply through the sudden introduction of new technologies, although they can help. It cannot be achieved simply through charity, although funding is indispensable and generosity is important. This article argues (and we agree) that progress for improved health and economic justice is best achieved by thinking small and taking small steps. It is also critically important to constantly monitor and evaluate a program to make improvements or change strategies.

One can think of the ongoing process of small improvements as "tinkering" as opposed to the idea of making "big ideas." Two important economists, William Easterly and Jeffrey Sacks, have argued about what is the best overall strategy. You can surmise their different perspectives from the titles of their books—Jeff Sachs's The End of Poverty: How We Can Make It Happen in Our Lifetime *as opposed to Bill Easterly's* The White Man's Burden: Why the West's Efforts to Aid the Rest Have Done So Much Ill and So Little Good. *This article critiques the Millennium Development Villages that grew out of the ideas promoted in Sachs's book; for more on this topic, the book* The Idealist *by Nina Munk is an interesting read.*

The title of this article is meant as a warning or a note of caution; it is not an invitation to complacency. On the contrary, global health and world poverty should be a concern of every citizen of the world, especially of those of us who have so much. There are all sorts of ways to contribute, but big plans and simple solutions often do not work.

It is your obligation as a global citizen to contribute, but you don't have to save the world today. You just have to do your own part, which may be a long-term project. It is important to remember that the world is always changing—it takes the effort and cooperation of many people to nudge the processes of change in the direction of social justice.

As you read this article, consider the following questions:

- **Can you think of a good example of "unintended consequences"? Do you think that those consequences were unpredictable?**
- **Explore what is meant by a "social business." In your opinion, how is a social business different from a regular business? What business skills and opportunities do you think that poor people need to get?**
- **Some of the projects described in this article, like the deworming project, are obviously good things that can improve local health. In your opinion, is the problem that the enthusiastic proponents of the project simply made exaggerated claims of its long-term effects?**
- **Have you ever thought about how you might contribute to the goals of Global Health and**

Michael Hobbes, "Stop Trying to Save the World." *New Republic,* November 17, 2014.

decrease in global poverty? What do you think you can do? What might your family members be able to do?

- **Go back to the introductory article and the box called "What's Your Major?" Do you think it is really true that everyone can contribute to global health and economic justice?**

CONTEXT

Michael Hobbes is a journalist whose specialty is International Development. He writes an excellent blog (www.rottenindenmark.wordpress.com) that brings the large complex issues of global health and poverty down to the personal level. This article appeared in the magazine *The New Republic*, and Hobbes publishes regularly in foreign policy journals about the world of NGOs. He recently wrote a blogpost entitled "I Live My Life One Professional Conference at a Time" in which he describes the experience of being critical in a world enmeshed in the culture of optimism. He lives in Berlin, Germany.

It seemed like such a good idea at the time: A merry-go-round hooked up to a water pump. In rural sub-Saharan Africa, where children are plentiful but clean water is scarce, the PlayPump harnessed one to provide the other. Every time the kids spun around on the big colorful wheel, water filled an elevated tank a few yards away, providing fresh, clean water anyone in the village could use all day.

PlayPump International, the NGO that came up with the idea and developed the technology, seemed to have thought of everything. To pay for maintenance, the elevated water tanks sold advertising, becoming billboards for companies seeking access to rural markets. If the ads didn't sell, they would feature HIV/AIDS-prevention campaigns. The whole package cost just $7,000 to install in each village and could provide water for up to 2,500 people.

The donations gushed in. In 2006, the U.S. government and two major foundations pledged $16.4 million in a public ceremony emceed by Bill Clinton and Laura Bush. The technology was touted by the World Bank and made a cameo in America's 2007 Water for the Poor Act. Jay-Z personally pledged $400,000. PlayPump set the goal of installing 4,000 pumps in Africa by 2010. "That would mean clean drinking water for some ten million people," a "Frontline" reporter announced.

By 2007, less than two years after the grants came in, it was already clear these aspirations weren't going to be met. A UNICEF report found pumps abandoned, broken, unmaintained. Of the more than 1,500 pumps that had been installed with the initial burst of grant money in Zambia, one-quarter already needed repair. *The Guardian* said the pumps were "reliant on child labour."

In 2010, "Frontline" returned to the schools where they had filmed children laughing on the merry-go-rounds, splashing each other with water. They discovered pumps rusting, billboards unsold, women stooping to turn the wheel in pairs. Many of the villages hadn't even been asked if they wanted a PlayPump, they just got one, sometimes replacing the handpumps they already had. In one community, adults were paying children to operate the pump.

Let's not pretend to be surprised by any of this. The PlayPump story is a sort of *Mad Libs* version of a narrative we're all familiar with by now: Exciting new development idea, huge impact in one location, influx of donor dollars, quick expansion, failure.

I came across the PlayPump story in Ken Stern's *With Charity For All*, but I could have plucked one from any of the dozen or so "development doesn't work" best-sellers to come out in the last ten years. In *The Idealist*—a kind of "where are they now?" for the ideas laid out in Jeffrey Sachs's *The End of Poverty*—Nina Munk discovers African villages made squalid by the hopes and checkbooks of Western do-gooders. Esther Duflo and Abhijit Banerjee's *Poor Economics* finds dozens of "common sense" development projects—food aid, crop insurance, microfinance—either don't help poor people or may even make them poorer.

International development is getting it from all sides. Governments and rich people ("major donors" in NGO-ese) are embracing terms like "philanthrocapitalism," "social entrepreneurship," and "impact bonds," arguing that donations are investments, not gifts. Australia and Canada have done away with their international development agencies altogether, absorbing them into mega-ministries covering foreign affairs and trade.

I am conflicted about this moment. I have worked at international development NGOs almost my entire career (primarily at two midsized human rights organizations—one you've probably heard of and one you probably haven't). I've been frustrated by the same inefficiencies and assumptions of my sector that are now getting picked apart in public. Like the authors, donors and governments attacking international development, I'm sometimes disillusioned with what my job requires me to do, what it requires that I demand of others.

Over the last year, I read every book, essay and roman à clef about my field I could find. I came out convinced that the problems with international development are real, they are fundamental, and I might, in fact, be one of them. But I also found that it's too easy to blame the PlayPumps of the world. Donors, governments, the public, the media, aid recipients themselves—they all contribute to the dysfunction. Maybe the problem isn't that international development doesn't work. It's that it can't.

In the late '90s, Michael Kremer, then an economics professor at MIT, was in Kenya working on an NGO project that distributed textbooks to schools in poor rural districts. Around that time, the ratio of children to textbooks in Kenya was 17 to 1. The intervention seemed obvious: Poor villages need textbooks, rich donors have the money to buy them. All we have to do is link them up.

But in the early stages of the project, Kremer convinced the researchers to do it differently. He wanted to know whether giving kids textbooks actually made them better students. So instead of handing out books and making a simple before-and-after comparison, he designed the project like a pharmaceutical trial. He split the schools into groups, gave some of them the "treatment" (i.e., textbooks) and the others nothing. Then he tested everyone, not just the kids who got the books but also the kids who didn't, to see if his intervention had any effect.

It didn't. The trial took four years, but it was conclusive: Some of the kids improved academically over that time and some got worse, but the treatment group wasn't any better off than the control.

Then Kremer tried something else. Maybe the kids weren't struggling in school because of what was going on in the classroom, but because of what was going on outside of it. So again, Kremer split the schools into groups and spent three years testing and measuring them. This time, the treatment was an actual treatment—medication to eradicate stomach worms. Worm infections affect up to 600 million children around the world, sapping their nutrition and causing, among other things, anemia, stomachaches and stunting.

Once more, the results were conclusive: The deworming pills made the kids noticeably better off. Absence rates fell by 25 percent, the kids got taller, even their friends and families got healthier. By interrupting the chain of infection, the treatments had reduced worm infections in entire villages. Even more striking, when they tested the same kids nearly a decade later, they had more education and earned higher salaries. The female participants were less likely to be employed in domestic services.

And compared with Kremer's first trial, deworming was a bargain. Textbooks cost $2 to $3 each. Deworming pills were as little as 49 cents. When Kremer calculated the kids' bump in lifetime wages compared with the cost of treatment, it was a 60-to-1 ratio.

This is perfect TED Talk stuff: Conventional wisdom called into question, rigorous science triumphing over dogma. As word of Kremer's study spread, he became part of a growing movement within international development to subject its assumptions to randomized controlled trials.

Dozens of books and articles (and yes, TED Talks) have tracked the rise of the randomistas, as they've come to be called. The most prominent of these, and the most fun to read, is *Poor Economics*, sort of the *Principia Mathematica* of "obvious" development interventions tested and found wanting.

If someone is chronically malnourished, to pick just one example, you should give them some food, right? Duflo and Banerjee describe dozens of projects finding that when you subsidize or give away food to poor people, they don't actually eat more. Instead, they just replace boring foods with more interesting ones and remain, in the statistics at least, "malnourished."

In Udaipur, India, a survey found that poor people had enough money to increase their food spending by as much as 30 percent, but they chose to spend it on alcohol, tobacco and festivals instead. Duflo and Banerjee interviewed an out-of-work Indonesian agricultural worker who had been under the food-poverty line for years, but had a TV in his house.

You don't need a Ph.D. to understand the underlying dynamic here: Cheap food is boring. In many developing countries, Duflo and Banerjee found that even the poorest people could afford more than 2,000 calories of staple foods every day. But given the choice between the fourth bowl of rice in one day and the first cigarette, many people opt for the latter.

Even in countries where development projects worked, where poor people went from hungry to nourished, they weren't more likely to get a job or make significantly more money. All the appealing metaphors of NGO websites and academo-best-sellers—"the poverty trap," "the ladder of development"—go limp under the magnifying glass of actually being tested.

Armed with his rigorously gathered results, Kremer founded an NGO, Deworm the World. He launched it at the 2007 World Economic Forum and committed to deworming ten million children. He was feted by the Clinton Global Initiative; GlaxoSmithKline, and Johnson & Johnson pledged $600 million worth of deworming treatments a year, enough for every infected primary school student in Africa. The World Health Organization issued a statement of support. Kenya asked him to help create a national program to deworm 3.6 million children. Two states in India initiated similar programs, aiming to treat millions more. The organization now claims to have helped 40 million children in 27 countries.

But wait a minute. Just because something works for 30,000 students in Kenya doesn't mean it will work for millions of them across Africa or India. Deworm the World's website talks a lot about its "evidence-based" approach. (It has now been folded into an NGO called Evidence Action.) Yet the primary evidence that deworming improves education outcomes is from Kremer's single Kenya case and a post-hoc analysis of deworming initiatives in the American South in 1910. In 2012, the organization said that it had treated 17 million children in India but didn't report whether their attendance, school performance or graduation rates improved.

I keep thinking I'm missing something really obvious, that I'm looking at the wrong part of their website. So I call up Evidence Action and ask Are you guys really not testing how deworming affects education anymore?

"We don't measure the effects on school attendance and school performance," says Alix Zwane, Evidence Action's executive director. At the scale they're going for in India, entire states at a time, splitting into control and treatment groups simply wouldn't be feasible.

Kremer tells me that enough trials have been done to warrant the upscaling. "There's more evidence for this than the vast majority of things that governments spend money on." Every time you want to build a new road, you can't stop to ask, Will this one really help people get from place to place?

"Meanwhile," he says, "there's a cohort of children that, if you don't implement the policy now, will go through years of schooling without treatment."

It's an interesting question—when do you have enough evidence to stop testing each new application of a development idea?—and I get that you can't run a four-year trial every time you roll out, say, the measles vaccine to a new country. But like many other aid projects under pressure to scale up too fast and too far, deworming kids to improve their education outcomes isn't the slam-dunk its supporters make it out to be.

In 2000, the *British Medical Journal* (*BMJ*) published a literature review of 30 randomized control trials of deworming projects in 17 countries. While some of them showed modest gains in weight and height, none of them showed any effect on school attendance or cognitive performance. After criticism of the review by the World Bank and others, the *BMJ* ran it again in 2009 with stricter inclusion criteria. But the results didn't change. Another review, in 2012, found the same thing: "We do not know if these programmes have an effect on weight, height, school attendance, or school performance."

Kremer and Evidence Action dispute the way these reviews were carried out, and sent me an upcoming study from Uganda that found links between deworming and improved test scores. But the evidence they cite on their own website undermines this data. Kremer's 2004 study reporting the results of the original deworming trial notes—in the abstract!—that "we do not find evidence that deworming improves academic test scores," only attendance. Another literature review cited on Deworm the World's website says, "When infected children are given deworming treatment, immediate educational and cognitive benefits are not always apparent."

Then there's the comparison to textbooks. Kenya, it turns out, is a uniquely terrible place to hand out textbooks to kids and expect better academic performance. When Kremer reported that textbooks had no overall effect, he also noted that they did actually improve test scores for the kids who were already at the top of the class. The main problem, it seems, was that the textbooks were in English, the second or third language for most of the kids. Of the third-graders given textbooks, only 15 percent could even read them.

In the 1980s and early '90s, a series of meta-analyses found that textbooks were actually effective at improving school performance in places where the language issues weren't as complex. In his own paper reporting the Kenya results, Kremer noted that, in Nicaragua and the Philippines, giving kids textbooks did improve their test scores.

But the point of all this is not to talk shit on Kremer—who has bettered the world more with his career than I ever have with mine—or to dismantle his deworming charity or to advocate that we should all go back to giving out free textbooks. What I want to talk shit on is the paradigm of the Big Idea—that once we identify the correct one, we can simply unfurl it on the entire developing world like a picnic blanket.

There are villages where deworming will be the most meaningful education project possible. There are others where free textbooks will. In other places, it will be new school buildings, more teachers, lower fees, better transport, tutors, uniforms. There's probably a village out there where a PlayPump would beat all these approaches combined. The point is, we don't know what works, where or why. The only way to find out is to test these models—not just before their initial success but afterward, and constantly.

I can see why it's appealing to think that, once you find a successful formula for development, you can just scale it up like a Model T. Host governments want programs that get more effective as they get bigger. Individual donors, you and me, we want to feel like we're backing a plucky little start-up that is going to save the world. No international institution wants to say in their annual report: "There's this great NGO that increased attendance in a Kenyan school district. We're giving them a modest sum to do the same thing in *one other district* in one other country."

The repeated "success, scale, fail" experience of the last 20 years of development practice suggests something super boring: Development projects thrive or tank according to the specific dynamics of the place in which they're applied. It's not that you test something in one place, then scale it up to 50. It's that you test it in one place, then test it in another, then another. No one will ever be invited to explain that in a TED talk.

The last NGO I worked for had 150 employees and a budget of more than $25 million. Employees were divided into "program staff" (the people researching, coordinating and implementing our mission) and "overhead staff" (the fund-raising, human resources and accounting departments helping them do it). Like most NGOs, we bragged to our donors that we had low overhead, that their dollars and euros and kroner and francs went to "the cause" and not to our rent or our heating bills. And this was, at least on the Excel sheets, true. Most of our money went to researcher and project manager salaries. The fund-raising, H.R. and accounting departments could have each fit comfortably in a minivan.

The problem is, those overhead tasks don't disappear just because you don't spend money on them. Someone has to monitor the accounts, find new donors, calculate taxes organize the holiday party. Centralizing these tasks in dedicated departments, hiring specialists, getting good at them, that would have looked like bureaucracy. So instead, we spun them out to the entire staff: We assigned researchers and project managers—anthropology majors mostly, some law school dropouts—to do our H.R., accounting, fund-raising and project evaluations.

The outcome was as chaotic as it sounds. Want to hire someone? You'll need to write your own job ad, find job boards to post it to and, in some cases, update the standard employment contract yourself. Want to issue a press release about the results of the study you just performed? Write it yourself and start sending it to journalists. Hopefully you know a few.

The downsides of this approach were most obvious in fund-raising. If there's one thing donors hate, it's paying us to find more donors. So every program staffer was responsible for raising (and accounting, and monitoring and reporting) funds for their own projects. Staff members spent days doing the same donor research ("which foundations fund work on water scarcity?") that a colleague across the hall did last week. Without a centralized staff to coordinate pitches, we contacted the same donors dozens of times with small-fry requests rather than combining them into one coherent "ask." (One employee, legend had it, asked Google if they could Google Translate our website as an in-kind donation.)

No one had any expertise in writing grant proposals, conducting impact assessments or managing high-maintenance funders like the European Commission—training courses would have counted as overhead spending. We missed opportunities for new funding, we bungled contracts we already had and we turned donors against us. Every staff meeting, one or two people announced they were leaving. "I wasn't hired to spend my day fund-raising" were the most common eight words at farewell parties.

My experience wasn't unique. Stern cites the example of the American Red Cross, which sent confused volunteers, clueless employees, and, bafflingly, perishable Danish pastries to the Gulf Coast after Hurricane Katrina because it hadn't invested in training its U.S. staff in actual crisis response. A buddy of mine works at an NGO with 150 staff where the H.R. department is exactly one person, and she's also the receptionist.

It's understandable that donors are paranoid about overhead. The last few years have seen charity after charity busted for blowing donations on corporate junkets, billboard advertising, and outright fraud. Some breast cancer charities pay telemarketing companies 90 cents of each dollar they raise just to raise it. Greg Mortenson, he of the *Three Cups of Tea* school-building empire, had to pay $1 million back to his own charity when a Jon Krakauer exposé revealed that he was spending donations on a never-ending book tour and pocketing the proceeds.

Dan Pallotta, who spent the '90s and 2000s running a $300 million breast cancer and AIDS charity, has produced two books arguing that this obsession with overhead keeps charities from reaching the scale required to take on large problems. Pallotta uses the example of two soup kitchens: One spends 60 cents of every donation dollar on "programs" (i.e., soup), while the other spends 90 cents.

According to the conventional wisdom of donors and charity rating agencies, your donation is better spent on the organization where only 10 percent of spending goes to overhead. But using this one number ignores much more important indicators of the charity's impact. Is the soup nutritious and warm? Is it getting to the right people? Does the kitchen open on time every day and have kind, professional staff? And, hang on, do free warm meals even help people escape poverty? Providing decent service, targeting handouts, testing these assumptions—these things cost money, whether donors like it or not.

So charities hide overhead, like we did, in overburdened program staff, untrained volunteers, and external consultants. Just as deworming millions of children is different in kind, not degree, from deworming a village of them, running a large, professional charity is completely different from running a new, start-uppy one. Small-scale projects (installing one PlayPump, say) can keep their overhead low through charismatic leaders, passionate staff, and long-standing relationships with the communities they're seeking to assist. Large-scale projects require stuff like budget managers, reporting frameworks, light bulbs, and, yes, a goddamn holiday party.

Pallotta's *Uncharitable* has a nice example of what this looks like. His first cross-country AIDS ride had 39 cyclists and almost zero overhead. The group was small enough to sleep in gymnasiums, to rely on churches and good samaritans to provide food and hot showers. If supplies fell short, they could knock on doors asking for help or, in a pinch, put up their tents in backyards. He raised $80,000.

By the 2000s, the rides were attracting an average of 3,000 riders. A group that size requires a logarithmic increase in organization and support—renting out whole campgrounds, professional catering, dedicated medical and legal staff. Overhead costs ballooned to 42 percent of each donation. But each ride raised $7 million.

As with the actual aid projects themselves, the success of a charity depends on specifics, not a single, one-size-fits-all indicator. Charities do all kinds of stuff—conduct research, train local NGOs, build infrastructure, give away goats. For donors to truly determine how well they're doing it, they'd need to come up with a customized report card for each charity.

For a soup kitchen, it would be the stuff I just mentioned: *Do they open on time? How's their soup?* For an NGO that, say, monitors government infrastructure projects for corruption, it would be things like, *What percentage of projects are they assessing? Are their assessments yielding correct information? Is this information being communicated to the communities affected by corruption?*

Judging charities like this, on the impacts of their work and whether they're addressing the problem they set out to solve, yields qualitative information, sentences, and observations that can't be compared across charities. Given the millions of international development NGOs with their upside-down hats out (the IRS, Stern notes, approves 99.5 percent of charity applications), it's faster and easier to measure them all by the same standard.

This is why donors love overhead. It's one number that allows you to compare the soup kitchen with the anti-corruption think tank. It smells all rigorous and objective, but it doesn't require any actual work. Charities provide their own overhead figures, after all, just like they write their own annual reports and produce their own little Kony 2012 fund-raising videos. International development NGOs aren't always obligated to issue audited accounts. Some of them report no overhead at all, the institutional equivalent of "I didn't inhale."

I'm not going to propose a cute little solution here to make this easier for donors, or suggest some "right" overhead percentage. For most charities, 10 percent overhead probably isn't enough, and 90 percent is just fucking around. But the whole point is that we shouldn't pick just one number to stand in for efficiency. We're always arguing that, if rich countries want to solve the problems of poor ones, they're going to have to spend time getting to know them. It's time we apply the same logic to the agencies we dispatch to do the job.

Dertu isn't a place very many people go on purpose. Located in northeastern Kenya, close to the Somali border, and next door to a sprawling refugee camp, in 2004 it was little more than a rest stop, a place for the local pastoralists to refresh their animals and catch up on local news. Its chief attraction was fresh water from a UNICEF-drilled borehole in the clay. Of the few thousand people living there permanently, more than 80 percent relied on food aid. Ninety percent were illiterate.

This is the "before" picture of Dertu that Jeffrey Sachs found when he initiated his Millennium Villages Project there in 2006. Sachs, a professor at Columbia University, became a Bono-approved development celebrity with his book *The End of Poverty*, a screed against the rich world's complacency in letting easily solvable problems—malaria, literacy, clean water—damn an entire continent to misery.

Sachs's book tour culminated in the establishment of the Millennium Villages Project, an ambitious plan to jump-start development with a huge influx of cash, in-kind support, and infrastructure to some of the poorest settlements in the world. Sachs's premise was that millions of people, dozens of countries, had fallen into the "poverty trap": Living in substandard housing leads to problems concentrating at school. Which leads to not graduating. Which leads to working in low-skilled jobs. Which leads to living in substandard housing. And on and on.

The only solution, Sachs argued, was to dramatically boost people to a level where they could start to develop themselves.

This is, it turns out, an incredibly persuasive idea, and in the two years after the book came out, Sachs raised $120 million (including $50 million from George Soros's personal checkbook) and identified 14 villages throughout sub-Saharan Africa to test his theory.

As described in Nina Munk's *The Idealist: Jeffrey Sachs and the Quest to End Poverty*, things looked promising in Dertu at first. Sachs convinced GE and Ericsson to donate medical equipment and cell phones. He hired local managers who knew the culture and language to ensure his project was responding to Dertu's needs. His teams built housing, schools, roads, health clinics. They set up a livestock market to attract farmers from all over the region.

But soon, the momentum faltered. Without electricity to run it or specialists to maintain it, the advanced medical equipment gathered dust—in Kenya, that means literally. The managers of the project, so knowledgeable about the local culture and mores, eventually succumbed to them, doling out benefits on the basis of tribal favoritism and tit-for-tat back-scratching. The borehole broke down and water had to be shipped in by truck.

The core of the problem, as Munk describes it, was that Dertu became a sort of company town, with the Millennium Villages Project providing the only reliable source of employment, benefits, and public services. Thousands of new residents came from the nearby refugee camp and other parts of Kenya, seeking jobs or handouts. Where Dertu was once a stopover for nomads, the influx of donor money, the improved infrastructure, the free housing and education and health care, had given people a reason to stay. Sachs's funding couldn't keep up. And eventually, it ran out.

In an interview about her book for *EconTalk*, Munk describes what Dertu looked like the last time she saw it, in 2011:

> They were now really living in a kind of squalor that I hadn't seen on my first visit. Their huts were jammed together; they were patched with those horrible polyurethane bags that one sees all over Africa. . . . There were streams of slop that were going down between these tightly packed huts. And the latrines had overflowed or were clogged. And no one was able to agree on whose job it was to maintain them. And there were ditches piled high with garbage. And it was just—it made my heart just sink.

This is the paradox: When you improve something, you change it in ways you couldn't have expected. You can find examples of this in every corner of development practice. A project in Kenya that gave kids free uniforms, textbooks, and classroom materials increased enrollment by 50 percent, swamping the teachers and reducing the quality of education for everyone. Communities in India cut off their own water supply so they could be classified as "slums" and be eligible for slum-upgrading funding. I've worked in places where as soon as a company sets up a health clinic or an education program, the local government disappears—why should they spend money on primary schools when a rich company is ready to take on the responsibility?

There's nothing avaricious about this. If anything, it demonstrates the entrepreneurial spirit we're constantly telling the poor they need to demonstrate.

My favorite example of unintended consequences comes, weirdly enough, from the United States. In a speech to a criminology conference, Nancy G. Guerra, the director of the Institute for Global Studies at the University of Delaware, described a project where she held workshops with inner-city Latina teenagers, trying to prevent them from joining gangs. The program worked in that none of the girls committed any violence within six months of the workshops. But by the end of that time, they were all, each and every one, pregnant.

"That behavior was serving a need for them," she says in her speech. "It made them feel powerful, it made them feel important, it gave them a sense of identity. . . . When that ended, [they] needed another kind of meaning in their lives."

The fancy academic term for this is "complex adaptive systems." We all understand that every ecosystem, each forest floor or coral reef, is the result of millions of interactions between its constituent parts, a balance of all the aggregated adaptations of plants and animals to their climate and each other. Adding a non-native species, or removing one that has always been there, changes these relationships in ways that are too intertwined and complicated to predict.

According to Ben Ramalingam's *Aid on the Edge of Chaos*, international development is just such an invasive species. Why Dertu doesn't have a vaccination clinic, why Kenyan schoolkids can't read, it's a combination of culture, politics, history, laws, infrastructure, individuals—all of a society's component parts, their harmony and their discord, working as one organism. Introducing something foreign into that system—millions in donor cash, dozens of trained personnel and equipment, U.N. Land Rovers—causes it to adapt in ways you can't predict.

A friend of mine works at an NGO that audits factories in India and China, inspecting them for child labor, forced labor, human-trafficking, everything celebrities are always warning us about. I asked him if, after ten years of inspections, conditions have gotten any better. "Yes and no," he said. "Anytime you set a standard, some companies will become sophisticated to meet it, and others will become sophisticated to avoid it."

So international development sucks, right? I've just spent thousands of words telling you all the ways the incentives of donors, recipients, and NGOs contradict each other. Why not just scrap it altogether?

Because I don't think that's the conclusion these examples suggest. I think they suggest something much less dramatic: It's not that development is broken, it's that our expectations of it are.

First, let's de-room this elephant: *Development has happened.* The last 50 years have seen about the biggest explosion of prosperity in human history. China, India, Taiwan, South Korea, Turkey, Mexico—these aren't the only countries where you'd rather be born now than 50 years ago. Even the poorest countries in the world—Burundi, Somalia, Zimbabwe—are doing way better on stuff like vaccinations and literacy than they did earlier in our own lifetimes.

You sometimes hear this Cambrian proliferation of well-being as an argument against development aid, like: "See? China got better *all by itself.*" But the rise of formerly destitute countries into the sweaters-and-smartphones bracket is less a refutation of the impact of development aid than a reality-check of its scale. In 2013, development aid from all the rich countries combined was $134.8 billion, or about $112 per year for each of the world's 1.2 billion people living on less than $1.25 per day. Did we really expect an extra hundred bucks a year to pull anyone, much less a billion of them, out of poverty?

Development, no matter how it happens, is a slow process. It wasn't until about 30 years after Mao's death that China's per capita GDP reached lower-middle-income status. The country's growth is arguably the fastest of any country's since we, as a species, started gathering economic statistics. Even in the most cartoonishly successful scenario imaginable, countries like the Central African Republic (per capita GDP: $700, adjusted for purchasing power), Burundi ($600), and the Democratic Republic of Congo ($400) will take decades just to reach the point where China is now.

The ability of international development projects to speed up this process is limited. Remember how I said the deworming project had a 60-to-1 ratio between the price of the pills and the increase in wages for the kids who got them? The increase was $30. Not $30 per year. The kids earned $30 more *over their lifetimes* as a result of the deworming treatment. You find this a lot in the development literature: Even the most wildly successful projects decrease maternal mortality by a few percent here, add an extra year or two of life expectancy there.

This isn't a criticism of the projects themselves. This is how social policy works, in baby steps and trial-and-error and tweaks, not in game changers. Leave the leaps and bounds to computing power. If a 49-cent deworming treatment really does produce a $30 increase in wages for some of the poorest people on Earth, we are assholes for not spending it.

And this is where I landed after a year of absorbing dozens of books and articles and speeches about international development: The arguments against it are myriad, and mostly logistical and technical. The argument for it is singular, moral, and, to me anyway, utterly convincing: *We have so much, they have so little.*

If we really want to fix development, we need to stop chasing after ideas the way we go on fad diets. Successful programs should be allowed to expand by degrees, not digits (direct cash payments, which have shown impressive results in Kenya and Uganda, are a great candidate for the kind of deliberate expansion I'm talking about). NGOs need to be free to invest in the kinds of systems and processes we're always telling developing countries to put in place. And rich countries need to spend less time debating how to divide up the tiny sliver of our GDP we spend on development and more time figuring out how to leverage our vast economic and political power to let it happen on its own.

As Owen Barder, a senior fellow at the Center for Global Development (from whom I stole many of the ideas in this essay), puts it:

> If we believe that trade is important, we could do more to open our own markets to trade from developing countries. If we believe property rights are important, we could do more to enforce the principle that nations, not illegitimate leaders, own their own natural resources. . . . If we believe transparency is important, we could start by requiring our own companies to publish the details of the payments they make to developing countries.

PlayPump International, the charity I started with, doesn't exist anymore. The pumps, however, are still being installed by Roundabout Water Solutions, an NGO that markets them as a "niche solution" that should only be installed at primary schools in poor rural areas. Four years ago, the same evaluations that so harshly criticized the rapid expansion of the project also acknowledged that, in some villages, under the right circumstances, they were fabulously helpful.

In 2010, "Frontline" interviewed the director of PlayPump about its failures, and he said, "It might have been a bit ambitious, but hey, you gotta dream big. Everyone's always said it's such a great idea."

And it was. But maybe when the next great idea comes along, we should all dream a little smaller.

SVEA CLOSSER AND PETER BROWN

49 GLOBAL HEALTH: YOUR LIFE, YOUR LIFE DECISIONS, YOUR MORAL OBLIGATIONS

The inequities and conditions of living and dying in the majority world are intolerable: that is why we are both passionate about the field of Global Health. While tremendous progress has been made in the last 25 years, there is much more to be done.

In our selection of readings for this book, we wanted to give students the big picture of the field, including both the severe challenges and the great successes. We want our students to learn to think critically about difficult questions, see multiple perspectives and make interesting and startling connections. College students, like most people, tend to live in a bubble of their own small world, their own problems, their own desires and their own complaints. We believe that education should help people break out of their bubble—or at the least become aware that they live a space confined by a narrow set of beliefs, attitudes and self-satisfaction. We want our students to become better world citizens. The opposite of being a world citizen, we believe, is to be narrow-minded, provincial, insular and unsophisticated. Becoming a world citizen does not mean that one must subscribe to a particular political point of view. Rather, we believe that becoming a world citizen is simply part of being a modern human being who recognizes the dignity and rights of our fellow humans.

Because we care so much about global health, we also want our students to be inspired and to make a personal commitment to the field. This commitment could be in their daily lives, or it could be bigger: continuing their studies or pursuing a career in global health.

Graduate programs in Global Health do not usually provide a historical background like the one we have emphasized in this book, nor do they focus on moral questions. The curricula often emphasize research methods and the development of skills necessary to work in existing Global Health programs. There are a lot of methods and skills to learn, and so there is seldom time to ponder the big issues, like the ethics of "just" saving lives described in Peter Redfield's analysis of MSF (Reading 33), the dynamics of power in aid programs described in James Pfeiffer's article on Mozambique (Reading 41), or the dangers of cost-effectiveness reasoning presented in the portrait of Paul Farmer in Haiti (Reading 12).

The curricula of MPH programs usually emphasize the "culture of optimism." Perhaps that is necessary. Global health programs need to hire people who are enthusiastic, hard-working, idealistic and ambitious to successfully complete projects. The saying is, "Hire an optimist for your staff but hire a pessimist as a consultant." Yet in this book we included both the optimistic and not-so-optimistic. Our goal is that you do not leave your course of study naïve.

Every student needs to have a pocketful of examples and facts on hand to counter pessimism about global health. While there are certainly inefficiencies and corruption that plague programs in global health, there are also dozens of impressive successes: you should be acquainted with both. When someone says that foreign aid represents wasted funds, you should have a response based on facts. When someone says we should not spend money on curing diseases in other countries because we have problems at home, you should be able to show that investments in global health protect our national security and can prevent pandemic diseases (Reading 42). When someone says that people in poor countries have too many children, you should be able to show that couples have fewer children when they know that their babies will probably survive. When talking with such pessimists, arguments about moral responsibilities or human rights may not be persuasive. To become an advocate for global health, it is very helpful to know how relatively small investments can have large returns on investment in terms of lives saved.

The world is complicated, and your study of global health should make you aware that there are no simple solutions to problems of disease and health inequities. These problems are rooted in legacies of colonialism and the structural violence inherent in globalization. If we turn

NEVER TOO LATE

It is never too late to learn nor too early to pursue an interest in global health. Understanding global health means understanding the variability in health and its relation to social, economic, and cultural determinants throughout the world. In turn, this perspective enriches our understanding of health in our own communities.

James Curran, MD, MPH
Emory University

the world upside down to see it from the views of the poorest, "we have so much, because they have so little" (Reading 39). We live at a time of multiple wars that threaten the health of populations (Reading 32), as well as at a time in which rapid intercontinental travel increases the chances of a pandemic. It may turn out to be the case that the global campaign to eradicate polio fails because of political instability. It may also turn out to be the case that rampant nationalism and intolerance result in greatly decreased funding for global health (Reading 42).

However, as in Bill Foege's understatement, "optimism is warranted" (see box "Is Optimism Warranted"). The progress that has been made in the last 30 years in terms of the UN's Millennium Development Goals is so stunning that all people should be proud of our collective achievements. Perhaps it is an impossible goal to "make poverty history," and improvements are never assured, but progress is possible, step by step.

Global Health Needs Everyone

We do not want to be preachy. Nevertheless, there are three personal moral obligations that are incumbent on every world citizen. First, you have an obligation to stay informed. Second, you have a moral obligation to take care of your own health so that you can educate others and be an example of healthy behavior. Third, you have an obligation to be actively involved in helping other people in the world. All three of these are life-long obligations, and they are, unfortunately, not so easy to do.

Stay Informed

We believe that the moral obligation to remain an informed world citizen involves one word: READ. In an age of partisan social media, reading widely, copiously and critically is more important than ever.

Be Healthy and Educate Others

In a world of stress and social pressures, taking care of yourself is an important part of improving global health. Nourish your body, eating plenty of healthy food. Take some time to do something active. Take stock of your alcohol and drug use and consider whether your choices reflect respect for both your own health and the health of those around you. Care for yourself by getting enough sleep. If you find yourself in an abusive relationship, reach out for the support you need to protect yourself and to leave. Take steps to make sure that you are not spreading infectious diseases. Wash your hands often. Get fully vaccinated: you will contribute to herd immunity and help protect those most vulnerable to infectious disease, like immunocompromised children.

As noted in the WHO definition, health is about more than your body. Consider your life priorities. What do you care about? Can you take a step back from the assignment due tomorrow and the social drama in your life this week to take a longer view of how you want to spend your time and what you want your priorities to be? Doing more of what is really important to you often involves saying no to other things.

As you support yourself, you can also more actively support and educate others. As Section 12 of this book explored in depth, educating others is a complicated endeavor. Most people do not like to be lectured to. (Maybe you are already getting annoyed by all the lecturing in this chapter.) A good life goal is to learn to engage in productive and respectful conversations with those you disagree with.

A good start to educating others is first to understand where they are coming from. For example, a growing number of people in the United States do not vaccinate their children. Too much of the talk about this issue in public health circles writes off these parents as selfish or uninformed. Neither is usually true, so the first steps in a respectful, thoughtful and evidence-based conversation around this issue are to find out why people made the choice that they did and to discuss the issues involved with honesty and caring.

Be Actively Involved

Being actively involved in Global Health starts at home. Be informed about health and social justice issues in your own community. Speak out about these issues. Vote for policies and people who will promote good health.

Volunteering can be a great way to support organizations whose mission you believe in. Long-term volunteering on a predictable schedule for a local organization is an effective way to make a real positive impact. Through this sort of long-term commitment, you are also likely to learn a lot about health issues in your community. One-off volunteering can also be helpful in certain circumstances, but consider whether you are really helping or whether you are engaging in resume-padding. Often, long-term commitments give the organization a more helpful and reliable source of labor and give you more opportunities to learn.

Volunteering in communities you are not familiar with—including those overseas—raises a complex set of issues and has the potential to be unhelpful or even in some cases damaging. This should not be thought of as volunteering; it is really a kind of tourism. Most undergraduates and many medical students do not yet have the skills required to do anything on a short-term basis more effectively than people who are already in the place they visit. In some cases, the cost of the foreign volunteer's plane ticket could have trained and hired multiple local staff with a stronger skill set. Sometimes, voluntourists do things, like give injections or assist in surgery, that they would not be permitted to do at home and that can carry potentially serious consequences.

This is not to say that voluntourism is necessarily a bad thing. The benefits to the tourist can be significant. They get some exposure to a new context and usually learn a lot in the process. Some students build deep and positive long-term relationships with the people they meet on their travels. Thus, this sort of tourism can have positive long-term impacts. But, like so much in global health, the ethics of voluntourism are complicated. Students who choose to embark on such travels should engage with, consider and learn from this complexity.

Longer-term positions for students overseas, like the Peace Corps, are affected by these issues to some extent, but because the student is in the area for much longer, the student both learns more and potentially contributes more. The language skills and understanding of other people's lives that Peace Corps volunteers gain often shape the course of the young Americans' lives in profound ways. These skills can also be built on a quality study abroad program, if that is something that is available to you.

Giving money to causes you care about is also an important part of being actively involved. If you are in an institution of higher education in the United States, you are almost surely relatively wealthy in a global context. How will you use that relative wealth?

Similarly, you can get involved in fundraising for global health organizations, using your connections to your community, your university and your family and friends to gather more funds to make an impact. Providing sustaining support to organizations—a recurring donation every month—is a meaningful way to provide long-term support. Even small amounts make a difference over time as you are part of creating a revenue stream that the organization can count on.

Choosing an organization to give to can be an opportunity to find out what's being done in an area you care about. There are many examples of great organizations in this book. Or, even better, choose one that you know from personal experience is doing quality work, maybe in your own community.

You don't need to be trained in health care to be important in global health. The key is remaining aware and informed and being generous with your wealth, time and talents.

Building a Career in Global Health

Some of you will choose a career in global health. Of course, devoting your life to the field is a powerful way to make a real difference.

Many people feel unprepared when they meet with their first failures in their careers in global health. Some people, frustrated by the real and seemingly intractable challenges they face, give up or become jaded.

But things generally do not become better when those who might change them just give up. Thoughtful people with an awareness of history make significant positive impacts all the time. Our personal heroes, people who have made deep and long-term contributions and lead

GLOBAL HEALTH WORK IN THE DOMESTIC SETTING

In the days after the 9/11 and anthrax terrorism attacks, in my job at the state department of health, I was often in a room with government officials and emergency responders. At one of those meetings, I was awed to realize that we *are* the ones solving this problem. A thought struck me: *if everyone in this room went home right now or quit, there would be no one left to work the problem.* It was a powerful moment.

Everyone in the room was worried about the safety of their families and fought the urge to just go home and hold loved ones close. But we inspired each other to work as hard as we needed to and shared a sense of duty to perform our tasks on behalf of the citizens who were counting on us. A sense of duty is both motivating and rewarding. It is a privilege to work alongside talented, educated professionals who have chosen public service over other possible paths.

I was never tempted to work internationally. I was motivated to serve my neighbors. Like many Americans, my ancestors, not too long ago, fled oppression and hardship in other places, and my parents made sure that I knew this. Watching the nightly news, my parents would often comment, "We're lucky to live in America." As I got older and learned more, I had trouble reconciling our health inequities with our identity as "the richest country in the world," one with "the world's best medical system." This country has serious problems, and it has citizens who are suffering unnecessarily. Why would I not want to help my own people? Those are the communities that I know and understand best and am therefore in the best position to serve.

We often hear people lambasting the government. When you *are* a part of the government, it is empowering to know that you are one of the people who can change things. If you observe that things cannot change at that particular moment in time, you can at least explain why to your fellow citizens. Inviting them into the process and engaging them in the work is what will ultimately lead to change.

You can engage in community-based work through many other organizations, of course. My volunteer work with local nonprofits has allowed me to both contribute and to learn. Public health experts are especially valuable at the local level, where it is hardest to reconcile community values and traditions with evidence-based practices and to delineate individual responsibility from the role of the government.

Civic engagement is powerful and gratifying, and therein lies the strength of public health. There is a human face on everything you do, and those faces—your neighbors and friends—hold you accountable. That is a reason to want to get out of bed in the morning and a reason to lie down proud of what you accomplished that day.

Pamela A. Berenbaum
Middlebury College

truly excellent health programs, share a few personal attributes that help them avoid becoming either a blindly optimistic Pollyanna or a cynical naysayer.

Humility

First, and above all, the people who make the most long-term positive impact in global health are humble. By this we don't mean that they are self-deprecating (though this is often the case). Rather, we mean that they start every endeavor assuming that they don't have the answers, that they will need to learn a lot by listening and asking a lot of questions. Humble people make adjustments as they fail. They don't just stumble in and tell others what they should be doing; rather, they listen. Their working assumption in everything they do is not that they are right; instead, it is that they probably have something to learn.

Recently, we asked a diverse group of global health practitioners, including executives, researchers and those just a few years out of college, What do undergraduates need to learn to be prepared for a career in global health? Their answer was clear, unanimous and simple: humility. They explained that skills like epidemiology could be learned. But for these people, a humble approach was a make-or-break proposition for effective work in global health.

Adaptability

The best global health programs are adaptable and run by adaptable people. Flexibility in method and approach is a hallmark of the highest-quality programs.

Succeeding in a global health project requires being flexible because what worked beautifully in one context often won't be ideal in another. Or there may be a

THE BENEFITS OF FAILURE

The field of global health is complex and rapidly changing, and yet our mission of equitable health improvement is meant to be long term and durable. Meaningful progress calls for personal attributes among practitioners and policy leaders that incorporate an appreciation for and commitment to working with this complexity and an attitude of resilience that can make use of failures as opportunities to learn, adjust and try a different tack. There are no overnight fixes.

My wife and I first went overseas—to West Africa—to work in global health when we got out of grad school several decades ago. We had taken a lot of courses and were good students, but our solutions-based curriculum did not prepare us for the real-world challenges we faced and the failures we experienced in our first job. And it certainly did not incorporate tools to understand the complex interplay of political dynamics among key actors.

In this first job, we failed in part because we were working with three very different institutions with three different very different aims. The national government wanted to use primary health care as a means to strengthen its visible presence in a border area with a minority tribal group. The academic institution that was our employer wanted to generate scholarly papers regardless of program impact. The funding organization wanted data to demonstrate quantifiable changes in health. None of these goals centered on a principal concern for the people in our project area themselves.

Because the aims differed and because the three institutions never worked on a common vision of the project, we—as the "worker bees" at the far end of the project pipeline, living in an unelectrified mud house in the middle of the Sahel—were continuously whipsawed with conflicting orders from the three headquarters. Train more community health workers, and quickly. Refine a manual that can be published and used as a showpiece in other countries. Set up a data system and generate reports that fit into a standardized framework. And on and on. A day doesn't go by that I don't think about what we learned from these failures and of the friendships and understanding we established with the local people with whom we worked. Not surprisingly, the latter were the more gratifying and enduring.

As we have seen repeatedly over our years in the field, most individual global health efforts end in partial or abject failure. If it was easy, it would already have been done. What we have learned is the importance of accepting failure, studying it as honestly as we can, and learning from it. And we have learned the importance of viewing those who are supposed to benefit from these efforts as active subjects rather than passive objects; if we fail to understand them, their life realities and their own perceived needs, our efforts cannot succeed. As Michael Hobbs writes (Chapter 48), people are often seduced into thinking they can address other people's problems and "save the world." This attitude leads to quick, misinformed action and disappointment. When we as educators sugarcoat global health work for our students, we do them a disservice.

These realities are rarely taught in academic programs that focus on epidemiology, disease burden, randomized controlled trials, and data analysis. And as a consequence, many people enter the field of global health sadly unprepared for the realities they will face. Some will learn by doing and will adjust and persevere. But all too often, I have seen bright and capable colleagues who have burned out, and other who have gotten locked in—two ends of the disappointment spectrum. Those who have burned out have become disillusioned and cynical about the petty agendas, the misuse of resources, the bureaucratic obstacles, and the level of politics involved in the process; they expected global health to somehow be cleaner and purer. Those who have gotten locked in have focused on a single key they have come across early in their careers and have put on blinders to the "extraneous factors" that perturb their intellectually elegant constructs; the real world need not apply.

There is no simple one-size-fits-all solution to the challenges of working in global health. The problems that global health practitioners face are complex and hard to solve, but step-by-step, they can be managed. When we learn from failures, good things happen, and over time we can help to build a critical mass that results in a seismic shift in the health and well-being of millions. It takes years to become an overnight success. To really make a difference, you have to be willing to make that investment.

Nils Daulaire
Harvard Global Health Institute

surprising better way. Smallpox eradication is an example of this. At the beginning of the program, mass vaccination was thought to be the only way to achieve eradication. But some people working in West Africa developed the surveillance-containment method (see Reading 4) when they were low on vaccine, and they were attentive enough to realize that this new method, initially developed as an emergency stopgap, could be better than mass vaccination. It was, and smallpox was eradicated.

Even when there is a proven solution, a lot of tinkering is often necessary to get a program right. The case of BRAC's dissemination of knowledge about how to prepare oral rehydration solution (ORS; Reading 5) is a great example. Even once the formula for ORS was developed, BRAC took years testing and retesting various approaches to teaching rural women about it. They tried different formulas, different measuring methods, and different supervision and incentive strategies for community health workers. They accepted trade-offs, using slightly less effective formulas because they were easier for rural women to carry out and remember. The reason they were so successful in teaching many millions of women about ORS is that they didn't try to do this education program on a large scale until they had tried many different approaches to find out what worked best.

Sometimes in global health programs, practitioners become tied to an approach that worked in one time and place (or many times and places) and try to force it to work in a context where it is not well suited. This approach can build resistance and resentment. Adaptability, coupled with the patience to find out what actually works, usually leads to much stronger programs in the long term.

Attentiveness to Project Recipients

The best health programs meet the needs of the people the program is serving. They ask people in target communities what their health needs are and what their major priorities are, and they seek to meet those needs and those priorities. These programs are clear about their orientation to those being served by a program, not to those funding it.

Some accountability to donors is usually necessary. But, the best projects don't sacrifice their accountability to the people they serve to please donors. Rather, they seek to educate donors about the importance of the health needs articulated by the populations they serve.

An example of a Global Health practitioner who lives this principle is Paul Farmer. Reading 12 describes Farmer's commitment to his patients. "It's through journeys to the sick," he says, "that we identify needs and problems." Farmer finds out what patients need and worries about donors later. While this sort of person may not be best suited to run an organization (good management, including budgeting, is often critical for sustaining programs in the long term), it is precisely this sort of person who should be the moral compass of an organization. It is often the

WORK IN PUBLIC HEALTH – WONDERFUL PEOPLE BUT DAUNTING COMPLEXITY

As I look back on nearly 30 years of work in public health and community health, I realise that one great advantage of this field is that it allows you to interact with an amazing range of people—across classes, social backgrounds, geographical areas and cultures. And it involves lots of team work. So if you like people, most probably you will like public health. One should not miss opportunities of interacting with diverse kinds of people, and one should also proactively learn to work as a team member and help build teams, which carry huge rewards in both personal and professional terms.

I also think that public health is a great way to combine professional work with social activism. This profession allows you to use your special knowledge to help people and support change in a direct manner and often on significant scale.

Public health is highly interdisciplinary; in fact, there are few areas of specialization that are as "unspecialized" (in the sense of avoiding narrow confines of a single discipline) as public health. This means you are learning and reaching across disciplinary boundaries all the time, which can be very exciting and fulfilling. It is also rewarding to switch between grasping the technical details of research and implementation and viewing the "big picture"—including the really big picture at the level of societies and ecosystems. To slightly rephrase what one of the founders of public health, Rudolf Virchow, said: Public health imperceptibly leads us into the social field and places us in a position of confronting directly the great problems of our time.

Finally, public health puts you face to face with complex systems all the time. You can learn to depart from linear, simplistic thinking, since you deal with processes that stretch across multiple levels, and you meet emergent phenomena around every corner. Instead of trying to predict with absolute precision, you can learn to dance with emergent reality. Working in public health and dealing with complexity on a daily basis involves moving from the desire for complete control to embracing evolving strategies for action, which can be a metaphor for living your life wisely in an increasingly complex world.

Dr. Abhay Shukla,
Senior Programme Coordinator, SATHI, and National Convenor, People's Health Movement, India

case that people living and working in a given community do in fact know the health needs of that community better than those examining data while sitting in air-conditioned conference rooms.

That said, there are times when asking project recipients what they want should not be the sole guiding principle of a global health project. People are very bad at assessing their risk for disease from various factors. For example, flu kills between 3,000 and 50,000 people every year in the United States. In comparison, the Ebola epidemic in 2015–2016 killed about 11,000 people globally and only 1 person in the United States. But while people in the United States were very worried about Ebola, many Americans neglected to get vaccinated for the flu.

While public health practitioners sometimes have good reason to make choices based on factors other than what people say they want, taking people's priorities into consideration is nonetheless extremely important. If the CDC had neglected Ebola control entirely in favor of pushing people to get flu vaccine (which, of course, they did not), you can imagine the public outcry that would result. People would lose trust in the CDC. Listening to the recipients of health projects, and building programs that meet their needs, is essential.

Respect

The most effective global health practitioners respect and listen to their colleagues, particularly those close to the communities they serve. There is a neocolonial aspect to many global health programs, where people from wealthy countries tell people from poor countries what to do (see Chapter 39). This dynamic can be lessened by respect and thoughtful listening—and by making sure that the tops of organizational structures aren't filled by people from rich countries but that instead, a real diversity of backgrounds is represented. "Turning the world upside down" allows space for the wisdom and insights of those from the "majority world."

Valuing the ideas and the labor of those at the community level goes beyond listening. The best projects understand that for ground-level staff like community health workers to be effective in the long term, they must be paid a living wage that supports their families and values their work. Paying people wages that reflect the value of their labor is an important part of respecting them. Providing

COMING FROM A BACKGROUND OF CONFLICT

My interest in global health is rooted in my personal experiences growing up in the conflict-afflicted Democratic Republic of the Congo (DRC). Growing up in the DRC, I saw the vast disparities that existed in the healthcare system, the lack of basic health services, and the lack of preventive measures. I also saw inadequate living conditions and inadequate access to basic needs such as clean water, sanitation, and essential nutrients.

Due to the conflict, I was forced to leave the DRC for Nairobi, Kenya, where I lived as refugee in a camp. While there, I saw many children and pregnant women dying from preventable diseases due to both a lack of resources and a lack of proper education on infectious diseases. I had the opportunity to visit many villages and cities where I witnessed first-hand the devastating impact of HIV/AIDS on families and communities. It was then that I realized that public health issues touch every family in sub-Saharan Africa and other developing regions around the world, and my family was no exception; I lost two young cousins to HIV/AIDS who left beautiful children.

This experience has induced in me an eagerness to contribute, even if in a small way, to the ensuring that healthcare is delivered to some of the world's most vulnerable people, particularly women and children. Reflecting on my journey from the DRC to the refugee camp in Kenya and what I have experienced along the way, I discovered a real passion—I would say a calling—for the field of global health, especially infectious diseases.

What advice would I give to students starting out in the field? Appreciate and respect different cultures and peoples. The best place to begin to do that is in your own community (or school). Be a friend to international students. They are great resources for understanding culture, health systems, and health issues.

Nadine Mushimbele
Mercy Health, Grand Rapids, Michigan

GRATEFUL FOR EMPOWERMENT

I wish I had known how grateful people in low-resource settings would be for the chance to take on tasks and to take over management of programs.

John E. McGowan, Jr.
Emory University

PERSONAL ADVICE

- People everywhere are people, we are more the same than we are different. This is true for your colleagues, be they "international" or "local" as well as the people you aim to help.
- I think it is important to always be aware of your own privilege, the biases you've inherited and how you are likely be perceived, be it warranted or not. That said, don't hold back! Speak your mind.
- Challenge yourself. Allow yourself to be uncomfortable. If at any point you feel that you are coasting, move on! There is too much to learn and so much potential for growth within the field.
- Global health has so many subfields and contexts you should never be bored or too confident. That said, I would recommend trying to carve out a niche of expertise and/or a very defined skill set so that you can contribute and not be "dead weight" to a given effort.

Kate Sabot
London School of Hygiene and Tropical Medicine

IDENTIFY YOUR OWN VALUES

During my first semester of graduate school as a student of public health I attended the American Public Health Association Annual Meeting. Sitting on the floor of a packed scientific session after 10 PM, I heard Jonathan Mann connect the stigma and discrimination experienced by people living with HIV/AIDS to the language and framework of human rights. It was in that moment that I found my calling to work at the intersection of health and human rights. One year later Dr. Mann passed away in a tragic plane crash, but his legacy lived on in me and many others. Soon after, I found myself in the foothills of the Himalayas working with adolescent Tibetan refugees—a community that because of Tibet's political situation is intimately aware of the importance human rights. In the two decades that have followed I have continued to integrate health and human rights into my work. Whether working with asylum seekers in Atlanta, on intimate partner violence in Brazil, or building capacity for Ebola response, the notion of a human right to health has always guided my work—independent of the geographic location or population focus. As you begin your career in global health my advice to you is simple: identify the core value that drives your passion for global health, and let that value guide your work.

Dabney P Evans
Emory University

opportunities for education and advancement within global health programs is very important too.

Hard Work and Long-Term Commitment

People who make significant positive impacts work hard, and they work hard for a long time. Planning, follow-through and long-term commitment take a lot of energy. Nothing worth achieving is easy, and well-funded, long-term programs are the best way to make a real difference in the long run. There are no cheap or quick fixes to the world's problems. But hard work over the long term can make a real difference.

Realism

The most effective Global Health practitioners think small. By taking on problems of a realistic size, rather than trying to save the world, they set themselves up for success. Once they make something work really well in one place, they may start to think bigger—but they are aware that "scaling up" is enormously hard. They work toward achieving what they can and trust that it will contribute to the broader picture of global health.

WHAT COLLEGE DIDN'T TEACH ME ABOUT GLOBAL HEALTH

In college, I discovered what I believed in. I took courses like African Politics and Human Ecology, and what I read changed me. The words of Dr. Paul Farmer in *Pathologies of Power* haunted me: "The idea that some lives matter less is the root of all that's wrong in the world."

My exposure to global health brought me back to the ground. It gave me a venue to put my values into action. It introduced me to a career and life path that was a concrete manifestation of what I believed in.

However, college didn't necessarily prepare me for what following that life path would be. I'm going to share with you two things that college did *not* prepare me for, just, you know, a little heads up.

1. It's Impossible to Get Straight As in the Real World

I strived—and generally succeeded—to fit into my college's culture of doing everything and doing it all perfectly: be the president of some extracurricular group, get As in all your classes, party on the weekends, eat only salad, and always be happy. I learned the hard way that outside of college, perfection can actually be the enemy of good. It's not realistic to have everything together all the time. Global health programs rarely go as smoothly or as quickly as planned, and this is ok (sometimes it's actually better, giving you time to learn from your mistakes and improve the building of the ship as you sail it). I've also learned that there is a fine line between being passionate about something and taking it all too personally. Self-worth is separate from the worth of the work you produce.

2. It's Not Always about Knowing, but Being Ok with What You Don't Know

Pretty early on during my time living in Togo I learned that I was the kind of person that liked things in neat little boxes of truths and answers and things that make sense. It did not take me long to realize that the certainty I craved was unattainable in a field like global health. I am beginning to understand that my part is not knowing. In my work in Togo, I am starting to embrace the fact that I'll never quite understand this culture and my place in it, but if that ignorance can lead to humility in my actions and my decisions, I might be on the right track.

Emily Bensen
Hope Through Health

EXPLORE AND ENGAGE

The journey of engaging in the field of public health is one that offers constant opportunities for growth. Consciously engage with all types of public health discourses; not only in your own country, but the world over. Public health does not only apply to health and disease. It is about complex systems and contexts. It is about health systems that are embedded within economies, politics and cultures. Engage with these nuances.

One of the best ways to do so is to explore multiple and diverse disciplines, from anthropology to economics. Try not to shy away from appreciating and understanding different fields, concepts and ideas. Establish and make connections and engage in networks. They are often made up of people from different fields and experiences. This will enable you to understand the complexities of the field. Read as much as you can beyond the traditional text book. Engage in newspapers, public debates, conferences—where you should be engaged in ways that really broaden your perspective.

Become an active participant. Assume the role of an advocate and an activist, because public health is about human rights and the rights to dignity and wellbeing. The field gives you the privilege and opportunity to effect and influence change at a population level as opposed to the individual. In one way or the other, the field goes beyond the abstract and academic. Immerse yourself in it. It is as exciting as it is sometimes depressing, but ultimately it becomes a calling.

Nonhlanhla Nxumalo
Wits University, Johannesburg, South Africa

Knowledge

Effective global health programs are designed with a deep understanding of context. The best practitioners have an awareness of history, politics, and power relations, so they are not surprised when historical and political forces affect their projects. Gaining this knowledge is a life-long project.

Note that here we are speaking of knowledge and not intelligence. This is a very deliberate choice. Some very smart people neglect to notice that they do not know everything. Wisdom frequently lies in knowing what it is that you don't know—and finding people who can teach you those things.

Optimism

The challenges facing global health practitioners are very real, and ignoring those challenges can doom projects. This is why optimism, by itself, can be dangerous.

However, when combined with humility, hard work, realism and the other attributes of effective health programs discussed here, optimism becomes critical. There is real reason for optimism: health has improved dramatically worldwide in recent years. And, a good dose of optimism is necessary when challenges present themselves. Optimism can breed a calm, balanced persistence in the face of challenge.

William Foege's message is clear: an optimistic view of what can be achieved in global health is warranted because of the successes of the past 40 years. However, there is more to be done. Throughout this book, we have included many different voices telling a great variety of stories about contemporary global health and its history. From young students to venerable heroes, we all have a part in understanding and grappling with the world's global health challenges. Armed with facts, informed

IS OPTIMISM WARRANTED?

The good news in global health is that—for all of our limited resources and support—we have applied the philosophy, skills, and required knowledge quite effectively in so many ways. The history of recent decades is amazing.

In this country, the United States, life expectancy has increased by seven hours a day for a century. Most of this increase is because of public health actions to protect against infectious diseases, provide safe water, and educate the public on issues like seat belts, helmets, smoking, and nutrition.

Smallpox has disappeared. It accounted for 300 million deaths in the 20th century. Guinea worm is about to disappear. Polio, that scourge that left parents holding their breaths, is down to a handful of cases in three countries. Measles deaths have decreased from over 3 million a year to less than 150,000 a year. Under-age-five mortality has fallen from 50,000 deaths a day when I became interested in global health 65 years ago to 15,000 deaths a day, a decline of two-thirds. And the World Bank says that 250,000 people leave the ranks of poverty every day.

Based on experience, then, optimism is absolutely justified. But, because of better tools, more resources, and more interest, you will be able to do far more than my generation. I regret that life is so short because I want to see what you accomplish!

There are problems, of course. Inequities continue between countries and within countries. Our bottom line objective can be condensed to three words: *global health equity.* It is not possible to leave out any of these three words, and an additional 200 words couldn't make it clearer.

We need to acknowledge a dysfunctional global system. For example, the WHO has been criticized, correctly, for its response to Ebola. But who mentions that the United States and other countries year after year told the WHO to reduce its budget?

Despite overwhelming evidence, we avoid adequate attention to the social determinants of health. They should be part of our daily agenda. Especially poverty— it is the slavery of today. How can we make reducing poverty an integral part of global health?

The major goals of global health training are, first, to impart a *philosophy,* which is eternal; second, to teach *skills,* which are for a lifetime; and third, to impart *knowledge,* which is ephemeral. Yet, this area is where we spend most of the academic time allotted.

First, philosophy. The basic philosophy of science is to discover truth. The basic philosophy of medicine is to use that truth for a patient. The basic philosophy of global health is to use that truth for everyone; the basic philosophy of global health is therefore social justice. As to your personal philosophy, as a student of global health, spend the time needed to understand your objectives, your aims, your purpose. What is most important, what do you want your obituary to say?

Next, skills. Skills you should master include epidemiology, statistics, and especially management. The difference between having knowledge that does or does not change health comes down to management.

And finally, knowledge. Knowledge is often specific to the problem at hand and must be sought to solve that problem. Knowledge changes so fast. The key, really, is knowing how to *get* knowledge, yet we spend so much of the curriculum time on providing knowledge that is soon out of date.

But there is another side. The late Yale professor Jaroslav Pelikan said that *good* scholarship often can be traced to mentors, the place of training, and the like, but that *great* scholarship is often the result of how much you know outside of your field. So seek knowledge—but especially general knowledge: How does the world work? What are the lessons of history? What are the conclusions of great minds from the past?

Are there any burning lessons in global health that keep coming back to me after more than 60 years of interest?

1. A career in public health will call on everything you ever learn.
2. A career in public health is built on your interest in equity rather than your interest in money.
3. Everything you do in the future will be done as part of a coalition. Leadership in public health is not dependent on a title; it goes to the person who can make a coalition function effectively. Some of my great memories of my 65 years working in global health involve sitting in meetings, around tables, or in the field, with diverse groups, realizing the importance of different perspectives. Different cultures lead to different perspectives. That diversity led to solutions because not one of us is as smart as all of us.
4. Remember to be a mentor. One study concludes that the best predictors of success after graduation are (i) having had a mentor and (ii) having internship experiences that allow the use of skills in real-life situations. Your goal in global health is a rational health future. To do this, remember that we live in a cause-and-effect world. Health improvement doesn't happen by chance. Know the truth.
5. But also, know the limits of science. Certainty, as physicist Feynman taught, is the Achilles' heel of science, religion, medicine, and politics. Better than science alone is science with a moral compass, science in the service of humanity, science serving equity.
6. Optimism is needed. Harland Cleveland said that the fuel of global health is unwarranted optimism. Never lose it.
7. Donald Trump likes to say, "America First." That is not a global health statement. The Earl of Shaftesbury said, "good" is having one's inclinations consistently directed toward the good of the group: the larger the group that inspires these feelings, the better. Global health, now and in the future, is as large as you can get!
8. Change social norms. Kierkegaard, the Danish philosopher and theologian, told the story of someone breaking into a jewelry store and taking nothing. All the intruder did was change the price tags. The world has distorted price tags. High prices are paid for athletes, Wall Street bankers, CEOs and the like while low prices go to schoolteachers, public health workers, physical therapists, and mental health workers. Help to change that.
9. Spend less time on a life plan and more time on a life philosophy. That will give you tools for making decisions at every fork in the road.

In the novel *Cutting for Stone* by Abraham Verghese, there is a line that says, "Home is not where you are from. Home is where you are needed." I hope you all find your way home.

Bill Foege

opinions and critical perspectives, we hope that you will continue to deepen your knowledge of and commitment to global health. Wherever your life takes you, we hope that you become a world citizen, mindful of the people throughout the globe who are living in economic and health contexts different than your own.

SECTION 13 CASES FOR TEACHING AND LEARNING

Visit the companion website, www.oup.com/us/brown-closser, for direct links to the featured online resources.

Ted Smalley Bowen and Kirsten Lundberg, *When BEST Intentions Go Awry: Arsenic Mitigation in Bangladesh*

This case introduces students to a project aimed at mitigating the health effects of arsenic contamination in groundwater in Bangladesh. Students consider what actions would be best to take when false rumors begin to fly that this arsenic-mitigation project is poisoning villagers. The case includes mini-biographies of the real people involved in this project.

Ruth Palmer, *The Elusive Tuberculosis Case: The CDC and Andrew Speaker*

This case explores a conflict between individual liberty and effective disease control. It follows the CDC's decision-making process regarding travel restrictions for a man with drug-resistant tuberculosis.

Vivek Srinavasan and Sudha Narayanan, *Food Policy and Social Movements: Reflections on the Right to Food Campaign in India*

This case engages the complicated relationships between activists advocating for food justice in Rajasthan, India, and the Indian government. Students consider a variety of policy options in working toward food justice.

SECTION 13 VIDEOS AND WEB RESOURCES

Visit the companion website, www.oup.com/us/brown-closser, for direct links to the featured online resources.

Satirical Websites

The following websites and videos, funny and cutting, are great for sparking class discussion around issues of representation and privilege.

Humanitarians of Tinder
Barbie Savior
6-Day Visit to Rural African Village Completely Changes Woman's Facebook Profile Picture
The Radi-Aid App: Change a Life with Just One Swipe
Who Wants to Be a Volunteer?

The Ethics of Philanthropy

Tiny Spark

Tiny Spark is an independent news source that investigates "the business of doing good." In addition to articles, the website includes an archive of a podcast. Many of the podcast episodes and articles are excellent foundations for discussion on ethics with topics including tracking aid dollars in Haiti; whether a business mindset has a place in philanthropy; and whether in-kind donations are a good idea. Students may particularly enjoy the podcast episode: "TOMS Shoes—Is It Good Aid?"

TED-Talk Reflections from Young Americans Working in Global Health

***Learning from Failure* – David Damberger**

This TedX Talk by an engineer working on water projects is an accessible introduction to the importance of accountability to communities rather than to donors. It also discusses Engineers Without Borders' decision to produce an annual "Failure Report." In addition, Engineers Without Borders has a small catalogue of failures in different NGOs at admittingfailure.org.

Poverty, Money, and Love – Jessica Jackley

The founder of kiva.org reflects on the ethics of giving.

Ethics Training

Ethics in Epidemics, Emergencies and Disasters: Research, Surveillance and Patient Care – Global Health Training Centre

This 10-hour course in Global Health Ethics is a useful resource for advanced self-study. It covers issues of ethics in public health surveillance, research and care provision.

First, Do No Harm: A Qualitative Research Documentary

This documentary, designed as a pretraining orientation for students engaging in overseas projects, explores the ethical issues involved in medical volunteer projects.

KEY TERMS

2×2 TABLE: The classic tool of **analytic epidemiology**, used to evaluate the relationship between an exposure to a given risk factor and a particular outcome.

ACQUIRED IMMUNE DEFICIENCY SYNDROME (AIDS): The final and most severe stage of an **HIV** infection, when the body's immune system is severely compromised, leading to secondary opportunistic infections. Untreated, AIDS is fatal.

AIR POLLUTION: Physical, chemical or biological contamination of the natural atmosphere. Air pollution can be both outdoor and indoor and can come from a range of sources, including vehicles, combustion, forest fires and industrial sites.

ALMA-ATA: In 1978, world leaders gathered in this city (now Almaty, Kazakhstan) for the International Conference on Primary Health Care and declared their goal of "Health for All by the Year 2000." The Alma-Ata conference is famous for marking a shift toward primary health care approaches.

ANALYTIC EPIDEMIOLOGY: A subdiscipline of **epidemiology** in which data about populations and exposure are collected to determine the cause of a disease. Frequently uses **2×2 tables**. Contrast with **descriptive epidemiology**.

ANTHROPOCENE: The geological age in which human activity is considered the most powerful influence on the environment and climate of the planet.

ANTI-RETROVIRAL THERAPY (ART): A multimedicine regime used for the treatment of people infected with **HIV**. ART does *not* cure HIV, but it slows the replication of the virus, preventing **AIDS** and decreasing likelihood of HIV transmission.

BIG FOOD: A nickname for the multinational food and beverage industry.

BILATERAL ORGANIZATIONS: Organizations that channel international aid from one government to another. Examples include the United States Agency for International Development (USAID) and DFID (the UK's Department for International Development).

BIOMEDICINE: A form of clinically oriented ethnomedicine often thought of as "scientific medicine." Biomedicine often views the body as a machine that can be cured through application of technologies.

BRAIN DRAIN: The process in which wealthy countries hire trained workers away from poorer countries, causing shortages in the sending countries.

BREASTFEEDING: Exclusive breastfeeding (only breastmilk) for the first 6 months of life and continued breastfeeding throughout the first 2 years of life (along with other foods) boosts child immune function and counters undernutrition and malnutrition in young children.

BUILDING BLOCKS: The **WHO**'s way of describing the components of a functioning health care system. The building blocks are leadership and governance, health-care financing, health workforce, medical products and technologies, information and research and service delivery.

BURDEN OF DISEASE: A measure of the impact of a given health issue on a population. Can be measured in **DALYs**.

CHAIN OF INFECTION: **A model of** the way infections spread from person to person. The chain includes an infectious agent, a mode of transmission and a host.

CHOLERA: An infectious disease caused by the bacteria *Vibrio cholera* that infects the small intestine and causes severe diarrhea and vomiting. Cholera can result in death by dehydration. *Vibrio cholera* can reside in marine or brackish waters or be spread by **fecal–oral transmission**.

CHRONIC DISEASES: **In general, risk of chronic** diseases (e.g., cancer and heart disease) comes from factors like diet and environment. However, the distinction between chronic disease and infectious disease is not always clear: for example, HIV infection can be a chronic condition in people with access to anti-retroviral therapy.

CIGARETTES: The largest single preventable cause of death in the world. Cigarettes are a highly profitable product that are promoted through advertising, especially in low- and middle-income countries.

CLIMATE CHANGE: The set of interconnected changes to the global climate resulying from human activities, particularly the burning of fossil fuels. These changes include increases in the frequency and severity of extreme weather events, an overall rise in average temperature, a rising sea level, and an increase in floods and droughts.

COLD CHAIN: A temperature-controlled supply system that keeps heat-sensitive drugs or vaccines cold from manufacture to delivery to the people who need them. A cold chain may include fridges, freezers, refrigerated transport, generators, fuel, coolers and ice.

COMMUNITY HEALTH WORKER (CHW): A lay health worker who is generally a member of the local community. With the right training and support, such workers can effectively carry out a wide variety of health treatments and preventive measures.

CONTROL (OR DISEASE CONTROL): When transmission of a disease has been brought down to a level deemed acceptable by decisionmakers.

COST-EFFECTIVE: A health intervention that provides a substantial health benefit per dollar spent.

DALY (DISABILITY-ADJUSTED LIFE YEARS): A way of measuring the burden of a given disease in a population. The DALY sums the number of years of life lost to illness, disability, injury or disease (a year of disability is calculated as a fraction of a year of life). Compare to **YLL**

DEMOGRAPHIC TRANSITION: The transition from high birth and death rates to lower birth and death rates that often accompanies industrialization.

DEMOGRAPHY: The science of counting people, or the study of statistics of fertility and death, and tracking changes in human populations.

DESCRIPTIVE EPIDEMIOLOGY: The field of study that describes the distribution of illness and disease in a population. It focuses on person, place and time. Compare with **analytic epidemiology**.

DETERMINANTS OF HEALTH: The factors that underlie people's good or poor health. These include social, economic and environmental factors.

DIRECTLY OBSERVED THERAPY (DOT): A strategy in which health workers or family members observe and record patients taking their medications to ensure that patients finish their treatments. An essential element of high-quality tuberculosis control programs, called DOTS or DOTS-plus.

DONOR-DRIVEN: Programs, initiatives or organizations whose activities or goals are driven more by the desires of donors than the needs of the people they serve.

DOUBLE BURDEN OF DISEASE: When both chronic and infectious diseases are significant contributors to morbidity and mortality for a particular population.

DOUBLE BURDEN OF MALNUTRITION: When undernutrition or micronutrient malnutrition co-exists with overnutrition. The double burden of malnutrition can happen at the country, family or individual level.

ELIMINATION: When a particular disease is completely gone from a certain area of the world. For example, polio has been eliminated from the Americas, although it remains in Nigeria, Afghanistan and Pakistan.

ENDEMIC: A disease that has existed for a long time in a population or region.

ENTERTAINMENT EDUCATION: Sometimes called "edu-tainment," a communications strategy where educational themes are translated into an entertaining format like soap operas or movies.

EPIDEMIC: A greater number of cases of a health issue than expected for a specific population

EPIDEMIOLOGICAL TRANSITION: Significant shifts in morbidity and mortality during human history. The first epidemiological transition occurred during the shift from hunter-gatherer lifestyle to agricultural (marking the rise of infectious disease), the second transition accompanied industrialization (marking the shift from infectious to chronic disease) and the third transition is the reemergence of infectious diseases in wealthy countries.

EPIDEMIOLOGY: The study of the prevalence, spread and possible control of health problems within populations. An epidemiologist is someone who studies epidemiology.

ERADICATION: To permanently and completely stop a disease from affecting humans. Samples of eradicated diseases may be kept in labs. As of 2017, only smallpox has been eradicated. Contrasted with **control** and **elimination.**

ETHNICITY: A group characterized by similarities within the group and differences from other groups. Ethnicities often share history, heredity, religion, culture, beliefs and variety of other traits. What we think of as "race" in the United States is better conceptualized as ethnicity.

ETHNOMEDICINE: The medical beliefs and practices of a particular group of people.

ENVIRONMENTAL HEALTH: The branch of public health that focuses on the factors of health that are determined by a person's environment, including physical, chemical, biological, social and psychosocial factors.

ENVIRONMENTAL JUSTICE: The efforts to counter the widespread effects of environmental racism or environmental injustice, in which particular populations (usually minorities) are disproportionately subjected to environmental hazards in relation to their representation in the larger population. For example, in the United States, African Americans are more likely than whites to be exposed to industrial pollution.

FALLACY OF EMPTY VESSELS: An incorrect assumption in many behavior-change programs in which populations targeted for health education are assumed to have no preexisting beliefs or knowledge.

FECAL–ORAL TRANSMISSION: A form of infectious disease transmission in which human feces infected with a virus, bacteria or parasite are ingested by another person, usually through contaminated food or water (e.g., cholera, polio, typhoid or ascariasis).

FEMALE GENITAL MODIFICATION (FGM): Sometimes also called female genital mutilation (FGM) or female genital cutting (FGC). A controversial set of procedures that involve the surgical modification or removal of external female genitalia for nonmedical reasons.

FOOD INSECURITY: The state of lacking reliable access to nutritious food. Food insecurity measures are relatively simple and include psychological variables and current access to adequate diet. Food insecurity can contribute to undernutrition, overnutrition and mental health problems.

FOUNDATION: A nongovernmental institution financed by donations that funds other groups, institutions, organizations or individuals through grants.

4FS: FLUIDS, FIELDS, FLIES AND FINGERS: The major pathways of **fecal–oral transmission**.

GENDER: A set of socially constructed categories encompassing social, cultural, economic and political ideas about what it means to be male, female or some other category. (These other categories vary by culture.)

GLOBAL HEALTH: A field of study that utilizes multiple disciplines to understand the extents and effects of global forces and population-level interventions on community health. Initially emerged as a rebranding of "International Health" but is based on somewhat different values.

GLOBAL NORTH: A nickname for high-income countries that tend to hold more political and economic power (sometimes also called the "developed world" or "first world").

GLOBAL SOUTH: Low-income countries with less political and economic power (sometimes also called the "developing world" or "third world").

GLOBALIZATION: The process by which countries are becoming more politically, economically and socially interconnected through media, technology and transportation.

GOBI-FFF: A package of health interventions associated with primary health care and recommended by UNICEF. GOBI-FFF stands for growth monitoring, **oral rehydration therapy**, **breastfeeding**, **immunization**, family planning, female education and food supplementation.

GREEN REVOLUTION: A period of significant agricultural change occurring between the 1940s and the 1960s in which new agricultural technologies, such as chemical fertilizers, harvesting technologies, irrigation methods and new crop varieties, led to a massive increase in food production globally.

HEALTH: According to the **WHO**, "a state of complete physical, mental, and social well-being and not merely the absence of disease or infirmity."

HEALTH BEHAVIORS: A broad term describing practices and actions of a person or group that affect health outcomes: for example, food practices, exercise habits, commuting patterns, or religious rituals.

HEALTH COMMUNICATION: The study and practice of relaying health messages to an individual or group. Can be through multiple forms, including media and interpersonal contact: for example, see **edu-tainment.**

HERD IMMUNITY: The population protection that comes from high percentages of people in a given community receiving vaccination.

HIGH INCOME: A way of describing countries that is more accurate than terms like "first world" or "developed." According to the World Bank's classification system as of July 2017, a high-income country has a gross national income of more than US$12,235 per person.

HUMAN IMMUNODEFICIENCY VIRUS (HIV): A virus spread through human bodily fluids that attacks the body's immune system. Without treatment, HIV leads to **AIDS**.

IMMUNIZATION: Also called **vaccination**, this is a technology can make person immune or resistant to an infectious disease, typically by the administration of a vaccine that stimulates antibody response. It is a safe and **cost-effective** method of preventing disease.

INDOOR AIR POLLUTION: The contamination of air inside of buildings by physical, chemical or biological means. Common sources include smoke from cooking fires, mold, tobacco and lead.

INFECTIOUS DISEASES: Diseases that can be transmitted from person to person, either directly or indirectly (such as through a **vector**). Caused by **pathogens** such as bacteria, viruses, fungi and parasites.

INJURY: Damage to the body. Injury can be accidental or intentional (including self-inflicted or inflicted by someone else).

INOCULATION: The practice of introducing a pathogen or antigen into an organism to stimulate the production of antibodies for that pathogen. Contrast with **immunization** or **vaccination**.

INTERNATIONAL HEALTH: A subfield of public health developed after World War II that focused on wealthier countries providing money and technical assistance to improve health in poor countries. The precursor to **Global Health**.

INTERNATIONAL MONETARY FUND (IMF): An international organization dedicated to stabilizing world currency flows, facilitating trade and assisting countries in financial crisis.

INTIMATE PARTNER VIOLENCE (IPV): Any form of intentional violence carried out by a current or former intimate partner toward the other. Includes sexual, physical and psychological violence.

LOW-INCOME: A way of describing countries that is more accurate than terms like "third world" or "developing." According to the World Bank's classification system as of July 2017, a low-income country has a gross national income of less than US$1,005 per person.

MACROPARASITES: Agents that cause disease through structural factors: for example, social inequality or poverty.

MALARIA: Disease caused by the Plasmodium parasite and transmitted by female Anopheles mosquitoes. Causes severe fever and is common in many countries in the Global South. A major cause of death in young children in many parts of sub-Saharan Africa.

MATERNAL MORTALITY: Death of a woman from pregnancy or childbirth-related causes.

MATERNAL MORTALITY RATE (MMR): The number of deaths of women from pregnancy or childbirth-related causes in relation to number of live births. Usually written in terms of deaths per 100,000 live births.

MDR-TB: Multidrug-resistant tuberculosis; a tuberculosis infection that is resistant to the standard tuberculosis drug treatment regime.

MEDICINE: The science and practice of curing and preventing health problems and attending to an individual's health. Compared with public health, the orientation of medicine is curative and focused on individuals.

MENTAL HEALTH: According to the **WHO**, "a state of well-being in which every individual realizes his or her own potential, can cope with the normal stresses of life, can work productively and fruitfully, and is able to make a contribution to her or his community."

MICRONUTRIENT MALNUTRITION: A form of malnutrition when someone is deficient in essential vitamins, minerals or other substances that the body only needs in small amounts, such as iodine, vitamin A or iron. Can manifest as a wide variety of symptoms.

MIDDLE-INCOME: According to the World Bank's classification system as of July 2017, a low-middle income country has a gross national income (GNI) of between US$1,006 and US$3,955 per person, and an upper-middle income country has a GNI between US$3,956 and US$12,235 per person.

MILLENNIUM DEVELOPMENT GOALS (MDGS): A set of eight goals with a series of quantifiable targets created in 2000 by the UN to improve the lives of the world's poorest people. After the 2015 deadline passed for the MDGs, they were replaced by the **Sustainable Development Goals (SDGs)**.

MINISTRY OF HEALTH: In most countries, the wing of the government that operates the country's health services.

MORBIDITY: Any departure from a state of health. Can be described for a population in terms of a morbidity rate. Contrast with **mortality.**

MORTALITY: Death. Can be described for a population in terms of a mortality rate.

MULTILATERAL ORGANIZATIONS: Consortiums that obtain and dispense funds from and to multiple actors, usually governments. The most prominent examples are the UN organizations.

NONGOVERNMENTAL ORGANIZATIONS (NGOs): In the broadest sense, an organizational entity that is not directly a part of a government. In most cases, the implication is that the organization is also nonprofit.

OPEN DEFECATION: Defecating in open spaces and not in any sort of latrine (e.g., in a field or a street)

OPEN SEWERS/DRAINS: Channels that carry storm or wastewater and are open to the air. Often contribute to fecal–oral disease spread or breeding of mosquitos.

OUTDOOR AIR POLLUTION: The contamination of outside air by physical, chemical or biological means. Common sources include motor vehicle emissions, garbage incineration and industrial processes.

OVERNUTRITION: The consumption of more calories or nutrients than is necessary for biological functioning. Can lead to obesity and cardiovascular diseases.

PAN AMERICAN HEALTH ORGANIZATION (PAHO): An international health agency that coordinates among countries in the Americas. The success of this organization served as the inspiration for the creation of the **WHO**.

PARTNERSHIP: Ideally, in global health, a partnership involves joining together the strengths and efforts of multiple actors, such as NGOs, private companies, institutions and universities, to promote health. Sometimes, the language of partnership can mask inequalities between donors and recipients.

PATHOGEN: An organism that causes disease, such as a virus, bacteria or parasite.

POSITIVE DEVIANCE: When an individual or group practices a positive health behavior or achieves a positive health outcome that differs from similar groups in spite of having the same obstacles.

PUBLIC HEALTH: The science and practice of monitoring and addressing health challenges of populations through an emphasis on prevention.

PRIMARY HEALTH CARE (PHC): The comprehensive provision of a broad range of basic health services, both preventive and curative, that address a wide range of health issues. PHC can be described as a horizontal approach because it provides accessible health services to all people. Compare with **vertical programs**.

RACE: A social grouping of people based on their ethnicity, physical appearance or geographical origin. The concept of "race" falsely assumes that racial categories match with biological categories. See **ethnicity.**

ROAD TRAFFIC ACCIDENTS: An event in which a motor vehicle hits another motor vehicle, person or object; most events are preventable and are not really "accidents." A major cause of morbidity and mortality in many parts of the world.

SELECTIVE PRIMARY HEALTH CARE: A group of vertical programs functioning in tandem. The philosophy of selective PHC is very unlike that of Primary Health Care. For an example of selective PHC, see **GOBI-FFF.**

SEXUALLY TRANSMITTED INFECTIONS (STIS): Sometimes also called sexually transmitted diseases (STDs). Infectious diseases that are spread through sexual contact.

SOCIAL DETERMINANTS OF HEALTH: The social, political and economic conditions that affect an individual's or a population's health outcomes.

SOCIAL MARKETING: A form of mass communication that uses the research and methods of business marketing to promote positive health behaviors or social beliefs.

SOCIAL MOBILIZATION: A process by which a wide range of stakeholders are mobilized to raise awareness of a particular development challenge.

SOCIAL VIOLENCE: Violence carried out by social groups: for example, gangs or nations.

SMOKING: The practice of breathing in smoke from a cigarette, cigar or other tobacco-burning device. Smoking is a major risk factor for many common diseases.

SOCIAL ENTREPRENEURSHIP: An ideology or approach in which business start-ups create innovative ideas that have the potential to solve social problems.

SOCIOECONOMIC GRADIENT: The range of wealth inequality from poor to wealthy. Groups on the higher end of the socioeconomic gradient have longer life expectancy and better health outcomes.

STRUCTURAL ADJUSTMENT PROGRAMS: Loans to countries from the International Monetary Fund (IMF) or World Bank with a set of conditions that frequently involve downsizing government, including government health services, and privatizing industries.

STRUCTURAL VIOLENCE: Social, economic and political structures that systematically disadvantage a group of people and lead to outcomes including disease and death.

STUNTING: A symptom of malnutrition in which children whose height for their age is significantly below what is expected for a healthy child their age. Stunting can be caused by chronic **undernutrition,** as well as infectious disease episodes that effect growth spurts.

SURVEILLANCE: The collection, analysis and interpretation of data on the status of a health problem or disease to use in planning, implementing and evaluating public health programs.

SUSTAINABLE DEVELOPMENT GOALS (SDGS): A set of goals adopted by the UN and its member nations in 2015 to alleviate poverty, protect the environment and ensure global peace and prosperity by 2030. Replaced the **Millennium Development Goals (MDGs)**.

TASK SHIFTING: The process of moving certain health care responsibilities from more highly trained staff (like doctors) to less trained yet competent staff, such as nurses or **community health workers**; this strategy is important in global mental health.

TRADITIONAL BIRTH ATTENDANTS: A pregnancy care or childbirth provider who was trained or operates outside of the biomedical system: for example, a traditional midwife.

TROPICAL MEDICINE: The health care system set up by colonial governments, intended to facilitate colonial goals by protecting troops and colonizers from the diseases of the nations they colonized, and ensuring the high economic productivity of colonized workers.

TUBERCULOSIS (TB): An infectious disease spread through the air by person-to-person contact. Caused by the bacteria *Mycobacterium tuberculosis*, TB most often infects the lungs.

UNDERNUTRITION: A form of malnutrition. Related to insufficient intake of food or nutrients.

UNICEF: The UN organization focused on children; it promotes child and maternal welfare globally.

VACCINATION: The act of inserting a substance into a body to stimulate the immune system to develop immunity against a specific disease. Also called **immunization**. The term derives from *vacca* (cow) because of Jenner's famous discovery that experience of mild cowpox causes protection to smallpox.

VECTOR: Any organism that transmits disease or parasites to humans: for example, *Anopheles* mosquitoes are vectors for malaria.

VERTICAL PROGRAM: A public health program that focuses on a single health-related goal or disease.

WASTING: A symptom of malnutrition in which children whose weight for their height is significantly below what is expected; often an indicator of acute food shortage.

WATER INSECURITY: When people do not have sufficient access to water.

WATER, SANITATION AND HYGIENE (WASH): A subfield of Global Health that focuses on the improvement of water and sanitation quality and access or hygiene behaviors to improve health outcomes. Focuses on prevention of fecal–oral disease transmission.

WATERBORNE (DISEASE): Pathogenic diseases caused by contact with or consumption of contaminated water.

WATER-WASHED (DISEASE): Diseases caused by poor hygiene or food contaminated with bacteria, generally resulting from lack of access to a sufficient quantity of water.

WORLD BANK: An international financial organization funded and managed by multiple countries, with the aim of reducing global poverty, usually through the provision of loans and the supply of technical assistance toward country governments.

WORLD HEALTH ORGANIZATION (WHO): A specialized agency of the United Nations, founded in 1947, who sets norms and standards for health-related issues, shapes the global research agenda, provides technical support to countries and monitors disease trends.

XDR-TB: A rare type of extreme multidrug-resistant tuberculosis (**MDR-TB**) that is impervious to most known drugs.

YLL (YEARS OF LIFE LOST): A form of measurement for the population burden of a health problem that calculates the years of life lost in a population owing to mortality from the health problem. YLL takes into account the age at which deaths occur, giving greater weight to deaths at younger ages. Unlike the **DALY**, the YLL does not take disability into account.

Printed in the USA/Agawam, MA
August 25, 2020

760343.144